Cancer Biomarkers: Developments, Applications and Therapies

Cancer Biomarkers: Developments, Applications and Therapies

Edited by **Karen Miles**

hayle medical

New York

Published by Hayle Medical,
30 West, 37th Street, Suite 612,
New York, NY 10018, USA
www.haylemedical.com

Cancer Biomarkers: Developments, Applications and Therapies
Edited by Karen Miles

International Standard Book Number: 978-1-63241-394-9 (Hardback)

Printed in China.

Contents

Preface

This book brings forth the emerging trends in the areas of diagnosis and treatment of Cancer. The ever growing need for advanced technology is the reason that has fuelled the research in the field of cancer biomarkers and targeted therapies in recent times. This book is a valuable compilation of topics, ranging from the basic to the most complex advancements in this field. Researchers and doctors around the world are studying cancer and devising new and effective therapies to cure it. Such studies and researches have been including in this text. It is a complete source of knowledge on the present status of this field. The extensive content of this book provides the readers with a thorough understanding of the subject.

Significant researches are present in this book. Intensive efforts have been employed by authors to make this book an outstanding discourse. This book contains the enlightening chapters which have been written on the basis of significant researches done by the experts.

Finally, I would also like to thank all the members involved in this book for being a team and meeting all the deadlines for the submission of their respective works. I would also like to thank my friends and family for being supportive in my efforts.

Editor

1

Hypoxic metabolism in human hematopoietic stem cells

Fatih Kocabas[1,2†], Li Xie[3,4†], Jingjing Xie[5†], Zhuo Yu[3,4], Ralph J. DeBerardinis[6], Wataru Kimura[1], SuWannee Thet[1], Ahmed F. Elshamy[7], Hesham Abouellail[8], Shalini Muralidhar[1], Xiaoye Liu[4], Chiqi Chen[3], Hesham A. Sadek[1], Cheng Cheng Zhang[9*] and Junke Zheng[3,4*]

Abstract

Background: Adult hematopoietic stem cells (HSCs) are maintained in a microenvironment, known as niche in the endosteal regions of the bone marrow. This stem cell niche with low oxygen tension requires HSCs to adopt a unique metabolic profile. We have recently demonstrated that mouse long-term hematopoietic stem cells (LT-HSCs) utilize glycolysis instead of mitochondrial oxidative phosphorylation as their main energy source. However, the metabolic phenotype of human hematopoietic progenitor and stem cells (HPSCs) remains unknown.

Results: We show that HPSCs have a similar metabolic phenotype, as shown by high rates of glycolysis, and low rates of oxygen consumption. Fractionation of human mobilized peripheral blood cells based on their metabolic footprint shows that cells with a low mitochondrial potential are highly enriched for HPSCs. Remarkably, low MP cells had much better repopulation ability as compared to high MP cells. Moreover, similar to their murine counterparts, we show that Hif-1α is upregulated in human HPSCs, where it is transcriptionally regulated by Meis1. Finally, we show that Meis1 and its cofactors Pbx1 and HoxA9 play an important role in transcriptional activation of Hif-1α in a cooperative manner.

Conclusions: These findings highlight the unique metabolic properties of human HPSCs and the transcriptional network that regulates their metabolic phenotype.

Keywords: Stem cells, Metabolism, Hypoxia, Hypoxic regulation of metabolism, Human hematopoietic progenitor and stem cells, HPSCs

Background

HSCs are defined by their inherent capacity for self-renewal and differentiation into all blood cell types. Adult HSCs reside in regions of the bone marrow challenged by low oxygen tension (hypoxia), which is termed "hypoxic niche" [1, 2]. We recently demonstrated that mouse HSCs in this hypoxic niche adopt a glycolytic metabolic profile, in which HSCs manifest lower rates of oxygen consumption, lower ATP content, and increased cytoplasmic glycolysis [3]. In addition, we and others showed that mouse HSCs demonstrate increased HIF-1α levels [3–5].

HIF-1 regulates various aspects of metabolism from the oxidant stress response to regulation of glycolysis and mitochondrial respiration [6–12]. HIF-1, a major mediator of transcriptional response to hypoxia, is composed of O_2 sensitive HIF-1α and constitutively active HIF-1β subunits [13–15]. Conditional deletion of HIF-1α in HSCs results in various defects such as loss of quiescence and progressive decline in HSC number following bone marrow transplantations and aging [4]. In addition hypoxic cultures promote the production of hematopoietic progenitors and enhance HSC expansion [1, 16, 17]. HIF-1α protein is mainly stabilized during hypoxia but normoxic upregulation of HIF-1α has also been reported [14, 18–25]. We recently demonstrated that Meis1 transactivates HIF-1α expression via a conserved

* Correspondence: alec.zhang@utsouthwestern.edu; zhengjunke@sjtu.edu.cn
†Equal contributors
[9]Departments of Physiology and Developmental Biology, UT Southwestern Medical Center at Dallas, 5323 Harry Hines Blvd, Dallas, TX 75390, USA
[3]Hongqiao International Institute of Medicine, Shanghai Tongren Hospital / Faculty of Basic Medicine, Shanghai Jiao Tong University School of Medicine, Shanghai 200025, China
Full list of author information is available at the end of the article

Meis1 binding motif located in the first intron of HIF-1α [3], and regulates mouse HSC metabolism [26].

Several reports suggest that homeobox protein Meis1 plays important roles in HPSC biology [27–32]. Homozygous mutant mice for Meis1 die during gestation with defects in hematopoiesis which results in decline in myeloid, lymphoid, and multipotent progenitors [33–35]. Meis1 is also associated with leukemogenesis in humans with a frequent up-regulation in primary acute myeloid leukemia (AML) [29, 30] and acute lymphoblastic leukemia (ALL) samples [36]. We recently showed that mouse LT-HSCs express Meis1 where a great majority of $Meis1^{+}$ HSCs coexpress Hif-1α [3]. Previous reports indicate that Meis1 interacts with the cofactors Pbx1 and HoxA9 in HSCs, which are known regulators of hematopoiesis [27, 28, 37–48]. However, the cooperative role of Meis1 and its cofactors in regulation of HIF-1 is unknown.

In the current report, we demonstrate that human HPSCs have a metabolic profile characterized by low mitochondrial oxidative phosphorylation, dependence on glycolytic metabolism, and upregulation of hypoxia-responsive pathways. We show that the metabolic phenotype of human HPSCs is mediated in part via transcriptional activation of Hif-1α by Meis1 and its cofactors Pbx1 and HoxA9.

Results

Metabolic profile of human HPSCs

HSCs have been reported to reside in hypoxic niches and this suggested that HSCs require adopting unique metabolic properties. Here, we demonstrate that human HPSCs ($Lin^{-}CD34^{+}CD38^{-}CD90^{+}$ cells) from G-CSF mobilized peripheral blood (MPB) have lower rates of mitochondrial respiration. The overall oxygen consumption by HPSCs is significantly lower compared to MPB mononuclear cells (Fig. 1a). Consistently, human HPSCs have lower ATP content (Fig. 1b). In addition, Fig. 1c shows that the rate of glycolysis is significantly higher in HPSCs compared to the MPB mononuclear cells, suggesting that human HPSCs rely primarily on glycolytic metabolism instead of mitochondrial oxidative phosphorylation.

Next we sought to profile human MPB HPSCs based on their mitochondrial proton gradient as an index of overall mitochondrial respiration. Similar to mouse HSCs, the majority of the human $Lin^{-}CD34^{+}CD38^{-}CD90^{+}$ cells (74 %) fell within a defined flow-cytometry gate which corresponds to 7–9 % of total G-CSF mobilized human peripheral blood cells (Fig. 1d and Additional file 1: Fig. S1a and b). Cells in this gate were characterized by low mitochondrial potential (low MP) while the majority of the remaining MPB populations fell within a high mitochondrial potential (high MP) (Fig. 1e-f). Furthermore, we determined percentages of different lineages within low and high MP cells of MPB (Fig. 1g and Additional file 1: Fig. S1c and d). The results showed the low MP cells only contained a few B cells (CD19, 7.9 %) and myeloid cells (Mac-1, 17.05 %). The high MP cells had lower percentage of B cells (CD19, 2.4 %), but much higher percentage of myeloid cells (Mac-1, 81.65 %). This result indicated that there were less differentiated cells in low MP cells compared to high MP cells, which was consistent with enrichment of HPSCs in low MP cells.

Low MP cells are primed for hypoxic niche

To characterize the metabolic properties of cells in the low and high MP gates, we performed a PCR array for hypoxia related gene expression in freshly isolated low and high MP cells. Under normoxic conditions, the low MP cells were characterized by significant upregulation of numerous hypoxia-inducible genes and regulatory glycolysis genes including Hif-1α (Fig. 2a). These results are not only supportive of the metabolic phenotype of low MP cells, but also suggest that the low MP cells are primed to handle hypoxic stresses. In addition, expression profile of the Hif-1α regulatory genes is in favor of stabilization of Hif-1α protein in low MP cells (Fig. 2b). PHD2, which is responsible for hydroxylation of Hif-1α resulting in its ubiquitination and degradation, was significantly ($p < 0.05$) downregulated in the low MP cells. Conversely, SIAH2 and VDU2, two stabilizers of Hif-1α were significantly ($p < 0.05$) upregulated in low MP cells compared to high MP cells. These results support the higher levels of Hif-1α and the higher expression of Hif-1α target genes in low MP cells.

Increased Hif-1α expression in low MP cells suggests that low MP cells could confer survival advantage at hypoxia. Thus, we measured the viability of low MP and high MP cells at normoxia and hypoxia (Fig. 2c). Survival of low MP cells at hypoxic condition, but not at normoxic condition, was much higher than that of high MP cells. The increased survival under hypoxic conditions by low MP cells in vitro suggested that low MP cells in physiological hypoxia could have higher survival ability. To further confirm this, we examined the apoptotic status of low and high MP cells at different conditions by staining with anti-Annexin V antibodies. Consistently, we demonstrated that there was a dramatic increase of apoptosis in high MP cells at hypoxic condition, but not at normoxic condition (Additional file 2: Fig. S2a). In addition, low MP cells consumed less oxygen compared to high MP cells at normoxia while there is no significant difference at hypoxia (Fig. 2d). Moreover, measurement of glycolysis rate of low MP and high MP cells showed that the glycolytic rate is significantly increased under hypoxia, which indicated the low MP cells preferred to glycolysis as the energy source in the physiologic niche (Fig. 2e). Moreover, we used the Seahorse XF96 extracellular flux analyzer to measure the oxygen consumption rate (OCR)

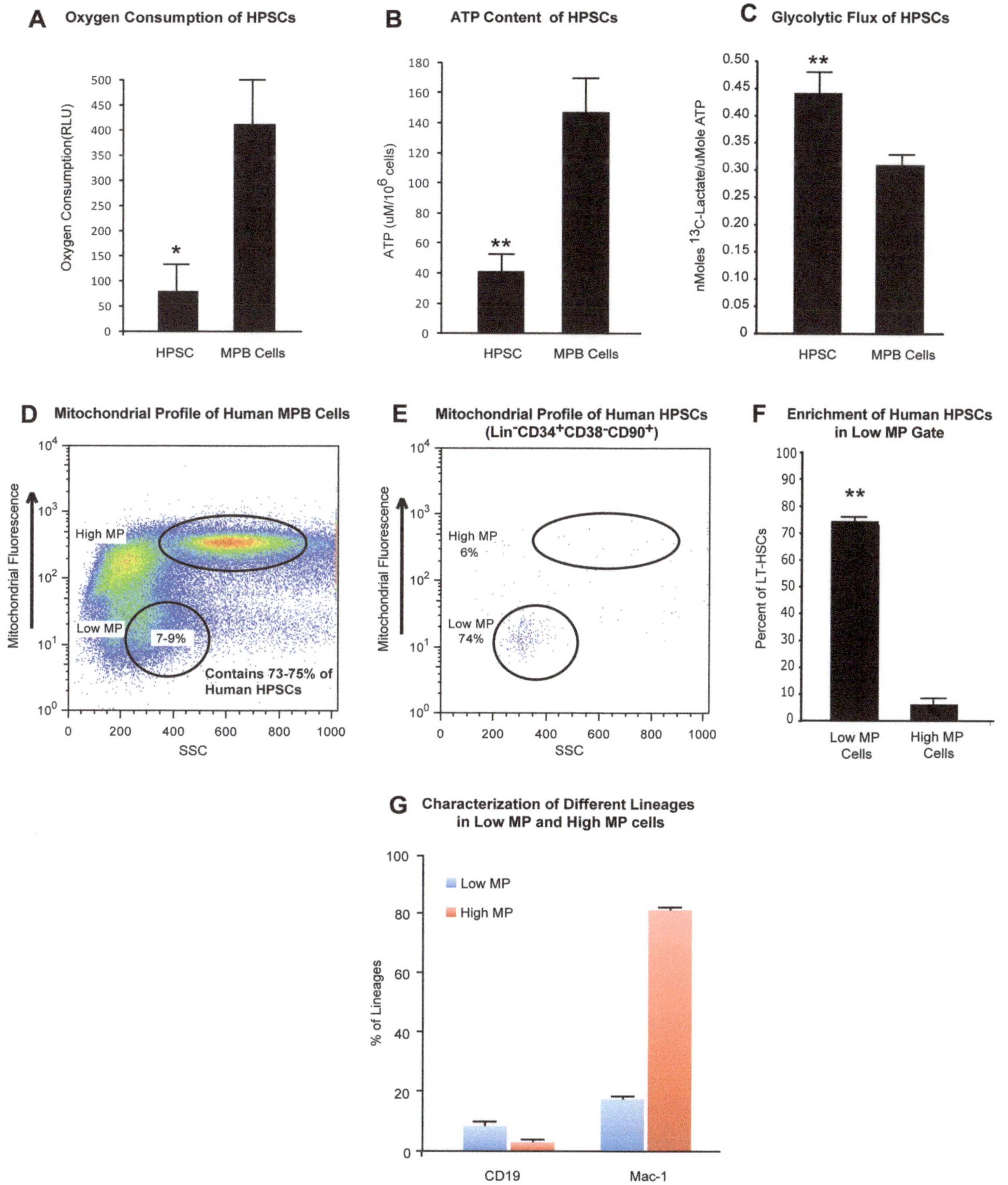

Fig. 1 (See legend on next page.)

(See figure on previous page.)
Fig. 1 Metabolic profile of human HPSCs. **a**) Oxygen consumption of $Lin^{-}CD34^{+}CD38^{-}CD90^{+}$ HPSCs and human mobilized peripheral blood cells (MPB Cells) demonstrating lower rates of oxygen consumption by HPSCs ($n = 3$). **b**) ATP level of HPSCs and MPB Cells demonstrating lower ATP levels in HPSCs ($n = 3$). **c**) Glycolytic flux of HPSCs and MPB Cells demonstrating higher rates of glycolysis in HPSCs ($n = 3$). **d**) Flow cytometry profile of MPB mononuclear cells stained with mitotracker. Note populations with different mitotracker fluorescence. **e**) Mitotracker profile of human HPSCs. The majority of human HPSCs (73–75 %) are localized to a unique population (7–9 %) of total human MPB mononuclear cells with low mitochondrial potential (low MP). **f**) Quantification of the percent of human HPSCs residing in low MP cells and high MP cells demonstrates significant enrichment of human HPSCs in low MP gate. **g**) Characterization of different lineages within low and high MP cells of MPB. The low MP cells only contained a few B cells (CD19, 7.9 %) and myeloid cells (Mac-1, 17.05 %). The high MP cells had lower percentage of B cells (CD19, 2.4 %), but much higher percentage of myeloid cells (Mac-1, 81.65 %) (n =3).$^{*}p < 0.05$, $^{**}p < 0.01$

indicative of oxidative phosphorylation, and the lactate production indicative of glycolysis (extracellular acidification rate, ECAR). As shown in Fig. 2f and g, low MP cells showed a significantly lower OCR rate as compared to high MP cells. In contrast, low MP cells showed a significantly higher ECAR rate, indicative of higher glycolytic metabolism. This data further revealed low MP cells using glycolysis as primary energy source.

Together, these results indicate that low MP cells are characterized by baseline upregulation of glycolytic and hypoxia inducible genes, which suggests adaptation of human HPSCs to glycolysis as the major source of energy production.

Characterization of stem cell profile of metabolically sorted cells

Given HSCs demonstrating distinct metabolic properties, we tested whether this metabolic footprint could enrich for HPSCs. Following flow cytometric separation of low and high MP cells, we utilized colony formation assay to test stem cell properties of low MP cells. Equal numbers of low and high MP cells were plated in methocult media for 12 days. Then, number and type of colonies were evaluated. Low MP cells had significantly ($p < 0.001$) higher colony formation compared to high MP cells (Fig. 3a). Additional classification of colony types showed that the low MP cells produced a higher percentage of CFU-GEMM type (mixed colonies) (Fig. 3b) with lower percentages of BFU-E (Fig. 3c) and CFU-GM (Fig. 3d) colonies than high MP cells. In addition to the *in vitro* assays, we also performed repopulation assays *in vivo* and demonstrated that low MP cells had much higher engraftment as compared to high MP cells. This provides the strong evidence that low MP cells are indeed enriched for HSPCs (Fig. 3e and Additional file 2: Fig. S2b). Furthermore, we evaluated the gene expression profile of low and high MP cells by PCR array. Similar to their mouse counterparts, low MP cells were characterized by enrichment of HPSC associated stem cell markers and diminished lineage differentiation markers when compared to high MP cells (Fig. 3f and g, respectively). These results indicate that low MP cells are enriched for human HPSCs.

Expression of Hif-1α and Meis1 in human HPSCs

In order to determine the molecular mechanism behind glycolytic phenotype of human HPSCs and the expression of Hif-1α in low MP MPB cells, we evaluated the expression pattern of Hif-1α and Meis1 in human MPB mononuclear cells and HPSCs. Meis1 is a transcription factor required for definitive hematopoiesis. We demonstrated that Meis1 transcriptionally regulates Hif-1α expression in mouse LT-HSCs [3]. However, whether Meis1 plays any role in the regulation of Hif-1α in human hematopoiesis was unknown. To address this question, we first determined the expression of Meis1 in human MPB mononuclear cells and HPSCs. Cells were fixed, permeabilized, and intracellularly stained by antibodies against Hif-1α and Meis1 followed by flow cytometry analysis. While about 5 % and 6 % of MPB mononuclear cells express Hif-1α and Meis1, respectively (Fig. 4a, Fig. 4d and Additional file 3: Fig. S3), a significantly higher percent of HPSCs express Hif-1α (47 %) (Fig. 4b-c and Additional file 4: Fig. S4) and Meis1 (48 %) (Fig. 4e-f and Additional file 4: Fig. S4). In addition, approximately 80 % of $Meis1^{+}$ MPB cells are Hif-1α positive (Fig. 4g-h and Additional file 3: Fig. S3). This expression pattern was obtained after hours of MPB harvest, which suggests that expression of Hif-1α in the MPB cells is not secondary to the *in vivo* hypoxic niche in the bone marrow.

Regulation of Hif-1α by Meis1

Given the confirmed conserved Meis1 consensus binding sequence in the Hif-1α intron [1] and the Meis1 expression in human hematopoietic cells, we sought to determine whether Meis1 is required for Hif-1α expression in HPSCs. To this end, we used siRNA to knockdown Meis1 in Kasumi-1 cells (a human myeloid progenitor cell line known to express Hif-1α at normoxic conditions [23]). Upregulation of Meis1 or Hif-1α in low MP cells and in Kasumi-1 cells was confirmed by real time PCR (Fig. 5a to 5c respectively) prior to siRNA experiments. Scrambled Meis1 siRNA was used as control. 50 nM Meis1 siRNA resulted in significant decrease of Meis1 mRNA levels (5.2 +/− 1.0 fold reduction) ($p < 0.05$). Conistently, the

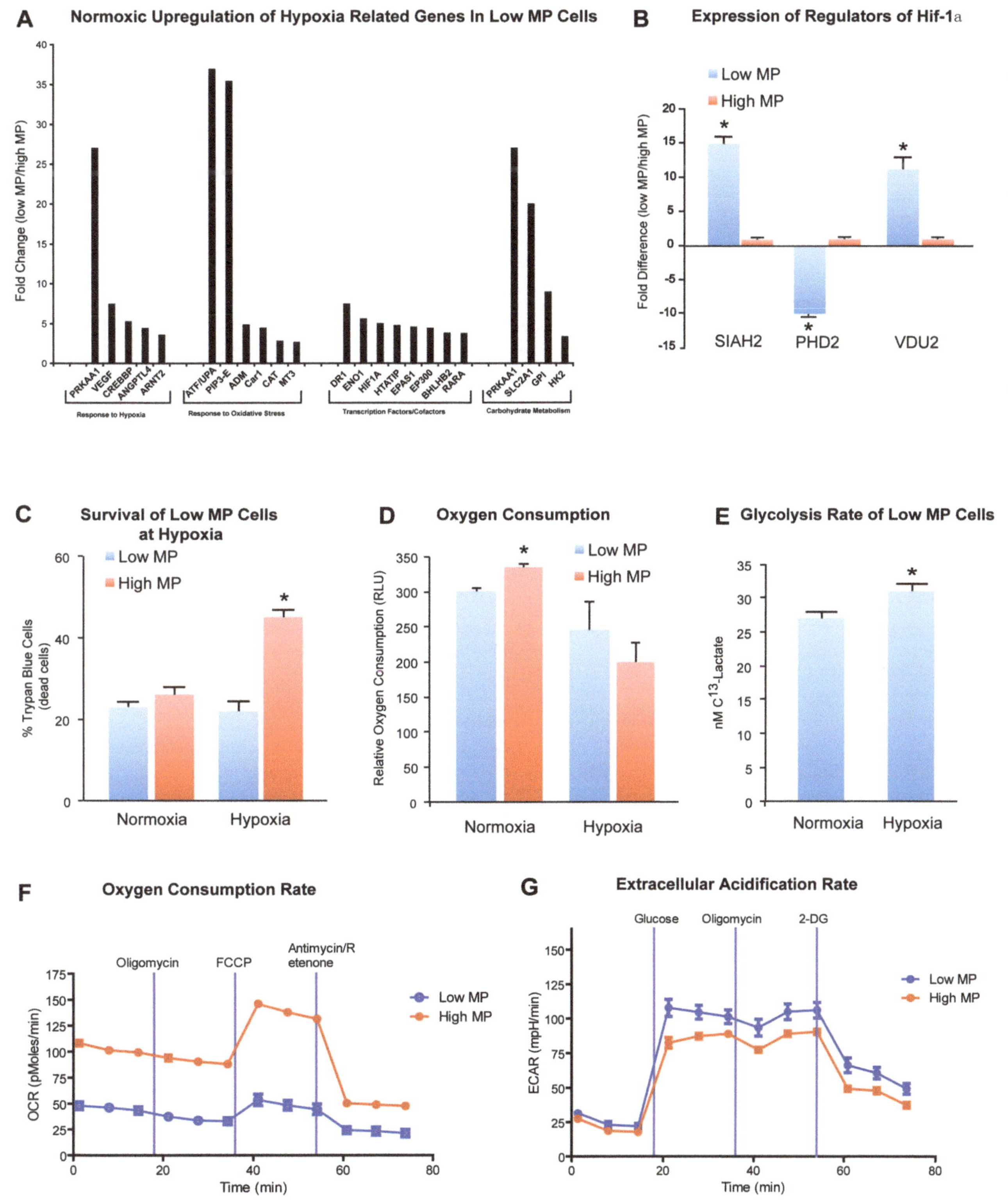

Fig. 2 (See legend on next page.)

(See figure on previous page.)
Fig. 2 Low MP Cells are primed for hypoxic niche. **a)** Real-time PCR array of low MP cells compared to high MP cells shows significant upregulation of a number of hypoxia inducible genes in the low MP cells at normoxia. **b)** Expression of regulators of Hif-1α in low and high MP cells by RT-PCR. Note the significant downregulation of the Hif-1α destabilizing enzyme PHD2 and the upregulation of two Hif-1α stabilizing enzymes SIAH2 and VDU2 in the low MP cells. **c)** Survival of low MP cells under hypoxia: The viability of low MP cells under hypoxic condition, but not normoxic condition, was much higher than that of high MP cells. **d)** Oxygen consumption by Low MP and High MP cells at normoxia and hypoxia. Low MP cells had lower rates of oxygen consumption at normoxia compared to high MP cells, but no significant difference at hypoxia. **e)** Increased glycolysis rate of low MP cells in vitro measured at hypoxia. Increased glycolytic rate under hypoxia by low MP cells suggest that low MP cells could respond to hypoxia via increasing glycolysis, which indicated the low MP cells prefer glycolysis as the energy source in the physiologic hypoxic niche. **f)** Plots of oxygen consumption rate (OCR) as a parameter of time in low MP cells and high MP cells. **g)** Extracellular acidification rate (ECAR) was plotted as a parameter of time in low MP cells and high MP cells (n =3).*$p < 0.05$

knockdown efficiency of Meis1 was further confirmed by western blotting (Additional file 5: Fig. S5). This was associated with a significant downregulation of Hif-1α mRNA (Fig. 5d), as well as reduced expression of glycolytic genes downstream of Hif-1α including lactate dehydrogenase (LDHA), Glut1 (SLC2A1), and phosphofructokinase (PFKL) (Fig. 5e) ($p < 0.05$). Furthermore, knockdown of Meis1 in Kasumi-1 cells demonstrated a relative metabolic shift towards increased oxidative phosphorylation in Kasumi-1 cells as shown by increased oxygen consumption and ATP levels (Fig. 5f) compared to negative control. These results demonstrate that Meis1 is required for optimal expression of Hif-1α and its downstream target genes in human hematopoietic cells.

Cooperation of Meis1 with Pbx1 and HoxA9 in the regulation of Hif-1α expression

In addition to Meis1 binding motif in the Hif-1α intron, we identified conserved putative Pbx1 ("TGAT") and HoxA9 ("ATAA") binding motifs in close proximity to consensus Meis1 binding site (Fig. 6a). Meis1, Pbx1 and HoxA9 pose interaction domains or motifs that facilitate cooperation in gene activation. Given that Meis1 is known to cooperate with Pbx1 and HoxA9 in gene activation, we tested the role of Pbx1 and HoxA9 in the activation of Hif-1α. Using Hif-1α-pGL2 luciferase reporter, which includes conserved Meis1, Pbx1 and HoxA9 sites, we demonstrate a dose dependent activation of Hif-1α by Pbx1 (Fig. 6b) and HoxA9 (Fig. 6c) in addition to Meis1 as we showed earlier [3]. This activation demonstrates dependence on binding of Pbx1 or HoxA9 to its consensus binding sequences in the Hif-1α reporter as mutation of the seed sequences (PbxMut-Hif-1α-pGL2 or HoxMut-Hif-1α-pGL2 reporters, respectively) completely abolished the activation of Hif-1α by Pbx1 or HoxA9 respectively. To test cooperation of Meis1 with Pbx1 and HoxA9 in the Hif-1α expression, we performed further luciferase assays using different combinations of Meis1, Pbx1, and HoxA9 vectors. Here we demonstrate that Meis1, Pbx1 and HoxA9 cooperate in the activation of Hif-1α (Hif-1α-pGL2 reporter) (Fig. 6d).

To further characterize the interaction of Meis1 with Pbx1 and HoxA9 proteins in the activation of Hif-1α, we generated mutant Meis1 protein lacking Pbx1 interaction Motifs (PIM) and HoxA9 protein lacking Meis1 interaction domain (MID) (Fig. 6e). As shown Additional file 6: Fig. S6, we could stably detect the expression of Meis1, Meis1ΔPIM, HoxA9 and HoxaΔMID, which indicated that deletion mutants of the proteins were stable in our system. These mutant proteins allowed us to demonstrate that protein-protein interaction between Meis1 and Pbx1 as well as Meis1 and HoxA9 are required for transcriptional activation of Hif-1α luciferase reporter by Meis1, Pbx1 and HoxA9 (Fig. 6f). In summary, Hif-1α expression is regulated by cooperative activation of Meis1, Pbx1 and HoxA9 (Fig. 6g). This activation is dependent on consensus binding motifs located at Hif-1α intronic region.

Discussion

Several studies indicated that human HPSCs reside in hypoxic niches and are capable of surviving upon hypoxic stress [1, 16, 17]. However, it is unclear if HPSCs are endowed with distinct metabolic properties that confer this hypoxic tolerance. In the current report, we show that human HPSCs are localized to a flow cytometry gate characterized by low mitochondrial potential (low MP). This population represents only 7–9 % of the G-CSF mobilized human peripheral blood cells, but is enriched for more than 70 % of human HPSCs as Lin^{-}CD34^{+}CD38^{-}CD90^{+} cells. Moreover, we confirm this metabolic profile by demonstrating that human HPSCs have lower ATP content, lower rates of oxygen consumption, and use cytoplasmic glycolysis instead of mitochondrial oxidative phosphorylation. Interestingly, here we demonstrated that the glycolytic phenotype of HPSCs persists in circulating cells, suggesting that the metabolic phenotype of HSCs is a product of intrinsic regulatory mechanisms and not just their environment. Similar to their murine counterparts, this unique metabolic profile is associated with upregulation of Hif-1α. It is noteworthy that we found human HPSCs are localized to the low MP gate even after G-CSF mobilization to the peripheral blood, which indicates that HPSCs may have

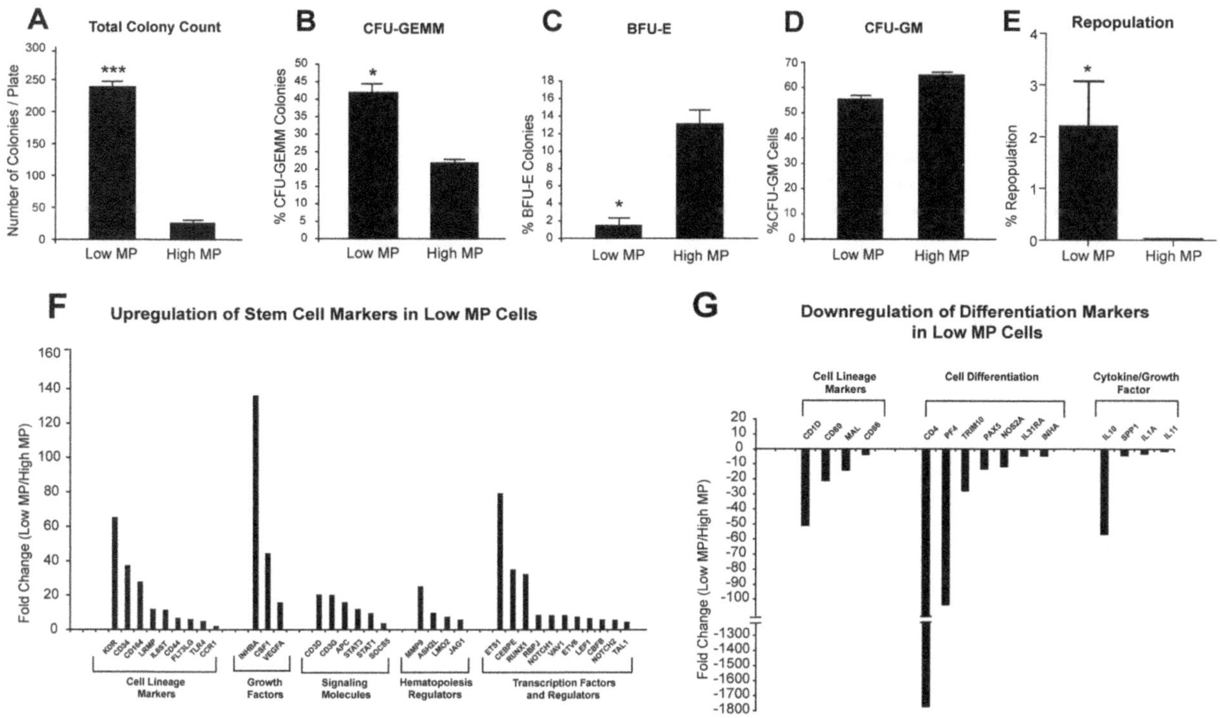

Fig. 3 Low MP Cells are enriched for hematopoietic stem cells. In vitro colony forming assay using low and high MP human MPB cells. Panel **a** to **d** shows the number of colonies derived from low and high MP cells after 12 days in methocult medium. Note the significantly higher number of colonies derived from the low MP population. ($n = 3$, $p < 0.001$) Different types of colonies derived from low and high MP cells were analyzed. **b**, **c** and **d** are the percentages of CFU-GEMM, BFU-E and CFU-GM respectively. **e**) FACS-sorted low MP cells and high MP cells were injected into the tibia of sublethally irradiated NOD/SCID mice. The donor repopulation was shown after 2 months. **f**) Real Time PCR array of HPSC markers comparing low MP cells to high MP cells. **g**) Real Time PCR array of differentiation markers comparing low MP to high MP cells. Note the enrichment of a number of markers for HPSCs and the downregulation of differentiation markers. *$p < 0.05$, ***$p < 0.001$

intrinsic mechanism for the regulation of their metabolic properties, other than their location in hypoxic niches.

Hif-1α as a master regulator of metabolism plays an essential role in various aspects of adaptation to hypoxic stress. Regulation of Hif-1α expression is well studied in terms of its posttranslational stabilization during hypoxia, however, little is known about its transcriptional regulation. Previous reports by our group and others indicate that Hif-1α is regulated at the transcription level not only at hypoxia but also normoxia [3, 22, 49–51]. Here we show that, the transcription factor Meis1 plays an important role in HPSC metabolism through transcriptional regulation of Hif-1α in cooperation with its cofactors Pbx1 and HoxA9. Meanwhile, we also noticed that anyone of Meis1, Pbx1 or HoxA9 was able to upregulate Hif-1α at transcription level (Fig. 6d). However, when one or more mutated factor(s) plus another WT factor did not transcriptionally upregulate Hif-1α (Fig. 6f). We speculated that the expression of mutant forms of the any protein might interrupt the action of any WT protein in transcriptional regulation of Hif-1α. This might indicate that normal expression levels of these factors play an important role in the synergistic effect in the expression of Hif-1α. Recently, our group recently demonstrated that Meis1 is an important regulator of postnatal cardiomyocyte cell cycle [52]. Intriguingly, we found that Pbx1 and HoxA9 were not expressed in postnatal cardiomyocytes, while other AbdB-like paralogue of Hox genes seem to have an expression pattern similar to Meis1. Therefore, it may be that the transcriptional activity of Meis1 in various compartments is regulated through differential expression pattern of its cofactors.

Conclusions

In summary, our findings demonstrate the unique metabolic properties of human HPSCs as compared to human MPB mononuclear cells, as well as the transcriptional network that regulates their metabolic phenotype. The transcriptional regulation of Hif-1α by Meis1 and its cofactors, and the metabolic shift that follows loss of Meis1 suggest that the metabolic profile of human HPSCs is an intrinsic characteristic of these cells and not only a product of their hypoxic microenvironment. It is therefore important for future studies to determine the role of these unique metabolic properties in vitro

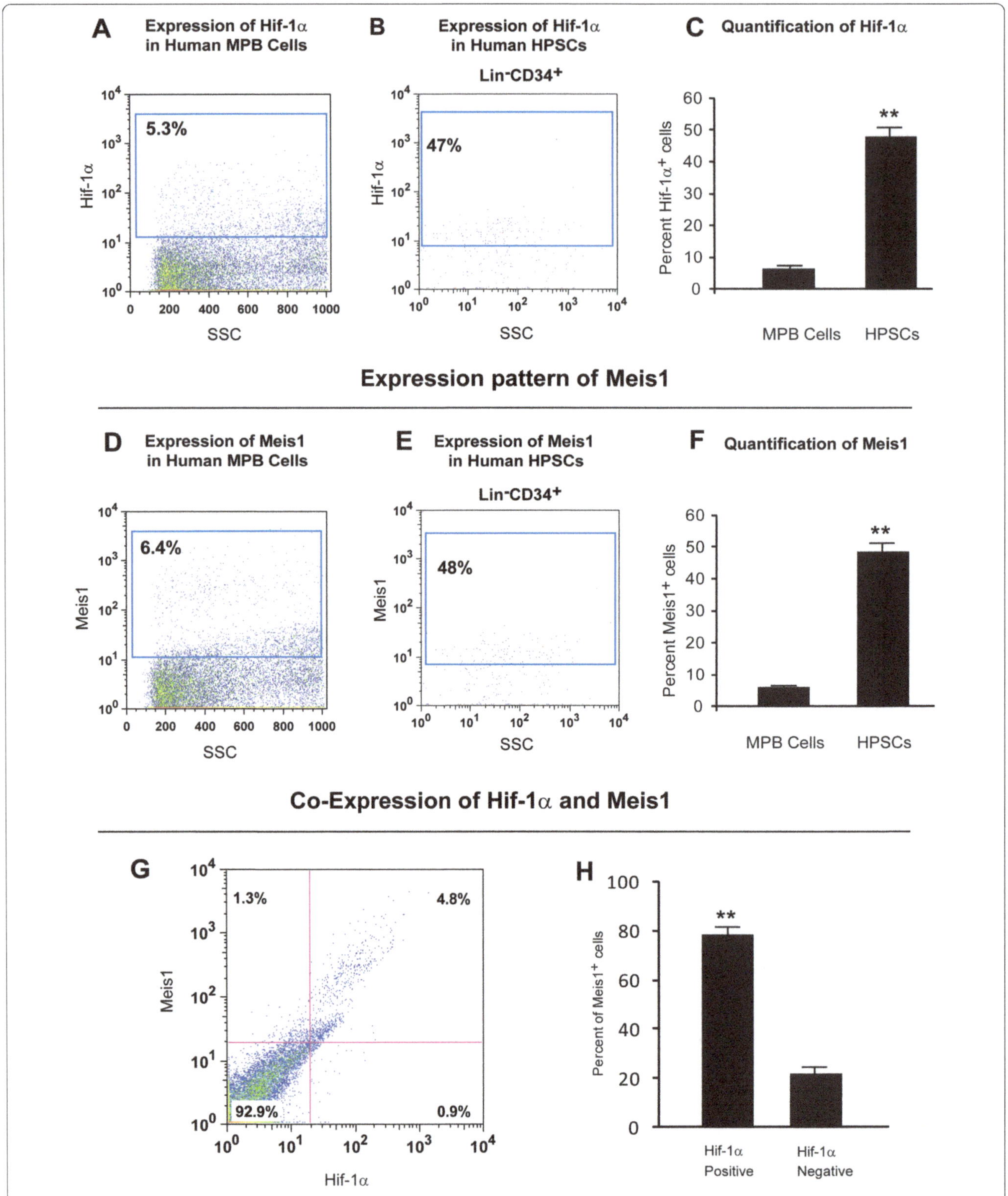

Fig. 4 (See legend on next page.)

(See figure on previous page.)
Fig. 4 Expression profile of Hif-1α and Meis1 in human HPSCs. Expression pattern of Hif-1α **a**) The left panel shows expression of Hif-1α in human MPB cells. **b**) Expression of Hif-1α in human HPSCs. **c**) Quantification of Hif-1α expression. Note that while 5.3 % of the human MPB cells express Hif-1α, the significantly higher percentage (47 %) of HPSCs express Hif-1α (~9 fold) ($n = 3$). Expression pattern of Meis1 **d**) The left panel shows expression of Meis1 in human MPB cells. **e**) Expression of Meis1 in HPSCs. **f**) The right panel shows quantification of Meis1 expression. Note that while 6.4 % of the human mobilized peripheral blood cells express Meis1, 48 % of HPSCs express Meis1 ($n = 3$) (~7.5 fold). Co-expression of Hif-1α and Meis1 **g**) Flow cytometric colocalization of Hif-1α and Meis1 in the human MPB cells. Left panel shows a representative flow cytometry profile of Hif-1α and Meis1 expression. **h**) Quantification of the percent of Meis1$^+$ cells. Note the majority of Meis1$^+$ cells coexpress Hif-1α. $^{**}p < 0.01$

human HPSC culture and expansion, as well as in designing therapeutic strategies for hematopoietic disorders.

Methods

Isolation of human mobilized peripheral blood (MPB) cells

Human G-CSF mobilized peripheral blood (MPB) was obtained from bone marrow transplant donors by plasmapheresis. Human cells were diluted and separated using ficoll to obtain the MPB mononuclear cell fraction. Then cells were suspended at $2–3 \times 10^6$ cells/mL in DMEM media with 10 % fetal bovine serum for flow cytometry. The study was approved by the Institutional Review Board of affiliated hospital of UT Southwestern Medical Center (Dallas, USA) and Shanghai JiaoTong University School of Medicine (Shanghai, China). Written informed consent was obtained from each donor for his enrollment. All clinical investigation was conducted in accordance with the principles expressed in the Declaration of Helsinki.

Flow cytometric profiling and separation of cells based on mitochondrial potential

Flow cytometric profiling and separation of human MPB cells based on their mitochondrial activity were performed by using mitotracker dyes as described previously [3]. Briefly, human MPB cells were enriched by lineage depletion using the BD IMag™ Human Lineage Cell Depletion Set (BD Biosciences) according to manufacturer's instructions. The whole MPB fraction and Lin$^-$CD34$^+$CD38$^-$CD90$^+$ cells (30 min incubation on ice) were then profiled based on their mitochondrial activity after 15 min staining with mitotracker dyes (MitoTracker Red FM Cat# M22425 and MitoTracker Green Cat# M7514, Invitrogen) at 37 °C (2×10^6 cells/mL, 200 nM mitotracker). Cell sorting based on high and low mitochondrial activity was performed using gates that separated the cells with those with the lowest 7–9 % of mitochondrial activity and equivalent number of cells with the high mitochondrial activity (named low and high mitochondrial potential (MP) cells).

Colony forming assay and *in vivo* transplantation

Based on mitochondrial profile, colony forming cell (CFC) assays were performed on human G-CSF MPB cells. Same numbers of human high and low MP cells (3×10^4 cells) were plated in each methocult plate (MethoCult® GF H4434, Stem Cell Technologies, USA). Viability was assessed with trypan blue as this is crucial that low MP gate often have dying cells with low mitochondrial activity. To minimize cell attachment, plates were precoated with 1 % agarose. After twelve days of culture, the total number of colonies (per plate) was counted and the types of colonies were quantified. Note CFU-GEMM colonies indicate mixed colonies whereas BFU-E and CFU-GM are measure of erythroid and myeloid progenitors, respectively. For *in vivo* transplantation, NOD-SCID mice were purchased from the Shanghai SLAC Laboratory Animal Co. Ltd. Five millions of FACS-sorted low MP or high MP cells in 50 μL of PBS were directly injected into the tibia as described previously [53]. Human engrafted cells in bone marrow were detected by using anti-human CD45 antibodies 2 months after transplantation.

Oxygen consumption

Oxygen consumption was determined using the BD Oxygen Biosensor System, 384 well (Cat#353,834) according to manufacturer's recommendations. MPB Cells and human HPSCs were separated as described above. Equal numbers of cells (5×10^4 cells/well in 50 μL volume) were incubated up to 6 h in the provided 384 well plate prior to measurement at Fluostar Optima plate reader (BMG Labtech). Culture media lacking cells was used as a negative control and sodium sulfite (100 mM) was used as a positive control. Oxygen consumption is presented as relative units.

ATP assay

HPSCs from human MPB Cells were isolated as described. Fifty thousand cells were used for each measurement. HPSCs and MPB Cells were centrifuged at 1200 g for 10 min. ATP standard curves were prepared using ATP concentrations between 10^{-6}-10^{-12} M. Then, 50 μl of ATP standards and 50 μl cell lysates were quantified using ATP Bioluminescence Assay Kit HS II (Roche) using Fluostar Optima plate reader (BMG Labtech) following manufacturer instructions. Finally, data were normalized to cell count.

Measurement of ^{13}C lactate production

Cells were cultured in DMEM (Sigma D5030) supplemented with L-glutamine (4 mM), $NaHCO_3$ (42.5 mM),

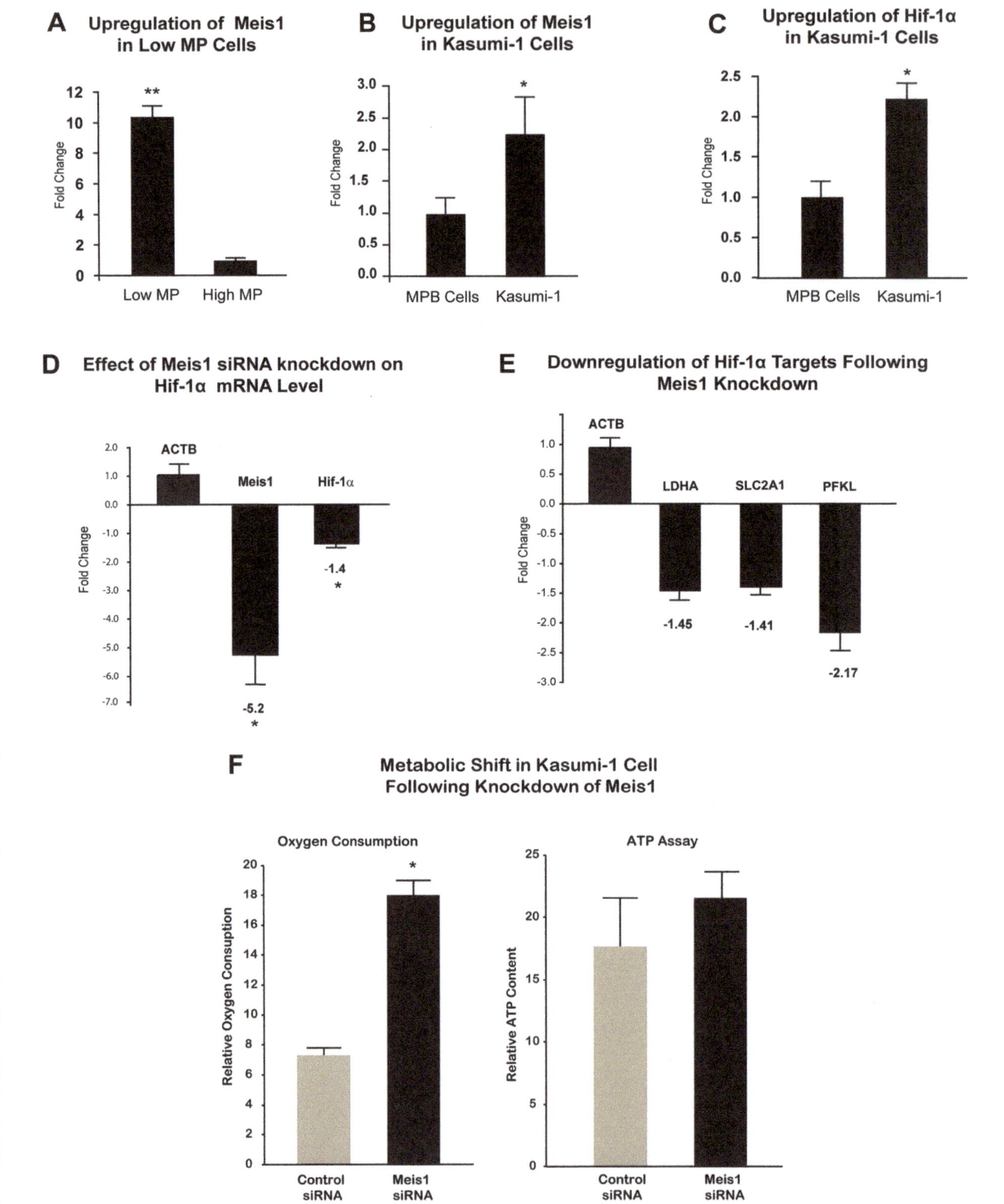

Fig. 5 (See legend on next page.)

(See figure on previous page.)
Fig. 5 Transcriptional regulation of Hif-1α by Meis1. **a**) Real Time PCR of Meis1 in low and high MP cells demonstrates significantly higher levels of Meis1 expression in low MP cells. **b**) Upregulation of Meis1 in Kasumi-1 cells compared to human MPB Cells and **c**) Upregulation of Hif-1α in Kasumi-1 cells compared to human MPB Cells. **d**) Real time PCR of Meis1 and Hif-1α in Kasumi-1 cells following siRNA knockdown of Meis1. **e**) Real time PCR of lactate dehydrogenase (LDHA), Glut1 (SLC2A1) and phosphofructokinase (PFKL) following siRNA knockdown of Meis1. Note the significant downregulation of Hif-1α mRNA and Hif-1α target genes following siRNA knockdown of Meis1. **f**) Relative metabolic shift towards increased oxidative phosphorylation in Kasumi-1 cells following Meis1 knockdown: There is increased oxygen consumption and ATP levels following knockdown of Meis1 in Kasumi-1 cells. $n = 3$, $^{*}p < 0.05$, $^{**}p < 0.01$

HEPES (25 mM), dialyzed fetal calf serum (10 % v/v), Penicillin/Streptomycin and no glucose per well of 96-well plate. The medium was supplemented with double labeled 10 mM D-[1-^{13}C, 6-^{13}C]-glucose (Cambridge Isotope Labs) to allow all of the glucose-derived lactate pool to be labeled on C-3. Fifty thousand cells (each well) were cultured in 40 μL of medium for 12 h. After the culture, the cells were pelleted and an aliquot of 25 μL of the medium was transferred to a glass test tube with the internal standard (17.9 nmol of Sodium L-[$^{13}C_3$]-Lactate, Cambridge Isotope Labs). Lactate was extracted by sequential addition of 1 mL of methanol, chloroform and water followed by vortexing and centrifugation at 2000 rpm for 5 min. The aqueous phase was evaporated, derivatized with 100 μL Tri-Sil reagent (Pierce) for 30 min at 42 °C, and analyzed by gas chromatography–mass spectrometry. A three-point standard curve was also prepared using mixtures of un-enriched lactate and L-[3-$^{13}C_3$]-lactate (Cambridge Isotope Labs). Lactate abundance was determined by monitoring m/z at 117 (un-enriched), 118 (lactate containing ^{13}C from glucose) and 119 (internal standard). The areas of 117 and 118 were summed and corrected against the 119 area to calculate total lactate abundance. To determine the atom percent excess (APE), the 117 and 118 areas were first corrected against the 119 abundance to account for inter-sample variability of extraction. Then the corrected ratio of 118/(117 + 118) was determined and compared to the standard curve. Finally, the APE was multiplied by the total nmoles lactate to determine the nmoles of ^{13}C-lactate produced. The final results were corrected for total cellular ATP concentration.

Metabolic assays with seahore XF96

Oxygen consumption and lactate generation were measured using the Seahorse XF96 extracellular flux analyzer as previously described [54]. Briefly, three replicate wells of 3×10^5 low MP or high MP cells per well were seeded overnight in 96-well XF96 well plates coated with BD Cell-Tak (BD Biosciences) in serum-free culture medium containing 20 ng/ml SCF and 20 ng/ml TPO. One hour prior to analysis, the medium was replaced by unbuffered DMEM and the well plates were incubated to 37°C for pH stabilization. Analyses were performed both at basal conditions and after injection of oligomycin (0.5 μM for OCR or 2 μM for ECAR), FCCP (2 μM), Antimycin A (0.5 μM), Glucose (10 mM), and 2-DG (100 mM).

Meis1 knockdown

Meis1 siRNA knockdown was carried out in Kasumi-1 cells (human myeloid progenitor cell line known to express Hif-1α at normoxic conditions [23]). Upregulation of Meis1 in low MP cells and Kasumi-1 cells compared to human MPB cells were confirmed by real time PCR. Kasumi-1 cells were diluted to a density of 200,000 cells per mL in RPMI media supplemented with 20 % FBS and antibiotics. The cells were centrifuged for 10 min at 1200 g at 4 °C and suspended in OPTIMEM (Invitrogen). The cells were then plated into 6-well plates. 12 μL of Hiperfect (Qiagen) and siRNA (50nM of siRNA per 750,000 cells/well) were incubated in 200 μL of OPTI-MEM (Invitrogen) for 20 min at RT. Silencer Select Pre-designed siRNAs (Applied Biosystems, Ambion) for Meis1 were diluted into 50nM stocks (siRNA ID# s8662: 5'-GGCAUCUACUCGUUCAGGAtt-3' and 5'-UCCUGAAC GAGUAGAUGCCgt-3'). siRNA were added to cells dropwise and incubated for 6 h. After 6 h incubation, 2.5 mL RPMI medium was added (20 % FBS and antibiotics) and plates were incubated under normal growth conditions for 48 h.

Expression profile of low and high MP cells

PCR arrays (HSC and hypoxia primer sets, SABiosciences) were performed to study HPSC and hypoxia inducible gene expression profile of low and high MP cells. RNA was isolated from low and high MP cells by TRIzol method (Invitrogen, Carlsbad, CA) following manufacturer instructions. cDNA was generated by using an RT-PCR kit (SA biosciences, Maryland, USA). Real-Time PCR was performed using Human Real-Time Syber Green PCR Mix (SuperArray) on an ABI Prism 7700 Sequence Detector (Applied Biosystems). The data was analyzed using the ΔΔCt method. Fold change was calculated as difference in gene expression between low and high MP cells.

Real time PCR for Meis1, Hif-1α and Hif-1α related genes

Total RNA was isolated using TRIzol reagent (Invitrogen). cDNA was generated by following the recommended

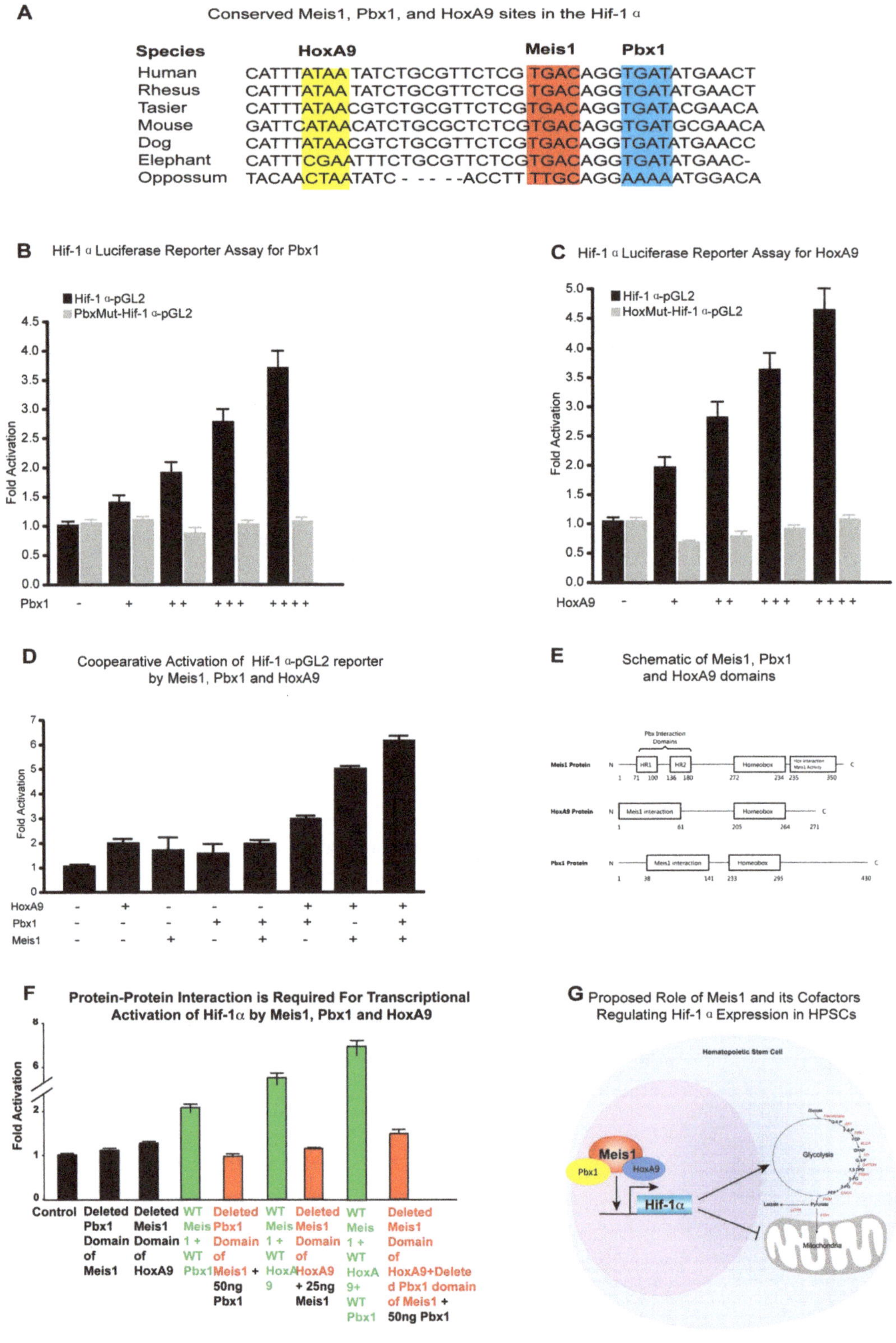

Fig. 6 (See legend on next page.)

(See figure on previous page.)
Fig. 6 Cooperative role of Pbx1, HoxA9, and Meis1 for transcriptional regulation of Hif-1α. **a**) Figure shows conserved consensus Meis1, Pbx1, and HoxA9 motifs found on Hif-1α gene. Note the binding motifs found next to each other in close proximity and highly conserved. **b**) Luciferase reporter assays demonstrate dose-dependent transcriptional activation of Hif-1α (Hif-1α-pGL2 reporter) by Pbx1 and mutation of Pbx1 bindings sites abolished Hif-1α activation (PbxMut-Hif-1α-pGL2 reporter) **c**) Luciferase reporter assays demonstrate dose-dependent transcriptional activation of Hif-1α (Hif-1α-pGL2 reporter) by HoxA9 and mutation of HoxA9 bindings sites abolish Hif-1α activation (HoxMut-Hif-1α-pGL2 reporter) **d**) Luciferase reporter assays with different combinations of Meis1, Pbx1, and HoxA9 demonstrates (additive) cooperation of Meis1, Pbx1 and HoxA9 for activation of Hif-1α (Hif-1α-pGL2 reporter) **e**) Schematic of Meis1, Pbx1 and HoxA9 domains **f**) Meis1, Pbx1 and HoxA9 protein interaction were assessed by deletion of pbx1 interaction domain at Meis1 (71-100aa HR1 and 136-180aa HR regions) and Meis1 interaction domain of HoxA9 (1-61aa). Transcriptional activation by WT vectors, and vectors with deleted domains were evaluated using Hif-1α-pGL2 construct. Luciferase measurements were calculated as firefly luciferase units versus b-gal units. **g**) Schematic of proposed model showing regulation of Hif-1α expression by a complex of Meis1/Pbx1/HoxA9 proteins in hematopoietic stem cells

protocol for SuperScript II Reverse Transcriptase (Invitrogen) using 2 μg total RNA. Real time PCR was performed with SyberGreen (Applied Biosystems) on ABI Prism 7700 Sequence Detector (Applied Biosystems) using primers at Table 1.

Intracellular detection of Hif-1α and Meis1 in HPSCs

Human MPB cells and human HPSCs underwent fixation with 4 % paraformaldehyde for 10 min at room temperature. After permeabilization (0.01 % Triton) and serum block, cells were incubated overnight with primary antibodies; 1:50 dilution of anti-Hif-1α (Cat#610958, BD Transcduction Laboratories) and 1:50 dilution of anti-Meis1 (sc-10599, Santa Cruz Biotechnology). Staining was assessed by flow cytometry after incubation with corresponding fluorophore-conjugated secondary antibody.

Generation of Meis1 lacking Pbx1 interaction motifs and HoxA9 lacking Meis1 interaction domain constructs

Meis1 and Pbx1 protein interaction were assessed by deletion of Pbx1 interaction domain of Meis1. For that purpose, we generated Meis1 lacking aminoacids for Pbx1 interaction domain (both 71–100 aa HR1 and 136-180aa HR regions) by polymerase chain reaction (PCR) from pCMV-SPORT6-Meis1 (MMM1013-7512739, Openbiosystems) using primers (NotI site were inserted for screening) Meis1dPIM(71–130)F: 5'- ATCTATcatgcggccg cAAAATGCCTATCGATTTGGTGATAG-3' and Meis1dPIM(71–130)R: 5'-ATCTATcatgcggccgcTAAAGCGTCAT TGACCGAGGAACCC-3'.

Meis1 and HoxA9 protein interaction were studied by co-tranfection of Meis1 with HoxA9 lacking Meis1 interaction domain (MID). HoxA9 lacking aminoacids for Meis1 interaction domain (1–61) were generated by PCR from pCMV-SPORT6-HoxA9 (MMM1013-9200573, Openbiosystems) using primers (BamHI site were inserted for screening) HoxA9dN(1–61)F: 5'-ATCTATcatggatccCA TTGCAGTAGCCCGCGCCTG GCCGG-3' and HoxA9 dN(1–61)R: 5'-ATCTATcatggatccGCGGTGTTTGGTGC CTCGTGGAACCC-3'.

Luciferase assays

Transcriptional activation of Hif-1α reporter by Meis1 (pCMV-SPORT6-Meis1, Cat#MMM1013-7512739,Open biosystems), Meis1 lacking Pbx1 interaction domain (Meis1ΔPIM), HoxA9 (pCMV-SPORT6-HoxA9, Cat# MMM1013-9200573, Openbiosystems), HoxA9 lacking Meis1 interaction domain (HoxaΔMID) and Pbx1 (pCMV-SPORT6-Pbx1, Cat# MMM1013-63227,Openbiosystems), were evaluated using Hif-1α-pGL2 or PbxMut-Hif-1α-pGL2 (having Pbx1 binding site mutated) or HoxMut-Hif-1α-pGL2 (having HoxA9 binding site mutated) reporter constructs as indicated in the figures. 0.8 μg of Hif-1α-pGL2 or PbxMut-Hif-1α-pGL2 or HoxMut-Hif-1α-pGL2 reporter construct were co-transfectedwith different doses of the Meis1, Meis1ΔPIM, HoxA9, HoxaΔMID and Pbx1 expression vectors and 0.2 μg of pCMV-LacZ (internal

Table 1 Primers used in this study

Gene [GenBank: Accession Numbers]	Forward Primer	Reverse Primer
Meis1 [NM_002398.2]	5'-ACGCTTTTTGTGACGCTTTT-3'	5'-TCACACAGTGGGGACAACAG-3'
Hif-1α [NM_001243084.1]	5'-GAAGTGGCAACTGATGAGCA-3'	5'-GCGCGAACGACAAGAAA-3'
LDHA [NM_001135239.1]	5'-GGAGATCCATCATCTCTCCC-3'	5'-GGCCTGTGCCATCAGTATCT-3'
SLC2A1 [NM_006516.2]	5'-GGCATTGATGACTCCAGTGTT-3'	5'-ATGGAGCCCAGCAGCAA-3'
PFKL [NM_001002021.2]	5'-GATGATGTTGGAGACGCTCA-3'	5'-GGTGCCAAAGTCTTCCTCAT-3'
SIAH2 [NM_005067.5]	5'-GTTTCTCCGTATGGTGCAGG-3'	5'-TCAGGAACCTGGCTATGGAG-3'
PHD2 [NM_022051.2]	5'-GTTCCATTGCCCGGATAAC-3'	5'-CGACCTGATACGCCACTGTA-3'
VDU2 [NM_001008563.4]	5'-TAGGGGTCTGGAGTGAGTGG-3'	5'-CTCTGAGCATTGGCGACC-3'

control) into COS cells using lipofectamine transfection reagent (Invitrogen). At 48 h after transfection, cell lysate were prepared and quantified for firefly luciferase activity using a luciferase reporter system (Promega). Luciferase measurements were calculated as firefly luciferase units versus b-gal units. Transcriptional activation was compared to basal luciferase levels in cells transfected with Hif-1α-pGL2 or PbxMut-Hif-1α-pGL2 or HoxMut-Hif-1α-pGL2 and empty pGL2. To test Pbx1 site specificity, Pbx1 binding site TGAT at Hif-1α-pGL2 reporter were mutated using site directed mutagenesis kit (Strategene) from Hif-1α-pGL2 vector with the following primers: PbxMut-Hif-1α-F:5'-CAATTTCTACAAACTTGTGTTTGCCG ACCCTG TCAGGAGAGCCCAGACGTTA-3' and PbxMut-Hif-1α-R: 5'-TAACGTCTGGGCTCTCCTGACAGGGTC GGCA AACACAAGTTTGTAGAAATTG-3'. Similarly, to test HoxA9 site specificity, HoxA9 binding site ATAA at Hif-1α reporter using site directed mutagenesis kit from Hif-1α-pGL2 vector with the following primers: HoxMu-Hif-1α-F: 5'-CCTGTCAGGAGAGCCCAGACGCCGCGTATCAA TATGTGGCTG CCTC-3' and HoxMut-Hif-1α-R: 5'-GAGGCAGCCACATATTGATACGCGGCGTCTG GG CTCTCCTGACAGG-3'.

Western blotting and apoptosis assay

Plasmids of pCMV-SPORT6-Meis1, Meis1ΔPIM, pCMV-SPORT6-HoxA9 and HoxaΔMID were transfected into 293 T cells. Whole cell lysates were electrophoresed on 8–10 % sodium dodecyl sulfate polyacrylamide gels and transferred onto polyvinylidene difluoride membranes (Millipore). The membranes were incubated with primary antibodies overnight at 4 °C followed by incubation with appropriate horseradish peroxidase-conjugated secondary antibodies. The following antibodies were used: anti-Meis1 (Abcam), anti-HoxA9 (Proteintech) and anti-β-actin (Calbiochem). For analysis of apoptosis, cells were stained with PE conjugated anti-annexin V and 7-AAD (BD Pharmingen) according to the manufacturer's instructions.

Statistical analysis

Results are expressed as mean ± SEM and a 2-tailed Student t test was used to determine the level of significance. $p < 0.05$ was considered statistically different.

Additional files

Additional file 1: Figure S1. Clustering and quantification of HSC frequency and lineages in Low or High MP cells. A) Quantification of HSC frequency in low MP and high MP cells: HSC ($Lin^-CD34^+CD38^-CD90^+$) frequency in low MP cells was 1.23 % (4.94 %*0.249 = 1.23 %), which was around 15-fold higher compared to high MP cells (0.332 %*0.252 = 0.084 %). B) Gating strategy showing clustering of human HPSCs into low and high MP gates. Human HPSCs clustered into low MP and high MP cells, where HSPCs were mostly located in low MP gate. C-D) Lineage distribution was measured in low and high MP cells by flow cytometric analysis with anti-CD19 and anti-Mac-1 antibodies. (PDF 711 kb)

Additional file 2: Figure S2. A) Quantification of the percentage of Annexin V^+ cells in low MP and high MP cells at normoxia or hypoxia. B) Representative flow cytometric analysis of repopulation of low MP and high MP cells. (PDF 324 kb)

Additional file 3: Figure S3. Gating stragegy for Meis1 and Hif-1α intracellular staining in human MPB Cells (Related to Fig. 4A, 4D, and 4G). (PDF 730 kb)

Additional file 4: Figure S4. Gating stragegy for Meis1 and Hif-1α intracellular staining in human HPSCs (Lin^-CD34^+) (Related to Fig. 4B and 4E). (PDF 442 kb)

Additional file 5: Figure S5. Knockdown efficiency of Meis1 by siRNA was examined by western blotting. (PDF 160 kb)

Additional file 6: Figure S6. WT and Deletion mutants (Meis1, Meis1ΔPIM, HoxA9 and HoxaΔMID) were overexpressed in 293T cells and detected by western blotting with anti-Meis1 and anti-HoxA9 antibodies. Both WT and deletion mutants of Meis1, HoxA9 were stably detected. (PDF 461 kb)

Abbreviations

HSCs: Hematopoietic stem cells; HPSCs: Human hematopoietic progenitor and stem cells; Hif-1α: Hypoxia-inducible factor 1-alpha; Meis1: Meis homeobox 1; MP: Mitochondrial potential; Pbx1: Pre-B-cell leukemia transcription factor 1; HoxA9: Homeobox A9.

Competing interests

The authors declare that they have no competing interests.

Authors' contributions

FK, HA, CCZ and JZ designed, performed experiments, interpreted data, and contributed to writing of the manuscript. LX, ZY, RJD, WK, ST, AFE, HA, SM, XL, CC and HAS contributed to experimental performance and interpretation. All authors read and approved the final manuscript.

Authors' information

JZ is a professor at Shanghai Jiao Tong University School of Medicine, working on the metabolic regulation of hematopoietic stem cells and leukemia stem cells as well as screening new growth factors for ex vivo expansion of hematopoietic stem cells.

Acknowledgments

This work is supported by grants from the American Heart Association (AHA Fellow to Faculty Award) (Sadek), the Gilead Research Scholars Program in Cardiovascular Disease (Sadek), NIH grant 1R01CA172268 (Zhang), CPRIT RP140402 (Zhang), March of Dimes Foundation Award #1-FY14-201 (Zhang), National Natural Science Foundation of China (81370654, 81471524 and 31171409), the Program for Professor of Special Appointment (Eastern Scholar) at Shanghai Institutions of Higher Learning and the Pujiang Program (13PJ1405600) (Zheng). We thank the support from CO-FUNDED Brain Circulation Scheme by The Scientific and Technological Research Council of Turkey (TÜBİTAK) and The Marie Curie Action COFUND of the 7th. Framework Programme (FP7) of the European Commission grant 115C039 (Kocabas), The Science Academy of Turkey Young Scientist Award Program (Kocabas), and funds provided by Yeditepe University, Istanbul, Turkey (Kocabas).

Author details

[1]Department of Internal Medicine, Division of Cardiology, UT Southwestern Medical Center at Dallas, Dallas, TX 75390, USA. [2]Department of Genetics and Bioengineering, Faculty of Engineering, Yeditepe University, Istanbul 34755, Turkey. [3]Hongqiao International Institute of Medicine, Shanghai Tongren Hospital / Faculty of Basic Medicine, Shanghai Jiao Tong University School of Medicine, Shanghai 200025, China. [4]Key Laboratory of Cell Differentiation and Apoptosis of Chinese Ministry of Education, Shanghai Jiao Tong University School of Medicine, Chongqing South Road 280, Shanghai 200025, China. [5]Bingzhou Medical University, Taishan Scholar Program, Yantai 264003, China. [6]Departments of Pediatrics and Genetics, UT Southwestern Medical Center at Dallas, Dallas, TX 75390, USA. [7]Department of Clinical Pathology, El

Galaa Hospital, Cairo, Egypt. [8]Faculty of Medicine Ain Shams University, El Abbaseya, Cairo, Egypt. [9]Departments of Physiology and Developmental Biology, UT Southwestern Medical Center at Dallas, 5323 Harry Hines Blvd, Dallas, TX 75390, USA.

References

1. Eliasson P, Jonsson JI. The hematopoietic stem cell niche: low in oxygen but a nice place to be. J Cell Physiol. 2010;222(1):17–22.
2. Wang LD, Wagers AJ. Dynamic niches in the origination and differentiation of haematopoietic stem cells. Nat Rev Mol Cell Biol. 2011;12(10):643–55.
3. Simsek T, Kocabas F, Zheng JK, DeBerardinis RJ, Mahmoud AI, Olson EN, et al. The distinct metabolic profile of hematopoietic stem cells reflects their location in a hypoxic niche. Cell Stem Cell. 2010;7(3):380–90.
4. Takubo K, Goda N, Yamada W, Iriuchishima H, Ikeda E, Kubota Y, et al. Regulation of the HIF-1alpha level is essential for hematopoietic stem cells. Cell Stem Cell. 2010;7(3):391–402.
5. Kim CG, Lee JJ, Jung DY, Jeon J, Heo HS, Kang HC, et al. Profiling of differentially expressed genes in human stem cells by cDNA microarray. Mol Cells. 2006;21(3):343–55.
6. Papandreou I, Cairns RA, Fontana L, Lim AL, Denko NC. HIF-1 mediates adaptation to hypoxia by actively downregulating mitochondrial oxygen consumption. Cell Metab. 2006;3(3):187–97.
7. Kim JW, Tchernyshyov I, Semenza GL, Dang CV. HIF-1-mediated expression of pyruvate dehydrogenase kinase: a metabolic switch required for cellular adaptation to hypoxia. Cell Metab. 2006;3(3):177–85.
8. Marin-Hernandez A, Gallardo-Perez JC, Ralph SJ, Rodriguez-Enriquez S, Moreno-Sanchez R. HIF-1alpha modulates energy metabolism in cancer cells by inducing over-expression of specific glycolytic isoforms. Mini Rev Med Chem. 2009;9(9):1084–101.
9. Zhang H, Gao P, Fukuda R, Kumar G, Krishnamachary B, Zeller KI, et al. HIF-1 inhibits mitochondrial biogenesis and cellular respiration in VHL-deficient renal cell carcinoma by repression of C-MYC activity. Cancer Cell. 2007;11(5):407–20.
10. Semenza GL. Regulation of cancer cell metabolism by hypoxia-inducible factor 1. Semin Cancer Biol. 2009;19(1):12–6.
11. Semenza GL. Regulation of oxygen homeostasis by hypoxia-inducible factor 1. Physiology (Bethesda). 2009;24:97–106.
12. Semenza GL. Oxygen homeostasis. Wiley Interdiscip Rev Syst Biol Med. 2010;2(3):336–61.
13. Semenza GL. HIF-1 and mechanisms of hypoxia sensing. Curr Opin Cell Biol. 2001;13(2):167–71.
14. Semenza GL. Hypoxia-inducible factor 1 (HIF-1) pathway. Sci STKE. 2007;2007(407):cm8.
15. Wang GL, Jiang BH, Rue EA, Semenza GL. Hypoxia-inducible factor 1 is a basic-helix-loop-helix-PAS heterodimer regulated by cellular O2 tension. Proc Natl Acad Sci U S A. 1995;92(12):5510–4.
16. Parmar K, Mauch P, Vergilio JA, Sackstein R, Down JD. Distribution of hematopoietic stem cells in the bone marrow according to regional hypoxia. Proc Natl Acad Sci U S A. 2007;104(13):5431–6.
17. Koller MR, Bender JG, Miller WM, Papoutsakis ET. Reduced oxygen tension increases hematopoiesis in long-term culture of human stem and progenitor cells from cord blood and bone marrow. Exp Hematol. 1992;20(2):264–70.
18. Salceda S, Caro J. Hypoxia-inducible factor 1alpha (HIF-1alpha) protein is rapidly degraded by theubiquitin-proteasome system under normoxic conditions. Its stabilization by hypoxia dependson redox-induced changes. J Biol Chem. 1997;272(36):22642–7.
19. Ivan M, Kondo K, Yang H, Kim W, Valiando J, Ohh M, et al. HIFalpha targeted for VHL-mediated destruction by proline hydroxylation: implications for O2 sensing. Science. 2001;292(5516):464–8.
20. Jaakkola P, Mole DR, Tian YM, Wilson MI, Gielbert J, Gaskell SJ, et al. Targeting of HIF-alpha to the von Hippel-Lindau ubiquitylation complex by O2-regulated prolyl hydroxylation. Science. 2001;292(5516):468–72.
21. Qi J, Nakayama K, Gaitonde S, Goydos JS, Krajewski S, Eroshkin A, et al. The ubiquitin ligase Siah2 regulates tumorigenesis and metastasis by HIF-dependent and -independent pathways. Proc Natl Acad Sci U S A. 2008;105(43):16713–8.
22. BelAiba RS, Bonello S, Zharinger C, Schmidt S, Hess J, Kietzmann T, et al. Transcriptional regulation of HIF-1alpha by NFkappaB in response to hypoxia. Circulation. 2006;114(18):182–3.
23. Pedersen M, Lofstedt T, Sun J, Holmquist-Mengelbier L, Pahlman S, Ronnstrand L. Stem cell factor induces HIF-1alpha at normoxia in hematopoietic cells. Biochem Biophys Res Commun. 2008;377(1):98–103.
24. Belaiba RS, Bonello S, Zahringer C, Schmidt S, Hess J, Kietzmann T, et al. Hypoxia up-regulates hypoxia-inducible factor-1alpha transcription by involving phosphatidylinositol 3-kinase and nuclear factor kappaB in pulmonary artery smooth muscle cells. Mol Biol Cell. 2007;18(12):4691–7.
25. Hagg M, Wennstrom S. Activation of hypoxia-induced transcription in normoxia. Exp Cell Res. 2005;306(1):180–91.
26. Kocabas F, Zheng J, Thet S, Copeland NG, Jenkins NA, DeBerardinis RJ, et al. Meis1 regulates the metabolic phenotype and oxidant defense of hematopoietic stem cells. Blood. 2012;120(25):4963–72.
27. Pineault N, Helgason CD, Lawrence HJ, Humphries RK. Differential expression of Hox, Meis1, and Pbx1 genes in primitive cells throughout murine hematopoietic ontogeny. Exp Hematol. 2002;30(1):49–57.
28. Argiropoulos B, Yung E, Humphries RK. Unraveling the crucial roles of Meis1 in leukemogenesis and normal hematopoiesis. Genes Dev. 2007;21(22):2845–9.
29. Eppert K, Takenaka K, Lechman ER, Waldron L, Nilsson B, van Galen P, et al. Stem cell gene expression programs influence clinical outcome in human leukemia. Nat Med. 2011;17(9):1086–93.
30. Becker MW, Jordan CT. Leukemia Stemness Signatures Step toward the Clinic. Cell Stem Cell. 2011;9(3):185–6.
31. Wang GG, Pasillas MP, Kamps MP. Meis1 programs transcription of FLT3 and cancer stem cell character, using a mechanism that requires interaction with Pbx and a novel function of the Meis1 C-terminus. Blood. 2005;106(1):254–64.
32. Wang GG, Pasillas MP, Kamps MP. Persistent transactivation by meis1 replaces hox function in myeloid leukemogenesis models: evidence for co-occupancy of meis1-pbx and hox-pbx complexes on promoters of leukemia-associated genes. Mol Cell Biol. 2006;26(10):3902–16.
33. Hisa T, Spence SE, Rachel RA, Fujita M, Nakamura T, Ward JM, et al. Hematopoietic, angiogenic and eye defects in Meis1 mutant animals. EMBO J. 2004;23(2):450–9.
34. Azcoitia V, Aracil M, Martinez-A C, Torres M. The homeodomain protein Meis1 is essential for definitive hematopoiesis and vascular patterning in the mouse embryo. Dev Biol. 2005;280(2):307–20.
35. Imamura T, Morimoto A, Takanashi M, Hibi S, Sugimoto T, Ishii E, et al. Frequent co-expression of HoxA9 and Meis1 genes in infant acute lymphoblastic leukaemia with MLL rearrangement. Br J Haematol. 2002;119(1):119–21.
36. Kawagoe H, Humphries RK, Blair A, Sutherland HJ, Hogge DE. Expression of HOX genes, HOX cofactors, and MLL in phenotypically and functionally defined subpopulations of leukemic and normal human hematopoietic cells. Leukemia. 1999;13(5):687–98.
37. Huang Y, Sitwala K, Bronstein J, Sanders D, Dandekar M, Collins C, et al. Identification and characterization of Hoxa9 binding sites in hematopoietic cells. Blood. 2011;119(2):388–98.
38. Ficara F, Murphy MJ, Lin M, Cleary ML. Pbx1 regulates self-renewal of long-term hematopoietic stem cells by maintaining their quiescence. Cell Stem Cell. 2008;2(5):484–96.
39. Calvo KR, Knoepfler P, McGrath S, Kamps MP. An inhibitory switch derepressed by pbx, hox, and Meis/Prep1 partners regulates DNA-binding by pbx1 and E2a-pbx1 and is dispensable for myeloid immortalization by E2a-pbx1. Oncogene. 1999;18(56):8033–43.
40. Hu YL, Fong S, Ferrell C, Largman C, Shen WF. HOXA9 modulates its oncogenic partner Meis1 to influence normal hematopoiesis. Mol Cell Biol. 2009;29(18):5181–92.
41. Cvejic A, Serbanovic-Canic J, Stemple DL, Ouwehand WH. The role of meis1 in primitive and definitive hematopoiesis during zebrafish development. Haematologica. 2011;96(2):190–8.
42. Pillay LM, Forrester AM, Erickson T, Berman JN, Waskiewicz AJ. The Hox cofactors Meis1 and Pbx act upstream of gata1 to regulate primitive hematopoiesis. Dev Biol. 2010;340(2):306–17.
43. Ferrell CM, Dorsam ST, Ohta H, Humphries RK, Derynck MK, Haqq C, et al. Activation of stem-cell specific genes by HOXA9 and HOXA10 homeodomain proteins in CD34+ human cord blood cells. Stem Cells. 2005;23(5):644–55.

44. Gwin K, Frank E, Bossou A, Medina KL. Hoxa9 regulates Flt3 in lymphohematopoietic progenitors. J Immunol. 2010;185(11):6572–83.
45. Lawrence HJ, Christensen J, Fong S, Hu YL, Weissman I, Sauvageau G, et al. Loss of expression of the Hoxa-9 homeobox gene impairs the proliferation and repopulating ability of hematopoietic stem cells. Blood. 2005;106(12):3988–94.
46. Thorsteinsdottir U, Mamo A, Kroon E, Jerome L, Bijl J, Lawrence HJ, et al. Overexpression of the myeloid leukemia-associated Hoxa9 gene in bone marrow cells induces stem cell expansion. Blood. 2002;99(1):121–9.
47. Yan J, Chen YX, Desmond A, Silva A, Yang Y, Wang H, et al. Cdx4 and menin co-regulate Hoxa9 expression in hematopoietic cells. PLoS One. 2006;1, e47.
48. Kirito K, Fox N, Kaushansky K. Thrombopoietin induces HOXA9 nuclear transport in immature hematopoietic cells: potential mechanism by which the hormone favorably affects hematopoietic stem cells. Mol Cell Biol. 2004;24(15):6751–62.
49. Laughner E, Taghavi P, Chiles K, Mahon PC, Semenza GL. HER2 (neu) signaling increases the rate of hypoxia-inducible factor 1 alpha (HIF-1 alpha) synthesis: Novel mechanism for HIF-1-mediated vascular endothelial growth factor expression. Mol Cell Biol. 2001;21(12):3995–4004.
50. Suda T, Takubo K, Semenza GL. Metabolic regulation of hematopoietic stem cells in the hypoxic niche. Cell Stem Cell. 2011;9(4):298–310.
51. Zhang CC, Sadek HA. Hypoxia and metabolic properties of hematopoietic stem cells. Antioxid Redox Signal. 2014;20(12):1891–901.
52. Mahmoud AI, Kocabas F, Muralidhar SA, Kimura W, Koura AS, Thet S, et al. Meis1 regulates postnatal cardiomyocyte cell cycle arrest. Nature. 2013;497(7448):249–53.
53. Anderson K, Lutz C, van Delft FW, Bateman CM, Guo Y, Colman SM, et al. Genetic variegation of clonal architecture and propagating cells in leukaemia. Nature. 2011;469(7330):356–61.
54. Varum S, Rodrigues AS, Moura MB, Momcilovic O, Easley CA, Ramalho-Santos J, et al. Energy metabolism in human pluripotent stem cells and their differentiated counterparts. PLoS ONE. 2011;6(6):e20914.

2

The actinin family of actin cross-linking proteins – a genetic perspective

Anita C.H. Murphy and Paul W. Young*

Abstract

Actinins are one of the major actin cross-linking proteins found in virtually all cell types and are the ancestral proteins of a larger family that includes spectrin, dystrophin and utrophin. Invertebrates have a single actinin-encoding *ACTN* gene, while mammals have four. Mutations in all four human genes have now been linked to heritable diseases or traits. *ACTN1* mutations cause macrothrombocytopenia, a platelet disorder characterized by excessive bleeding. *ACTN2* mutations have been linked to a range of cardiomyopathies, and *ACTN4* mutations cause a kidney condition called focal segmental glomerulosclerosis. Intriguingly, approximately 16 % of people worldwide are homozygous for a nonsense mutation in *ACTN3* that abolishes actinin-3 protein expression. This *ACTN3* null allele has undergone recent positive selection in specific human populations, which may be linked to improved endurance and adaptation to colder climates. In this review we discuss the human genetics of the *ACTN* gene family, as well as *ACTN* gene knockout studies in several model organisms. Observations from both of these areas provide insights into the evolution and cellular functions of actinins.

Keywords: Actinin, Alpha-actinin, ACTN1, ACTN2, ACTN3, ACTN4, Actin cross-linking, Actin binding proteins

Introduction

Actinins are dimeric actin filament cross-linking proteins. At their amino terminus two adjacent calponin homology (CH) domains comprise an actin-binding domain (ABD) [1]. Anti-parallel dimerisation of actinin monomers, mediated by the central spectrin-like repeats (SLRs) [2], positions the actin-binding domains at either end of the rod shaped dimer and facilitates cross-linking of actin filaments (Fig. 1). The carboxyl terminal calmodulin-like (CaM) domain, made up of two pairs of EF-hand motifs (EF1/2 and EF3/4), plays a regulatory role. EF1/2 can bind Ca^{++} in some actinins, disrupting actin binding at high Ca^{++} concentrations [1]. A postulated interaction of EF3/4 with the "neck" region between the ABD and first SLR of the opposing monomer [3] has been confirmed by the recently determined X-ray crystallographic structure of the human actinin-2 dimer [4]. This structure reveals actinin to be in a "closed" conformation. Phospholipid binding to the ABD causes a conformational change, resulting in the "opening" of the structure that allows EF3/4 to bind the sarcomeric organizer protein titin [5, 6] – a potential mechanism to regulate titin and actinin integration into the muscle Z-disk. More broadly though, this structure presents a picture of the intimate interactions between the subunits in the actinin dimer, providing a framework to better understand the molecular details of actin cross-linking and its regulation in all actinins and perhaps in spectrins too.

Actinins would appear to have first evolved in a common ancestor of amoebas, fungi and yeast [7, 8]. Thus, they were a component of early eukaryotic actin-based cytoskeletons, though notably, they are not found in plants. Actinin is also thought to be the ancestor of the spectrin and dystrophin families of actin-binding proteins, with spectrins probably evolving in the immediate ancestors of metazoans, based on their presence in choanoflagellates [9, 10], and the dystrophins arising in early metazoans [11]. As eukaryotic cells evolved, cross-linking of microfilaments, and anchoring them to membranes and other subcellular structures, were probably key to effective actin-based force generation, whether by myosin, or through actin polymerization [12]. In particular, actinins seem to have collaborated successfully with myosin II motors to assemble the actin-based contractile

* Correspondence: p.young@ucc.ie
School of Biochemistry and Cell Biology, University College Cork, Cork, Ireland

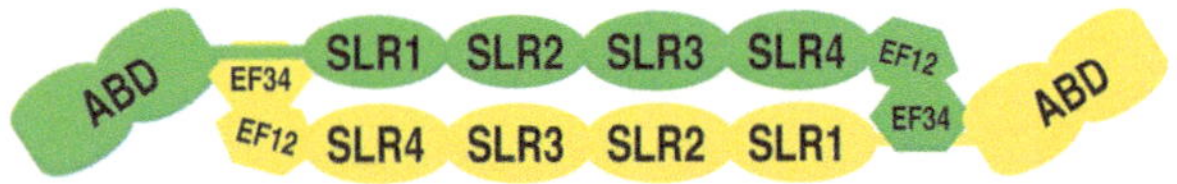

Fig. 1 Schematic representation of the actinin dimer. The domain organization of the anti-parallel actinin dimer is depicted schematically in the closed conformation as observed in the X-ray crystallographic structure of the human actinin-2 [4]. In each subunit two calponin homology (CH) domains make up the N-terminal actin-binding domain (ABD). The rod domain composed of four spectrin-like repeats (SLR1-4) makes up the bulk of the dimer interface. The carboxyl terminal calmodulin-like (CaM) domain is made up of two pairs of EF-hand motifs (EF1/2 and EF3/4). EF1/2 binds Ca^{++} in some actinins [1]. EF3/4 from one subunit interacts with the "neck" region between the ABD and first SLR of the opposing monomer (depicted as a line) [3]. This interaction clamps the protein into a closed conformation that is thought to be opened up by phospholipid binding to the ABD [4, 3]

systems required for diverse cellular processes, such as cytokinesis, cell motility and muscle contraction. Reflecting these fundamental functions, the basic domain organization of actinins has remained unchanged through evolution, with the exception of some variability in the number of SLRs (two in most fungal actinins versus four in virtually all other taxa) [8]. A multiple sequence alignment of the actinin proteins discussed in this review is provided as additional information [Additional file 1]. Invertebrates generally have a single *ACTN* gene, while vertebrates usually have three (or more), presumably as a result of the two rounds of large-scale gene, or whole-genome, duplication that are thought to have occurred early in the vertebrate lineage (2R hypothesis) [13]. Vertebrate actinins can be classified as either Ca^{++}- sensitive or -insensitive with respect to actin binding. This arises from alternative splicing of two variants of exon 19, which encodes part of the first EF-hand motif. Alternative splicing of this exon seems to have arisen in chordates [14]. The exon 19a and 19b variants can generate Ca^{++}- sensitive and -insensitive actinin isoforms respectively. Of the four mammalian actinins, alternative splicing of exon 19 has been retained in *ACTN1* and *ACTN4* to generate Ca^{++}-sensitive variants that are widely-expressed, and Ca^{++}-insensitive variants that are found predominantly in smooth muscle and the central nervous system (CNS) [1, 15]. In contrast, *ACTN2* and *ACTN3* exclusively encode exon 19b-containing Ca^{++}-insensitive proteins that are expressed in electrically excitable cells (cardiac and skeletal muscle cells, as well as neurons) [16, 17].

Here we review genetic studies of actinin function, summarizing findings both from model organisms (ranging from yeast to mice) and from human disease-association studies. This survey highlights the multiple functions of this versatile actin cross-linker, some of which are evolutionarily conserved, and others that probably represent specialized roles acquired in particular phyla or species.

Genetic studies of actinins in non-vertebrate model organisms

Yeast

Fission yeast (*Schizosaccharomyces pombe*), but not budding yeast (*Saccharomyces cerevisiae*), possess an actinin protein. It has only two spectrin-like repeats and is thought to be Ca^{++}-insensitive with respect to actin binding [18]. *S. pombe* actinin has mainly been studied with regard to contractile ring assembly during cytokinesis. The contractile ring forms from complexes termed nodes in the middle of the cell during interphase. Actinin is not essential for cytokinesis under normal growth conditions, but actinin null yeast show severe cytokinesis defects under stressful conditions of low temperature and high salt [19]. While actinin null cells do complete cytokinesis under normal growth conditions, the formation of the contractile ring is delayed [20]. This is because the actin network is more dynamic during node condensation, and the cytokinesis nodes frequently condense into clumps before eventually recovering to form a contractile ring. In cells over expressing actinin, actin filament structures are stabilized, inhibiting myosin-dependent movements of nodes that are essential for node condensation [20]. This results in a delayed ring assembly, but for reasons different to those in actinin null cells. Not surprisingly, there is considerable redundancy in the machinery of cytokinesis. Fimbrin is another actin cross-linker involved in this process. It seems to be able to compensate to a large extent for loss of actinin (and vice versa), since cells null for both these proteins have more severe defects in contractile ring formation than single mutants [20, 19]. Overall, it appears that in yeast, a balance between actin cross-linking and myosin motor activity must be achieved in order for cytokinesis to proceed in a controlled fashion – a concept that seems to hold true in mammalian cells too [21].

Slime molds

The mycetozoan *Dictyostelium discoideum* is an excellent unicellular model in which to study the role of the cytoskeleton in cell biological processes that are shared with multi-cellular animals. Actinin null *D. discoideum* strains are largely normal, but exhibit slow growth under hyper-osmotic conditions [22]. However, much more severe defects are seen in double mutants lacking actinin and either of the actin-bundling proteins filamin (ABP120, gelation factor) or ABP34. These double mutants show decreased growth at normal osmolarity, deficient pinocytosis, motility defects and abnormal morphogenesis of the multi-cellular fruiting body structure [22]. A study which employed more natural growth conditions revealed further deficiencies in the ability of actinin single null mutants to efficiently complete development and form viable spores [23]. These observations point to important roles for actinin in several dynamic processes in *D. discoideum,* but with significant though not complete, functional redundancy between actinin and other actin cross-linking proteins – a similar conclusion to the studies in fission yeast.

Flies and worms

Drosophila melanogaster has a single *ACTN* gene that is alternatively spliced within the region encoding the ABD. This alternative splicing generates isoforms that are differentially expressed in non-muscle, larval muscle and adult muscle tissues [24]. Embryos harboring null *ACTN* alleles that eliminate all isoforms can complete embryogenesis, but larvae die within two days of hatching [25]. These larvae are capable of some degree of movement, but have severely disrupted myofibrils, show muscular degeneration, and experience paralysis that is ultimately lethal [26]. Nevertheless, the initial stages of sarcomere assembly do not seem to require actinin, an observation confirmed in more recent studies using RNA interference targeting actinin [27, 28]. These studies suggest that in flies, actinin functions to stabilize the forming sarcomeric Z-disk, rather than initiating its assembly. In addition, other non-muscle aspects of embryogenesis in actinin null *D. melanogaster* seemed to proceed normally in the absence of actinin [24], and in mosaic flies, in which patches of eye tissue lacked actinin, the morphology of ommatidial rhabdomeres was normal [26].

Studies in *Caenorhabditis elegans* yield quite similar conclusions to those in flies. Worms harboring a deletion of the sole *C. elegans ACTN* gene (*ATN-1*) exhibit structural abnormalities of the focal adhesion-like dense bodies in the body wall muscle, though the dense bodies still accumulate integrin, talin and vinculin [29]. Muscle cells exhibit actin striations, but with some actin disorganization and abnormal accumulations of actin in bundles at cell boundaries. Nevertheless, the mutant worms show nearly normal movement in several assays, though a deficiency in the amplitude of body bending was discernible by video-microscopy [29]. Similar to flies, non-muscle aspects of development seem to proceed normally in actinin null *C. elegans*, suggesting that actinin is not absolutely required for many fundamental processes, such as cytokinesis, cell-cell adhesion or cell motility. The apparent absence of non-muscle phenotypes in flies and worms suggests that either actinin does not play an important role in such processes in these species, or that its absence can be compensated for to a significant extent by other proteins.

Genetic studies of actinins in mammals

Mammals have four ACTN genes. *ACTN1* and *ACTN4,* through alternative splicing, encode widely-expressed Ca^{++}-sensitive isoforms, as well as Ca^{++}-insensitive variants that are found predominantly in smooth muscle and in the central nervous system (CNS) [30]. *ACTN2* and *ACTN3* encode Ca^{++}-insensitive proteins only, expressed predominantly in cardiac and skeletal muscle, but also in the CNS in the case of *ACTN2* [16, 17]. Mutations in all four human ACTN genes have now been linked to heritable diseases or traits. In addition, knockout mice lacking actinin-3 and actinin-4 have been described [31, 32]. Genetic studies of each mammalian actinin are discussed in turn below.

Actinin-1

In many cell types, actinin-1 cross-links actin filaments and anchors them to structures such as cell:cell and cell:-matrix junctions, playing an important role in processes such as cytokinesis, cell adhesion and cell migration [33]. The International Mouse Phenotyping Consortium has performed initial phenotyping of mice heterozygous for an *ACTN1* knockout allele [34]. Presumably heterozygotes were used because homozygous mice were not viable, though there is little background information available about these mice. In any case, it would not be surprising if *ACTN1* were an essential gene, given its ubiquitous expression and many described functions.

A role for actinin-1 in a human genetic disorder has become apparent in the past two years, with three independent studies showing *ACTN1* to be one of many causative genes implicated in dominantly-inherited congenital macrothrombocytopenia (CMTP) [35–37]. This is a rare blood disorder characterized by a reduced number of platelets in the peripheral vascular system along with increased platelet size [38]. Initially, Kunishima et al. [37] identified six *ACTN1* variants that co-segregated with affected individuals in six Japanese families suffering with CMTP. Expression of these variants in Chinese hamster ovary cells and primary mouse fetal liver-derived megakaryocytes lead to abnormal alterations in actin cytoskeleton organization [37]. Gueguen et al. [36] subsequently reported an ACTN 1 variant, Arg46Gln, to be co-segregating with CMTP in a French family. This missense mutation had already been reported by Kunishima et al., but its appearance in an independent patient cohort supplies reliable evidence for the definite involvement of *ACTN1* in CMTP. Most recently, Bottega et al. reported 8 new *ACTN1* variants in families from Italy and the United Kingdom [35]. Expression of corresponding mutant actinin-1 proteins in human fibroblast cultured cells caused actin cytoskeleton disorganization. It has been suggested that a possible cause for macrothrombocytopenias is a deficiency in the regulation of platelet production [39]. In support of this, primary mouse fetal liver-derived megakaryocytes transfected with *ACTN1* variants displayed altered pro-platelet formation and size [37]. This finding is compatible with the increased platelet size that is characteristic of CMTP.

Intriguingly, all of the actinin-1 mutations linked to CMTP map within the ABD and CaM domains, or to regions that link these domains to the central rod domain (Table 1). No CMTP-associated mutations have been found within the rod domain itself, even though the rod encompasses half of the actinin protein sequence. This observation, together with the cytoskeletal abnormalities seen upon heterologous expression, suggests that these actinin-1 variants may have altered actin-binding properties. However, this has not been directly examined to date, and the location of these mutations on the three-dimensional structure of the actinin dimer does not provide obvious clues as to how they might affect actin-binding properties [4]. Individuals heterozygous for these mutations display relatively mild macrothrombocytopenia, apparently in the absence of other pathologies. This finding points to a specific role for actinin-1 in platelet formation, possibly through its actin binding and bundling ability, that is exquisitely sensitive to mutational perturbation and cannot be compensated for by other actinin isoforms.

Table 1 Human actinin mutations and associated diseases or phenotypes

Protein	Mutation	Domain	Disease/Phenotype	Reference
Actinin-1	Asp22Asn	ABD	CMTP	[35]
	Gln32Lys	ABD, CH1	CMTP	[37]
	Arg46Gln	ABD, CH1	CMTP	[36, 37]
	Arg46Trp	ABD, CH1	CMTP	[35]
	Val105Ile	ABD, CH1	CMTP	[37]
	Glu225Lys	ABD, CH2	CMTP	[37]
	Gly251Arg	ABD/Neck	CMTP	[35]
	Thr737Asn	Rod/CaM	CMTP	[35]
	Arg738Trp	Rod/CaM	CMTP	[37]
	*Arg752Gln	CaM, EF12	CMTP	[37]
	Gly764Ser	CaM, EF12	CMTP	[35]
	Glu769Lys	CaM, EF12	CMTP	[35]
Actinin-2	Gln9Arg	ABD	DCM	[41]
	Gly111Val	ABD, CH1	HCM	[42]
	Ala119Thr	ABD, CH1	HCM, DCM, IVF, LVNC, SUD	[45, 44]
	Met228Thr	ABD, CH2	HCM + Atrial Arrhythmias	[46]
	Thr495Met	Rod, SLR2	HCM	[44, 42]
	Glu583Ala	Rod, SLR3	HCM	[44]
	Glu628Gly	Rod, SLR3	HCM	[44]
	*Arg759Thr	CaM, EF12	HCM	[42]
Actinin-3	Arg577X	Rod, SLR3	Altered muscle metabolism	[50]
Actinin-4	Trp59Arg	ABD, CH1	FSGS	[77]
	Ile149del	ABD, CH1	FSGS	[77]
	Lys255Glu	ABD, CH2	FSGS	[76]
	Thr259Ile	ABD, CH2	FSGS	[76]
	Ser262Pro	ABD, CH2	FSGS	[76]

Mutations in the four human actinin proteins that are associated with diseases or phenotypic traits are listed.
The protein domain and subdomain (e.g. ABD, CH1) in which each mutation occurs is indicated in the third column. A forward slash (e.g. Rod/CaM) indicates a mutation within a region linking the two domains indicated. The asterisk indicates that these are equivalent Arg residues in a sequence alignment of actinin-1 and −2. A multiple sequence alignment highlighting the postions of disease-causing mutations is provided as additional information [Additional file 1].
Abbreviations: *IVF* Idiopathic ventricular fibrillation, *LVNC* Left ventricular non-compaction, *SUD* Sudden unexplained death, *CMTP* Congenital macrothrombocytopenia, *HCM* Hypertrophic cardiomyopathy, *DCM* Dilated cardiomyopathy, *FSGS* Focal segmental glomerulosclerosis

Actinin 2

Actinin-2 is expressed in skeletal and cardiac muscle fibers [16], as well as in the brain [17]. In muscle, it is a highly abundant protein and is the major Z-disk protein that cross-links anti-parallel actin filaments from neighboring sacromeres. Actinin-2 also serves as a scaffold to which many other Z-disk components are anchored, and may be involved in mechanical strain sensing and signaling through interacting proteins such as CSRP3/MLP, PDLIM3/ALP and LDB3/ZASP/cypher [40]. A number of investigations have now linked dominantly-inherited *ACTN2* missense mutations to a range of myopathies. An *ACTN2* mutation was reported in a patient with dilated cardiomyopathy (DCM), a condition characterized by dilation of the left ventricle of the heart and a reduction in the heart's ability to contract [41]. This Gln9Arg mutation is found in the ABD of actinin-2 and abrogates an interaction of actinin-2 with the Z-disk component MLP [41]. Examining patients with hypertrophic cardiomyopathy (HCM), Theis et al. identified thirteen mutations in five Z-disk proteins, including three in actinin-2 [42]. HCM is a chronic heart muscle disease that affects about 0.2 % of people, and is characterized by a thickened wall of the left ventricle in the heart [43]. Semsarian and coworkers found one of these same mutations (Thr495Met), as well as three novel mutations in Australian families affected by HCM and other heterogeneous cardiac conditions [44, 45]. Similarly an actinin-2 Met228Thr mutation was found to segregate with affected individuals in a large Italian family that had a history of HCM and juvenile atrial arrhythmias [46]. Eight *ACTN2* mutations have thus far been linked to HCM, DCM and/or other cardiac abnormalities. These mutations do not map to a particular region of actinin-2, with some located in the ABD, some in the central rod and one in the CaM domain (Table 1). While mutations that map to the ABD and CaM domains may affect actin-binding properties, those in the rod domain are more likely to affect the binding of other Z-disc proteins to α-actinin. However the consequences of these mutations have not been examined experimentally for the most part. Given the distribution of the mutations, it would appear unlikely that there is a unifying molecular mechanism linking them. In some of the studies, individuals from a family carrying the same *ACTN2* mutation experience profound clinical and phenotypic heterogeneity [44]. For example the Ala119Thr substitution was identified in a family with a history of DCM, left ventricular non-compaction, idiopathic ventricular fibrillation and unexplained sudden death [44]. This suggests that factors other than genetics, such as diet, exercise and environmental conditions, are also likely to influence clinical outcome [47]. The availability of a high resolution actinin-2 crystal structure will be useful to further our understanding of how these mutations affect actinin-2 function and ultimately cause disease [4].

Actinin 3

Actinin-3 seems to be the most specialized of the mammalian actinins based on its restricted expression in type 2 fast glycolytic skeletal muscle fibers, the fibers responsible for the generation of rapid and forceful contractions [16, 48, 49]. Surprisingly, an *ACTN3* polymorphism, causing the nonsense mutation p.Arg577X, was found to be very prevalent in many human populations [50]. Approximately 16 % of the world's population are homozygous for this sequence change that completely prevents the production of the actinin 3 protein, meaning that more than one billion people lack actinin-3 expression [51]. This null genotype is not associated with any disease, suggesting that *ACTN3* is a non-essential gene in humans and its loss compensated for by actinin-2 [50]. Though absent in birds, the *ACTN3* gene is conserved in most other vertebrates, including fish, suggesting that it arose by gene duplication early in vertebrate evolution [52]. Actinin-3 must have had non-redundant functions through the course of vertebrate evolution in most lineages to explain its sequence conservation. In early humans however, it appears that the p.Arg577X mutation arose, was not detrimental, and was maintained for some time, before expanding under positive selection to achieve a very high frequency in specific populations (e.g. European and Asian), but not others (e.g. African) [49]. What is the basis for this highly unusual, positive selection for a null allele?

Yang et al. [53] initially reported an overrepresentation of the wild type *ACTN3* allele (p.Arg577Arg) in elite Australian sprint athletes, suggesting that its presence is advantageous in sprint and power activities. They also found the homozygous p.Arg577X genotype to be more common in female endurance athletes when compared to power athletes. This suggested that *ACTN3* genotype is linked to normal variation in muscle function, with each genotype possibly conferring an advantage for different types of athletic performance. Numerous other studies have subsequently investigated the association between *ACTN3* genotype and athletic performance, in both normal populations and various groups of elite athletes. Some studies support the basic findings of Yang et al. [53], while others do not find significant associations. A complete discussion of this literature is beyond the scope of this review but is covered quite comprehensively by Eynon et al. [54]. However, it can be concluded that at least in some populations (e.g. Caucasians), the association of the wildtype allele with sprint and power performance seems to hold true, while the association of the p.Arg577X variant with enhanced endurance is not as clear cut [54, 55]. Notably though, in African populations, where the frequency of the p.Arg577X variant is very low, no association of *ACTN* genotype with elite athlete status was found [56], despite Kenyans and Ethiopians having dominated long–distance running in recent years [57]. This suggests that we must consider not only the *ACTN3* genotype but also other polymorphisms that may be working in combination with, or independently of, *ACTN3* to dictate athletic performance [55]. In addition, athletic performance depends not just on an individual's genetic make-up, but also on environmental factors, training regimes and coaching expertise [54, 55].

Studies of *ACTN3* knockout mice provide further insights [58]. These mice are viable and healthy. They do exhibit slight decreases in muscle mass and muscle strength, but these values are regarded as within the normal range and are not a sign of muscle dysfunction [59]. More significantly, these mice display muscle metabolism conversion from the anaerobic pathway, typically utilized in fast muscle fibers, to the oxidative aerobic pathway, which is generally seen in slow muscle fibers [58]. Activity of key enzymes associated with oxidative metabolism, such as citrate synthase and succinate dehydrogenase, and glycolysis, such as hexokinase, are increased, while indicators of anaerobic metabolism, namely glycogen phosphorylase, show decreased activity. These metabolic changes have a positive effect on endurance; knockout mice have a much greater running distance prior to experiencing fatigue compared to wild-type controls [58]. The function of glycogen phosphorylase is to break down glycogen. In humans, activities such as sprinting rely on glycogen as a main source of energy, a reduction in glycogen breakdown would therefore be unfavorable to sprint athletes [59]. However, a reduced ability to breakdown glycogen might be beneficial to endurance athletes, as it allows them to utilize other fuels and conserve glycogen [60]. Thus, metabolic changes observed in *ACTN3* knockout mice provide plausible explanations for the association of *ACTN3* genotypes with sprint/power versus endurance performance in humans. More efficient aerobic muscle metabolism may be the trait associated with the p.Arg577X genotype that has been positively selected for in specific human populations. The frequency of this allele in human ethnic groups is correlated with latitude, with the p.Arg577X mutation more prevalent further from the equator [61]. Latitude-associated environmental variables, such as mean temperature or species diversity, may have influenced positive selection for this *ACTN3* allele [61]. Indeed, recently described alterations in the calcium kinetics in skeletal muscles of *actinin-3* knockout mice are consistent with cold acclimatization and thermogenesis [62, 60].

What molecular mechanisms might mediate these powerful effects of actinin-3 on multiple aspects of muscle metabolism and physiology? Actinin-2 and actinin-3 serve as a scaffold to anchor many signaling proteins and metabolic enzymes to the Z-disk [63]. Most of these interactions are probably shared by both muscle actinin isoforms, though this has often not been explicitly tested, nor have actual binding affinities been compared. Assuming there are some differential interactions of signaling proteins with actinin-2 versus actinin-3, then alterations in sarcomeric signal transduction in humans or mice lacking actinin-3 could drive a program of gene expression resulting in the actinin-3 null muscle phenotype. Calsarcin-2 (CALS-2, Myozenin-1, FATZ), a regulator of calcineurin signaling, displays just such a differential interaction [64]. Actinin-3 deficient muscle in both mice and humans show enhanced calcineurin signaling, probably as a result of increased binding of calsarcin-2 to actinin-2 in the absence of actinin-3 [64]. Calcineurin signaling is known to shift muscle fibers towards an oxidative phenotype [65–67], providing a potential mechanism to explain the changes in muscle metabolism in actinin-3 knockout mice [64]. Whether alterations in other signaling pathways are also involved remains to be seen.

Actinin-4

Actinin-4 is regarded as a non-muscle isoform that is expressed widely, in a pattern that largely overlaps actinin-1 expression. These two isoforms show a high degree of sequence homology and have similar actin binding properties [15]. Three significant functional differences between actinin-1 and actinin-4 are apparent however. Firstly, aberrant actinin-4 expression has been described in many tumor types and has been linked to infiltrative phenotypes and poor outcomes in several cancers [68–75]. By contrast, over-expression of actinin-1 in tumor tissues has not been widely reported. Secondly, human studies have identified five dominant *ACTN4* mutations that cause the kidney disease focal segmental glomerulosclerosis (FSGS) [76, 77] (Table 1), while actinin-4 knockout mice exhibit altered podocyte morphology, develop glomerular disease, and finally, experience kidney failure [31]. In humans a kidney-specific role for actinin-4 can be simply explained by the lack of actinin-1 expression in the kidney [76], however in mice both actinin-1 and –4 are expressed in podocytes, yet actinin-1 cannot compensate for a loss of actinin-4 [31]. Thirdly, actinin-4 can translocate to the nucleus and play a role in transcriptional regulation [78–84]. This ability may be shared by actinin-2 [85], but a similar, "non-canonical" role for actinin-1 has not been reported. The diverse cell biological roles of actinin-1 and actinin-4 have recently been reviewed [30], and the roles of actinin-4 in cancer and kidney physiology are described in detail in other reviews in this special issue [86, 87]. For these reasons actinin-4 is not discussed further here.

Conclusions

The *ACTN* gene family presents a fascinating case study in genetics. Through the course of evolution, from their origin in early eukaryotes, actinins have performed a core function as actin cross-linking proteins in cells. As more complex multi-cellular metazoan species evolved, actinin's cross-linking activity was required in an increasing number of cell biological contexts in different cell and tissue types. Alternative splicing in the ABD and CaM domains arose, most likely to tweak actin-binding properties for tissue-specific functions. In vertebrates, gene duplications facilitated sub-functionalization compared to the ancestral invertebrate actinin, as well as neo-functionalization. In mammals, actinin-1 probably retained the broadest range of ancestral protein functions. Sub-functionalization saw actinin-2 specialize as the major thin filament cross-linker of the sarcomeric Z-disk in heart and skeletal muscle, as well as playing a role at neuronal synapses. Actinin-3 assumed an even more specific role in fast muscle fibers, where it is required for maintenance of the anaerobic metabolic phenotype of these fibers. Actinin-4 has largely overlapping expression and functions with actinin-1, except in the kidney. It has acquired, probably through neo-functionalization, a role in the cell nucleus as a transcriptional regulator and a unique ability to promote an aggressive cancer phenotype when over-expressed. Missense mutations in *ACTN1*, *ACTN2* and ACTN4 cause dominantly inherited platelet, cardiac and renal disorders respectively, while a nonsense mutation in *ACTN3* seems to have been beneficial during the recent evolution of some human populations. Still our understanding of molecular mechanisms linking these mutations to their respective phenotypes is incomplete and represents an ongoing challenge to researchers in this field.

Additional file

Additional file 1: Multiple sequence alignment of selected actinin protein sequences. An alignment prepared using ClustalX of human actinin-1, −2, −3 and −4, as well as actinin sequences from select model organisms. Sequence conservation is plotted beneath the alignment and conserved residues marked and color-coded according to the default CustalX settings. Locations of PFAM protein domains as identified in the Protein Data Bank for human actinin-2 (PDB ID: 4D1E) are indicated in red below the alignment. Known disease/phenotype associated mutations for the human actinins are identified in red text above the alignment. Accession numbers for sequences are as follows: *Hs*ACTN1 = NP_001093.1; *Hs*ACTN2 = NP_001094.1; *Hs*ACTN3 = NP_001095.2; *Hs*ACTN4 = NP_004915.2; *Dd*ACTN = XP_646979; *DmACTN* = NP_477484; *Ce*ACTN = NP_506127; *Sp*ACTN = NP_594295. Hs = *Homo sapiens;* Dm = *Drosophila melanogaster;* Ce = *Caenorhabditis elegans;* Dd = *Dictyostelium discoideum;* Sp = *Schizosaccharomyces pombe.* (PDF 3345 kb)

Abbreviations

CH: Calponin homology; ABD: Actin-binding domain; SLR: Spectrin-like repeats; CaM: Calmodulin-like; CNS: Central nervous system; CMTP: Congenital macrothrombocytopenia; HCM: Hypertrophic cardiomyopathy; DCM: Dilated cardiomyopathy; FSGS: Focal segmental glomerulosclerosis.

Competing interests

The authors declare that they have no competing interests.

Authors' contributions

PWY and ACHM co-wrote this review article. Both authors read and approved the final manuscript.

Acknowledgements

We gratefully acknowledge the Irish Research Council for their support of our work on actinin through a Government of Ireland Postgraduate Scholarship to ACHM. We thank Kellie Dean for proof-reading the manuscript.

References

1. Blanchard A, Ohanian V, Critchley D. The structure and function of alpha-actinin. J Muscle Res Cell Motil. 1989;10(4):280–9.
2. Djinovic-Carugo K, Young P, Gautel M, Saraste M. Structure of the alpha-actinin rod: molecular basis for cross-linking of actin filaments. Cell. 1999;98(4):537–46.
3. Young P, Gautel M. The interaction of titin and alpha-actinin is controlled by a phospholipid-regulated intramolecular pseudoligand mechanism. Embo J. 2000;19(23):6331–40.
4. Ribeiro Ede Jr A, Pinotsis N, Ghisleni A, Salmazo A, Konarev PV, Kostan J, et al. The structure and regulation of human muscle alpha-actinin. Cell. 2014;159(6):1447–60.
5. Atkinson RA, Joseph C, Kelly G, Muskett FW, Frenkiel TA, Nietlispach D, et al. Ca2 + -independent binding of an EF-hand domain to a novel motif in the alpha-actinin-titin complex. Nat Struct Biol. 2001;8(10):853–7.
6. Young P, Ferguson C, Bañuelos S, Gautel M. Molecular structure of the sarcomeric Z-disk: two types of titin interactions lead to an asymmetrical sorting of alpha-actinin. EMBO J. 1998;17(6):1614–24.
7. Pollard TD, Wu JQ. Understanding cytokinesis: lessons from fission yeast. Nat Rev Mol Cell Biol. 2010;11(2):149–55.
8. Virel A, Backman L. A comparative and phylogenetic analysis of the alpha-actinin rod domain. Mol Biol Evol. 2007;24(10):2254–65.
9. Baines AJ. Evolution of spectrin function in cytoskeletal and membrane networks. Biochem Soc Trans. 2009;37(Pt 4):796–803.
10. King N, Westbrook MJ, Young SL, Kuo A, Abedin M, Chapman J, et al. The genome of the choanoflagellate Monosiga brevicollis and the origin of metazoans. Nature. 2008;451(7180):783–8.
11. Jin H, Tan S, Hermanowski J, Bohm S, Pacheco S, McCauley JM, et al. The dystrotelin, dystrophin and dystrobrevin superfamily: new paralogues and old isoforms. BMC Genomics. 2007;8:19.
12. Richards TA, Cavalier-Smith T. Myosin domain evolution and the primary divergence of eukaryotes. Nature. 2005;436(7054):1113–8.
13. Meyer A, Schartl M. Gene and genome duplications in vertebrates: the one-to-four (–to-eight in fish) rule and the evolution of novel gene functions. Curr Opin Cell Biol. 1999;11(6):699–704.
14. Lek M, MacArthur DG, Yang N, North KN. Phylogenetic analysis of gene structure and alternative splicing in alpha-actinins. Mol Biol Evol. 2010;27(4):773–80.
15. Foley KS, Young PW. An analysis of splicing, actin-binding properties, heterodimerization and molecular interactions of the non-muscle alpha-actinins. Biochem J. 2013;452(3):477–88.
16. Beggs AH, Byers TJ, Knoll JH, Boyce FM, Bruns GA, Kunkel LM. Cloning and characterization of two human skeletal muscle alpha-actinin genes located on chromosomes 1 and 11. J Biol Chem. 1992;267(13):9281–8.
17. Wyszynski M, Kharazia V, Shanghvi R, Rao A, Beggs AH, Craig AM, et al. Differential regional expression and ultrastructural localization of alpha-actinin-2, a putative NMDA receptor-anchoring protein, in rat brain. J Neurosci. 1998;18(4):1383–92.
18. Jayadev R, Kuk CY, Low SH, Murata-Hori M. Calcium sensitivity of alpha-actinin is required for equatorial actin assembly during cytokinesis. Cell Cycle. 2012;11(10):1929–37.
19. Wu JQ, Bahler J, Pringle JR. Roles of a fimbrin and an alpha-actinin-like protein in fission yeast cell polarization and cytokinesis. Mol Biol Cell. 2001;12(4):1061–77.
20. Laporte D, Ojkic N, Vavylonis D, Wu JQ. alpha-Actinin and fimbrin cooperate with myosin II to organize actomyosin bundles during contractile-ring assembly. Mol Biol Cell. 2012;23(16):3094–110.
21. Mukhina S, Wang YL, Murata-Hori M. Alpha-actinin is required for tightly regulated remodeling of the actin cortical network during cytokinesis. Dev Cell. 2007;13(4):554–65.
22. Rivero F, Furukawa R, Fechheimer M, Noegel AA. Three actin cross-linking proteins, the 34 kDa actin-bundling protein, alpha-actinin and gelation factor (ABP-120), have both unique and redundant roles in the growth and development of Dictyostelium. J Cell Sci. 1999;112(Pt 16):2737–51.
23. Ponte E, Rivero F, Fechheimer M, Noegel A, Bozzaro S. Severe developmental defects in Dictyostelium null mutants for actin-binding proteins. Mech Dev. 2000;91(1–2):153–61.
24. Roulier EM, Fyrberg C, Fyrberg E. Perturbations of Drosophila alpha-actinin cause muscle paralysis, weakness, and atrophy but do not confer obvious nonmuscle phenotypes. J Cell Biol. 1992;116(4):911–22.
25. Fyrberg E, Kelly M, Ball E, Fyrberg C, Reedy MC. Molecular genetics of Drosophila alpha-actinin: mutant alleles disrupt Z disc integrity and muscle insertions. J Cell Biol. 1990;110(6):1999–2011.
26. Fyrberg C, Ketchum A, Ball E, Fyrberg E. Characterization of lethal Drosophila melanogaster alpha-actinin mutants. Biochem Genet. 1998;36(9–10):299–310.
27. Rui Y, Bai J, Perrimon N. Sarcomere formation occurs by the assembly of multiple latent protein complexes. PLoS Genet. 2010;6(11):e1001208.
28. Clark KA, Kadrmas JL. Drosophila melanogaster muscle LIM protein and alpha-actinin function together to stabilize muscle cytoarchitecture: a potential role for Mlp84B in actin-crosslinking. Cytoskeleton (Hoboken). 2014;70(6):304–16.
29. Moulder GL, Cremona GH, Duerr J, Stirman JN, Fields SD, Martin W, et al. alpha-actinin is required for the proper assembly of Z-disk/focal-adhesion-like structures and for efficient locomotion in Caenorhabditis elegans. J Mol Biol. 2010;403(4):516–28.
30. Foley KS, Young PW. The non-muscle functions of actinins: an update. Biochem J. 2014;459(1):1–13.
31. Kos CH, Le TC, Sinha S, Henderson JM, Kim SH, Sugimoto H, et al. Mice deficient in alpha-actinin-4 have severe glomerular disease. J Clin Invest. 2003;111(11):1683–90.
32. MacArthur DG, Seto JT, Chan S, Quinlan KG, Raftery JM, Turner N, et al. An Actn3 knockout mouse provides mechanistic insights into the association between alpha-actinin-3 deficiency and human athletic performance. Hum Mol Genet. 2008;17(8):1076–86.
33. Otey CA, Carpen O. Alpha-actinin revisited: a fresh look at an old player. Cell Motil Cytoskeleton. 2004;58(2):104–11.
34. The International Mouse Phenotyping Consortium. https://www.mousephenotype.org/data/genes/MGI:2137706#order.

35. Bottega R, Marconi C, Faleschini M, Baj G, Cagioni C, Pecci A, et al. ACTN1-related thrombocytopenia: identification of novel families for phenotypic characterization. Blood. 2015;125(5):869–72.
36. Gueguen P, Rouault K, Chen JM, Raguenes O, Fichou Y, Hardy E, et al. A Missense Mutation in the Alpha-Actinin 1 Gene (ACTN1) Is the Cause of Autosomal Dominant Macrothrombocytopenia in a Large French Family. PLoS One. 2013;8(9):e74728.
37. Kunishima S, Okuno Y, Yoshida K, Shiraishi Y, Sanada M, Muramatsu H, et al. ACTN1 mutations cause congenital macrothrombocytopenia. Am J Hum Genet. 2013;92(3):431–8.
38. Kunishima S, Saito H. Congenital macrothrombocytopenias. Blood Rev. 2006;20(2):111–21.
39. Thon JN, Italiano Jr JE. Does size matter in platelet production? Blood. 2012;120(8):1552–61.
40. Gautel M. The sarcomeric cytoskeleton: who picks up the strain? Curr Opin Cell Biol. 2011;23(1):39–46.
41. Mohapatra B, Jimenez S, Lin JH, Bowles KR, Coveler KJ, Marx JG, et al. Mutations in the muscle LIM protein and alpha-actinin-2 genes in dilated cardiomyopathy and endocardial fibroelastosis. Mol Genet Metab. 2003;80(1–2):207–15.
42. Theis JL, Bos JM, Bartleson VB, Will ML, Binder J, Vatta M, et al. Echocardiographic-determined septal morphology in Z-disc hypertrophic cardiomyopathy. Biochem Biophys Res Commun. 2006;351(4):896–902.
43. Maron BJ. Cardiology patient pages. Hypertrophic cardiomyopathy. Circulation. 2002;106(19):2419–21.
44. Chiu C, Bagnall RD, Ingles J, Yeates L, Kennerson M, Donald JA, et al. Mutations in alpha-actinin-2 cause hypertrophic cardiomyopathy: a genome-wide analysis. J Am Coll Cardiol. 2010;55(11):1127–35.
45. Bagnall RD, Molloy LK, Kalman JM, Semsarian C. Exome sequencing identifies a mutation in the ACTN2 gene in a family with idiopathic ventricular fibrillation, left ventricular noncompaction, and sudden death. BMC Med Genet. 2014;15(1):99.
46. Girolami F, Iascone M, Tomberli B, Bardi S, Benelli M, Marseglia G, et al. Novel alpha-actinin 2 variant associated with familial hypertrophic cardiomyopathy and juvenile atrial arrhythmias: a massively parallel sequencing study. Circ Cardiovasc Genet. 2014;7(6):741–50.
47. Kelly M, Semsarian C. Multiple mutations in genetic cardiovascular disease: a marker of disease severity? Circ Cardiovasc Genet. 2009;2(2):182–90.
48. MacArthur DG, North KN. ACTN3: A genetic influence on muscle function and athletic performance. Exerc Sport Sci Rev. 2007;35(1):30–4.
49. Mills M, Yang N, Weinberger R, Vander Woude DL, Beggs AH, Easteal S, et al. Differential expression of the actin-binding proteins, alpha-actinin-2 and −3, in different species: implications for the evolution of functional redundancy. Hum Mol Genet. 2001;10(13):1335–46.
50. North KN, Yang N, Wattanasirichaigoon D, Mills M, Easteal S, Beggs AH. A common nonsense mutation results in alpha-actinin-3 deficiency in the general population. Nat Genet. 1999;21(4):353–4.
51. Lek M, Quinlan KG, North KN. The evolution of skeletal muscle performance: gene duplication and divergence of human sarcomeric alpha-actinins. Bioessays. 2010;32(1):17–25.
52. Holterhoff CK, Saunders RH, Brito EE, Wagner DS. Sequence and expression of the zebrafish alpha-actinin gene family reveals conservation and diversification among vertebrates. Dev Dyn. 2009;238(11):2936–47.
53. Yang N, MacArthur DG, Gulbin JP, Hahn AG, Beggs AH, Easteal S, et al. ACTN3 genotype is associated with human elite athletic performance. Am J Hum Genet. 2003;73(3):627–31.
54. Eynon N, Ruiz JR, Femia P, Pushkarev VP, Cieszczyk P, Maciejewska-Karlowska A, et al. The ACTN3 R577X polymorphism across three groups of elite male European athletes. PLoS One. 2012;7(8):e43132.
55. Alfred T, Ben-Shlomo Y, Cooper R, Hardy R, Cooper C, Deary IJ, et al. ACTN3 genotype, athletic status, and life course physical capability: meta-analysis of the published literature and findings from nine studies. Hum Mutat. 2011;32(9):1008–18.
56. Yang N, MacArthur DG, Wolde B, Onywera VO, Boit MK, Lau SY, et al. The ACTN3 R577X polymorphism in East and West African athletes. Med Sci Sports Exerc. 2007;39(11):1985–8.
57. Larsen HB. Kenyan dominance in distance running. Comp Biochem Physiol A Mol Integr Physiol. 2003;136(1):161–70.
58. MacArthur DG, Seto JT, Raftery JM, Quinlan KG, Huttley GA, Hook JW, et al. Loss of ACTN3 gene function alters mouse muscle metabolism and shows evidence of positive selection in humans. Nat Genet. 2007;39(10):1261–5.
59. Berman Y, North KN. A gene for speed: the emerging role of alpha-actinin-3 in muscle metabolism. Physiology (Bethesda). 2010;25(4):250–9.
60. Quinlan KG, Seto JT, Turner N, Vandebrouck A, Floetenmeyer M, Macarthur DG, et al. Alpha-actinin-3 deficiency results in reduced glycogen phosphorylase activity and altered calcium handling in skeletal muscle. Hum Mol Genet. 2010;19(7):1335–46.
61. Friedlander SM, Herrmann AL, Lowry DP, Mepham ER, Lek M, North KN, et al. ACTN3 allele frequency in humans covaries with global latitudinal gradient. PLoS One. 2013;8(1):e52282.
62. Head SI, Chan S, Houweling PJ, Quinlan KG, Murphy R, Wagner S, et al. Altered Ca2+ kinetics associated with alpha-actinin-3 deficiency may explain positive selection for ACTN3 null allele in human evolution. PLoS Genet. 2015;11(2):e1004862.
63. Sjoblom B, Salmazo A, Djinovic-Carugo K. Alpha-actinin structure and regulation. Cell Mol Life Sci. 2008;65(17):2688–701.
64. Seto JT, Quinlan KG, Lek M, Zheng XF, Garton F, MacArthur DG, et al. ACTN3 genotype influences muscle performance through the regulation of calcineurin signaling. J Clin Invest. 2013;123(10):4255–63.
65. Chin ER, Olson EN, Richardson JA, Yang Q, Humphries C, Shelton JM, et al. A calcineurin-dependent transcriptional pathway controls skeletal muscle fiber type. Genes Dev. 1998;12(16):2499–509.
66. Delling U, Tureckova J, Lim HW, De Windt LJ, Rotwein P, Molkentin JD. A calcineurin-NFATc3-dependent pathway regulates skeletal muscle differentiation and slow myosin heavy-chain expression. Mol Cell Biol. 2000;20(17):6600–11.
67. Long YC, Glund S, Garcia-Roves PM, Zierath JR. Calcineurin regulates skeletal muscle metabolism via coordinated changes in gene expression. J Biol Chem. 2007;282(3):1607–14.
68. Barbolina MV, Adley BP, Kelly DL, Fought AJ, Scholtens DM, Shea LD, et al. Motility-related actinin alpha-4 is associated with advanced and metastatic ovarian carcinoma. Lab Invest. 2008;88(6):602–14.
69. Fukushima S, Yoshida A, Honda K, Maeshima AM, Narita Y, Yamada T, et al. Immunohistochemical actinin-4 expression in infiltrating gliomas: association with WHO grade and differentiation. Brain Tumor Pathol. 2013;31(1):11–6.
70. Honda K, Yamada T, Endo R, Ino Y, Gotoh M, Tsuda H, et al. Actinin-4, a novel actin-bundling protein associated with cell motility and cancer invasion. J Cell Biol. 1998;140(6):1383–93.
71. Kikuchi S, Honda K, Tsuda H, Hiraoka N, Imoto I, Kosuge T, et al. Expression and gene amplification of actinin-4 in invasive ductal carcinoma of the pancreas. Clin Cancer Res. 2008;14(17):5348–56.
72. Miyanaga A, Honda K, Tsuta K, Masuda M, Yamaguchi U, Fujii G, et al. Diagnostic and prognostic significance of the alternatively spliced ACTN4 variant in high-grade neuroendocrine pulmonary tumours. Ann Oncol. 2012;24(1):84–90.
73. Quick Q, Skalli O. Alpha-actinin 1 and alpha-actinin 4: contrasting roles in the survival, motility, and RhoA signaling of astrocytoma cells. Exp Cell Res. 2010;316(7):1137–47.
74. Welsch T, Keleg S, Bergmann F, Bauer S, Hinz U, Schmidt J. Actinin-4 expression in primary and metastasized pancreatic ductal adenocarcinoma. Pancreas. 2009;38(8):968–76.
75. Yamamoto S, Tsuda H, Honda K, Takano M, Tamai S, Imoto I, et al. ACTN4 gene amplification and actinin-4 protein overexpression drive tumour development and histological progression in a high-grade subset of ovarian clear-cell adenocarcinomas. Histopathology. 2012;60(7):1073–83.
76. Kaplan JM, Kim SH, North KN, Rennke H, Correia LA, Tong HQ, et al. Mutations in ACTN4, encoding alpha-actinin-4, cause familial focal segmental glomerulosclerosis. Nat Genet. 2000;24(3):251–6.
77. Weins A, Kenlan P, Herbert S, Le TC, Villegas I, Kaplan BS, et al. Mutational and Biological Analysis of alpha-actinin-4 in focal segmental glomerulosclerosis. J Am Soc Nephrol. 2005;16(12):3694–701.
78. An HT, Kim J, Yoo S, Ko J. sLZIP negatively regulates skeletal muscle differentiation via interaction with alpha-actinin-4. J Biol Chem. 2013;289(8):4969–79.
79. Chakraborty S, Reineke EL, Lam M, Li X, Liu Y, Gao C, et al. Alpha-actinin 4 potentiates myocyte enhancer factor-2 transcription activity by antagonizing histone deacetylase 7. J Biol Chem. 2006;281(46):35070–80.

80. Goffart S, Franko A, Clemen CS, Wiesner RJ. Alpha-actinin 4 and BAT1 interaction with the cytochrome c promoter upon skeletal muscle differentiation. Curr Genet. 2006;49(2):125–35.
81. Khurana S, Chakraborty S, Cheng X, Su YT, Kao HY. The actin-binding protein, actinin alpha 4 (ACTN4), is a nuclear receptor coactivator that promotes proliferation of MCF-7 breast cancer cells. J Biol Chem. 2011;286(3):1850–9.
82. Khurana S, Chakraborty S, Zhao X, Liu Y, Guan D, Lam M, et al. Identification of a novel LXXLL motif in alpha-actinin 4-spliced isoform that is critical for its interaction with estrogen receptor alpha and co-activators. J Biol Chem. 2012;287(42):35418–29.
83. Kumeta M, Yoshimura SH, Harata M, Takeyasu K. Molecular mechanisms underlying nucleocytoplasmic shuttling of actinin-4. J Cell Sci. 2010;123 (Pt 7):1020–30.
84. Poch MT, Al-Kassim L, Smolinski SM, Hines RN. Two distinct classes of CCAAT box elements that bind nuclear factor-Y/alpha-actinin-4: potential role in human CYP1A1 regulation. Toxicol Appl Pharmacol. 2004;199(3):239–50.
85. Huang SM, Huang CJ, Wang WM, Kang JC, Hsu WC. The enhancement of nuclear receptor transcriptional activation by a mouse actin-binding protein, alpha actinin 2. J Mol Endocrinol. 2004;32(2):481–96.
86. Honda K. The biological role of actinin-4 ACTN4 in malignant phenotypes of cancer. Cell Bioscie. DOI:10.1186/s13578-015-0031-0
87. Feng D, DuMontier C, Pollak MR. The role of alpha-actinin-4 in human kidney disease. Cell Biosci. in press.

3

Tip110 binding to U6 small nuclear RNA and its participation in pre-mRNA splicing

Ying Liu[1*], Jinfeng Liu[1,2], Zenyuan Wang[1,3] and Johnny J He[1]

Abstract

Background: RNA–protein interactions play important roles in gene expression control. These interactions are mediated by several recurring RNA-binding motifs including a well-known and characterized ribonucleoprotein motif or so-called RNA recognition motif (RRM).

Results: In the current study, we set out to identify the RNA ligand(s) of a RRM-containing protein Tip110, also known as p110^{nrb}, SART3, or p110, using a RNA-based yeast three-hybrid cloning strategy. Six putative RNA targets were isolated and found to contain a consensus sequence that was identical to nucleotides 34–46 of U6 small nuclear RNA. Tip110 binding to U6 was confirmed to be specific and RRM-dependent in an electrophoretic mobility shift assay. Both in vitro pre-mRNA splicing assay and in vivo splicing-dependent reporter gene assay showed that the pre-mRNA splicing was correlated with Tip110 expression. Moreover, Tip110 was found in the spliceosomes containing prespliced pre-mRNA and spliced mRNA products. Nonetheless, the RRM-deleted mutant (ΔRRM) that did not bind to U6 showed promotion in vitro pre-mRNA splicing, whereas the nuclear localization signal (NLS)-deleted mutant ΔNLS that bound to U6 promoted the pre-mRNA splicing both in vitro and in vivo. Lastly, RNA-Seq analysis confirmed that Tip110 regulated a number of gene pre-mRNA splicing including several splicing factors.

Conclusions: Taken together, these results demonstrate that Tip110 is directly involved in constitutive eukaryotic pre-mRNA splicing, likely through its binding to U6 and regulation of other splicing factors, and provide further evidence to support the global roles of Tip110 in regulation of host gene expression.

Keywords: Tip110, Small nuclear RNA, U6, RNA binding, Pre-mRNA, Splicing

Background

In eukaryotic cells, gene expression begins in nucleus with transcription of protein-coding genes to primary RNA transcripts, or so-called pre-messenger RNA (pre-mRNA) or heterogeneous nuclear RNA (hnRNA) [1]. The pre-mRNA are processed to become mature mRNA through a series of post-transcriptional modifications [2]. One of them is the precise excision of noncoding sequences (introns) from pre-mRNA in the spliceosomes [2]. The spliceosomes are formed through assembly of spliceosomal small nuclear ribonucleoprotein (snRNP) and recruitment of numerous splicing factors to pre-mRNA [1, 2]. Efficient and proper pre-mRNA splicing is a critical step in gene expression control [3, 4]. Dysregulation of splicing elements or splicing regulators and subsequent abnormal pre-mRNA splicing result in expression of aberrant protein products and development of diseases [3, 4]. For example, overexpression of splicing factor SF2/ASF has been shown to trigger malignant transformation [5].

snRNP are important components of the spliceosomes in which the pre-mRNA splicing occurs [6]. There are five major snRNP U1, U2, U4, U5, and U6 in the spliceosomes containing small nuclear RNA (snRNA) U1 snRNA, U2 snRNA, U4 snRNA, U5 snRNA, and U6 snRNA, respectively [6]. Those snRNA are transcribed in the nucleus and exported to the cytoplasm after acquiring a m7G-cap [1, 2]. The core snRNP are initially assembled in the cytoplasm to contain snRNA, survival motor neuron protein, Gem-associated proteins, and Sm proteins, followed

*Correspondence: ying.liu@unthsc.edu
[1] Department of Cell Biology and Immunology, Graduate School of Biomedical Sciences, University of North Texas Health Science Center, 3500 Camp Bowie Blvd., Fort Worth, TX 76107, USA
Full list of author information is available at the end of the article

by nuclear import [7]. Once the core snRNP get into the nucleus, they enter the Cajal body, undergo further modifications such as RNA-targeted ribose methylation and pseudouridylation, recruit additional proteins to complete its final assembly for pre-mRNA splicing [7]. One group of the best-defined proteins that snRNP recruit in the Cajal body are serine-/arginine-rich repeat (RS domain)-containing splicing factors called SR proteins [8]. SR proteins are characterized by the presence of RNA recognition motifs (RRM) in the N terminus and the presence of RS domain in the C terminus. Most of the serine/arginine-rich (SR) proteins are found in the nucleus, specifically in nuclear speckles, and are known for their roles in alternative and constitutive pre-mRNA splicing [9, 10]. Besides SR proteins, there are a number of other pre-mRNA splicing factors in the nuclear speckles. Those pre-mRNA splicing factors are constantly moving between nuclear speckles and the nucleoplasm or other nuclear substructures [11]. Nevertheless, nuclear speckles are often regarded as the sites for storage, assembly, and modification of the splicing factors as well as the supply sources of splicing factors for active transcription sites [12–14]. In addition, nuclear speckles have been shown to be directly involved in the pre-mRNA splicing [15].

Tip110, also known as $p110^{nrb}$, SART3, or p110, has been proposed to serve several important biological functions. These include tumor antigen function [16–18], control of gene transcription [19–21], regulation of protein stability [22, 23], and stem cell pluripotency and differentiation [24–26]. In addition, Tip110 has been proposed to be directly involved in pre-mRNA splicing through interaction with RNPS1 [16], U4/U6 snRNP [27, 28], YB-1 [29], and C-MYC [26]. In agreement with Tip110 roles in pre-mRNA splicing, Tip110 has two RNA recognition domains [16] and has been detected in the nuclear substructures Cajal bodies and nuclear speckles [14, 30, 31]. Further supporting Tip110 roles in pre-mRNA splicing is the recent findings that Tip110 directly binds to unphosphorylated C-terminal domain (CTD) of RNA polymerase II in the direct manner [21]. In the current study, we set out to identify specific RNA targets, if any, that might be involved in interaction with Tip110 and account for Tip110 function in pre-mRNA splicing. We took advantage of the RNA–protein binding-based yeast three hybrid screening strategy and identified snRNA U6 from a hybrid RNA library as putative Tip110-binding partner. We then characterized the interaction and its role in pre-mRNA splicing.

Methods

Cell lines and cell transfection

293T and Hela cells were purchased from American Tissue Culture Collection (ATCC, Manassas, VA, USA) and maintained in Dulbecco's modified Eagle's medium supplemented with 10% fetal bovine serum, in a 37°C, 5% CO_2 incubator. Cells were transfected using the standard calcium phosphate precipitation method.

Plasmids

Plasmids pTip110.His, pTip110s.His, and deletion mutants ΔNLS and ΔRRM, and pGEX-Tip110, pGEX-Tip110s, and deletion mutants ΔNLS and ΔRRM, and pAD.Tip110 were described elsewhere [20]. The standard PCR cloning technique was used to construct pTip110ΔLSM, with pTip110.His as the templates and primers 5′-GGA ATT CAC CAT GGC GAC TGC GGC CGA A-3′ and 5′-CCG CTC GAG TCA ATG ATG ATG ATG ATG ATG GGC AAC TGC AGG AGC CG-3′ (the restriction enzyme sites underlined). The Tip110 siRNA expression plasmid was constructed in the backbone of pSHAG-1 by annealing oligonucleotides 5′-CGG GAT CCG ACT CAG CCT CGG GTT CTG AA-3′ and 5′-CGG GAT CCA AAA AAT TGG ACT CAG CCT CA-3′, and inserting the annealed DNA at the Bam HI site of pSHAG-1. All recombinant plasmids and deletion mutants were verified by sequencing. The sources of the other plasmids used in the study are: pGEX-4T-3 from Amersham (Piscataway, NJ, USA), pSHAG-1 from Dr. Gregory Hannon, pIIIA.MS2 from Dr. Marvin Wickens, pT7.U6 from Dr. Iain Mattaji, pDM138 from Dr. Thomas Hope, pcRev from Dr. Bryan Cullen, and pSP64-Hβδ6 from Dr. Adrian Krainer.

Construction of a hybrid RNA library and yeast three-hybrid screening

A hybrid RNA library and yeast three-hybrid screening were performed as previously described [32], with some modifications. Briefly, genomic DNA was isolated from 293T cells and digested by Mse I, Tsp509I, Alu I and Rsa I, and then by T4 DNA polymerase in the presence of 100 μM dNTP. Digested DNA was fractionated on a 2% agarose gel to obtain DNA fragments of 50–150 bp. These small DNA fragments were then ligated into SmaI-linearized and calf intestine phosphatase-treated pIIIA.MS2 plasmid. The ligation mixture was transformed into GC5 competent bacteria for propagation and isolation of the library DNA. Yeast strain L40coat stably expressing LexA-MS2 coat fusion protein was first transformed with pAD-Tip110 plasmid and then with the RNA expression library. The selection of transformed yeast was performed on synthetic complete plates containing 0.5 mM 3-aminotriazole and no tryptophan, leucine, uracil and histidine, followed by X-gal filter assay for β-galactosidase expression. β-galactosidase-positive colonies were further cultured to isolate the hybrid RNA plasmids.

Recombinant protein purification

GST-Tip110, GST-Tip110s, Tip110 deletion mutants ΔNLS and ΔRRM, and GST proteins were expressed in and purified from *E. coli* BL21, as previously described [20]. Briefly, expression plasmids were transformed into BL21 and induced with 1 mM isopropyl-D-thiogalactopyranoside for 2 h at 37°C. GST fusion proteins were purified using a Pierce GST fusion protein purification kit (Rockford, IL, USA). When necessary, GST was removed by treating the eluted protein with thrombin protease (10 units) (Invitrogen, Carlsbad, CA, USA) at room temperature for 18 h. The digested protein solution was dialyzed overnight in 4 l of phosphate-buffered saline and cleared of GST protein by additional incubations with fresh glutathione beads. The purified proteins were electrophoresed on a 8% SDS-polyacrylamide gel and stained with Gold–Blue (Pierce) to ensure the complete removal of GST protein as well as undigested fusion protein and other contaminated proteins.

RNA–protein gel mobility shift assay

U6 RNA was synthesized using an Ambion in vitro transcription kit (Austin, TX, USA). Briefly, pT7-U6 plasmid was linearized with Dra I and incubated with ATP, CTP, GTP and ^{32}P-labeled UTP in the presence of T7 RNA polymerase at 30°C for 1 h, followed by removal of free nucleotides by an CentriSpin column (Princeton Separation, Princeton, NJ, USA). ^{32}P-labeled-U6 RNA was then mixed with purified GST-Tip110 or its mutant proteins in a total volume of 20 μl containing 1 mM HEPES, pH 7.6, 1 μM $MgCl_2$, 16 mM KCl, 2.5% glycerol (v/v), and 10 nM DTT. The mixture was incubated on ice for 15 min and then subjected to 5% nondenaturing polyacrylamide gel electrophoresis (acrylamide-bisacrylamide, 80:1) in the 0.5× TBE buffer. The gel was dried and exposed for autoradiography.

Preparation of pre-mRNA and in vitro splicing assay

Human β-globin minigene pre-mRNA was synthesized using an Ambion in vitro capped RNA transcription kit (Ambion). Briefly, pSP64-Hßδ6 plasmid was linearized with BamH I and incubated with ATP, CTP, GTP, cap anolog and ^{32}P-labeled UTP at 37°C for 2 h. ^{32}P-labeled pre-mRNA was then purified on a 5% denaturing polyacrylamide gel and suspended in 10 mM Tris.HCl, pH 7.9. The ^{32}P-labeled pre-mRNA was then aliquoted and stored at −80°C. Splicing reactions were carried out in a 25 μl volume containing 12.8 μM $MgCl_2$, 500 μM ATP, 20 mM creatine phosphate, 2.7% (w/v) polyvinyl alcohol, 1,000 U/ml RNasin, 12.8 mM HEPES, pH 8.0, 14% (v/v) glycerol, 62 mM KCl, 0.12 mM EDTA, and 0.7 mM DTT at 30°C for 2 h. The reactions contained 6 μl Hela nuclear extract (Promega, Madison, WI, USA) and 12.5 ng ^{32}P-labeled pre-mRNA prepared above.

Monoclonal antibody production

Anti-Tip110 monoclonal antibodies were produced by Promab Biotechnologies, Inc. (Albany, CA, USA). Briefly, purified GST-Tip110 protein was used to immunize BALB/c mice. The mice were given an additional boost immunization after 3 weeks. Three days after the boost, the spleen cells were isolated from the immunized mice and fused with SP20 cells (ATCC) using polyethylene glycol (Sigma, St. Louis, MO, USA). Resulting hybridoma were screened to be specific anti-Tip110 antibody using ELISA. To purify the monoclonal antibody, the hybridoma cells were cultured in a production module of the miniPERM device (Viva Science, Inc.), and the antibody was further purified from the culture supernatant using a Protein A column and a AKTA prime-automated liquid chromatography system (Amersham, Piscataway, NJ, USA). The antibody protein purity was determined to be IgG_2 with a purity of higher than 99%.

Tip110 immunodepletion

Purified Tip110 monoclonal antibody (20 μg) was incubated with 50 μl of 50% slurry protein A-Sepharose (Amersham) in a buffer containing 20 mM HEPES, pH 8.0, 100 mM KCl, 0.2 mM EDTA, 20% (v/v) glycerol, 0.5 mM PMSF, 1 mM DTT at 4°C for 4 h with continuous mixing. The protein A beads were then recovered by centrifugation and repeated washes with the same incubation buffer to remove excess anti-Tip110 antibody. An aliquot of the beads were then incubated with Hela nuclear extract at 4°C for 2 h with continuous mixing, and the supernatant was used as Tip110-depleted Hela nuclear extract. Tip110 protein on the immunoabsorbed beads was eluted by adding 20 μl of 4× SDS sample buffer, followed by boiling 5 min. The eluent and aliquot of the Tip110-depleted Hela nuclear extract were subjected to 10% SDS-PAGE gel and Western blot analysis to ensure efficient Tip110 depletion.

Pre-mRNA splicing-dependent CAT reporter gene assay

293T cells were plated in a 6-well plate at a density of 0.72 × 10^6 cells/well and 1 day later transfected with 1 μg pDM138, 1 μg pcRev, 1–5 μg pTip110.His or pTip110.siRNA. In all transfections, a CMVβGal plasmid was included to normalize transfection variations, and pcDNA3 was used to equalize the amount of transfected DNA. Forty-eight hours after transfection, the cells were harvested and subjected to 3 rounds of freeze–thaw in 0.25 M Tris.HCl, pH 8.0, and the lysates were collected for β-galactosidase and CAT activities. β-galactosidase was determined using a colorimtric assay [20], while CAT was determined by one-step simple phase extraction and scintillation counting as described [33].

Preparation of cell lysates and Western blot analysis

Cells were washed twice with ice-cold phosphate-buffered saline (PBS), and cell pellets were suspended in two volumes of whole cell lysis buffer containing10 mM $NaHPO_4$, 150 mM NaCl, 1% Triton X-100, 0.1% SDS, 0.2% sodium azide, 0.5% sodium deoxycholate, 0.004% sodium fluoride, and 1 mM sodium orthovanadate and incubated on ice for 10 min. Cell lysates were obtained by centrifugation, removal of the cell debris, and electrophoretically separated on 10% SDS-PAGE and analyzed by immunoblotting. Anti-His antibody was from Qiagen (Valencia, CA, USA), while β-actin was from Santa Cruz Biotech. (Santa Cruz, CA, USA). The blots were first probed with primary antibodies, followed by appropriate horseradish peroxidase-conjugated secondary antibodies, and then visualized with the ECL system (Amersham).

RNA isolation and RNA-Seq

Hela were transfected with human Tip110 siRNA or the universal control siRNA. Total RNA was purified from transfected cells using Trizol according to the manufacturer's instructions (Life Technologies, Grand Island, NY, USA) and used for RNA-Seq. The RNA-Seq was performed at the Genomic Core of UT Southwestern Medical Center, Dallas, TX, USA. The RNA-Seq reads were aligned to the human genome sequences for further differential and spliceosome pathway analysis using the Panther Pathway Analysis software.

qRT-PCR

Total RNA was extracted using Trizol and used to synthesize cDNA using a ScriptII RT reagent kit (Promega). cDNAs were used for qPCR using a Power Sybr®Green PCR kit (Life Technologies) according to the manufacturer's instructions. The qPCR program consisted of one cycle of 95°C for 10 min, 40 cycles of 95°C for 15 s and 60°C for 1 min.

Results

Identification of Tip110 RNA ligands by the yeast three-hybrid cloning

To determine if Tip110 bound to specific RNAs, we took advantage of a RNA–protein interaction-based yeast three-hybrid cloning strategy [34]. This genetic assay was initially developed to study RNA–protein interactions and later adapted to identify RNA ligands of an RNA binding protein [32]. It is based on the transcriptional activation of separable domains of transcriptional factors such as GAL4 and LexA, and is composed of two hybrid proteins and one hybrid RNA (Figure 1a). One hybrid protein consists of the DNA binding domain of transcriptional activator LexA fused to a known RNA binding protein bacteriophage MS2 coat protein. The hybrid RNA is a RNA library expressing a MS2 coat protein RNA binding sequence. The other hybrid protein consists of the activation domain of transcriptional activator Gal4 fused to a bait protein, in our case Tip110. Binding of the bait protein Tip110 to the target RNA in the RNA hybrid brings closer the Gal4 activation domain and the LexA DNA binding domain and subsequently activates expression of the reporter genes LacZ/His. We constructed a hybrid RNA library from 50 to 150 bp fragments of genomic DNA isolated from 293T cells and transformed it into the L40coat strain containing both LexA-MS2 and Gal4 AD-Tip110. We then plated the transformants on synthetic media lacking uracil, leucine, tryptophan, and histidine, which are used to select for the presence of these three hybrids and activation of the His reporter gene. We also include 0.5 mM 3-aminotriazole to reduce a background level of His gene expression. Among an estimate of 11.4 million yeast transformants, about 450 colonies were formed after 1 week. Of these, 156 were found to be β-galactosidase-positive. We then cultured these colonies in rich media to lose the Gal4 AD-Tip110 plasmid and tested them for their ability to activate reporter genes. The results showed that of these 156 colonies only 6 were no longer β-galactosidase-positive, while other 150 appeared to activate LacZ gene expression in

a

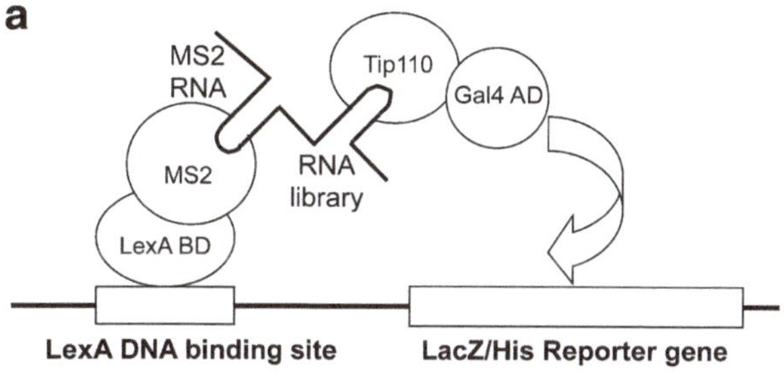

b

```
 auucggc gaacgauacagag ccggauuagu
     cca gaucguaacagac ggcuauacagauuc
 ugcguua gaacgauagagag agguccggug
      gg gaaccauagagau uuaggccaaccuagu
  aguuac aaacgauacagag uccuaggccuu
gguuaucc gaacgauacagag cggauauu
Consensus gaacgauacagag
```

Figure 1 Identification of U6 as a Tip110 binding RNA target. **a** Scheme of the yeast three-hybrid cloning strategy. LexA BD-MS2: LexA DNA binding domain fused with phage coat protein MS2; MS2 RNA–RNA library: the target RNA sequence of MS2 protein was fused to a pool of RNAs transcribed from human genomic DNA; Gal4 AD-Tip110: Gal4 activation domain fused to Tip110 protein. Respective binding of MS2 protein to MS2 target RNA and Tip110 protein to its putative RNAs leads to activation of LacZ and His reporter genes. **b** Sequences of RNA hits obtained from the yeast three-hybrid screening using Tip110 as the bait. The consensus sequence was matched to small nuclear U6 RNA at nucleotides 34–46.

the absence of Gal4 AD-Tip110. Sequence analysis of these RNA inserts revealed a consensus of 13 nucleotides (nt.): gaacgauacagag (Figure 1b). We performed a BLAST search with the sequence, and found it to be identical to small nuclear RNA U6 at nt. 34–46.

Binding of Tip110 protein to U6 RNA

To ascertain Tip110 binding to U6 RNA, we synthesized U6 RNA in vitro in the presence of α-^{32}P-UTP and used the ^{32}P-labeled U6 RNA as a probe. We then incubated 1, 5, 10 and 50 ng purified recombinant GST-Tip110 protein with ^{32}P-labeled U6 RNA and determined Tip110-U6 complex formation using a gel mobility shift assay. The same amounts of purified GST protein were included as a control in the experiments. Complex formation between Tip110 and U6 became evident when 5 ng Tip110 was added and increased significantly when more Tip110 protein was present (Figure 2a). There was no complex formation between GST and U6 in all reactions. To determine the specificity of Tip110 binding to U6, we incubated 10 ng GST-Tip110 protein with ^{32}P-labeled U6 RNA in the presence of 1-, 10-, and 100-fold excess amount of unlabeled U6 RNA, yeast tRNA and poly(I.C) and determined Tip110-U6 complex formation using the same assay. Increasing amounts of unlabeled U6 effectively competed out ^{32}P-labeled U6 for Tip110 binding, as Tip110 and ^{32}P-labeled U6 no longer formed a complex in the presence of unlabeled U6 RNA (Figure 2b). In contrast, inclusion of U6-unrelated yeast tRNA and poly(I.C) had little effects on the complex formation between Tip110 and ^{32}P-labeled U6 RNA. There are two RRMs at the C-terminal of Tip110, one at aa700–778 and the other at aa802–874, and one nuclear localization signal (NLS) at aa601–650 [20]. To determine the role of the RRM domains in Tip110 binding to U6 RNA, we constructed, expressed and purified recombinant GST-Tip110 mutant that had both RRMs deleted (ΔRRM) and determined its ability to bind to U6RNA. Similarly, we also expressed, purified and included in these experiments recombinant Tip110 mutant ΔNLS containing no NLS and a naturally occurring small splicing variant that only encodes the N-terminal 365 amino acids of Tip110 (Tip110s) [20]. Compared to Tip110, both ΔRRM and Tip110s showed no binding to U6 RNA, while ΔNLS retained the U6 binding activity (Figure 2c), suggesting that RRMs were directly involved in Tip110 binding to U6 RNA. Collectively, these results confirm the finding from the yeast three-hybrid cloning that Tip110 binds to U6 RNA in a specific manner.

Promotion of pre-mRNA splicing by Tip110

Small nuclear U6 RNA directly participates in pre-mRNA splicing [35]. Our early studies have shown that Tip110 is localized in the spliceosome-rich "speckles" subnuclear structure [20]. Thus, the finding of Tip110 binding to U6 prompted us to determine the possible

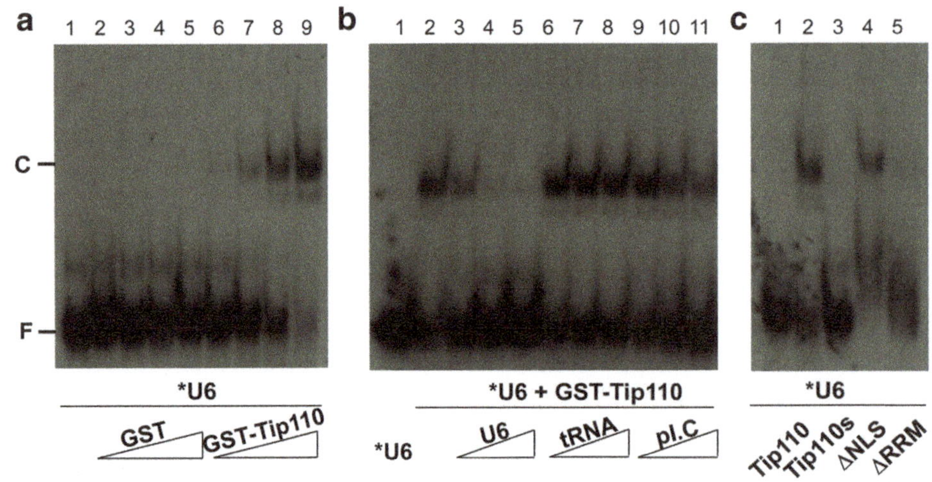

Figure 2 Specific binding of Tip110 protein to U6 RNA. **a** Complex formation between Tip110 and U6 RNA. ^{32}P-labeled U6 RNA (*U6) was incubated with 1, 5, 10, and 100 ng recombinant GST (*lanes 2–5*) or GST-Tip110 (*lanes 6–9*). The reaction containing no recombinant protein was included to show free ^{32}P-labeled U6 RNA (*lane 1*). The RNA–protein complex formation was determined using the electrophoretic mobility shift assay (EMSA). **b** Specificity of Tip110 binding to U6 RNA. ^{32}P-labeled U6 RNA (*U6) was incubated with 10 ng recombinant GST-Tip110 in the presence of 5, 10, and 50 ng unlabeled U6 RNA (*lanes 3–5*), yeast tRNA (*lanes 6–8*), or polyinosinic:polycytidylic acid (poly I.C) (*lanes 9–11*). The complex formation of Tip110 and U6 RNA was determined using the EMSA. The binding reactions containing *U6 only (*lane 1*) and *U6 and GST-Tip110 (*lane 2*) were also included. **c** Binding of Tip110 mutants to U6 RNA. ^{32}P-labeled U6 RNA (*U6) was incubated with 10 ng recombinant GST-Tip110s (*lane 3*), GST-ΔNLS (*lane 4*), or GST-ΔRRM (*lane 5*). The RNA–protein complex formation was determined using the EMSA. The binding reactions containing *U6 RNA only (*lane 1*) or *U6 RNA and GST-Tip110 (*lane 2*) were also included. *C* RNA–protein complex; *F* unbound free RNA.

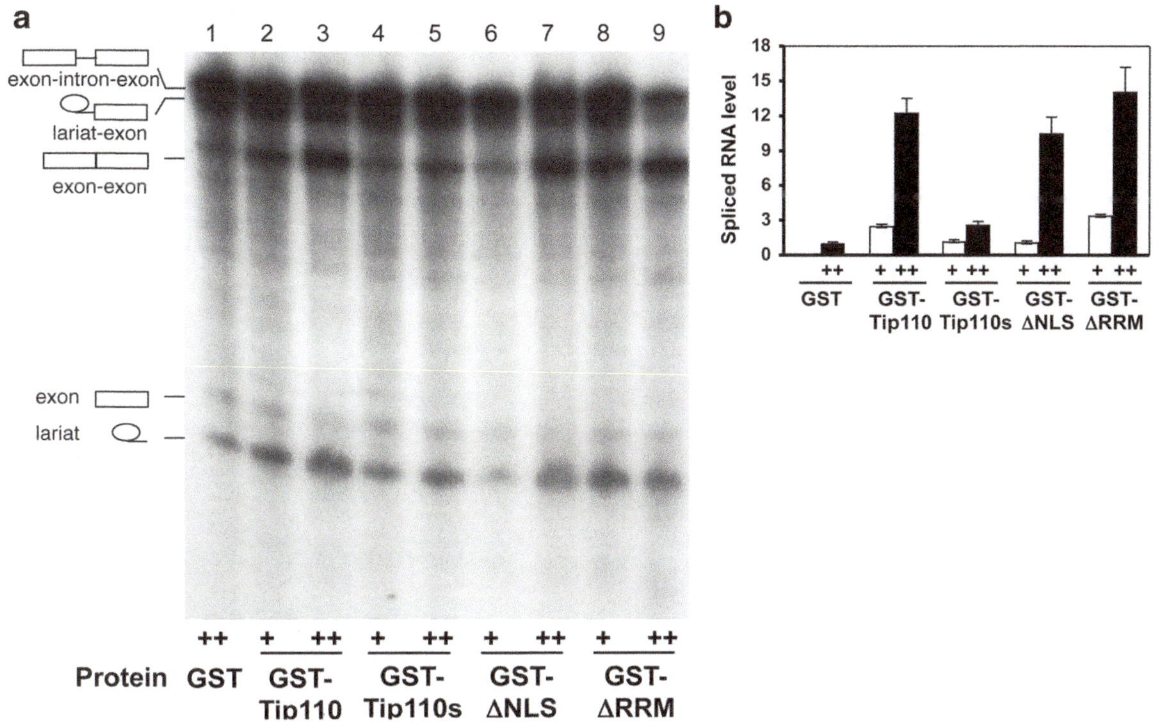

Figure 3 Human β-hemaglobin pre-mRNA splicing by Tip110 and its mutants. ^{32}P-labeled human β-hemaglobin minigene pre-mRNA was incubated with Hela nuclear extract in the presence of 10 (+) or 50 ng (++) recombinant GST-Tip110 (*lanes 2* and *3*), GST-Tip110s (*lanes 4* and *5*), GST-ΔNLS (*lanes 6* and *7*), or GSTΔRRM (*lanes 8* and *9*). Recombinant GST protein (50 ng) was included as a control (*lane 1*). The reaction mixtures were separated on 8% denaturing PAGE (**a**). The *symbols on the left* are pre-mRNA and its splicing products. Splicing was quantitated by densitometric scanning of the intronless spliced RNA product on the autoradiography, the spliced RNA product in the reaction containing GST (*lane 1*) was set as the reference to calculate the relative level of pre-mRNA splicing (**b**).

role of Tip110 in eukaryotic pre-mRNA splicing. We then performed an in vitro splicing assay using a human β-globin minigene pre-mRNA as a substrate. This minigene encodes the first exon, the first intron, and a major part of the second exon of human β-globin and has been well characterized and widely used in the in vitro splicing assay [36, 37]. We added 10 and 100 ng purified GST-Tip110 protein in the splicing reaction and determined its effects on the β-globin pre-mRNA splicing (Figure 3a). We also included 100 ng GST protein as a control. Compared to the GST control, 10 and 100 ng GST-Tip110 increased the splicing efficiency by about 3-fold and 12-fold, respectively (Figure 3b). We also added GST-Tip110s, GST-ΔNLS and GST-ΔRRM in the splicing reaction. GST-Tip110s only showed a very modest increase in splicing, while both GST-ΔNLS and GST-ΔRRM enhanced the pre-mRNA splicing similarly to that of the GST-Tip110 (Figure 3b). These results demonstrate that Tip110-mediated pre-mRNA splicing and that the domain responsible for this function was located at the C terminus of the protein. In addition, promotion of pre-mRNA splicing by GST-ΔRRM suggest that Tip110 might function in other steps of pre-mRNA splicing, at least in the context of the in vitro splicing assay.

Inhibition of pre-mRNA splicing by Tip110 depletion and its reversal by Tip110 add-back

To determine the significance of Tip110 function in pre-mRNA splicing, we decided to immunodeplete Tip110 protein from the Hela nuclear extract that was used in the in vitro splicing assay. Thus, we first generated anti-human Tip110 monoclonal antibodies using recombinant GST-Tip110. We then incubated Hela nuclear extract with anti-human Tip110 antibodies and protein-A agarose beads. Tip110-depleted Hela nuclear extract was recovered by brief centrifugation, followed by removal of the beads. An isotype-matched IgG was included as a control. Western blot analysis showed that immunodepletion efficiently removed Tip110 protein from Hela nuclear extract (Figure 4a). We used these extracts and performed the pre-mRNA splicing assay (Figure 4b). Compared to the IgG control, little splicing products were detected in anti-Tip110 antibody-depleted Hela nuclear extract (Figure 4c). To ascertain Tip110 function

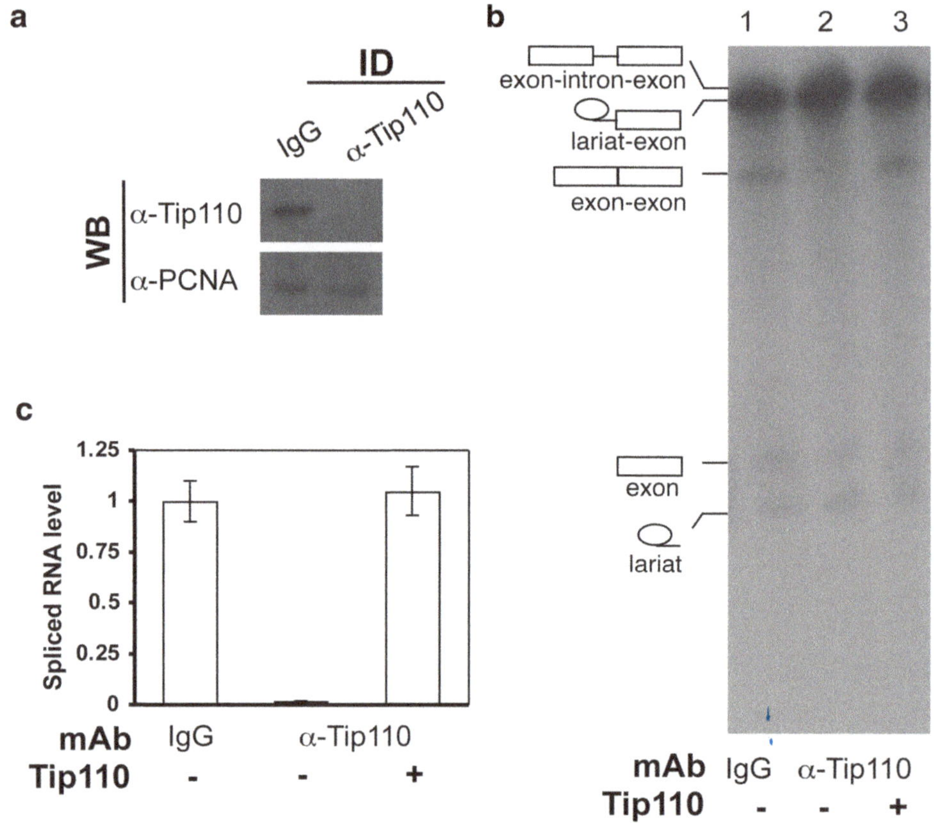

Figure 4 Effects of Tip110 immunodepletion and add-back on pre-mRNA splicing. Hela nuclear extract was pre-incubated with Tip110 mAb-conjugated protein-A beads to deplete endogenous Tip110 protein, as determined by Western blot analysis (**a**), and then used for pre-mRNA splicing reaction (**b**). An isotype-matched immunoglobulin control (IgG) was included as an immunodepletion control. Tip110-depleted nuclear extract was supplemented with recombinant Tip110 (100 ng) for the splicing reaction (**b**). Splicing was quantitated by densitometric scanning of the intronless spliced RNA product on the autoradiography, the spliced RNA product in the reaction containing the control IgG-immunodepleted Hela nuclear extract was set as the reference to calculate the relative level of pre-mRNA splicing (**c**).

in pre-mRNA splicing, we performed the splicing assay by adding back GST-Tip110 protein into Tip110-depleted Hela nuclear extract. The results showed that Tip110 add-back restored the splicing activity. Taken together, these results show that Tip110 is indispensible for constitutive pre-mRNA splicing.

Correlation between Tip110 expression and pre-mRNA splicing-dependent reporter gene expression

Although pre-mRNA splicing mainly occurs in the nucleus, some processes involve both cytosol and nucleus [38]. It is clear that the in vitro splicing assay is likely not representative some aspects of in vivo splicing process. Thus, we decided to further determine Tip110 function in pre-mRNA splicing in vivo. We took advantage of a HIV-1 Rev-dependent reporter gene DM138 (Figure 5a) and determined the relationship between Tip110 expression and pre-mRNA splicing. The chloramphenicol acetyltransferase (CAT) reporter gene in DM138 is under the control of the CMV promoter, is flanked by introns containing splice donor and acceptor sites, and has the CAT gene linked to a DNA sequence encoding HIV-1 Rev responsive element (RRE) [39, 40]. The construct is designed in such a manner that the CAT pre-mRNA transcripts contain the introns and RRE, which will not be exported into the cytosol from the nucleus for CAT protein translation unless HIV-1 Rev is provided *in trans*. We reasoned that if Tip110 enhanced pre-mRNA splicing, Tip110 expression would negate HIV-1 Rev-dependent expression of intron-containing pre-mRNA. Thus, we transfected 293T cells with DM138 alone, or in combination with HIV-1 Rev plasmid and increasing amount of Tip110 expression plasmid. We then determined CAT activity. As expected, Rev expression significantly improved CAT gene expression (Figure 5b). On the other hand, Tip110 expression decreased Rev-dependent CAT gene expression, and the decrease appeared to be dose-dependent. Furthermore, we also knocked down

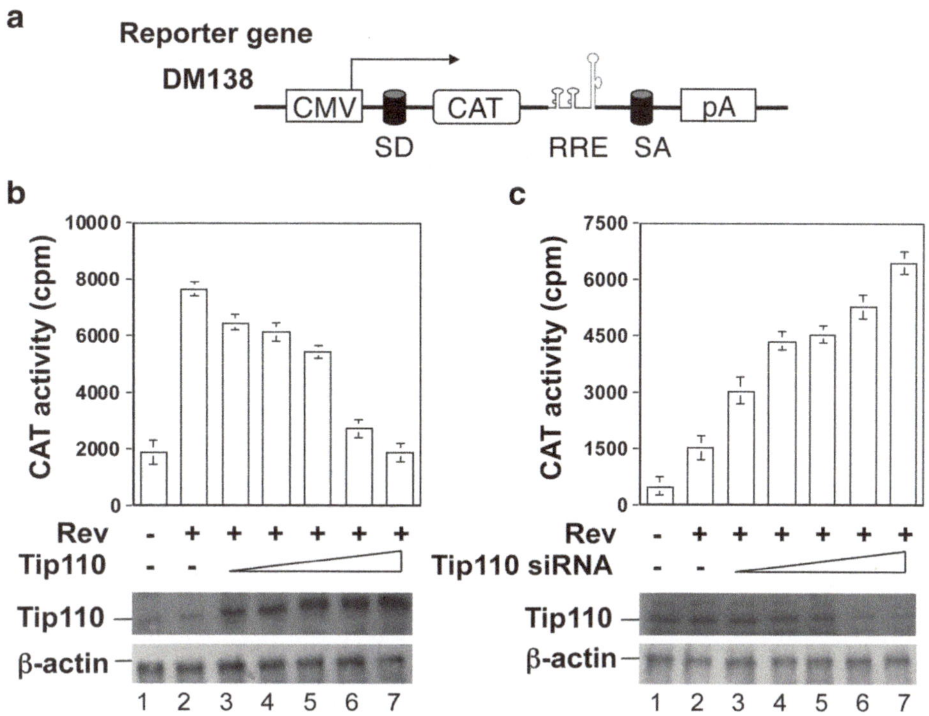

Figure 5 Effects of Tip110 expression on pre-mRNA splicing-dependent CAT reporter gene expression. A. Scheme of the HIV-1 Rev protein-dependent intron-containing CAT reporter DM138. the CAT gene expression requires nuclear export of intron-containing (unspliced) CAT transcript through the interaction between HIV-1 Rev protein and Rev responsive element (RRE) within the CAT transcript. *SD* splice donor, *SA* splice acceptor. **b** 293T cells were transfected with DM138 (*lane 1*), DM138 and Rev (*lane 2*), or DM138, Rev and increasing amounts of Tip110 (*lanes 3–7*). The cells were harvested 48 h after transfection for CAT assay (*top panel*) or Western blot for Tip110 (*bottom panel*). **c** 293T cells were transfected with DM138 (*lane 1*), DM138 and Rev (*lane 2*), or DM138, Rev and increasing amounts of Tip110 siRNA expression plasmids (*lanes 3–7*). The cells were harvested 48 h after transfection for CAT assay (*top panel*) or Western blot for Tip110 (*bottom panel*). The amount of total DNA in all transfections was equalized with pcDNA3 plasmid. A CMVβGal plasmid was included to normalize the transfection variations for CAT assay, while β-actin was included to show equal loading (**b**, **c**). Compared to Figure 5b, c only used one fifth of DM138 reporter plasmid in the transfections.

constitutive Tip110 expression using a Tip110 siRNA expression plasmid and determined its effects on CAT gene expression. In contrast to Tip110 over-expression, Tip110 knockdown increased CAT gene expression, and the increase was also dose-dependent (Figure 5c). The inverse correlation between Tip110 expression and pre-mRNA splicing dependent CAT reporter gene expression confirm that Tip110 is directly involved in eukaryotic pre-mRNA splicing.

Requirement of Tip110 domains and pre-mRNA splicing

Next, we performed the same reporter gene assay using different Tip110 deletion mutants and further examined the structure–function relationship of Tip110 in terms of pre-mRNA splicing. We transfected 293T cells with DM138 alone, or in combination with HIV-1 Rev plasmid, and Tip110s, ΔNLS, or ΔRRM expression plasmid. We also included full-length Tip110 and Tip110 siRNA expression plasmids in these experiments. In agreement with previous results (Figure 5), Tip110 over-expression decreased CAT gene expression (Figure 6a). As expected, Tip110 siRNA expression increased CAT gene expression. On the other hand, over-expression of Tip110 or ΔRRM showed no effects on CAT gene expression. Interestingly, over-expression of ΔNLS inhibited CAT gene expression, but to a lesser extent than that of full-length wild-type Tip110. In addition, we also constructed a mutant ΔLSM lacking the Lsm motif located between aa942–963, which has been postulated to interact with Lsm proteins to promote U4/U6 formation [41]. Similar to Tip110s and ΔRRM, ΔLSM over-expression had no effects on CAT gene expression. We also performed a Western blot analysis to ensure comparable protein expression of Tip110 and its mutants (Figure 6b). These results suggest that the U6-binding domain RRM, the Lsm proteins-interacting domain LSM, and NLS are all important for Tip110 function in pre-mRNA splicing.

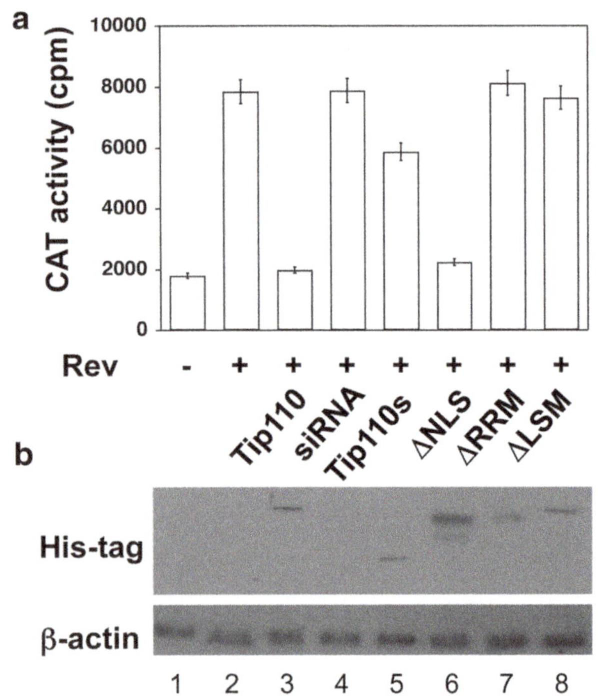

Figure 6 Effects of Tip110 mutants on pre-mRNA splicing-dependent CAT reporter gene expression. 293T cells were transfected with DM138 (*lane 1*), DM138 and Rev (*lane 2*), or DM138, Rev, and Tip110 (*lane 3*), Tip10 siRNA (*lane 4*), Tip110s (*lane 5*), ΔNLS (*lane 6*), ΔRRM (*lane 7*), or ΔLSM (*lane 8*). The cells were harvested 48 h after transfection for CAT assay (**a**) or Western blot for expression of Tip110 and its mutants (**b**). The amount of total DNA in all transfections was equalized with pcDNA3 plasmid. A CMVβGal plasmid was included to normalize the transfection variations for CAT assay, while β-actin was included to show equal loading.

Presence of Tip110 in the splicing complexes

To test whether Tip110 is physically associated with active spliceosomes, we incubated an in vitro splicing reaction with immobilized anti-Tip110 antibody, immunoprecipitated the labeled RNA species in the splicing reaction, and analyzed the immunoprecipitated RNA species. An isotype-matched IgG was included as a control. In addition, the splicing reaction without any IgG was also included as a mock control. Compared to the mock control, no significant RNA species were detected in the IgG control immunoprecipitates (lane 2, Figure 7), whereas more unspliced β-globin pre-mRNA and less intron-spliced β-globin mRNA were detected in the anti-Tip110 immunoprecipitates (lane 3, Figure 7). Of note was that released lariat RNA species was also detected in the anti-Tip110 immunoprecipitates. These results confirmed that Tip110 was associated with active spliceosomes and provide further support for Tip110 function in pre-mRNA splicing.

Effects of Tip110 on global pre-mRNA splicing

We next determined whether Tip110 expression would globally affect pre-mRNA splicing. We transfected Hela with Tip110-specific siRNA or control siRNA, isolated mRNA and performed the next generation RNA sequencing (RNA-Seq). The cells transfected with Tip110 siRNA and control siRNA were compared for the alternative gene spliced transcripts. Bioinformatics analysis of the RNA transcripts indicated that Tip110 knockdown led to changes of alternative spliced RNA transcripts of 17,498 genes with statistical significant difference ($p < 0.05$). Using the Panther pathways analysis, those genes were mainly grouped as the following categories: protein-binding transcription factors (37%), catalytic molecules (35%), nucleic acid-binding transcription factors (9%), structural molecules (6%), and receptors (4%) (Figure 8a). Of particular note were four pre-mRNA splicing factors snRNP polypeptide B (SNRPB2), zinc finger RNA-binding motif and serine/arginine-rich 2 (ZRSR2), pre-mRNA processing factor 4 (PRPF4) and pre-mRNA processing factor 38b (PRPF38b) that showed all down-regulation in Tip110 siRNA-transfected cells (Figure 8b). qRT-PCR was then performed to quantify the mRNA expression of these four genes in Tip110 siRNA-transfected Hela as well as in Tip110-transfected Hela. The results showed the positive association between Tip110 and mRNA levels of these four genes (Figure 8c). Similar results were obtained in 293T. Taken together, these results showed that Tip110 exhibited global effects on expression of host genes including the pre-mRNA splicing factors and suggest that Tip110-induced changes in pre-mRNA splicing factors may provide additional regulatory control of Tip110-mediated pre-mRNA splicing.

Discussion

In this study we aimed to identify the RNA targets for Tip110 binding. We demonstrated that Tip110 specifically interacted with small nuclear U6 RNA through the yeast 3-hybrid screen and RNA EMSA (Figures 1, 2). Tip110 promoted pre-mRNA splicing in vitro (Figure 3) and in a pre-mRNA splicing-dependent reporter gene assay (Figure 5). Corroborated with these findings were that depletion of Tip110 from nuclear extract led to inhibition of pre-mRNA splicing and that add-back Tip110 restored pre-mRNA splicing (Figure 4). Moreover, RRM domain of Tip110 was shown to be important for U6 RNA binding; RRM, LSM, and NLS domains were all important for Tip110 function in pre-mRNA splicing (Figures 2, 6). Furthermore, Tip110 was detected in association with pre-mRNA- and spliced RNA-containing spliceosomes (Figure 7). Lastly, RNA-Seq analysis showed that Tip110 expression was linked to alternate pre-mRNA splicing of the majority of genes in human

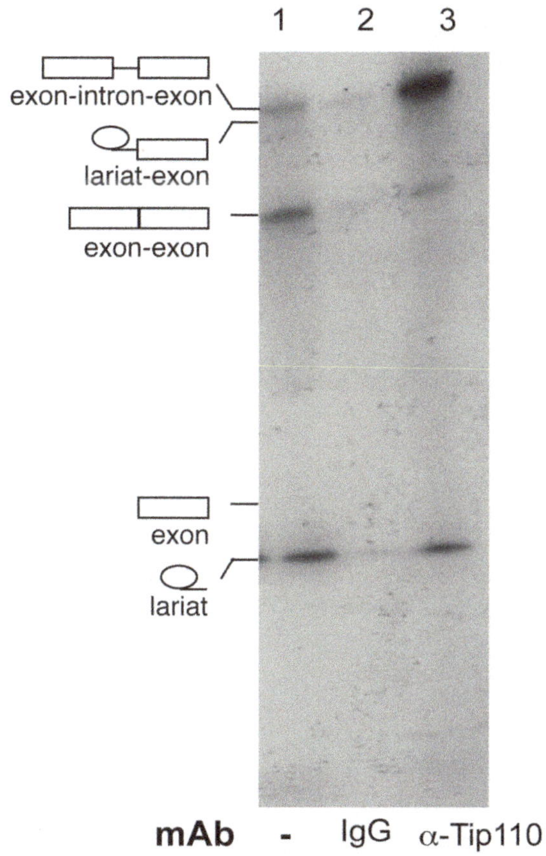

Figure 7 Tip110 association with pre-mRNA and spliced RNA products in the spliceosomes. ^{32}P-labeled human β-hemaglobin minigene pre-mRNA was first incubated with Hela nuclear extract (*lane 1*). The splicing reaction was then immunoprecipitated with an anti-Tip110 monoclonal antibody (*lane 3*), or an isotype-mached IgG control (*lane 2*). The immunprecipitates were subjected to 8% denaturing PAGE. The *symbols on the left* are pre-mRNA and its splicing products.

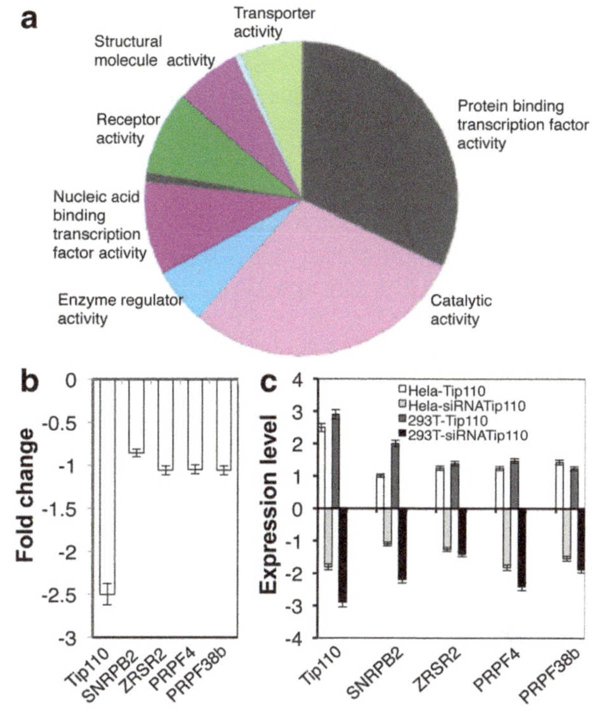

Figure 8 Tip110 global regulation on alternate pre-mRNA splicing and validation of Tip110-regulated four splicing factors. **a** Hela were transfected with Tip110-specific siRNA and the control siRNA. Cells were harvested for RNA isolation, the RNA was used for RNA-Seq. Panther pathway analysis was performed to group the total of 17,498 genes with changes in alternate pre-mRNA splicing. **b** Four splicing factors were down-regulated at the mRNA level from RNA-Seq. **c** qRT-PCR was performed to validate these four mRNA expression from Hela and 293T that were either transfected with Tip110 expression vector and siRNA for Tip110. cDNA3 was included as the control for Tip110; siRNA control was included as the control for Tip110 siRNA. The fold changes were calculated using the control as the reference (**b**, **c**).

genome including several splicing factors (Figure 8). These results demonstrated that Tip110 regulated global pre-mRNA splicing likely through interaction with snRNA U6 and other splicing factors.

Biogenesis of the snRNP U1, U2, U4, U5, and U6 is a complex process. Newly synthesized snRNP undergo various modification and assembly, and then export from nuclear to cytoplasm where they mature and transport back into the Cajal bodies in the nucleus. snRNA/snRNP then recruit other splicing factors, undergo further assembly and maturation in the Cajal bodies [42–44]. Our current study identified U6 snRNA to be the putative Tip110-binding target through the yeast three hybrid cloning (Figure 1) and further confirmed the binding specificity through the gel shift mobility assay (Figure 2). These results are consistent with the previous reports that the U6 snRNP is targeted to the CB by specific binding to Tip110, followed by Tip110-induced assembly of U4/U6 snRNP for recycling of U4 and U6 snRNPs [27, 28, 41, 45]. Tip110 has been shown to localize not only in Cajal bodies, and is also required for the induction of CB formation as well [14, 31, 46]. These studies together suggest that Tip110 not only targets U6 snRNP to Cajal bodies through direct interaction, but also is required for snRNP U6 assembly into mature U4/U6.U5 tri-snRNP to exit Cajal bodies. When we further defined the Tip110 regions that were responsible for the snRNA U6 binding, we made a series of deletion mutants which including the C-terminal (1–350aa), deletion of NSL (Δ600–670aa), deletion of two RRM (Δ740–850aa). The C-terminal truncated protein had no binding activity at all, the deletion of NSL didn't affect the binding, but deletion of the two RRM could abort the binding activity to about 80% (Figures 2, 6). Thus, the two RRM domains are very important to maintain the U6 binding activity of Tip110.

After exiting Cajal bodies, mature snRNP enter nuclear speckles. Nuclear speckles are sites for pre-mRNA splicing that serve as storage and/or modification sites for splicing factors [47]. Our previous digital fluorescence microscopic imaging revealed that Tip110 was detected within the nuclear speckle structure [20]. Tip110 may shuttle from Cajal bodies to nuclear speckles, likely along with the mature spliceosomes for pre-mRNA splicing, as both Cajal bodies and nuclear speckles are enriched in the snRNP U1, U2, U4, U5, and U6 [48]. Tip110 was shown to bind to RNPS1 at its C terminus and could be involved in constitutive and alternative pre-mRNA splicing [16]. RNPS1 is expressed in nuclear speckles and found in the active spliceosomes and functions as a general activator of pre-mRNA splicing [49, 50]. Our current study showed that Tip110 played important functions in pre-mRNA splicing (Figures 3, 4, 5) and was present in the spliceosomes (Figure 7). Therefore, it is likely that Tip110 interaction with RNPS1 and co-localization in nuclear speckles structure are also important for Tip110 function in pre-mRNA splicing. Transcription and pre-mRNA splicing are believed to be coupled by the C-terminal domain (CTD) of the large subunit of RNA polymerase II (Pol II) [1]. CTD phosphorylation is required for the stimulatory effect of the CTD on splicing [51, 52]. We have previously shown that Tip110 bound to the C-terminal domain of unphosphorylated RNA polymerase II in a direct and specific manner and Tip110 expression was associated with increased phosphorylation of serine 2 of the heptapeptide repeats within the RNAPII C-terminal domain [21]. Thus, Tip110 association with unphosphorylated RNAPII CTD provides another line of evidence to support direct involvement and function of Tip110 in pre-mRNA splicing.

To further determine the significance of Tip110 involvement in pre-mRNA splicing, we performed RNA-Seq analysis of the alternate pre-mRNA splicing transcripts. As expected, Tip110 knockdown led to alterations in a large number of the gene transcripts including four known genes in pre-mRNA splicing (Figure 8). Tip110 knockdown significantly decreased expression of PRPF4, PRPF38b, SNRPB2, and ZRSR2. PRPF4 is a component of the U4/U6 di-snRNP and the U4/U6.U5 tri-snRNP and is important for maintaining the pre-mRNA splicing efficiency [53]. SNRPB2 is also important for maintaining the pre-mRNA splicing efficiency [54]. ZRSR2 is a splicing factor engaged in the initial steps of pre-mRNA splicing, including 3′ splice-site recognition [55]. PRPF38b interacts (directly or indirectly) with at least one of the U6 snRNA-containing snRNP complexes and is required for pre-mRNA splicing [56]. These findings suggest that Tip110 regulation of these key pre-mRNA splicing factors, is, if not more, as important as its interaction with snRNA U6 in pre-mRNA splicing. Tip110 is barely detectable in normal tissue and cells and highly elevated in tumors and differentiating stem cells [20, 25]. Thus, it is possible that Tip110 function in pre-mRNA splicing is evident only in cancerous cells and tumors through which elevated Tip110 expression causes changes in pre-mRNA splicing and gene expression and subsequent stem cell differentiation and malignant transformation.

Authors' contributions

YL, JF and ZW performed experiments; YL and JH designed experiments and analyzed data; YL and JH wrote the manuscript. All authors read and approved the final manuscript.

Author details

[1] Department of Cell Biology and Immunology, Graduate School of Biomedical Sciences, University of North Texas Health Science Center, 3500 Camp Bowie Blvd., Fort Worth, TX 76107, USA. [2] Department of Infectious Diseases, The First Affiliated Hospital of Medical College, Xi'an Jiaotong University, Xi'an 710061, Shaanxi, China. [3] Department of Forensic Science, College of Medicine, Xi'an Jiaotong University, Xi'an 710061, Shaanxi, China.

Acknowledgements

We would like to thank Dr. Marvin Wickens for pIIIA.MS2 plasmid, Dr. Iain Mattaji for pT7.U6 plasmid, Dr. Thomas Hope for pDM138 plasmid, Dr. Bryan Cullen for pcRev, Dr. Adrian Krainer for pSP64-Hβδ6 plasmid, and Dr. Gregory Hannon for pSHAG-1 plasmid.

Compliance with ethical guidelines

Competing interests

The authors declare that they have no competing interests.

References

1. Lee KM, Tarn WY. Coupling pre-mRNA processing to transcription on the RNA factory assembly line. RNA Biol. 2013;10:380–90.
2. Moore MJ, Proudfoot NJ. Pre-mRNA processing reaches back to transcription and ahead to translation. Cell. 2009;136:688–700.
3. Cooper TA, Wan L, Dreyfuss G. RNA and disease. Cell. 2009;136:777–93.
4. Garcia-Blanco MA, Baraniak AP, Lasda EL. Alternative splicing in disease and therapy. Nat Biotechnol. 2004;22:535–46.
5. Karni R, de Stanchina E, Lowe SW, Sinha R, Mu D, Krainer AR. The gene encoding the splicing factor SF2/ASF is a proto-oncogene. Nat Struct Mol Biol. 2007;14:185–93.
6. Gornemann J, Kotovic KM, Hujer K, Neugebauer KM. Cotranscriptional spliceosome assembly occurs in a stepwise fashion and requires the cap binding complex. Mol Cell. 2005;19:53–63.
7. Matera AG, Shpargel KB. Pumping RNA: nuclear bodybuilding along the RNP pipeline. Curr Opin Cell Biol. 2006;18:317–24.
8. Sharma A, Markey M, Torres-Munoz K, Varia S, Kadakia M, Bubulya A, et al. Son maintains accurate splicing for a subset of human pre-mRNAs. J Cell Sci. 2011;124:4286–98.
9. Mintz PJ, Patterson SD, Neuwald AF, Spahr CS, Spector DL. Purification and biochemical characterization of interchromatin granule clusters. EMBO J. 1999;18:4308–20.
10. Saitoh N, Spahr CS, Patterson SD, Bubulya P, Neuwald AF, Spector DL. Proteomic analysis of interchromatin granule clusters. Mol Biol Cell. 2004;15:3876–90.
11. Spector DL, Lamond AI. Nuclear speckles. Cold Spring Harb Perspect Biol. 2011;3. doi:10.1101/cshperspect.a000646.

12. Kurogi Y, Matsuo Y, Mihara Y, Yagi H, Shigaki-Miyamoto K, Toyota S, et al. Identification of a chemical inhibitor for nuclear speckle formation: implications for the function of nuclear speckles in regulation of alternative pre-mRNA splicing. Biochem Biophys Res Commun. 2014;446:119–24.
13. Spector DL, Schrier WH, Busch H. Immunoelectron microscopic localization of snRNPs. Biol Cell. 1983;49:1–10.
14. Stanek D, Neugebauer KM. Detection of snRNP assembly intermediates in Cajal bodies by fluorescence resonance energy transfer. J Cell Biol. 2004;166:1015–25.
15. Hall LL, Smith KP, Byron M, Lawrence JB. Molecular anatomy of a speckle. Anat Rec A Discov Mol Cell Evol Biol. 2006;288:664–75.
16. Harada K, Yamada A, Yang D, Itoh K, Shichijo S. Binding of a SART3 tumor-rejection antigen to a pre-mRNA splicing factor RNPS1: a possible regulation of splicing by a complex formation. Int J Cancer. 2001;93:623–8.
17. Koga M, Komatsu N, Kawamoto N, Shichijo S, Itoh K, Yamada A. Analysis of cellular localization of SART3 tumor antigen by a newly established monoclonal antibody: heterotopic expression of SART3 on the surface of B-lineage leukemic cells. Oncol Rep. 2004;11:785–9.
18. Ono T, Harada M, Yamada A, Tanaka M, Takao Y, Tanaka Y, et al. Antitumor effects of systemic and local immunization with a CTL-directed peptide in combination with a local injection of OK-432. Clin Cancer Res. 2006;12:1325–32.
19. Liu Y, Kim BO, Kao C, Jung C, Dalton JT, He JJ. Tip110, the human immunodeficiency virus type 1 (HIV-1) Tat-interacting protein of 110 kDa as a negative regulator of androgen receptor (AR) transcriptional activation. J Biol Chem. 2004;279:21766–73.
20. Liu Y, Li J, Kim BO, Pace BS, He JJ. HIV-1 Tat protein-mediated transactivation of the HIV-1 long terminal repeat promoter is potentiated by a novel nuclear Tat-interacting protein of 110 kDa, Tip110. J Biol Chem. 2002;277:23854–63.
21. Zhao W, Liu Y, Timani KA, He JJ. Tip110 protein binds to unphosphorylated RNA polymerase II and promotes its phosphorylation and HIV-1 long terminal repeat transcription. J Biol Chem. 2014;289:190–202.
22. Timani KA, Liu Y, Suvannasankha A, He JJ. Regulation of ubiquitin-proteasome system-mediated Tip110 protein degradation by USP15. Int J Biochem Cell Biol. 2014;54:10–9.
23. Long L, Thelen JP, Furgason M, Haj-Yahya M, Brik A, Cheng D, et al. The U4/U6 recycling factor SART3 has histone chaperone activity and associates with USP15 to regulate H2B deubiquitination. J Biol Chem. 2014;289:8916–30.
24. Liu Y, Lee MR, Timani K, He JJ, Broxmeyer HE. Tip110 maintains expression of pluripotent factors in and pluripotency of human embryonic stem cells. Stem Cells Dev. 2012;21:829–33.
25. Liu Y, Timani K, Mantel C, Fan Y, Hangoc G, Cooper S, et al. TIP110/p110nrb/SART3/p110 regulation of hematopoiesis through CMYC. Blood. 2011;117:5643–51.
26. Liu Y, Timani K, Ou X, Broxmeyer HE, He JJ. C-MYC controlled TIP110 protein expression regulates OCT4 mRNA splicing in human embryonic stem cells. Stem Cells Dev. 2013;22:689–94.
27. Bell M, Schreiner S, Damianov A, Reddy R, Bindereif A. p110, a novel human U6 snRNP protein and U4/U6 snRNP recycling factor. EMBO J. 2002;21:2724–35.
28. Medenbach J, Schreiner S, Liu S, Luhrmann R, Bindereif A. Human U4/U6 snRNP recycling factor p110: mutational analysis reveals the function of the tetratricopeptide repeat domain in recycling. Mol Cell Biol. 2004;24:7392–401.
29. Timani KA, Liu Y, He JJ. Tip110 interacts with YB-1 and regulates each other's function. BMC Mol Biol. 2013;14:14.
30. Stanek D, Rader SD, Klingauf M, Neugebauer KM. Targeting of U4/U6 small nuclear RNP assembly factor SART3/p110 to Cajal bodies. J Cell Biol. 2003;160:505–16.
31. Novotny I, Malinova A, Stejskalova E, Mateju D, Klimesova K, Roithova A, et al. SART3-dependent accumulation of incomplete spliceosomal snRNPs in cajal bodies. Cell Rep. 2015;10:429–40.
32. Sengupta DJ, Wickens M, Fields S. Identification of RNAs that bind to a specific protein using the yeast three-hybrid system. RNA. 1999;5:596–601.
33. He J, Furmanski P. Sequence specificity and transcriptional activation in the binding of lactoferrin to DNA. Nature. 1995;373:721–4.
34. SenGupta DJ, Zhang B, Kraemer B, Pochart P, Fields S, Wickens M. A three-hybrid system to detect RNA–protein interactions in vivo. Proc Natl Acad Sci USA. 1996;93:8496–501.
35. McKeown M. The role of small nuclear RNAs in RNA splicing. Curr Opin Cell Biol. 1993;5:448–54.
36. Mayeda A, Ohshima Y. Short donor site sequences inserted within the intron of beta-globin pre-mRNA serve for splicing in vitro. Mol Cell Biol. 1988;8:4484–91.
37. Krainer AR, Maniatis T. Multiple factors including the small nuclear ribonucleoproteins U1 and U2 are necessary for pre-mRNA splicing in vitro. Cell. 1985;42:725–36.
38. Uemura A, Oku M, Mori K, Yoshida H. Unconventional splicing of XBP1 mRNA occurs in the cytoplasm during the mammalian unfolded protein response. J Cell Sci. 2009;122:2877–86.
39. Zolotukhin AS, Tan W, Bear J, Smulevitch S, Felber BK. U2AF participates in the binding of TAP (NXF1) to mRNA. J Biol Chem. 2002;277:3935–42.
40. Hope TJ, Huang XJ, McDonald D, Parslow TG. Steroid-receptor fusion of the human immunodeficiency virus type 1 Rev transactivator: mapping cryptic functions of the arginine-rich motif. Proc Natl Acad Sci USA. 1990;87:7787–91.
41. Rader SD, Guthrie C. A conserved Lsm-interaction motif in Prp24 required for efficient U4/U6 di-snRNP formation. RNA. 2002;8:1378–92.
42. Spector DL. SnapShot: cellular bodies. Cell. 2006;127:1071.
43. McCracken S, Fong N, Yankulov K, Ballantyne S, Pan G, Greenblatt J, et al. The C-terminal domain of RNA polymerase II couples mRNA processing to transcription. Nature. 1997;385:357–61.
44. Shpargel KB, Matera AG. Gemin proteins are required for efficient assembly of Sm-class ribonucleoproteins. Proc Natl Acad Sci USA. 2005;102:17372–7.
45. Trede NS, Medenbach J, Damianov A, Hung LH, Weber GJ, Paw BH, et al. Network of coregulated spliceosome components revealed by zebrafish mutant in recycling factor p110. Proc Natl Acad Sci USA. 2007;104:6608–13.
46. Novotny I, Blazikova M, Stanek D, Herman P, Malinsky J. In vivo kinetics of U4/U6.U5 tri-snRNP formation in Cajal bodies. Mol Biol Cell. 2011;22:513–23.
47. Fong KW, Li Y, Wang W, Ma W, Li K, Qi RZ, et al. Whole-genome screening identifies proteins localized to distinct nuclear bodies. J Cell Biol. 2013;203:149–64.
48. Hu Y, Ericsson I, Doseth B, Liabakk NB, Krokan HE, Kavli B. Activation-induced cytidine deaminase (AID) is localized to subnuclear domains enriched in splicing factors. Exp Cell Res. 2014;322:178–92.
49. Mayeda A, Badolato J, Kobayashi R, Zhang MQ, Gardiner EM, Krainer AR. Purification and characterization of human RNPS1: a general activator of pre-mRNA splicing. EMBO J. 1999;18:4560–70.
50. Kataoka N, Dreyfuss G. A simple whole cell lysate system for in vitro splicing reveals a stepwise assembly of the exon–exon junction complex. J Biol Chem. 2004;279:7009–13.
51. Hirose Y, Tacke R, Manley JL. Phosphorylated RNA polymerase II stimulates pre-mRNA splicing. Genes Dev. 1999;13:1234–9.
52. Millhouse S, Manley JL. The C-terminal domain of RNA polymerase II functions as a phosphorylation-dependent splicing activator in a heterologous protein. Mol Cell Biol. 2005;25:533–44.
53. Linder B, Hirmer A, Gal A, Ruther K, Bolz HJ, Winkler C, et al. Identification of a PRPF4 loss-of-function variant that abrogates U4/U6.U5 tri-snRNP integration and is associated with retinitis pigmentosa. PLoS One. 2014;9:e111754.
54. Zanetti S, Meola M, Bochud A, Puoti A. Role of the C. elegans U2 snRNP protein MOG-2 in sex determination, meiosis, and splice site selection. Dev Biol. 2011;354:232–41.
55. Yoshida K, Ogawa S. Splicing factor mutations and cancer. Wiley Interdiscip Rev RNA. 2014;5:445–59.
56. Blanton S, Srinivasan A, Rymond BC. PRP38 encodes a yeast protein required for pre-mRNA splicing and maintenance of stable U6 small nuclear RNA levels. Mol Cell Biol. 1992;12:3939–47.

4

Hypoxia induces calpain activity and degrades SMAD2 to attenuate TGFβ signaling in macrophages

Wei Cui[1,2], Jie Zhou[1], Nathalie Dehne[2] and Bernhard Brüne[2*]

Abstract

Background: Under inflammatory conditions or during tumor progression macrophages acquire distinct phenotypes, with factors of the microenvironment such as hypoxia and transforming growth factor β (TGFβ) shaping their functional plasticity. TGFβ is among the factors causing alternative macrophage activation, which contributes to tissue regeneration and thus, resolution of inflammation but may also provoke tumor progression. However, the signal crosstalk between TGFβ and hypoxia is ill defined.

Results: Exposing human primary macrophages to TGFβ elicited a rapid SMAD2/SMAD3 phosphorylation. This early TGFβ-signaling remained unaffected by hypoxia. However, with prolonged exposure periods to TGFβ/hypoxia the expression of SMAD2 declined because of decreased protein stability. In parallel, hypoxia increased mRNA and protein amount of the calpain regulatory subunit, with the further notion that TGFβ/hypoxia elicited calpain activation. The dual specific proteasome/calpain inhibitor MG132 and the specific calpain inhibitor 1 rescued SMAD2 degradation, substantiating the ability of calpain to degrade SMAD2. Decreased SMAD2 expression reduced TGFβ transcriptional activity of its target genes thrombospondin 1, dystonin, and matrix metalloproteinase 2.

Conclusions: Hypoxia interferes with TGFβ signaling in macrophages by calpain-mediated proteolysis of the central signaling component SMAD2.

Keywords: Hypoxia, TGFß, phospho-SMAD2, SMAD2 degradation, Calpain, Macrophages

Introduction

Macrophages are found throughout the body, where they contribute to tissue homeostasis and orchestrate innate as well as adaptive immune responses. They display a remarkable plasticity, which allows them to change their functional repertoire with regard to the environment they are facing. Numerous sub-phenotypes are described. Based on distinct functional roles and marker expression profiles an operative useful but over-simplifying nomenclature categorizes classical, i.e., pro-inflammatory and alternatively activated macrophages [1]. An alternatively activated macrophage phenotype is elicited by interleukin-4 (IL-4), IL-10, or transforming growth factor ß (TGFß), which are produced by helper 2 or regulatory T cells, tumor cells, or macrophages themselves during late stage immune responses and tumor cells. Monocyte-derived macrophages and tissue resident macrophages are found in tumors. These tumor-associated macrophages are known to support cancer progression rather than mounting anti-cancer responses. This tumor-supporting phenotype is elicited by cytokines like TGFß [2].

TGFß controls proliferation, differentiation, and fosters fibrosis. TGFß binds to transforming growth factor receptor 2 (TGFBR2), which recruits and phosphorylates transforming growth factor receptor 1 (TGFBR1), thereby activating downstream signaling [3]. SMAD proteins mediate canonical TGFß signaling, while the PI3K-AKT, MAPK pathway conveys non-canonical signals [4]. The canonical pathway phosphorylates regulatory SMADs via receptor activation. In macrophages stimulation with TGFβ predominantly activates the regulatory SMAD2 and −3 but activation of SMAD1 and −5 was also observed [5]. Phosphorylated SMAD2 and SMAD3 share high affinity

* Correspondence: b.bruene@biochem.uni-frankfurt.de
[2]Institute of Biochemistry I, Faculty of Medicine, Goethe-University Frankfurt, 60590 Frankfurt, Germany
Full list of author information is available at the end of the article

for SMAD4 and show oligomerization, which is necessary for nuclear translocation and activation of transcription [3]. SMAD7 is an inhibitory SMAD, which negatively controls this pathway.

TGFß plays a substantial role in tumor progression, acting both as a tumor suppressor and tumor promoter [6]. Early in tumorigenesis, TGFß arrests the cell-cycle, which is SMAD-dependent. With tumor progression, tumor cells often harbor inactivating mutations in the TGFß pathway, allowing them to overcome these growth-inhibitory effects. In the tumor microenvironment, TGFß responsive cells secret cytokines and enzymes to promote EMT (epithelial mesenchymal transition), angiogenesis, tumor invasion, and metastasis. Besides, TGFß also recruits and activates immune cells [7]. Of particular interest is the induction of an alternatively activated macrophage phenotype, which promotes tumor development [8, 9]. TGFß-recruited macrophages are highly phagocytic for aberrant cells and thereby decrease the ability of tumor antigens to be delivered to the adaptive immune system [10]. Inhibition of NF-κB in TGFß-polarized macrophages accounts for their reduced ability to produce pro-inflammatory cytokines [7, 11].

At sites of inflammation, like in tumors, macrophages face hypoxia. Hypoxia promotes angiogenesis, fibrosis, and immune suppression [12]. Activation of the hypoxia-inducible factor (HIF) conveys many responses to hypoxia, by altering transcriptional outputs. HIF is a heterodimeric transcription factor composed of an ubiquitously expressed β-subunit and an oxygen-sensitive α-subunit [13, 14]. Three HIF-α subunits are identified in the human genome (HIF-1α, HIF-2α or EPAS1, and HIF-3α), which all share the oxygen-dependent degradation domain (ODD). In well-oxygenated tissue specific prolyl hydroxylases hydroxylate the ODD of the α-subunit, allowing their recognition by the von Hippel-Lindau tumor suppressor and subsequent proteosomal degradation [13, 14]. Under hypoxic conditions HIF-α is stabilized, translocates to the nucleus and thus, promotes transcription of target genes to induce angiogenesis, ensures cell survival, restores oxygen homeostasis but also promotes fibrosis [15]. These functions overlap with TGFß-signaling, indicating some signal crosstalk [6, 12, 16]. In renal epithelial cells and prostate cancer cells TGFß provokes HIF-1α accumulation, which in turn enhances expression of common target genes [17, 18]. In contrast, TGFß alone failed to accumulate HIF-1α in macrophages [19] even though the prolyl-hydroxylase-2 and −3 (PHD2/3) mRNA were decreased [20]. Although macrophages play an important role in fibrosis and immune suppression the impact of hypoxia on TGFß-signaling in macrophages is poorly understood. We provide evidence that TGFß-signaling under hypoxia is impaired, due to calpain-mediated SMAD2 degradation in macrophages.

Results

Hypoxia attenuates TGFß-induced SMAD2 activation in macrophages

Macrophages in the tumor microenvironment are exposed to hypoxia and TGFß but their signaling crosstalk has not been explored in detail. Therefore, we time-dependently stimulated primary human macrophages with 10 ng/mL TGFß under normoxia vs. hypoxia and followed phosphorylation of SMAD2 (p-SMAD2) and SMAD3 (p-SMAD3) by Western blot analysis. Resting macrophage did not show SMAD2 phosphorylation (Fig. 1a, b), whereas TGFß provoked a rapid SMAD2 phosphorylation within 15 min. Phospho-SMAD2 reached its maximum after 1 h both under normoxia and hypoxia. After 4 h, the level of p-SMAD2 gradually declined under hypoxia compared to normoxia. These differences became significant after 8 h (Fig. 1a, b). In contrast, the amount of p-SMAD3 rapidly increased upon TGFß addition, with phosphorylation not being affected by hypoxia. Although we noticed declining levels of p-SMAD3 at 4 to 8 h, this occurred irrespective to the presence or absence of oxygen (Fig. 1c, d). Apparently, in TGFβ-stimulated macrophages, only SMAD2, but not SMAD3, was sensitive to hypoxia. To explore this response for longer incubation times, we stimulated cells with TGFβ for 8 to 24 h at 20 % or 1 % O_2. We observed decreased SMAD2 phosphorylation comparing 8 to 16 or 24 h, an effect drastically enhanced by hypoxia (Fig. 1e, f). Using an antibody to detect total SMAD2 protein showed a progressively reduced expression under hypoxia from 8 to 24 h (Fig. 1e, g). Apparently, hypoxia reduced phosphorylation of SMAD2 at 8 to 24 h following TGFβ-stimulation because of reduced SMAD2 protein expression.

A decrease in SMAD2 under hypoxia is unrelated to TGFBR2 or SMAD7

Several publications link SMAD activation to its subsequent degradation [21, 22]. Therefore, we started to validate TGFBR2 and SMAD7 as potential HIF target genes that were previously identified by ChIP-Seq and mRNA array experiments [23]. TGFBR2 is the receptor subunit that binds TGFß and phosphorylates the co-receptor TGFBR1 to initiate intracellular signaling. An altered expression level of TGFBR2 will alter the ratio of TGFβ to its receptor, thereby modulating downstream signaling. SMAD7 is an inhibitory SMAD, which competes with SMAD2/3 at the TGFß receptor to control TGFß signal transmission. Increased expression under hypoxia may reduce SMAD2 activation. First, we validated microarray data by quantitative PCR 8 h after TGFß and/or hypoxia stimulation and verified hypoxic

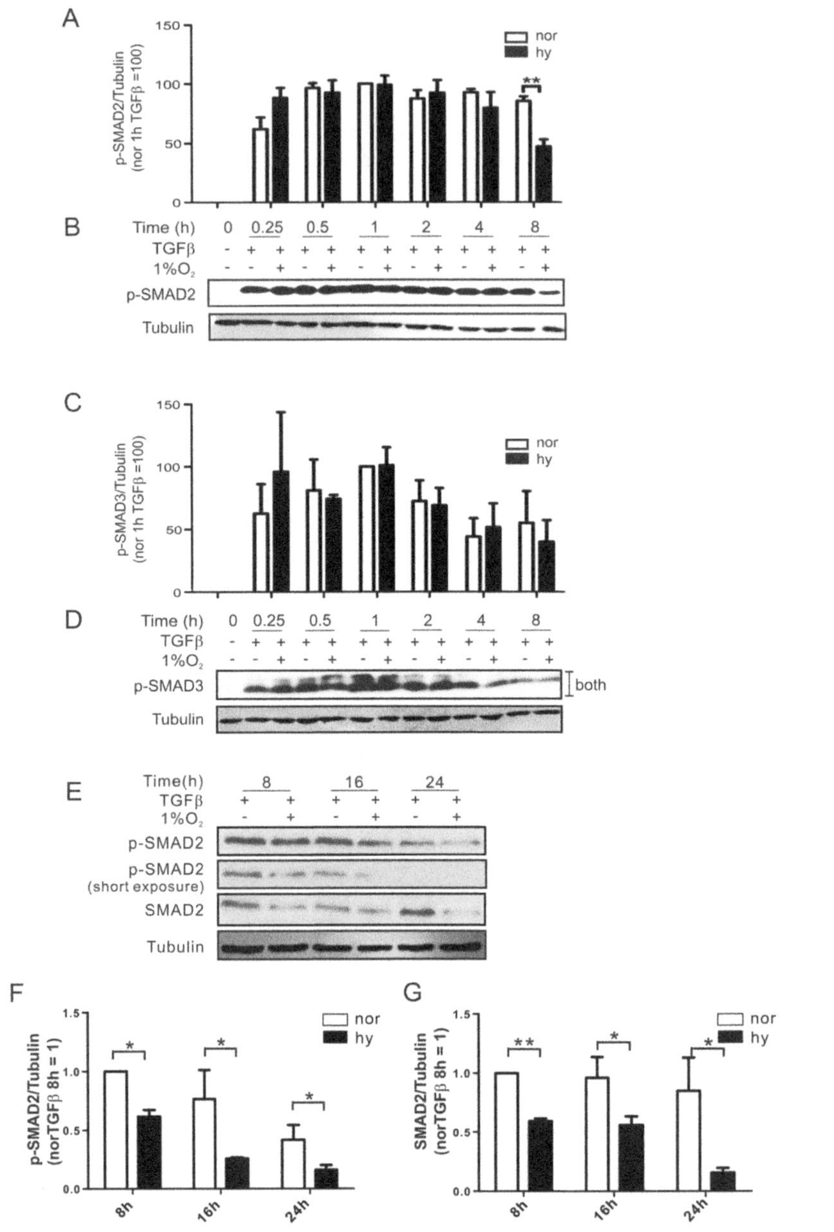

Fig. 1 Hypoxia attenuates TGFß-induced SMAD2 phosphorylation in macrophages. Time-dependent Western blot analysis **b**, **d** and the corresponding statistical evaluation **a**, **c** of SMAD2 **a**, **b** and SMAD3 **c**, **d** phosphorylation in human primary macrophages exposed to TGFß under normoxia (–; nor) or hypoxia (1 % O_2; hy). Macrophages were exposed to TGFß under normoxia vs. hypoxia for 8, 16, and 24 h, followed by (**e**) Western blot analysis of total SMAD2 and SMAD2 phosphorylation and corresponding statistical analysis **f**, **g**. Tubulin served as a loading control

induction of TGFBR2 mRNA (Fig. 2a). The knockdown of HIF-1α or HIF-2α, which was verified by Western blot analysis (Additional file 1: Figure S1A, B), reduced hypoxic TGFBR2 mRNA induction. mRNA expression of TGFBR2 under hypoxia/TGFß was lower compared to the hypoxic response. In contrast, SMAD7 was predominantly induced by TGFß, with the signal not being altered by a HIF-knockdown (Fig. 2b). Hypoxia only showed a small mRNA induction of SMAD7, while induction by hypoxia/TGFß was comparable to TGFß alone. A knockdown of either HIF-1α or HIF-2α slightly reduced hypoxic induction of SMAD7 and significantly reduced induction by hypoxia/TGFß, suggesting the involvement of HIF in hypoxic SMAD7 mRNA regulation.

To determine the impact of hypoxia on TGFBR2 protein expression, we examined its surface appearance after 8 h by flow cytometry (Fig. 2c, d). TGFBR2 expression was neither altered by TGFß nor by the

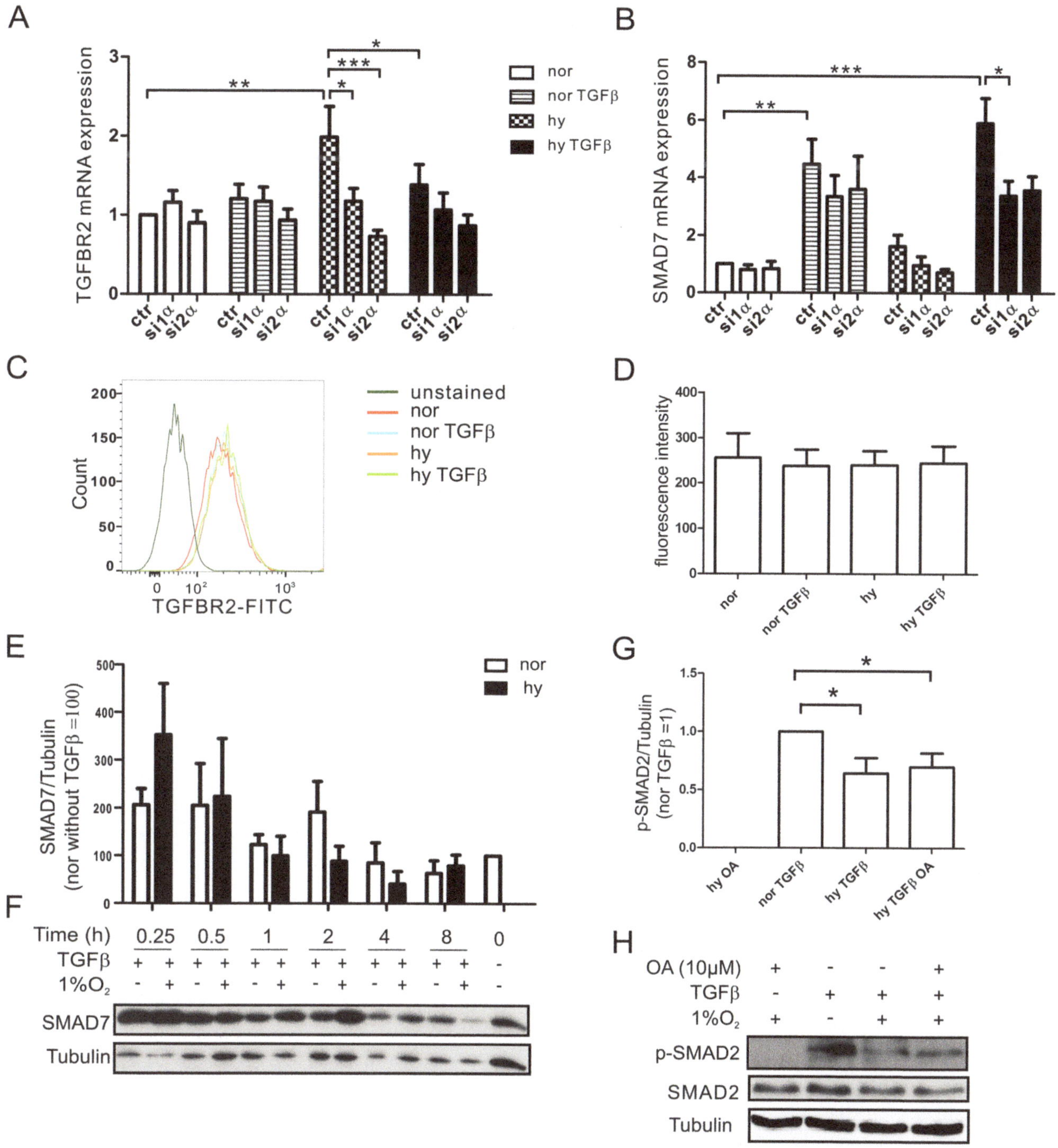

Fig. 2 Expression of TGFBR2 and SMAD7 in response to TGFß/hypoxia. Macrophages were transfected with non-targeting siRNA constructs (ctr), siRNA-HIF1α (si1α), or siRNA-HIF2α (si2α) and mRNA expression of TGFBR2 **a** or SMAD7 **b** were analyzed by quantitative PCR after treatments with TGFß under normoxia (nor) or hypoxia (hy) for 8 h. **c** Cell surface expression of TGFBR2 was followed by flow cytometry after stimulation of macrophages with TGFß under normoxia (nor) vs. hypoxia (hy) for 8 h and **d** mean fluorescence intensity was calculated from 4 individual experiments. **e, f** Time-dependent Western blot analysis and statistical evaluation of SMAD7 expression in macrophages exposed to TGFß under normoxia or hypoxia. **g, h** Macrophages were exposed to the phosphatase inhibitor okadaic acid (OA) 1 h prior to adding TGFß for 8 h. Phosphorylation and total protein expression of SMAD2 was followed by Western blot analysis, using tubulin as a loading control

combination of hypoxia/TGFß, indicating that the SMAD2 decrease is unrelated to TGFBR2 expression. In addition, Western blot analysis verified that the expression of SMAD7 increased by TGFß at 15 to 30 min, decreased after 1–2 h and remained low up to an 8 h incubation period. However, SMAD7 protein expression was similarly affected by TGFß supplied under normoxia and hypoxia (Fig. 2e, f). Thus, it appears that neither the expression of TGFBR2 nor of SMAD7 account for the specific effects of hypoxia seen at the level of SMAD2.

Next, we considered phosphatases to decrease SMAD2 phosphorylation. It was reported that PP2A dephosphorylates p-SMAD3 under hypoxia [24]. Supplying the PP2A inhibitor okadaic acid (OA) 1 h prior to addition of TGFß for 8 h failed to rescue the decrease of phoshorylated or total SAMD2 under TGFß/hypoxia (Fig. 2h). Excluding SMAD2 activation or dephoshorylation as an explanation for its decreased protein amount, we went on to analyze SMAD2 mRNA. In general, protein expression is either regulated by an altered mRNA expression, reduced translation, and/or enhanced degradation. SMAD2 mRNA expression was slightly induced but not reduced by hypoxia (Fig. 3a). Therefore, we examined protein stability by suppressing translation using 10 μg/ml cycloheximide (CHX). SMAD2 was degraded faster, comparing hypoxia to normoxia (Fig. 3b). The half-life of SAMD2 under normoxia/TGFß was calculated to be 8.9 ± 1.2 h, while it was reduced to 5.1 ± 0.6 h under hypoxia/TGFß (Fig. 3c). In conclusion, SMAD2 is destabilized under hypoxia in TGFß-stimulated macrophages.

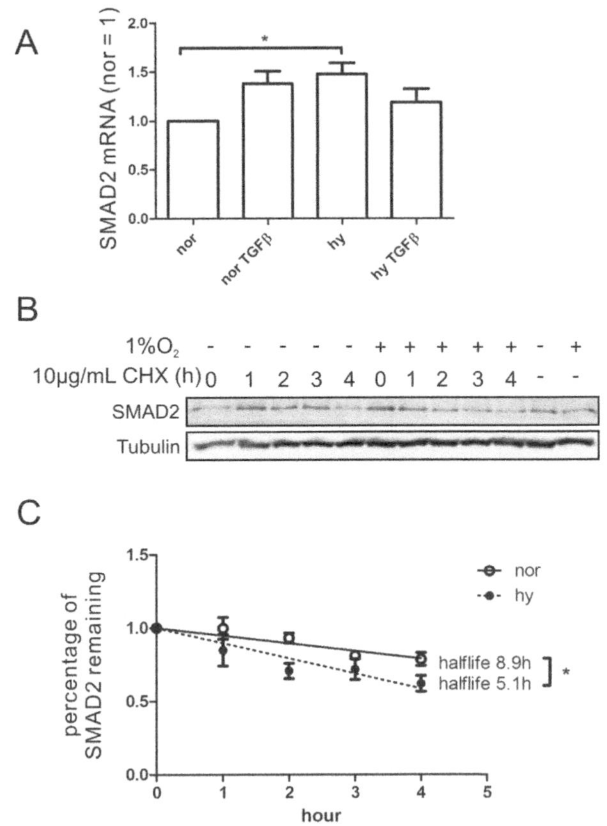

Fig. 3 SMAD2 protein stability is reduced in response to TGFß/hypoxia. **a** mRNA expression of SMAD2 followed by quantitative PCR in macrophages stimulated for 8 h with TGFß under normoxia (nor) vs. hypoxia (hy). **b** Macrophages were stimulated with TGFß for 4 h, followed by the addition of cycloheximide for 0 h to 4 h and subsequent Western blot analysis of SMAD2 expression. **c** Half-life determination of SMAD2 in TGFß-stimulated macrophages under normoxia (nor) vs. hypoxia (hy) as a result of experiments performed in Fig. 3b

SMAD2 degradation under hypoxia is facilitated by calpain

Considering increased degradation of SMAD2 under TGFß/hypoxia, we analyzed pathways being involved. Using bafilomycin A1 to inhibit lysosomal functions, SMAD2 degradation remained unaffected thus, ruling the involvement of the lysosomal compartment out (Fig. 4a, b). We then used MG132 to block proteasomal- and calpain-dependent degradation systems. MG132 rescued SMAD2 degradation in response to TGFß/hypoxia, while lactacystin, a more specific proteasomal inhibitor, not affecting calpain, failed to restore SMAD2 expression under these conditions (Fig. 4c-f). Calpain is a calcium-dependent non-lysosomal cysteine proteolytic system that comprises a small regulatory subunit (CAPNS1, also known as calpain reg) and a large catalytic subunit (μ-calpain/m-calpain, also known as CAPN). We tested mRNA expression of CAPNS1 in macrophages stimulated with TGFß under normoxia and hypoxia. CAPNS1 mRNA was significantly upregulated by hypoxia or hypoxia/TGFß compared to normoxia or TGFß-stimulation (Fig. 4g). The mRNA increase became also apparent at the protein level (Fig. 4h). Expression of the catalytic subunit (CAPN1) was not affected by TGFβ or hypoxia nor their combination (Fig. 4i). Following macrophage activation with hypoxia/TGFß, holo-calpain (80KD) is proteolytically processed and the removal of 14 or 28 amino acids forms active calpain. Western blot analysis detected active calpain in macrophages stimulated with TGFß/hypoxia but not with TGFβ or hypoxia alone (Fig. 4j). Experiments with the specific calpain inhibitor 1 CPI (10 μM), showed that decreased SMAD2 expression seen under hypoxia/TGFß was fully recovered when calpain activity was blocked (Fig. 4k). Conclusively, in TGFß-stimulated macrophages hypoxia promotes degradation of SMAD2 by increasing calpain activity.

To explore how hypoxia affects TGFß-induced transcriptional activity, we used a SMAD-specific reporter assay. Due to difficulties in transfecting primary human macrophages we used the J774A.1 mouse macrophage cell line, which responded with SMAD2 phosphorylation in

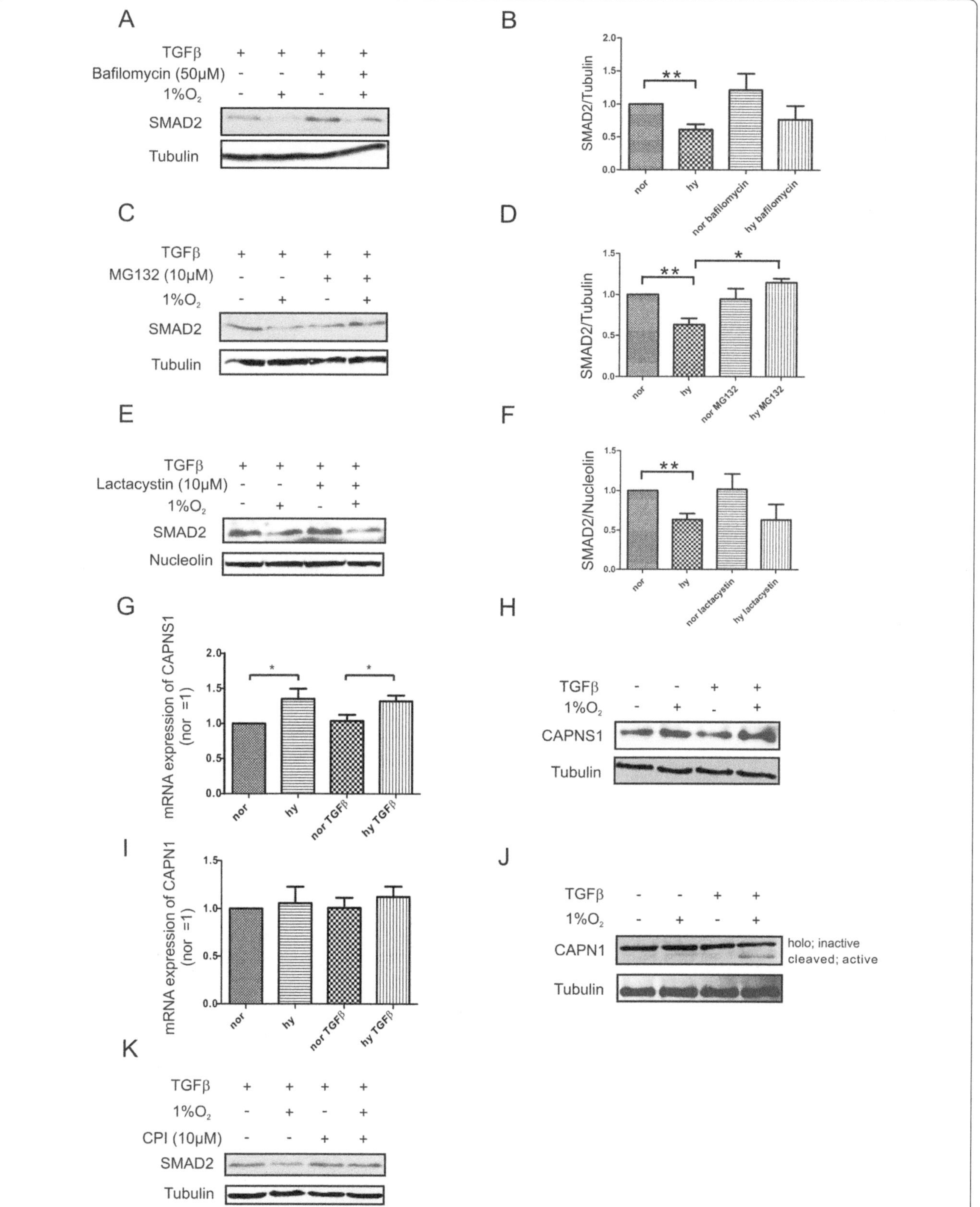

Fig. 4 (See legend on next page.)

(See figure on previous page.)

Fig. 4 SMAD2 degradation under hypoxia is facilitated by calpain. **a-f** Macrophages were stimulated with TGFß under normoxia vs. hypoxia for 8 h in the presence of bafilomycin **a**, **b**, MG132 **c**, **d**, or lactacystin **e**, **f**. 2 h after TGFß, inhibitors were added and incubations went on for 6 h. Western blot analysis and statistical evaluation is presented. **g** mRNA expression of the calpain regulatory subunit (CAPNS1) was analyzed by quantitative PCR in macrophages exposed for 8 h to TGFß under normoxia (nor) vs. hypoxia (hy). **h** Western blot analysis of the calpain regulatory subunit after exposure to TGFß and/or hypoxia for 8 h. **i** mRNA expression of the calpain 1 catalytic subunit (CAPN1) was analyzed by quantitative PCR in macrophages exposed for 8 h to TGFß under normoxia (nor) vs. hypoxia (hy). **j** Proteolytic cleavage of CAPN1 under TGFß/hypoxia was followed in macrophages by Western blot analysis after 8 h. **k** Macrophages were exposed to the calpain inhibitor 1 (CPI) to follow SMAD2 degradation after stimulating cells for 8 h with TGFß under normoxia vs. hypoxia

response to TGFß, also showing a decrease in SMAD2 expression with TGFß/hypoxia under longer exposure times (Additional file 1: Figure S1C, D). Stimulation of J774A.1 cells, transfected with the SMAD reporter plasmid SEB4-Luc, with TGFß under hypoxia significantly reduced transcriptional activity compared to TGFß supplied under normoxia (Fig. 5a). We then analyzed expression of SAMD2 and SMAD3 target genes in primary human macrophages. Thrombospondin 1 (TSP1), dystonin (DST), and matrix metalloproteinase 2 (MMP2) were reported to be selectively regulated by SMAD2 [25–27] and we confirmed their responsiveness to TGFβ (Fig. 5b, c, d). Induction was significantly reduced in macrophages stimulated with TGFβ at 1 % O_2, reflecting the reduced expression of

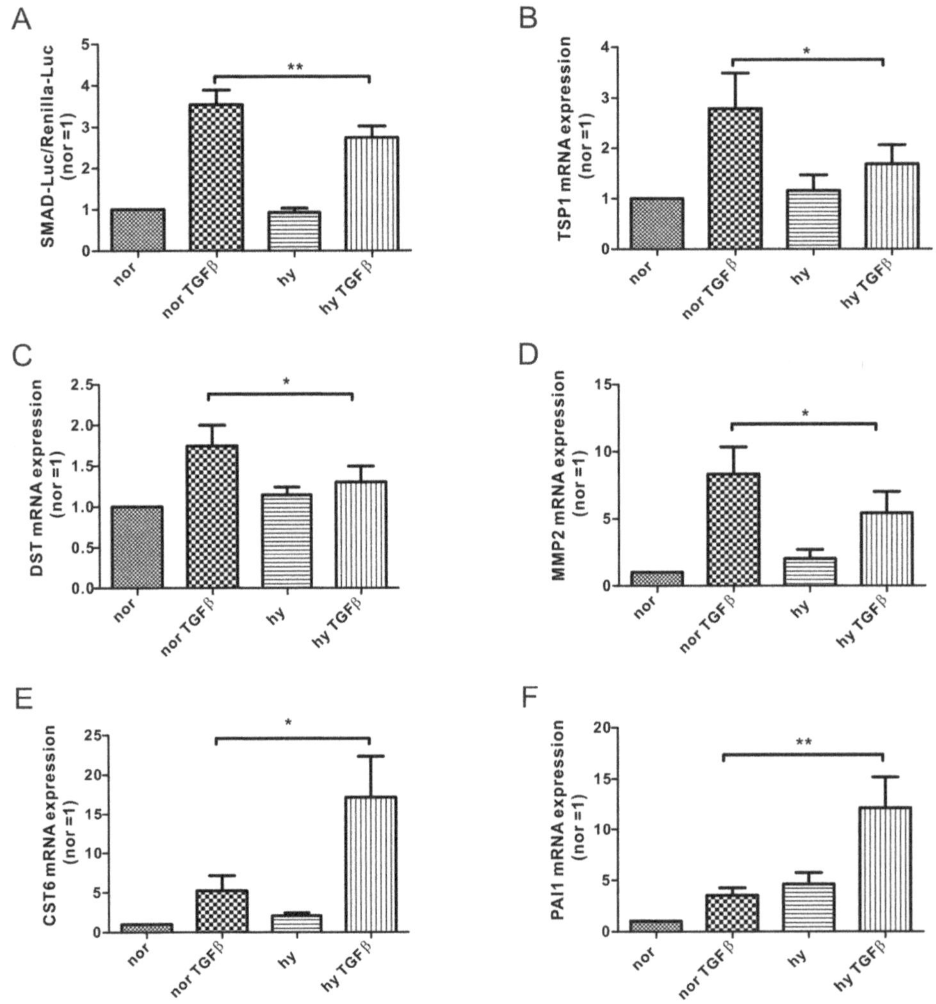

Fig. 5 Hypoxia reduces SMAD2-dependent transcription. **a** TGFß-induced transcriptional activity in J774A.1 cells transfected with a SBE4-Luc (4xSMAD binding element coupled to luciferase) as well as a Renilla-Luc plasmid. Stimulation was with TGFß under normoxia (nor) vs. hypoxia (hy) for 8 h. mRNA expression of **b** thrombospondin1 (TSP1), **c** dystonin DST, **d** matrix metalloproteinase (MMP2), **e** cystatin (CST6), and **(f)** plasminogen activator inhibitor 1 (PAI1) was analyzed by quantitative PCR in macrophages exposed for 8 h to TGFß under normoxia (nor) vs. hypoxia (hy)

SMAD2. In contrast induction of SMAD3 target genes such as cystatin (CST6) and plasminogen activator inhibitor 1 (PAI1) [25] was not reduced under hypoxia (Fig. 5e, f). Apparently, only transcriptional responses of SMAD2 are selectively reduced by hypoxia in TGFβ-stimulated human macrophages.

Discussion

In human macrophages, in contrast to epithelial and parenchymal cells [17, 18], periods of 8 h hypoxia or longer reduced TGFß-induced SMAD2 activation. Decreased phosphorylation of SMAD3, but not SMAD2, under hypoxia was noticed in HeLa cells and attributed to protein phosphatase 2A (PP2A) directly interacting with SMAD3 [24]. In macrophages the decrease of p-SMAD2 was not due to PP2A activation, altered TGFBR2 receptor activation, or inhibitory SMAD7 expression, but rather resulted from hypoxia-evoked destabilization of SMAD2. Regulation of SMAD2 degradation is complex. Smurf2 is an E3 ubiquitin ligase, directly interacting with activated SMAD2 and promoting its proteasomal degradation. Neural precursor cell expressed developmentally down-regulated protein 4–2 (NEDD4-2), another E3 ubiquitin ligase like Smurf1 or 2, binds SMAD2 and SMAD3 but exclusively degrades SMAD2 [21]. In addition, TGFβ-induced factor homeobox 1 (TGIF) interacting ubiquitin ligase 1 (Tiul1), induces SMAD2 to bind TGIF, which triggers SMAD2 degradation [22]. Our data add proteolysis by the calpain system also to account for alterations in the SMAD2 protein amount. Interestingly, Lo and coworkers studied the proteasomal degradation of SMAD2 [28]. Along our observations, their results suggested that lactacystin cannot rescue a SMAD2 decrease to the same extent as MG132, although they did not consider the calpain system.

The calpain system consists of a catalytic subunit (μ-calpain/m-calpain) and a common regulatory subunit CAPNS1 as well as the inhibitory subunit calpastatin. After calcium binding, calpastatin detaches from the protein complex and calpain is activated by autolysis [29]. The calpain system plays important roles in macrophages. IFNγ induces calpain mRNA and protein expression in U937 and THP1 cells [30]. Calpain cleaves iNOS and thus, affects inflammatory responses [31]. There are several reports that calpain activity is upregulated under hypoxia, with platelets being one typical example [32–35]. Hypoxia-induced thrombogenesis is associated with CAPNS1-dependent calpain activation in the platelet activation cascade [35]. In line, we noticed increased calpain activity under TGFβ/hypoxia by upregulating CAPNS1 in macrophages. The calpain regulatory subunit functions like a chaperone, assisting the catalytic subunit to fold properly [36]. We showed that combining TGFß and hypoxia is necessary to activate calpain in human macrophages as indicated in Fig. 4j, while hypoxia alone did not activate calpain. This is in line with findings showing that ischemia/hypoxia provokes an influx of Ca^{2+} into the cell [32, 35], but the Ca^{2+} increase is not sufficient to activate calpain [29, 37]. It is well established that TGFß could also increase the influx of Ca^{2+} into cells [38]. Presumably, a high expression of CAPNS1 and the influx of Ca^{2+} by the combined stimulation, hypoxia plus TGFß, promotes activation of calpain. Calpain digests proteins at a limited number of cleavage sites producing large polypeptide fragments rather than small peptides or amino acid [29]. Early studies suggested that preferred residues of the cleavage P_2 position are Leu, Thr, and Val, and in the P_1 position are Lys, Thr, and Arg [39]. Following the P_2-P_1 rule, SMAD2 has 17 potential cleavage sites. In addition, calpain prefers small hydrophilic Ser residue at the P_1' position. Considering this preference, there are still 4 possible cleavage sites at K46, Y101, R108, Y266 for calpain in SMAD2. On the other hand, there are indications that the specificity for calpain is not exclusively governed by amino acid but rather by the 3D conformation of the substrates [29, 39]. Using currently available online tools at http://calpain.org for calpain substrates, amino acids at sites 166, 395, and 6 are the top 3 predicted cleavage sites with a score of 0.39, 0.39, 0.37 respectively [40]. For the identification of the accurate cleavage sites more experiments are needed that would be beyond the scope of this work.

Our experimental conditions aimed to simulate conditions macrophages are facing when entering the tumor microenvironment, facing hypoxia and TGFß [41]. SMAD2 and SMAD3 have distinct transcriptional roles in the tumor [27, 42, 43]. SMAD2 provokes secretion of anti-angiogenetic factors, such as thrombospondin 1 (TSP1, Fig. 5) as well as the VEGF-A antagonist sFlt-1, whereas SMAD3 induces the secretion of pro-angiogenetic factor, i.e., VEGF-A or plasminogen activator inhibitor 1 (PAI1, Fig. 5), promoting angiogenesis when SMAD2 is inactive [26, 44]. In addition, TSP1 overexpression in tumor cells enhances the recruitment of pro-inflammatory macrophages and reduces tumor growth [45]. Conditional medium of SMAD2 knockdown fibroblast induces proliferation and *in vivo* deletion of SMAD2 in tumor cells generates a more aggressive phenotype compared to controls [26]. The decrease of SMAD2 under TGFβ/hypoxia in tumor-associated macrophages may add to their roles supporting angiogenesis and tumor progression.

Angiogenesis influences tumor growth but also enables metastasis [46]. Metastasis is a complex process requiring invasive growth of tumor cells, epithelial to mesenchymal transition (EMT), induction of angiogenesis, intra- and extravasation, and tumor growth at the secondary sites [47]. Matrix metalloproteases (MMPs) like MMP2 coordinate multiple steps of this process. In general they promote metastasis by allowing extracellular matrix remodeling and releasing growth factors like VEGF from the matrix. MMP2 was also implicated in endothelial cell apoptosis [46, 48]. As full activation of MMP2 by the membrane type (MT)1-MMP provokes endothelial cell death and expression of MMP2 in endothelial cells and macrophages is reduced in acute hypoxia (Fig. 5d), one might speculate that this reduction prevents endothelial cell death under hypoxia when angiogenesis is usually enhanced [48, 49]. Other TGFß-induced genes involved in metastasis are enhanced under hypoxia since SMAD3 target genes like PAI-1 or CST6 (Fig. 5) are regulated by the hypoxia-inducible factor (HIF) as well [16, 50]. In a previous study we used ChIP-seq technology to identify HIF-1 and HIF-2 binding sites in primary human macrophages and identified, amongst others, CST6 and PAI-1 [23]. Apparently, in these cases TGFß/hypoxia enhances rather than decreases gene expression in macrophages. Thus, specifically attenuating SMAD2 under TGFß/hypoxia might have functional roles on macrophages biology and tumor progression.

Conclusion

Our results indicate that hypoxia attenuates SMAD2 activation in TGFβ-stimulated macrophages (Fig. 6). Mechanistically, this results from degradation of SMAD2 by calpain.

Material and methods

Cell culture and incubation procedures

If not indicated otherwise, all chemicals were purchased from Sigma (Steinheim, Germany), while cell lines came from ATCC (LGC Promochem, Wesel, Germany). J774A.1 cells were cultured in Dulbecco's Modified Eagle Medium with 10 % fetal calf serum, 100 U/ml penicillin, and 100 μg/ml streptomycin (PAA Laboratories, Cölbe, Germany). Primary human monocytes were isolated from 50 ml buffy coats (DRK Blutspendedienst Baden-Württemberg-Hessen, Frankfurt, Germany). Blood was layered on a Ficoll-Isopaque gradient ($P = 1077$ g ml^{-1}). The interphase containing peripheral blood mononuclear cells was obtained after centrifugation (800 × g, 20 min). Cells were recovered, washed twice in PBS, and left to adhere on culture dishes

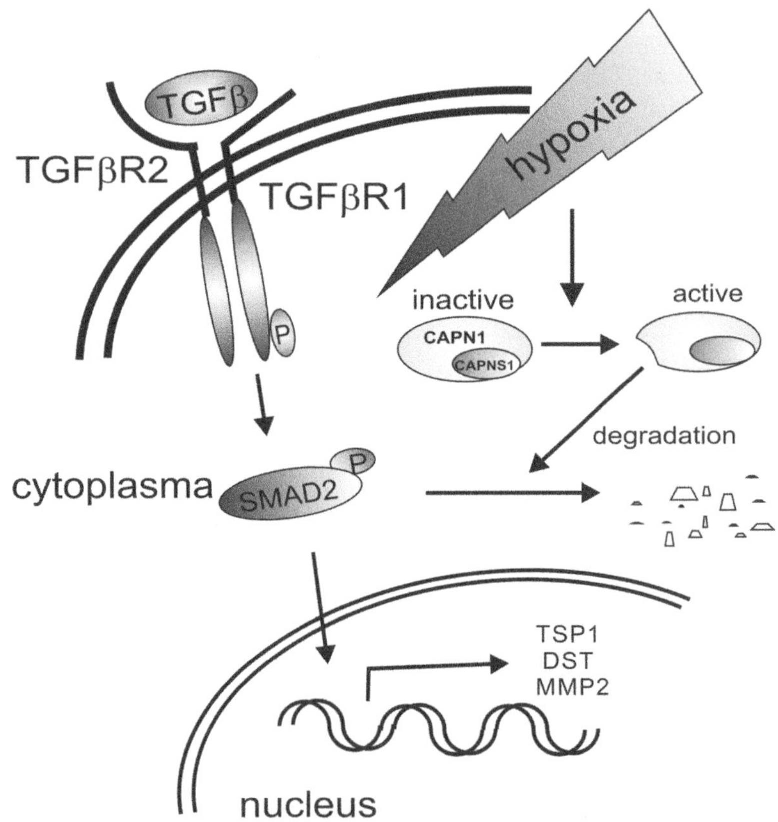

Fig. 6 Graphical abstract. TGFβ binds to its receptor (TGFβR1 and TGFβR2), induces phosphorylation of TGFβR1 and downstream signaling molecules like SMAD2. Active SMAD2 translocates to the nucleus to provoke expression of target genes, i.e., TSP1, DST, and MMP2. Hypoxia in combination with TGFβ activates calpain to degrade SMAD2, which in turn attenuates SMAD2-dependent transcriptional activation and thus, diminishes the induction of TSP1, DST, and MMP2

(Sarstedt, Nümbrecht, Germany) for 90 min at 37 °C. Non-adherent cells were removed. The medium was changed to fresh RPMI 1640 medium, supplemented with 3 % (v/v) human plasma (HP), 2 mM L-glutamine, 100 U/ml penicillin, and 100 μg/ml streptomycin (PAA Laboratories, Cölbe, Germany). Cells were kept at 37 °C in a humidified atmosphere with 5 % CO_2. Monocytes were differentiated with human plasma for 6–8 days before they were treated with 10 ng/ml TGFß. Purity of macrophage cultures was about 90 %. To establish hypoxic conditions cells were incubated in a hypoxic workstation with 1 % O_2, 94 % N_2, 5 % CO_2 (Invivo2 400, Ruskinn Technology, Leeds U.K.). Protein stability was assessed by stimulating macrophage with TGFß for 4 h, followed by 10 μg/mL cycloheximide (CHX). Samples were harvested after additional 1, 2, 3, or 4 h. Degradation of SMAD2 was followed by the addition of 10 μM lactacystin, 10 μM MG132 (Z-Leu-Leu-Leu-al), or 50 μM bafilomycin A1. After 2 h incubations with TGFß co-incubations with TGFß and inhibitors went on for 6 h. Phosphatase PP2A was inhibited by 10 μM okadaic acid (OA), preincubated for 1 h. 10 μM calpain inhibitor 1 was added simultaneously together with TGFß to macrophages.

Transfection of primary human macrophages

For siRNA transfections human macrophages were seeded in 6-well plates as described above. 50 nM siRNA against HIF-1α (ON-TARGETplus SMART pool, Human HIF1A, Thermo Scientific, Karlsruhe, Germany), HIF-2α (ON-TARGETplus SMART pool, Human EPAS1, Thermo Scientific), or non-targeting siRNA pool (GE Healthcare Dharmacon) was used with 16.8 μl HiPerfect (Qiagen, Hilden, Germany) in 500 μl medium with penicillin and streptomycin for each well. After adding the mix, cells were incubated for 24 h. Then medium was removed and replaced by medium containing penicillin, streptomycin and human serum to start experiments.

Western blot analysis

Cells were lysed in lysis-buffer (6.65 M urea, 10 % glycerol, 1 % SDS, 10 mM Tris/HCl pH 6.8, pH was adjusted to 7.4) and sonicated. After centrifugation (16.000 × g, 10 min) the protein content in the supernatants was determined by a protein assay kit (Bio-Rad, Munich, Germany), 70 μg total protein was separated on 10 % SDS gels and blotted on nitrocellulose membranes. The following antibodies were used: human pSMAD2 (#3108, Cell Signaling Technology), human pSMAD3 (ab52903, Abcam), human SMAD7 (ab124890 Abcam), human SMAD2/3 (#3102 Cell Signaling Technology), human calpain regulatory subunit (sc-32785, Santa Cruz), CAPN1 (C5736, Sigma), nucleolin (sc-13057, Santa Cruz), and ß-tubulin (T4026, Sigma). Horseradish peroxidase-conjugated goat anti-rabbit or anti-mouse IgG (Sigma) were used as secondary antibodies. Densitometry was performed using image J software (http://rsbweb.nih.gov/ij/). Briefly, rectangles were used to assess signal strength of each individual band and the background was measured by using the baseline tool and subtracted from individual values. Target protein expression was normalized to the loading control i.e., tubulin or nucleolin.

Luciferase reporter activity

The SBE4-Luc reporter plasmid was a gift from Bert Vogelstein (Addgene plasmid # 16495) [51], while the renilla control vector pRL-SV40 was bought from Promega (Frankfurt, Germany). J774A.1 cells were transiently transfected with 0.2 μg plasmid using JetPrime™ transfection reagent (Polyplus transfection, Illkirch, France) according to the manufacturer's protocol. After 16 h, medium was changed and cells were starved for 2 h prior to stimulation. Afterwards, cells were lysed and firefly as well as renilla luciferase activities were determined using a Dual Luciferase kit assay (Promega) on a Mithras LB 940 luminometer (Berthold, Bad Wildbad, Germany).

Flow cytometry (FACS)

For TGFBR2 surface expression, single cell suspensions were generated from detached macrophages by digestion with accutase (PAA) for 10 min at 37 °C. 10^5 cells were transferred to new tubes. Before staining, non-specific antibody binding to Fcγ receptors was blocked with Fcγ Block Receptor Binding Inhibitor (eBioscience, Frankfurt, Germany) for 15 min on ice, followed by staining with human TGFBR2 fluorescein-conjugated antibody (FAB241F,R&D Systems, Germany) using standard protocols. We used an LSRFortessa Cell Analyzer (BD, US) and results were analyzed using FlowJo software 7.6.1 (Treestar, Ashland, OR, USA). To discriminate macrophages from other non-leukocyte cells, samples were stained with CD45 (BD Bioscience). For daily instrument calibration we used Cytometer Setup and Tracking beads (BD Biosciences).

mRNA isolation and quantitative PCR

Isolation of mRNA and quantitative PCR was performed as described in [52]. Primers are:

SMAD2, forward: CCGACACACCGAGATCCTAAC,
reverse: GAGGTGGCGTTTCTGGAATATAA;
SMAD7, forward: CCAGGCTCCAGAAGAAGTTG,
reverse: CCAACTGCAGACTGTCCAGA;
TGFBR2, forward: GGAAACTTGACTGCACCGTT,
reverse: CTGCACATCGTCCTGTGG;
CAPNS1, forward:
GACACCCTGATCTGAAGACTGA,
reverse: GCCTGCCACCTTTTGATGTT;

CAPN1, forward: ACATGGAGGCCATCACTTTC
reverse: GGTCCACGTTGTTCCACTCT
TSP1, forward: CCAGATCAGGCAGACACAGA
reverse: AGTTGTCCCGTTCATTGAGG.
DST, forward: GATGCAGATCCGAAAACCCCT
reverse: CTCAGTGCGGTCCAGTTGTA
MMP2, forward: AGGGCACATCCTATGACAGC
reverse: ATTTGTTGCCCAGGAAAGTG
CST6, forward: CTACTTCCGAGACACGCACA
reverse: GGAACCACAAGGACCTCAAA
PAI1, forward: AGCTCCTTGTACAGATGCCG
reverse: ACAACAGGAGGAGAAACCCA
TBP, forward: GGGCCGCCGGCTGTTTAACT,
reverse: AGCCCTGAGCGTAAGGTGGCA.

Statistics

Experiments for mRNA expression and flow cytometry were performed in duplicate and repeated at least 3 times. Western blot analysis was performed at least 3 times. Data are expressed as means ± SEM. Multigroup statistically significant differences were calculated after analysis of one-way variance (ANOVA) and Bonferroni's test. A statistically significant difference between two groups was calculated by paired T test. Individual P values are given in the figures ($^*P < 0.05$, $^{**}P < 0.01$, $^{***}P < 0.001$).

Competing interests

The authors declare that they have no competing interests.

Authors' contributions

WC performed experiments; WC and ND designed experiments and analyzed data; WC, ND, BB wrote the manuscript; JZ revised the paper. All authors read and approved the final version of the manuscript. BB supervised the project.

Authors' information

Nathalie Dehne and Bernhard Brüne shared senior authorship.

Acknowledgements

This work was supported by the Deutsche Forschungsgemeinshaft (SFB 815, project A8), Deutsche Krebshilfe (111578), and Sander Foundation (2013.036.1).
Thanks to China Scholarship Council granting a stipend to Wei Cui.

Author details

[1]College of Life Sciences, Beijing Normal University, 100875 Beijing, China.
[2]Institute of Biochemistry I, Faculty of Medicine, Goethe-University Frankfurt, 60590 Frankfurt, Germany.

References

1. Murray PJ, Allen JE, Biswas SK, Fisher EA, Gilroy DW, Goerdt S, et al. Macrophage activation and polarization: nomenclature and experimental guidelines. Immunity. 2014;41(1):14–20.
2. Weigert A, Brüne B. Nitric oxide, apoptosis and macrophage polarization during tumor progression. Nitric Oxide. 2008;19(2):95–102.
3. Shi Y, Massagué J. Mechanisms of TGF-β signaling from cell membrane to the nucleus. Cell. 2003;113(6):685–700.
4. Derynck R, Zhang YE. Smad-dependent and Smad-independent pathways in TGF-β family signalling. Nature. 2003;425(6958):577–84.
5. Nurgazieva D, Mickley A, Moganti K, Ming W, Ovsyi I, Popova A, et al. TGF-β1, but not bone morphogenetic proteins, activates Smad1/5 pathway in primary human macrophages and induces expression of proatherogenic genes. J Immunol. 2015;194(2):709–18.
6. Pickup M, Novitskiy S, Moses HL. The roles of TGFβ in the tumour microenvironment. Nat Rev Cancer. 2013;13(11):788–99.
7. Flavell RA, Sanjabi S, Wrzesinski SH, Licona-Limón P. The polarization of immune cells in the tumour environment by TGFβ. Nat Rev Immunol. 2010;10(8):554–67.
8. Gong D, Shi W, Yi S-j, Chen H, Groffen J, Heisterkamp N. TGFβ signaling plays a critical role in promoting alternative macrophage activation. BMC Immunol. 2012;13(1):31.
9. Gigante M, Gesualdo L, Ranieri E. TGF-beta: a master switch in tumor immunity. Curr Pharm Des. 2012;18(27):4126–34.
10. Byrne SN, Knox MC, Halliday GM. TGFβ is responsible for skin tumour infiltration by macrophages enabling the tumours to escape immune destruction. Immunol Cell Biol. 2007;86(1):92–7.
11. Mantovani A, Sica A. Macrophages, innate immunity and cancer: balance, tolerance, and diversity. Curr Opin Immunol. 2010;22(2):231–7.
12. Harris AL. Hypoxia — a key regulatory factor in tumour growth. Nat Rev Cancer. 2002;2(1):38–47.
13. Ratcliffe PJ. Oxygen sensing and hypoxia signalling pathways in animals: the implications of physiology for cancer. J Physiol. 2013;591(8):2027–42.
14. Brüne B, Dehne N, Grossmann N, Jung M, Namgaladze D, Schmid T, et al. Redox control of inflammation in macrophages. Antioxid Redox Signal. 2013;19(6):595–637.
15. Nath B, Szabo G. Hypoxia and hypoxia inducible factors: diverse roles in liver diseases. Hepatology. 2012;55(2):622–33.
16. Ueno M, Maeno T, Nomura M, Aoyagi-Ikeda K, Matsui H, Hara K, et al. Hypoxia-inducible factor-1α mediates TGF-β-induced PAI-1 production in alveolar macrophages in pulmonary fibrosis. Am J Physiol Lung Cell Mol Physiol. 2011;300(5):L740–52.
17. Basu RK, Hubchak S, Hayashida T, Runyan CE, Schumacker PT, Schnaper HW. Interdependence of HIF-1α and TGF-β/Smad3 signaling in normoxic and hypoxic renal epithelial cell collagen expression. Am J Physiol Renal Physiol. 2011;300(4):F898–905.
18. Chae K, Kang M, Lee J, Ryu B, Lee M, Her N, et al. Opposite functions of HIF-α isoforms in VEGF induction by TGF-β1 under non-hypoxic conditions. Oncogene. 2011;30(10):1213–28.
19. Herr B, Zhou J, Werno C, Menrad H, Namgaladze D, Weigert A, et al. The supernatant of apoptotic cells causes transcriptional activation of hypoxia-inducible factor−1α in macrophages via sphingosine-1-phosphate and transforming growth factor-β. Blood. 2009;114(10):2140–8.
20. Dehne N, Tausendschön M, Essler S, Geis T, Schmid T, Brüne B. IL-4 reduces the proangiogenic capacity of macrophages by down-regulating HIF-1α translation. J Leukoc Biol. 2014;95(1):129–37.
21. Kuratomi G, Komuro A, Goto K, Shinozaki M, Miyazawa K, Miyazono K, et al. NEDD4-2 (neural precursor cell expressed, developmentally down-regulated 4–2) negatively regulates TGF-beta (transforming growth factor-beta) signalling by inducing ubiquitin-mediated degradation of Smad2 and TGF-beta type I receptor. Biochem J. 2005;386:461–70.
22. Seo SR, Lallemand F, Ferrand N, Pessah M, L'Hoste S, Camonis J, et al. The novel E3 ubiquitin ligase Tiul1 associates with TGIF to target Smad2 for degradation. EMBO J. 2004;23(19):3780–92.
23. Tausendschön M, Rehli M, Dehne N, Schmidl C, Döring C, Hansmann M-L, et al. Genome-wide identification of hypoxia-inducible factor-1 and-2 binding sites in hypoxic human macrophages alternatively activated by IL-10. Biochim Biophys Acta. 2015;1849(1):10–22.

24. Heikkinen PT, Nummela M, Leivonen SK, Westermarck J, Hill CS, Kahari VM, et al. Hypoxia-activated Smad3-specific Dephosphorylation by PP2A. J Biol Chem. 2009;285(6):3740–9.
25. Koinuma D, Tsutsumi S, Kamimura N, Taniguchi H, Miyazawa K, Sunamura M, et al. Chromatin immunoprecipitation on microarray analysis of Smad2/3 binding sites reveals roles of ETS1 and TFAP2A in transforming growth factor β signaling. Mol Cell Biol. 2009;29(1):172–86.
26. Nakagawa T, Li JH, Garcia G, Mu W, Piek E, Böttinger EP, et al. TGF-β induces proangiogenic and antiangiogenic factorsvia parallel but distinct Smad pathways1. Kidney Int. 2004;66(2):605–13.
27. Piek E, Ju WJ, Heyer J, Escalante-Alcalde D, Stewart CL, Weinstein M, et al. Functional characterization of transforming growth factor β signaling in Smad2-and Smad3-deficient fibroblasts. J Biol Chem. 2001;276(23):19945–53.
28. Lo RS, Massagué J. Ubiquitin-dependent degradation of TGF-β activated Smad2. Nat Cell Biol. 1999;1(8):472–8.
29. Goll DE, Thompson VF, Li H, Wei W, CONG J. The calpain system. Physiol Rev. 2003;83(3):731–801.
30. Deshpande RV, Goust J-M, Chakrabarti AK, Barbosa E, Hogan EL, Banik NL. Calpain expression in lymphoid cells increased mRNA and protein levels after cell activation. J Biol Chem. 1995;270(6):2497–505.
31. Walker G, Pfeilschifter J, Otten U, Kunz D. Proteolytic cleavage of inducible nitric oxide synthase (iNOS) by calpain I. Biochim Biophys Acta. 2001;1568(3):216–24.
32. Zheng X, Zhou A-X, Rouhi P, Uramoto H, Borén J, Cao Y, et al. Hypoxia-induced and calpain-dependent cleavage of filamin A regulates the hypoxic response. Proc Natl Acad Sci. 2014;111(7):2560–5.
33. Iwamoto H, Miura T, Okamura T, Shirakawa K, Iwatate M, Kawamura S, et al. Calpain inhibitor-1 reduces infarct size and DNA fragmentation of myocardium in ischemic/reperfused rat heart. J Cardiovasc Pharmacol. 1999;33(4):580–6.
34. Zhang J, Patel JM, Block ER. Hypoxia-specific upregulation of calpain activity and gene expression in pulmonary artery endothelial cells. Am J Physiol Lung Cell Mol Physiol. 1998;275(3):L461–8.
35. Tyagi T, Ahmad S, Gupta N, Sahu A, Ahmad Y, Nair V, et al. Altered expression of platelet proteins and calpain activity mediate hypoxia-induced prothrombotic phenotype. Blood. 2014;123(8):1250–60.
36. Zimmerman UJP, Boring L, Pak UH, Mukerjee N, Wang KK. The calpain small subunit gene is essential: its inactivation results in embryonic lethality. IUBMB Life. 2000;50(1):63–8.
37. Zhou J, Köhl R, Herr B, Frank R, Brüne B. Calpain mediates a von hippel-lindau protein–independent destruction of hypoxia-inducible factor-1α. Mol Biol Cell. 2006;17(4):1549–58.
38. Muldoon LL, Rodland K, Magun B. Transforming growth factor beta and epidermal growth factor alter calcium influx and phosphatidylinositol turnover in rat-1 fibroblasts. J Biol Chem. 1988;263(35):18834–41.
39. Tompa P, Buzder-Lantos P, Tantos A, Farkas A, Szilágyi A, Bánóczi Z, et al. On the sequential determinants of calpain cleavage. J Biol Chem. 2004;279(20):20775–85.
40. Ono Y, Sorimachi H, Mamitsuka H. Calpain cleavage prediction using multiple kernel learning. PLoS One. 2011;6(5):e19035.
41. Whiteside T. The tumor microenvironment and its role in promoting tumor growth. Oncogene. 2008;27(45):5904–12.
42. LaGamba D, Nawshad A, Hay ED. Microarray analysis of gene expression during epithelial–mesenchymal transformation. Dev Dyn. 2005;234(1):132–42.
43. Kretschmer A, Moepert K, Dames S, Sternberger M, Kaufmann J, Klippel A. Differential regulation of TGF-β signaling through Smad2, Smad3 and Smad4. Oncogene. 2003;22(43):6748–63.
44. Petersen M, Pardali E, Van Der Horst G, Cheung H, Van Den Hoogen C, Van Der Pluijm G, et al. Smad2 and Smad3 have opposing roles in breast cancer bone metastasis by differentially affecting tumor angiogenesis. Oncogene. 2009;29(9):1351–61.
45. Martin-Manso G, Galli S, Ridnour LA, Tsokos M, Wink DA, Roberts DD. Thrombospondin 1 promotes tumor macrophage recruitment and enhances tumor cell cytotoxicity of differentiated U937 cells. Cancer Res. 2008;68(17):7090–9.
46. Deryugina EI, Quigley JP. Tumor angiogenesis: MMP-mediated induction of intravasation-and metastasis-sustaining neovasculature. Matrix Biol. 2015. doi:10.1016/j.matbio.2015.04.004.
47. Jiang W, Sanders A, Katoh M, Ungefroren H, Gieseler F, Prince M, et al. Tissue invasion and metastasis: molecular, biological and clinical perspectives. Semin Cancer Biol. 2015. doi: 10.1016/j.semcancer.2015.03.008.
48. Shapiro S, Khodalev O, Bitterman H, Auslender R, Lahat N. Different activation forms of MMP-2 oppositely affect the fate of endothelial cells. Am J Physiol Cell Physiol. 2010;298(4):C942–51.
49. Ben-Yosef Y, Lahat N, Shapiro S, Bitterman H, Miller A. Regulation of endothelial matrix metalloproteinase-2 by hypoxia/reoxygenation. Circ Res. 2002;90(7):784–91.
50. Chowdhury UR, Samant RS, Fodstad O, Shevde LA. Emerging role of nuclear protein 1 (NUPR1) in cancer biology. Cancer Metastasis Rev. 2009;28(1-2):225–32.
51. Zawel L, Le Dai J, Buckhaults P, Zhou S, Kinzler KW, Vogelstein B, et al. Human Smad3 and Smad4 are sequence-specific transcription activators. Mol Cell. 1998;1(4):611–7.
52. Jennewein C, Kuhn A-M, Schmidt MV, Meilladec-Jullig V, von Knethen A, Gonzalez FJ, et al. Sumoylation of peroxisome proliferator-activated receptor γ by apoptotic cells prevents lipopolysaccharide-induced NCoR removal from κB binding sites mediating transrepression of proinflammatory cytokines. J Immunol. 2008;181(8):5646–52.

5

Ferulic acid combined with aspirin demonstrates chemopreventive potential towards pancreatic cancer when delivered using chitosan-coated solid-lipid nanoparticles

Arvind Thakkar*, Sushma Chenreddy, Jeffrey Wang and Sunil Prabhu

Abstract

Background: The overall goal of this study was to demonstrate potential chemopreventive effects of ferulic acid (FA), an antioxidant, combined with aspirin (ASP), a commonly used anti-inflammatory drug for pancreatic cancer chemoprevention, using a novel chitosan-coated solid lipid nanoparticles (c-SLN) drug delivery system encapsulating FA and ASP.

Results: Our formulation optimization results showed that c-SLNs of FA and ASP exhibited appropriate initial particle sizes in range of 183 ± 46 and 229 ± 67 nm, encapsulation efficiency of 80 and 78 %, and zeta potential of 39.1 and 50.3 mV, respectively. In vitro studies were conducted to measure growth inhibition and degree of apoptotic cell death induced by either FA or ASP alone or in combination. Cell viability studies demonstrated combinations of low doses of free FA (200 μM) and ASP (1 mM) significantly reduced cell viability by 45 and 60 % in human pancreatic cancer cells MIA PaCa-2 and Panc-1, respectively. However, when encapsulated within c-SLNs, a 5- and 40-fold decreases in dose of FA (40 μM) and ASP (25 μM) was observed which was significant. Furthermore, increased apoptosis of 35 and 31 % was observed in MIA PaCa-2 and Panc-1 cells, respectively. In vivo studies using oral administration of combinations of 75 and 25 mg/kg of FA and ASP c-SLNs to MIA PaCa-2 pancreatic tumor xenograft mice model suppressed the growth of the tumor by 45 % compared to control, although this was not statistically significant. In addition, the immunohistochemical analysis of tumor tissue showed significant decrease in expression of proliferation proteins PCNA and MKI67, and also increased expression of apoptotic proteins p-RB, p21, and p-ERK1/2 indicating the pro-apoptotic role of the regimen.

Conclusion: Combination of FA and ASP delivered via a novel nanotechnology-based c-SLN formulation demonstrates potential for pancreatic cancer chemoprevention and could be a promising area for future studies.

Keywords: Chemoprevention, Pancreatic cancer, Ferulic acid, Aspirin, Chitosan, Solid lipid nanoparticles

Background

Cancer of the pancreas is the fourth leading cause of cancer in the US affecting about 44,000 Americans each year. It has become increasingly apparent that despite more than 20 years of intensive research on treatment, the survival rate continues to be a dismal <5 % within 5 years of diagnosis [1]. Current treatment modalities are largely ineffective, thus bringing to the forefront the development of alternative strategies to tackle this disease [2]. A viable strategy could be the use of chemopreventive agents to suppress, delay or even reverse the onset of the disease [3–5]. Our group has been interested in the use of novel chemopreventive agents and their combinations for pancreatic cancer prevention. Recently, we have also demonstrated the importance of delivering these agents using novel nanotechnology-based drug delivery systems

*Correspondence: thakkara@westernu.edu
Department of Pharmaceutical Sciences, College of Pharmacy, Western University of Health Sciences, 309 E Second Street, Pomona, CA 91766, USA

wherein high efficacy has been achieved at very low doses [3, 6–9].

Pancreatic carcinoma arises from a heterogeneous molecular pathogenesis involving several oncogenic pathways and defined genetic mutations. In the last few years, however, oxidative stress and inflammation have emerged as important risk factors in pancreatic carcinogenesis [10–13]. The reports on the role of reactive oxygen species (ROS) in tumor initiation have proved that oxidative stress acts as a DNA-damaging agent, effectively increasing the mutation rate within cells and thus promoting oncogenic transformation [14]. Additionally, oxidative stress acts by further recruiting inflammatory cells to the site of damage and producing more reactive species. This sustained inflammatory/oxidative environment leads to a loop effect, which can damage healthy neighboring epithelial and stromal cells and over a prolonged time period lead to carcinogenesis [15]. Based on this information, the hypothesis of this study was to combine chemopreventive agents ferulic acid (FA) and aspirin (ASP) encapsulated in c-SLNs for the synergistic chemoprevention of pancreatic cancer.

FA is one of the most abundant antioxidants found in plants. FA has a high antioxidant potential due to its resonance-stabilized phenoxyl radical structure, allowing it to be an effective scavenger of free radicals to show its anti-cancer effects [16]. Recently many researchers have focused their attention on the anti-cancer activity of FA on skin, colon, liver and breast cancers [17–19]. However, no other group has investigated its potential in pancreatic cancer chemoprevention. Non-steroidal anti-inflammatory drugs (NSAIDs) such as ASP are currently the best studied chemopreventive agents for many cancers, and have been demonstrated to modulate the NF-κB pathway [20]. Clinical studies associated with the long term use of ASP for pancreatic cancer prevention, however, have met with mixed results thus far [21–23]. Given these conflicting reports on the use of ASP in pancreatic cancer but, simultaneously, realizing the proven benefits of ASP as a chemopreventive in cancer, it reaffirms the need for further study of this drug in pancreatic cancer prevention.

Solid-lipid nanoparticles (SLNs) were developed over a decade ago but have never before been considered extensively for chemoprevention of pancreatic cancer. For the current study, we are proposing a novel SLN delivery system coated with chitosan (c-SLN). Our previous research in chitosan-based drug delivery systems combined with the current research on SLNs enables us to design an effective hybrid system for chemoprevention. Chitosan is a nontoxic, biodegradable and biocompatible polysaccharide derived from the shells of crustaceans, with proven in vivo safety profile [24, 25]. c-SLNs are biodegradable, bioadhesive and have permeation enhancing properties thus acting as promising vehicles for oral drug delivery with wide range of pharmaceutical applications [26]. The primary amino group in chitosan offers some special properties such as water-solubility, hemocompatibility, and cationic groups which could react with a big number of anions or other negatively charged molecules [27]. And also based on the cationic property, chitosan-based nanoparticles exhibit a mucoadhesive feature because of their positive charge, thereby capable of prolonging their residence time in the negatively charged epithelia in small intestine [28], thus increasing the drug concentration at the site of absorption. Moreover, chitosan can mediate the opening of tight junctions between neighboring epithelial cells reversibly, facilitating the paracellular transport of drug molecules ultimately leading to improved bioavailability of the drugs [29]. Thus, c-SLN combines the advantages of SLN with the biological properties of chitosan as a drug delivery vehicle.

In this study, we have used a novel c-SLN technology for the oral delivery of combinations of FA and ASP for pancreatic cancer to evaluate their combined chemopreventive efficacy in two different human pancreatic cancer cells, MIA PaCa-2 and Panc-1. Additionally, a pancreatic tumor xenograft mouse model was used to determine the efficacy of the chemopreventive regimen.

Results

Physical characterization of FA and ASP encapsulated c-SLNs

Based on the methodology described earlier [3, 9], c-SLNs of FA and ASP exhibited initial particle sizes in the nanometer range of 183 ± 46 and 229 ± 67, respectively. All the c-SLNs showed optimal particle size with low variability. The c-SLNs exhibited 80 and 78 % encapsulation efficiency of the FA and ASP respectively within the lipid nanoparticles. The zeta potential of FA particles were −8.0 and 39.1 mV before and after coating with chitosan, respectively. The surface charge on ASP nanoparticles were −6.0 and 50.3 mV before and after coating with chitosan, respectively. The polydispersity index (PDI) was 0.25 and 0.19 for FA and ASP c-SLN, respectively (Table 1).

In vitro evaluation of FA and ASP drug release from c-SLNs

The ability of nanoparticles to deliver drugs was examined by determining the drug release in PBS solution (pH 6.8) and acidic conditions (pH 1.6), as shown in Fig. 1. The percentage of drug released from c-SLN was plotted as a function of time. The release of the drug from nanoparticles prepared using stearic acid as lipid was conducted over a period of 96 h. As shown in Fig. 1a, the release of FA in PBS solution was faster compared to ASP at initial time point up to 12 h. A cumulative drug release of approximately 98 % of ASP was observed within 48 h

Table 1 Particle size and encapsulation efficiency of drug loaded chitosan-solid lipid nanoparticles

Drug	Particle size (nm)	Encapsulation efficiency (%)	Zeta potential (mV)	Polydispersity index (PDI)
Ferulic acid c-SLN	183 ± 46	80	39.1 ± 3.4	0.25 ± 0.06
Aspirin c-SLN	229 ± 67	78	50.3 ± 7.3	0.19 ± 0.05

c-SLN chitosan solid lipid nanoparticle

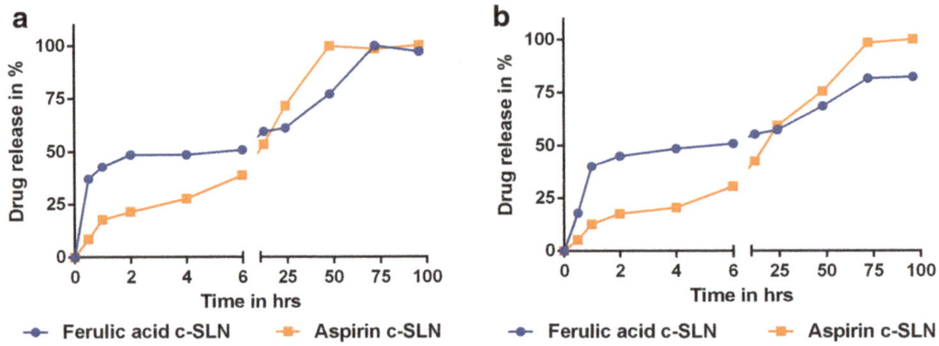

Fig. 1 In vitro drug release from chitosan solid lipid nanoparticle (c-SLN). **a** In vitro drug release from c-SLNs over a period of 96 h in phosphate buffered saline (PBS), pH 6.8; and **b** in vitro drug release from c-SLNs over a period of 96 h in acidic medium, pH 1.6. The drug release was analyzed using a HPLC system

of the study, and then showed constant release up to 96 h. The FA c-SLN showed approximately 98 % drug release at 72 h, even though it showed a faster release pattern in initial time points compared to ASP. Both the formulations exhibited slow sustained release of the drug. The release profile was similar in acidic condition at pH 1.6 compared to PBS solution at pH 6.8 (Fig. 1b).

Determination of IC_{50} concentration of free and c-SLN encapsulated FA and ASP

In order to evaluate the combined effects of FA and ASP on pancreatic cancer, we first treated MIA PaCa-2 and Panc-1 cells with various individual concentrations (5–5000 µM) of FA and ASP for 72 h, and cell growth was measured by the MTS assay. Our observations show that there was a dose-dependent inhibition of the growth of MIA PaCa-2 and Panc-1 cells. In case of MIA PaCa-2, the IC_{50} values for FA and ASP observed were 1.7 and 2.6 mM, respectively (Fig. 2a); whereas in Panc-1 cells, the IC_{50} values for FA and ASP were 1.9 and 2.4 mM, respectively (Fig. 2b).

As shown in Fig. 2, cell viability assay was performed with serial dilutions (1–1000 µM) of FA and ASP c-SLN nanoparticle formulations. In MIA PaCa-2 cells, the IC_{50} concentrations for FA c-SLN, ASP c-SLN, and blank c-SLN observed were 81.15, 34.66, and 362 µM, respectively (Fig. 2c); whereas in Panc-1 cells, the IC_{50} values for FA c-SLN, ASP c-SLN, and blank c-SLN were 66.6, 58.32, and 341.8 µM respectively (Fig. 2d).

Effect of the combination of FA and ASP c-SLN on pancreatic cancer cells

To examine the effect of combined regimen on cell proliferation, MIA PaCa-2 and Panc-1 cells were treated with low and ineffective concentrations of free form FA (200 µM) and ASP (1 mM) for 72 h. As shown in Fig. 3a, single agents did not show significant change in cell viability at these concentrations. However, when used in combination at identical concentrations, FA + ASP showed a significant effect with a reduction in cell viability of MIA PaCa-2 cells by as much as 45 % ($P < 0.01$), whereas FA + ASP combination in Panc-1 cells showed a remarkable decrease of 60 % ($P < 0.001$) cell viability.

In case of c-SLNs, after determining the dose response curves individually and obtaining the IC_{50} value for FA and ASP c-SLNs, ineffective and low concentrations were selected for FA c-SLN (40 µM) and ASP c-SLN (25 µM) showing minimal inhibitory response on the cell lines (Fig. 3b). When combined together (FA + ASP c-SLNs), the cell viability was reduced to 70 % for MIA PaCa-2 and Panc-1 cells, respectively ($P < 0.001$). Thus, the combination of FA and ASP c-SLN administered at low concentrations showed a significant reduction in cell viability compared to unmodified, free form combinations of FA and ASP. The blank c-SLN at same concentration did not show reduction in cell viability, hence demonstrating that c-SLN formulation excipient has no significant effect on cell viability of pancreatic cancer cells (Fig. 3b).

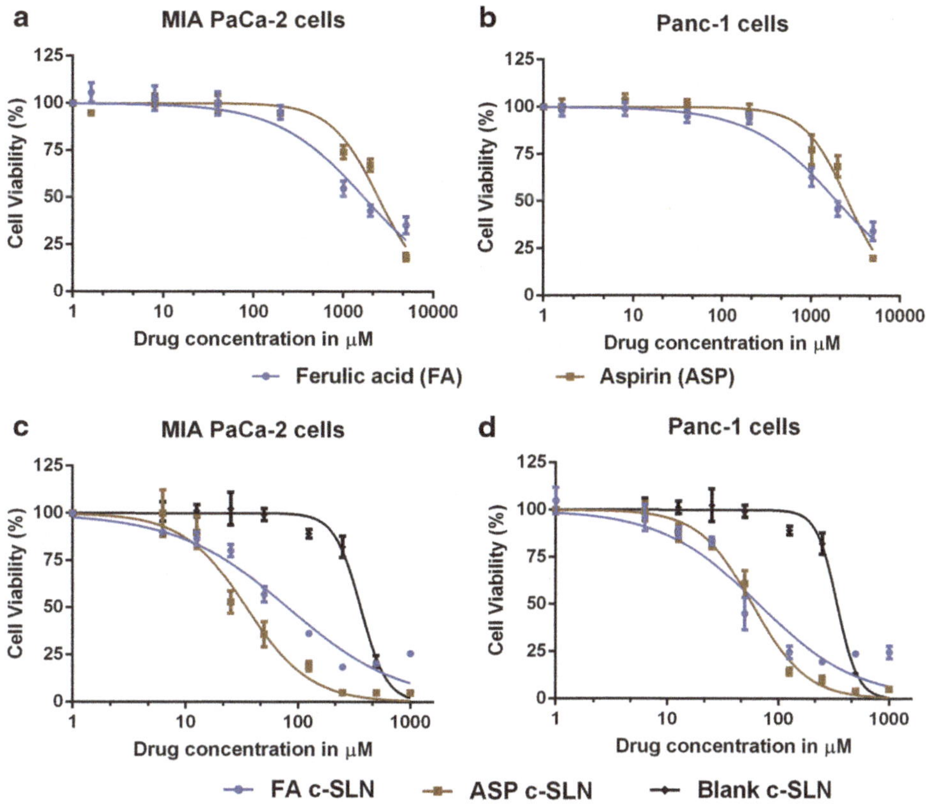

Fig. 2 Dose dependent inhibition of cell viability in pancreatic cancer cells. **a, c** MIA PaCa-2 and **b, d** Panc-1 cells were treated with unmodified ferulic acid (FA), unmodified aspirin (ASP), FA encapsulated in chitosan-solid lipid nanoparticles (c-SLNs), and ASP c-SLNs. MTS assay was performed to determine the cell viability of MIA PaCa-2 and Panc-1 cells after treating with a range of concentrations of free and c-SLN modified FA and ASP for 72 h. The IC_{50} values were then determined using nonlinear regression using graph pad prism software. Each data point represents the mean percent viable cells measured in three parallel but independent experiments

FA and ASP combination induces apoptosis in pancreatic cancer cells

The induction of apoptosis was measured by flow cytometry for all individual drugs and their combinations on MIA PaCa-2 and Panc-1 cells. Individual concentrations of FA c-SLN (40 μM) and ASP c-SLN (25 μM) showed minimal apoptotic cells (data not shown). In case of MIA PaCa-2 cells (Fig. 3c), FA and ASP c-SLN combinations demonstrated approximately 35 % apoptotic cells ($P < 0.01$). In case of Panc-1 cells (Fig. 3d), c-SLN combined FA + ASP showed 31 % of apoptotic cells ($P < 0.01$). Overall, our studies confirmed that FA + ASP combinations were significantly effective in inducing apoptosis of cancer cells.

FA and ASP combination modulates proliferation proteins in pancreatic cancer cells

From our previously published studies, aspirin was reported to modulate proliferation proteins and ERK pathway [6, 7], hence we wanted to determine whether the proliferation proteins like PCNA, MKI67, RB and ERK1/2 are involved in growth inhibition. The MIA PaCa-2 and Panc-1 protein lysates were analyzed by western blot analysis. We observed that incubation of MIA PaCa-2 and Panc-1 cells with combination FA + ASP inhibits PCNA and MKI67 proteins, and produced higher phosphorylation of ERK1/2 and RB proteins compared with the control and individual drugs (Fig. 3e).

FA and ASP c-SLN in a pancreatic xenograft tumor model

In vivo studies using a xenograft mouse model was subsequently conducted to determine whether oral administration of FA + ASP c-SLN combinations could suppress the growth of pancreatic tumor. MIA PaCa-2 cells were implanted subcutaneously in SCID mice. The treatment by oral gavage started 1 day after tumor implantation and continued as per protocol for 5 weeks (Fig. 4a). The FA and ASP c-SLN were administered at the dose of 75 and 25 mg/kg daily via oral gavage. During the experiment, all mice were monitored to investigate possible adverse effects caused by drug treatment. The FA and ASP c-SLN treatment did not cause any significant weight loss of the mice (Fig. 4b). These results suggested that no noticeable side

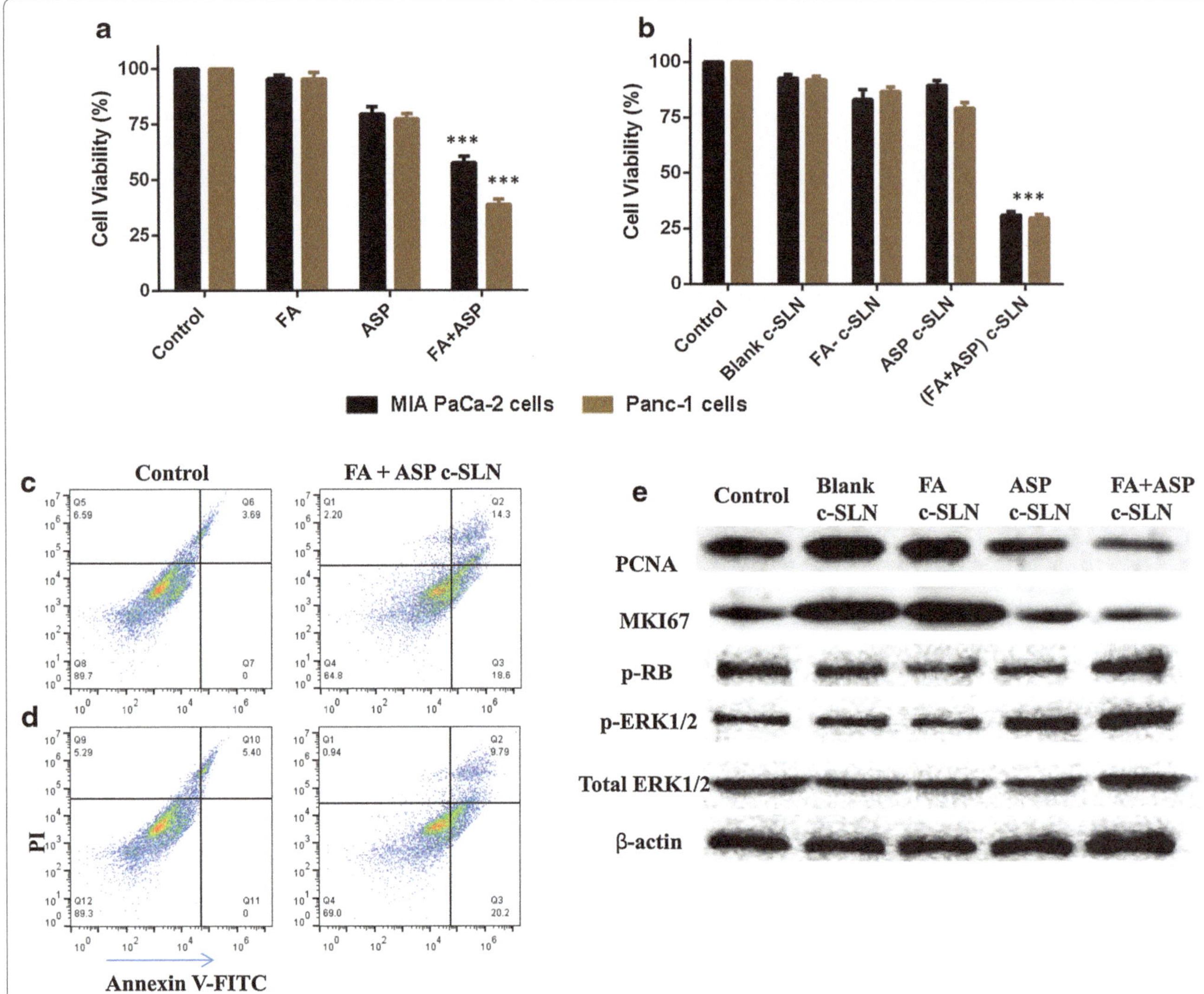

Fig. 3 Synergistic effect of ferulic acid (FA) and aspirin (ASP) combination on cell viability and apoptosis. MTS assay was performed to determine the cell viability of **a** free FA + ASP and **b** chitosan-solid lipid nanoparticle (c-SLN) encapsulated FA + ASP combination. MIA PaCa-2 and Panc-1 cells were treated with free FA (200 μM), with ASP (1 mM) and c-SLN FA (40 μM) with c-SLN ASP (25 μM) individually and in combination for 72 h. Each *bar* represents the mean percent viable cells measured in three parallel but independent experiments. **c** MIA PaCa-2 and **d** Panc-1 cells were treated with c-SLN encapsulated FA (40 μM) with c-SLN ASP (25 μM) for 48 h and stained with Annexin V-PI apoptosis detection kit. **e** Panc-1 cells were treated with FA (40 μM) with c-SLN ASP (25 μM) alone or in combination for 24 h. The expression of PCNA, MKI67, phospho-RB, and phospho-ERK1/2 proteins were evaluated by western blot analysis. The equal loading was confirmed by using an anti-β-actin antibody. Statistical significance was determined by one-way ANOVA followed by Dunnett's multiple comparison test post hoc *analysis*. ***P < 0.001 represents statistical significance of differences between control and treatment group

effects or toxicity were caused by the treatment regimen. Furthermore, no gross signs of toxicity were observed during visible inspections of general appearance and macroscopic examinations of individual organs.

In an effort to establish the efficacy of a combined therapy compared with single-agent treatment, we determined the mean tumor volume in all treated groups. For instance, at day 36 the mean tumor volume (mean ± SEM) in control and blank c-SLN (vehicle control) mice were 2576 ± 530 and 2513 ± 352 mm^3 respectively, as compared with 2235 ± 244 mm^3 in FA c-SLN and 2713 ± 736 mm^3 in ASP c-SLN treated mice. However, mean tumor volume in FA + ASP c-SLN group was 1424 ± 402 mm^3 (Fig. 4c). The administration of FA and ASP c-SLN combination treatment resulted in 45 % reduction in the mean tumor volume compared with vehicle control group, though this reduction was statistically non-significant.

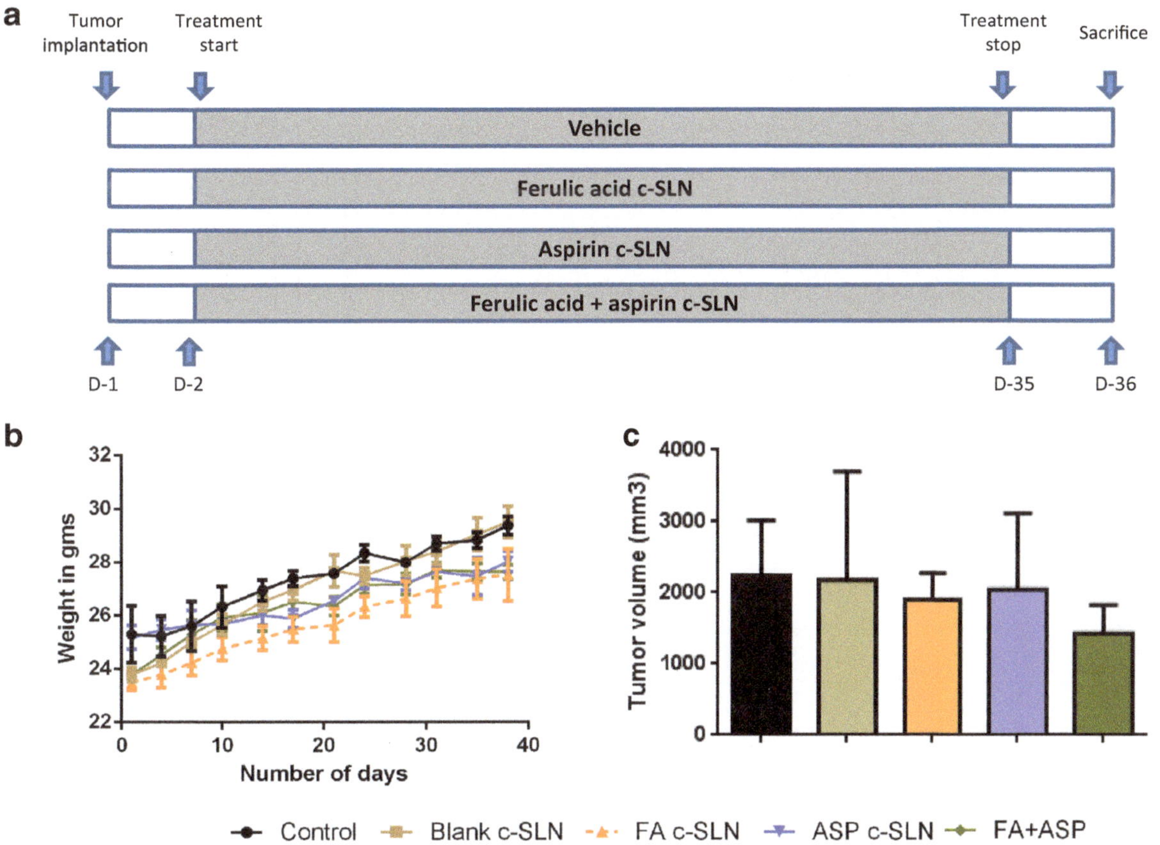

Fig. 4 In vivo effect of ferulic acid (FA) and aspirin (ASP) c-SLNs on MIA PaCa-2 xenograft SCID mice. **a** Flow chart representation of experimental design for in vivo studies. **b** Body weight variations of xenograft SCID mice during the FA and ASP c-SLNs treatment period. Average body weight transitions of mice over the 35 days treatment period. **c** Average tumor growth of pancreatic cancer cells MIA PaCa-2 over a period of 35 d after treatment. FA and ASP c-SLNs were administered via oral gavage for 35 days. Statistical significance was determined by one-way ANOVA followed by Dunnett's multiple comparison test post hoc *analysis*

FA and ASP inhibits expression of proliferation markers in pancreatic tumor tissues

In order to evaluate the effect of FA + ASP chemopreventive regimens on tumor cell proliferation, immunohistochemistry (IHC) was performed to measure the expression of cell proliferation markers proliferating cell nuclear antigen (PCNA; Fig. 5a, c) and MKI67 (Fig. 5b, d) on pancreatic tissues. The protein expression was evaluated by IHC scores as described in the methods section. The results in Fig. 5 showed that FA c-SLN in combination with ASP c-SLN showed 46 and 43 % down-regulation in the expression of PCNA and MKI67 proliferation proteins respectively in tumor tissues compared with the blank c-SLN control group ($p < 0.001$). Together, our results suggest that FA and ASP c-SLN combination treatment down regulates expression of proliferation proteins.

FA and ASP c-SLN combination inhibits apoptotic and cell cycle proteins in pancreatic tumor tissues

Important families of proteins that are involved in the regulation of apoptosis are mammalian mitogen activated protein kinases (MAPK) that can be subdivided in extracellular signal-regulated kinases (ERKs) that regulate cell growth and differentiation [30, 31]. Also anti-carcinogenic effect of FA has been linked to down-regulation of an anti-apoptotic p21 protein [32]. Based on this information, we evaluated the expression of phosphorylated retinoblastoma (p-RB) protein, phospho-ERK1/2 and p21 protein expression using IHC. As shown in Fig. 6, the FA + ASP c-SLN combination group showed 220 and 178 % up-regulation of p21 and p-RB proteins compared to vehicle control, which are anti-apoptotic and tumor suppressor protein, respectively. The FA + ASP c-SLN treatment group also showed 363 % upregulation

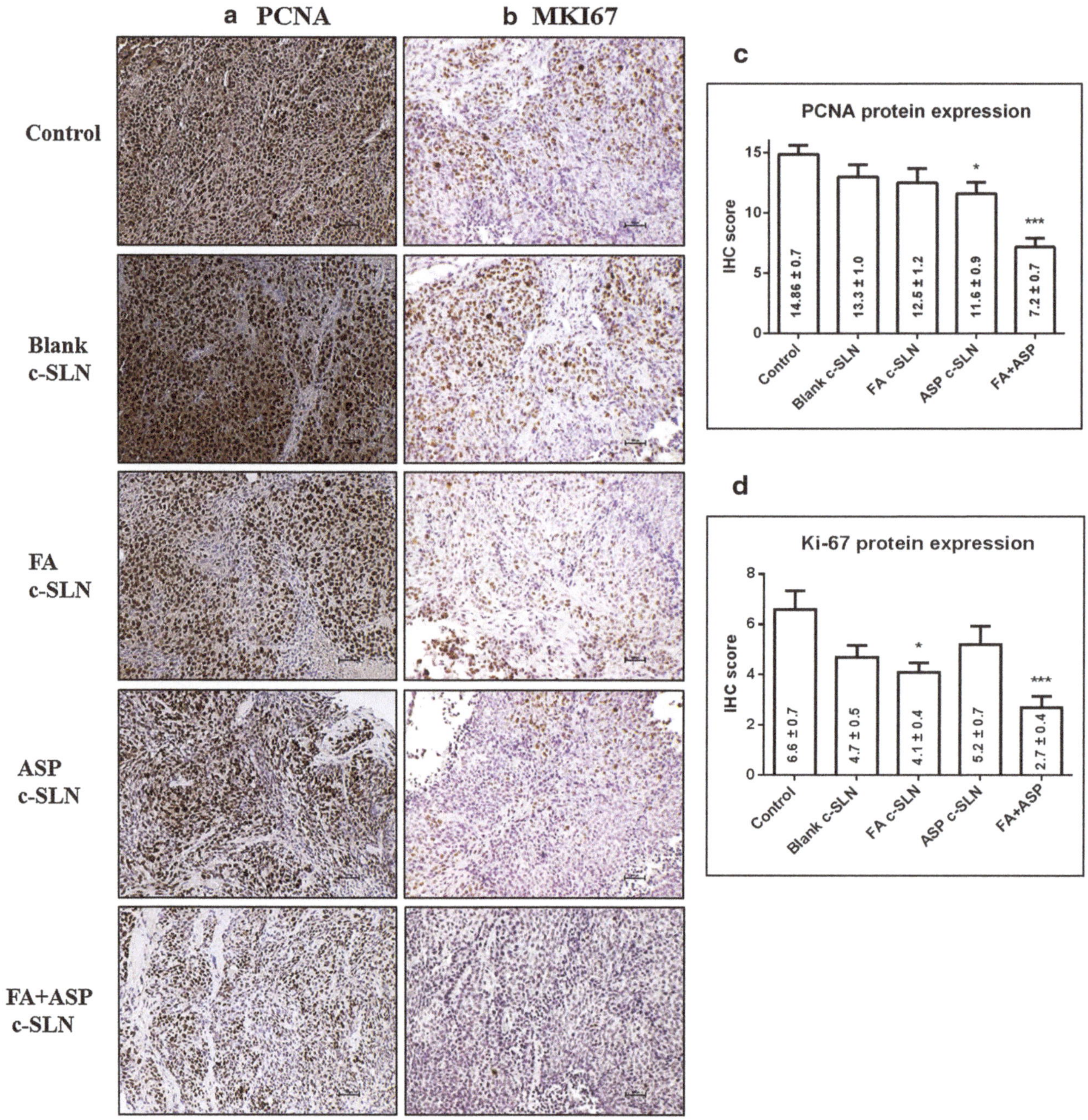

Fig. 5 Effect of ferulic acid (FA) and aspirin (ASP) chemopreventive regimen on tumor cell proliferation and apoptosis. Immunohistochemical analysis was performed on paraffin-embedded and micro-sectioned pancreatic tissues as described in methods section. **a**, **b** Representative images showing effect of modified FA and ASP c-SLN combination on PCNA and MKI67 (marker of proliferation Ki-67) expressions in pancreatic tissue. **c**, **d** A significant decrease in the PCNA and MKI67 expression was observed in modified FA + ASP treatment groups compared to blank c-SLN vehicle control group. All the pictures were taken at ×200 magnification. Statistical significance was determined by one-way ANOVA followed by Dunnett's multiple comparison test post hoc *analysis*. *$p < 0.05$; ***$p < 0.001$ represents statistical significance between blank c-SLN vehicle control and FA + ASP c-SLN treatment

of p-ERK1/2 protein compared to vehicle control, which correlated with our published chemoprevention studies of ASP combinations, suggests activation of p-ERK1/2 as a mechanism of action of ASP [6].

Discussion

Pancreatic carcinoma arises from a heterogeneous molecular pathogenesis involving several oncogenic pathways and defined genetic mutations. Studies have

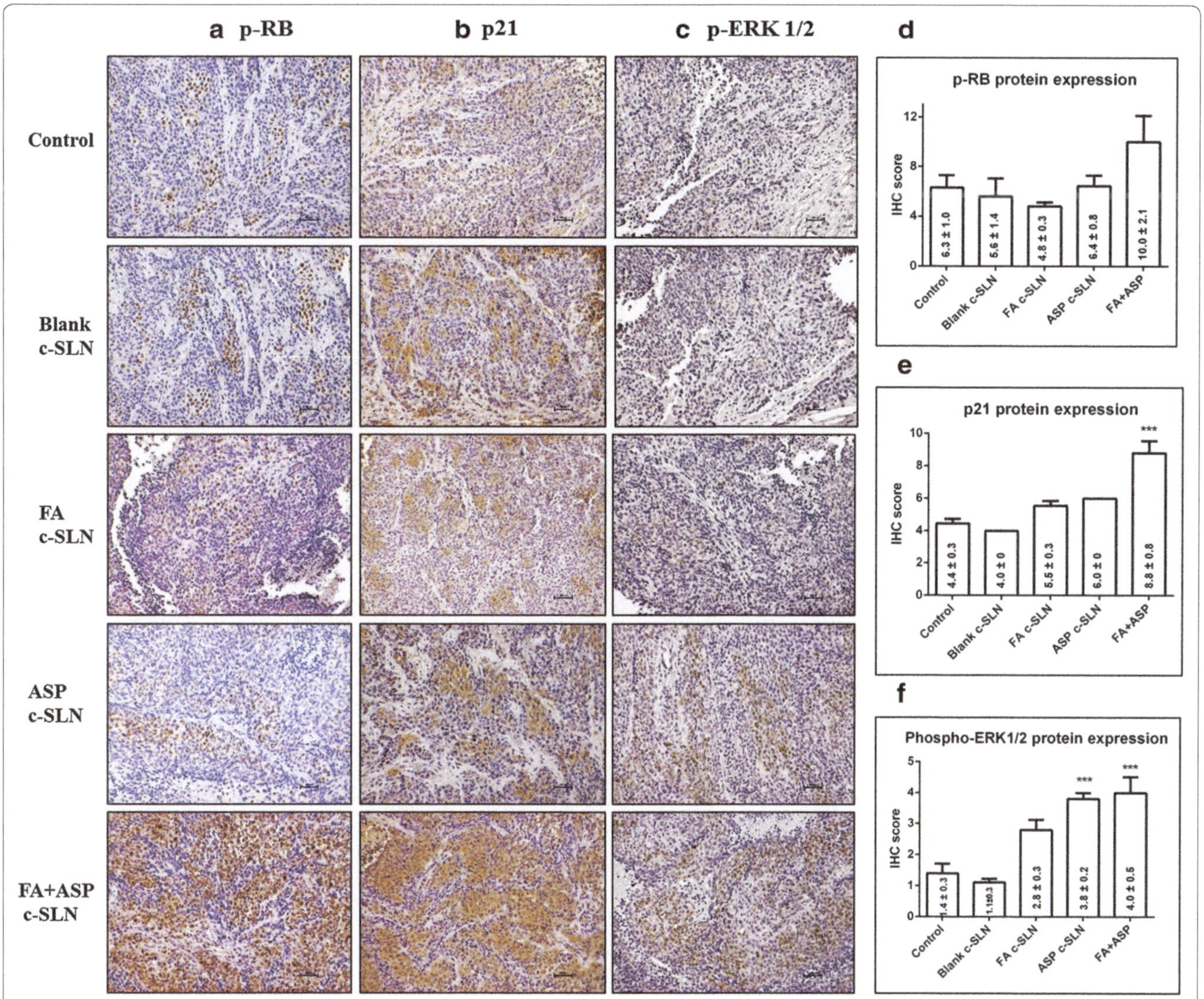

Fig. 6 Effect of ferulic acid (FA) and aspirin (ASP) chemopreventive regimen on apoptotic proteins. Immunohistochemical analysis was performed on paraffin-embedded and micro-sectioned pancreatic tissues as described in methods section. **a**–**c** Representative images showing effect of modified FA and ASP c-SLN combination on p-RB, p21, and p-ERK1/2 protein expressions in pancreatic tissue, respectively. **d**–**f** An increase in the p-RB, p21 and p-ERK1/2 protein expressions was observed in FA + ASP c-SLN treated groups compared to the vehicle control group. All the pictures were taken at ×200 magnification. Statistical significance was determined by one-way ANOVA followed by Dunnett's multiple comparison test post hoc *analysis*. ***$p < 0.001$ represents statistical significance between blank c-SLN vehicle control and FA + ASP c-SLN treatment

suggested that chronic oxidative stress, particularly from chronic inflammation, is associated with carcinogenesis [33, 34]. For example, ulcerative colitis has long been linked with high incidence of colorectal cancer; and chronic gastrititis, such as from infection with *H. pylori*, has been associated with a high incidence of gastric cancer [35, 36]. Recent studies have shown an important role for ROS in tumor development [37, 38]. ROS can be produced from endogenous sources, such as from mitochondria, peroxisomes, and inflammatory cell activation [34, 39]; and exogenous sources, including environmental agents. This oxidative stress then, in turn, may cause DNA, protein, and/or lipid damage, leading to changes in chromosome instability, genetic mutation, and/or modulation of cell growth that may result in cancer. The potential outcomes of oxidative stress occur when not counter-balanced by antioxidant defenses of the cell.

Previous studies in literature show the uptake of SLNs from the intestinal lymphatic system thus bypassing first pass metabolism in the liver, increasing circulation time, reducing dosage and ensuring high bioavailability of the drugs [40–43]. The addition of chitosan also provides steric stabilization of nanoparticles thus reducing their uptake by the reticulo-endothelial (RES) system in the blood [44, 45]. Moreover, chitosan can mediate the opening of tight junctions between epithelial cells reversibly, facilitating the paracellular transport of drug molecules ultimately leading to improved bioavailability of the drugs [29]. Thus, c-SLN combines the advantages of SLN with the biological properties of chitosan as a drug delivery vehicle.

The effect of FA and ASP was initially evaluated by calculating the IC_{50} values and then by combining the ineffective concentrations to exhibit an additive or synergistic effect against the pancreatic cancer cells proving to be more efficacious at lower concentrations. When free FA and ASP were combined at ineffective concentrations of 200 μM and 1 mM respectively, showed 45–60 % inhibition of cell growth. The cell viability assay on FA and ASP entrapped c-SLNs was carried out using FA (40 μM) and ASP (25 μM) as individual concentrations. Individually, they showed little or no decrease in the cell viability, but when combined, a significant reduction by 70 % was observed in MIA PaCa-2 and Panc-1 cells. However, a comparative study between the two forms of the drugs i.e., the free form and c-SLN form showed approximately 5 and 40-fold reductions in FA c-SLN and ASP c-SLN respectively in comparison to the free form of the drugs. Studies have been reported where drug loaded c-SLNs have exhibited better cytotoxicity profile in comparison to the free drug [3, 9]. This has been mainly attributed to the smaller particle size of the nanoparticles which increases the overall uptake of the drug. In order to validate the efficacy of the combination regimen, apoptosis assay was conducted which determined the progression of a cancer cell from four different phases after the addition of the drug: living cell, early apoptotic cell, late apoptotic cell and necrotic cells. These results are consistent with our findings in the cell viability assay.

Pancreatic tumor growth inhibition in in vivo xenograft mice model was observed by the oral administration of 75 and 25 mg/kg FA and ASP c-SLN combination, respectively, even though the effect was not statistically significant. In our previously published study [7], we used SLN encapsulated aspirin at a dose range of 2–20 mg/kg, which demonstrated to be effective in suppressing the progression to pancreatic cancer in a hamster model. In this study, we used a conversion factor to calculate the dose given to the hamster to mouse which resulted in 25 mg/kg of ASP for the current study [46]. For FA, dose of 75 mg/kg used for these experiments were deduced from publications demonstrating the use of higher doses than the proposed dose for the current studies [19, 47, 48]. Other in vivo studies have found elevated levels of detoxifying enzymes in liver and colonic mucosa in rats fed with FA at the dose of 100 mg/kg [17]. In the same study, FA reduced the incidence and multiplicity of intestinal azoxymethane-induced tumors after 35 weeks of oral administration of 250 mg FA/kg body weight/day.

IHC was performed to evaluate the molecular effect of FA + ASP chemopreventive regimens on tumor reduction. This study showed decreased proliferation as documented by PCNA and MKI67 immunostaining, and increased apoptosis as documented by increased p21 expression within tumors. Moreover, our results demonstrate that the upregulation of p-ERK1/2 and p-RB proteins in FA + ASP treatment group compared to vehicle control group. A number of studies have shown the importance of ERK signaling pathway in regulating apoptosis [6, 49, 50]. Although ERK pathway delivers a survival signal, recent studies and our previously published article on chemoprevention of aspirin have linked the activation of p-ERK with induction of apoptosis [51–53]. Our published study also presents a plausible mechanism by which aspirin, curcumin, sulforaphane (ACS) in combination can induce apoptosis in pancreatic cancer cells through activation of the p-ERK1/2 signaling system. The ACS combination initiated p-ERK1/2 induction at 8 h, and the activity remained highly elevated through the remaining time period examined (48 h). It is important to note that there are different mechanisms of ERK activation, such as induction by growth factors could be rapid (occurring within minutes) and transient, which leads to cell proliferation and survival [54]. But persistent or sustained p-ERK1/2 activation that lasts more than 12 h is involved in cell differentiation and death [55]. Our results support the pro-apoptotic role of p-ERK1/2 during FA + ASP treatment and are in agreement with previous studies [6, 51–53].

Conclusions

This study investigated the potential chemopreventive effects of a combination of free FA and ASP as well as c-SLN encapsulated FA and ASP. We demonstrated for the first time that the FA and ASP c-SLN combination showed a synergistic inhibition of cell viability and induced apoptosis in MIA PaCa-2 and Panc-1 human pancreatic cancer cells. Further in vivo studies demonstrated the tumor shrinking capability of this c-SLN combination, even though this was not statistically significant. Immunohistochemical studies indicate the pro-apoptotic role of the regimen from significantly elevated protein expression. In conclusion, the preliminary data obtained from these studies provide a baseline on which further research is warranted to confirm this nanotechnology-based combination regimen as a potentially viable chemopreventive tool in the fight against pancreatic cancer.

Methods

Cell lines and cell culture

Human pancreatic cancer cell lines MIA PaCa-2 and Panc-1 were obtained from American Type Culture Collection (ATCC, Manassas, VA, USA). Cells were cultured in Dulbecco's modified eagle medium (DMEM) supplemented with 10 % fetal bovine serum (FBS), and 1 % penicillin–streptomycin at 37 °C in a 5 % CO_2 humidified environment.

Reagents and antibodies

FA and ASP were purchased from Sigma-Aldrich (St. Louis, MO, USA). Stearic acid, Poloxamer 188, chitosan and lecithin was obtained from Spectrum Chemicals (Gardena, CA, USA). Dichloromethane (DCM) was obtained from Fisher Scientific (Houston, TX, USA). Sodium chloride was purchased from ChemCruz (Santa Cruz, CA, USA). Hydrochloric acid was purchased from Ricca Chemicals (Arlington, TX, USA). The primary antibodies against PCNA, p-ERK1/2 (Thr202/Tyr204), and p-RB were obtained from Cell Signaling Technologies (Danvers, MA, USA). The MKI67 and p21 primary antibodies were purchased from Abcam (Cambridge, MA, USA).

Preparation of chitosan solid lipid nanoparticles (c-SLNs)

FA and ASP c-SLNs were prepared using a hot melt oil-in-water (o/w) emulsion technique (Fig. 7). Stearic acid was used as the lipid to make nanoparticle formulations. Briefly, 1 g of stearic acid was melted by heating at 70 °C. The drug (250 mg) was dissolved in 5 ml of DCM. The drug solution was then added to the melted stearic acid and heated until all DCM was evaporated. The water phase consisted of 2 % poloxamer solution which was heated to the same temperature as that of the oil phase. The volume ratio of oil phase to water phase was kept at 1:10. The oil phase was then added to the poloxamer solution drop wise using continuous high sheer homogenization and the mixture was further sonicated for 30 s using an ultra-sonicator (Los Angeles, CA, USA) to create an o/w emulsion. The emulsion so formed was mixed with equal volume of 0.1 % chitosan dissolved in 0.1 % acetic acid. The mixture of SLNs with chitosan was stirred for 2 h. The resulting chitosan-SLNs were centrifuged and pellet was collected. The c-SLNs were lyophilized in a freeze dryer (Labconco, Kansas City, MO, USA) and subjected to particle size and encapsulation efficiency determination.

Measurement of particle size, encapsulation efficiency and zeta potential

The mean particle size (z-average) and polydispersity index (PDI) as a measure of the width of particle size and distribution was determined by photon correlation spectroscopy using Zetasizer (Nano ZS 90, Malvern Instruments, Malvern, UK) at 25 °C and 90° scattering angle. The c-SLN formulation was diluted with nano-pure water to weaken opalescence before measurements. The surface charge was assessed by measuring zeta potential of c-SLNs based on the Smoluchowski equation, using the same equipment at 25 °C with electric field strength of 23 V/cm [54].

Determination of percentage encapsulation efficiency of FA and ASP c-SLNs

Encapsulation efficiency was determined by dissolving 10 mg of the c-SLN formulation in 10 ml acetonitrile. The drug was released from the lipid into acetonitrile and allowed to dissolve freely for 10 min in a sonicator after which it was filtered through a 0.45 μm filter. The resulting solution was further diluted with acetonitrile and was analyzed by using a Shimadzu LC-20 binary HPLC system (Columbia, MD, USA). Caffeine was used as the

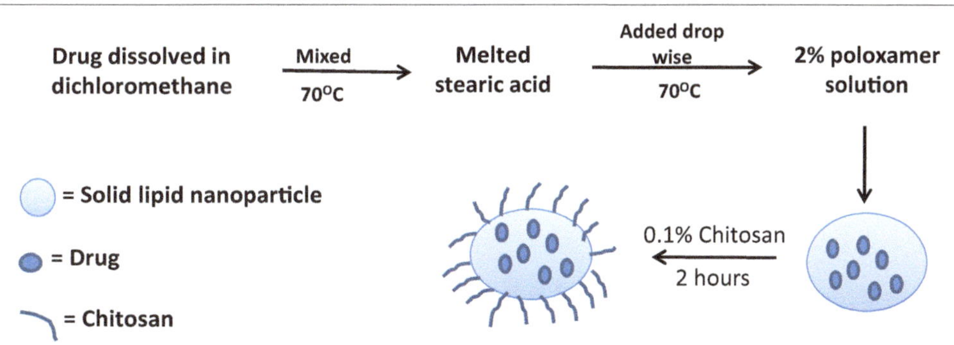

Fig. 7 Schematic representation of chitosan solid lipid nanoparticle (c-SLN) formulation development

internal standard. The entrapment efficiency was calculated using the following formula:

$$EE\,(\%) = \left[Amount\,(mg)\ of\ drug\ per\ HPLC\ method\ /\ theoretical\ yield\,(mg)\right] \times 100.$$

In vitro drug release from FA and ASP c-SLNs

The cumulative release of ASP and CUR from c-SLNs was determined in both phosphate buffered saline (PBS), pH 6.8 and acidic medium, pH 1.6. Briefly, acidic medium composed of a mixture of sodium chloride (34.2 mM), lecithin (20 μM) and hydrochloric acid with pH adjusted to 1.6. Five mg of the c-SLNs were suspended in 50 ml of PBS/acidic medium and placed in an incubator at 37 °C with a shaking speed of 100 rpm. At predetermined time intervals (0, 0.5, 1, 2, 4, 6, 12, 24, 48, 72, 96 h), 1 ml of the buffer was withdrawn and replaced with equivalent volume of fresh buffer. All samples are centrifuged at 5000 rpm for 10 min. The amount of released drug was analyzed using HPLC. The analysis was carried out in triplicate.

Cell viability assay

The cell viability assay was performed according to the manual included with the Promega Cell Titre 96 Aqueous MTS reagent (Madison, WI, USA). Briefly, 7.5×10^3 cells were seeded in 96 well plates and treated with FA and ASP alone and in combination for a period of 72 h. On the last day of the incubation period, 20 % MTS and 1 % of phenazine methosulfate (PMS) were added to the medium and incubated for 2 h at 37 °C and absorbance was measured at 490 nm. All the assays were performed in triplicate.

Flow cytometric analysis for apoptosis

The detection was performed according to the manual included with the Annexin V-fluorescein isothiocyanate (FITC) Vybrant Apoptosis assay kit #3 (Invitrogen, Grand Island, NY). Approximately 1×10^5 MIA PaCa-2 and Panc-1 cells were seeded in six-well plates and treated with c-SLN modified FA and ASP alone and in combination at concentrations of 40 and 25 μM, respectively. After incubation for 48 h, cells were harvested, washed twice with ice-cold phosphate buffer saline (PBS), and then subjected to 5 μl of FITC Annexin V and 1 μl of the 100 μg/ml PI. The samples were analyzed using Beckman Coulter Cytomics FC500.

Western blot analysis

MIA PaCa-2 and Panc-1 cells were treated with FA and ASP alone and in combination for 24 h. Cells were lysed in RIPA buffer and were fractionated on SDS–PAGE gels and then transferred to nitrocellulose membranes. The membranes were blocked with 2 % bovine serum albumin (BSA) in tris-buffered saline (TBS)-Tween 20 and probed with primary antibodies (1:1000 dilution) followed by horseradish peroxidase (HRP)–labeled secondary antibodies (1:5000 dilutions). The blots were probed with the Super Signal West Pico Chemiluminescent substrate (Thermo Scientific, Pittsburgh, PA, USA) to visualize the immunoreactive bands.

Tumor xenograft model

The study was conducted on male severe combined immunodeficient (SCID) mice, 6 weeks old with an average body weight of ~20 g. All animals were maintained in pathogen-free sterile isolators and in a controlled atmosphere with a 12 h light to 12 h dark cycle according to institutional guidelines. All studies were conducted as per protocol approved by the Western University of Health Sciences Institutional Animal Care and Use Committee and conformed to the "Principles of Laboratory Animal Care". Mice were gavage daily with the chemopreventive regimen and weighed twice a week throughout the experimental period. The human pancreatic cancer cells MIA PaCa-2 were grown in DMEM media containing 10 % FBS and harvested in HyQTase cell detachment solution (Hyclone). Cells were resuspended in saline at 1×10^6 cells/0.1 ml volume, and placed on ice. SCID mice were injected with 0.1 ml of the cell suspension subcutaneous on the right flank and observed daily for tumor growth. After transplantation, tumor size was measured using calipers, and the tumor volume was estimated according to the following formula: tumor volume (mm^3) = $L \times W^2$, where L is the length and W is the width. After 5 weeks, mice were sacrificed and tumors were excised immediately.

FA + ASP c-SLN treatment regimen

As indicated in Table 2, this set consisted of five groups (T1–T5) of 4 mice per group. The treatment groups T3-T5 received FA c-SLN, ASP c-SLN alone and a combination of FA + ASP c-SLN regimen daily via oral gavage,

Table 2 Treatment plan showing group of mice treated with c-SLN modified FA, and ASP

Groups	Number of mice	Treatment plan	Dose (mg/kg)
T1	4	Saline (control)	0
T2	4	Blank c-SLN (vehicle control; no drug)	100
T3	4	FA c-SLN	75
T4	4	ASP c-SLN	25
T5	4	FA + ASP c-SLN combination	75 + 25

ASP aspirin, *FA* ferulic acid, *c-SLN* chitosan solid lipid nanoparticle respectively. Treatment started the day after tumor cell implantation and continued every 24 h for 5 weeks. The T1 group served as control and received 0.1 ml PBS, and T2 group received blank c-SLN serving as vehicle control. The dose selected for FA c-SLN and ASP c-SLN regimens were 75 and 25 mg/kg respectively, which was determined based on current evidence in literature [19, 48, 55].

Histological examination

All organs of the thoracic and abdominal cavities were carefully examined in situ macroscopically after euthanization. The MIA PaCa-2 tumor tissue was fixed in 10 % phosphate-buffered formalin for 24 h. The formalin-fixed pancreatic tumor was cut into small pieces at 2 cm intervals, and 5 μm thick sections were processed.

Immunohistochemistry (IHC)

Paraffin-embedded sections of pancreatic tumor tissue were deparaffinized, rehydrated, and heated in citrate buffer (pH 6.0) for 20 min for antigen retrieval. Endogenous peroxidase activity was quenched by incubating the slides in 3 % hydrogen peroxide, followed by washing in PBS-Tween 20. Subsequently, 5 % normal goat serum blocking buffer was applied. The blocking buffer was removed after 1 h of incubation in humidified chamber and primary antibody was added to the slides, incubated overnight at 4 °C. The horseradish peroxidase (HRP)-labelled secondary antibody (Cell Signaling Technologies) was then added and incubated for 90 min at room temperature. The section was developed with ImmPACT DAB peroxidase substrate kit (Vector Labs, Burlingame, CA, USA).

Evaluation of staining

Antibody stained tissues were assessed using scoring system based on the Quickscore method [56]. For IHC staining, the protein stained in brown color was considered labeled/positive and nuclear staining in blue as unlabeled/negative staining. Briefly, the proportion of positive cells were estimated and given a score on a scale of 1–4 (1 = 0–10 %; 2 = 11–30 %; 3 = 31–59 %; 4 = 60–100 %). The intensity of the staining was estimated and given a score from 1–4 (1 = no staining; 2 = weak; 3 = intermediate; and 4 = strong staining). A score was then calculated by multiplying the percentage of positive cells score by the intensity score, to yield a minimum value of 1 and a maximum value of 16.

Statistical analysis

Results were expressed as mean ± SEM. A one-way ANOVA followed by Dunnett's multiple comparison test post hoc *analysis* using Graphpad prism software (La Jolla, CA, USA) was done to analyze and compare the results. A probability value of ≤0.05 % was considered significant.

Abbreviations

FA: ferulic acid; ASP: aspirin; c-SLN: chitosan-solid-lipid nanoparticle; NSAIDs: non-steroidal anti-inflammatory drugs; ROS: reactive oxygen species; DCM: dichloromethane; PDI: polydispersity index; PMS: phenazine methosulfate; FITC: fluorescein isothiocyanate; PCNA: proliferation cell nuclear antigen; ERK1/2: extracellular signal-regulated kinases; RB: retinoblastoma; IHC: immunohistochemistry; HRP: horseradish peroxidase; RES: reticuloendothelial system; MAPK: mitogen activated protein kinases.

Authors' contributions

AT designed the study and carried out most of the experiments and drafted the manuscript; SC assisted in in vitro and in vivo studies; JW was involved in the revising the manuscript; SP conceived the studies, coordinated the experiments and was involved in the drafting the manuscript and revising it. All authors read and approved the final manuscript.

Compliance with ethical guidelines

Competing interests

The authors declare that they have no competing interests.

References

1. Siegel R, Ma J, Zou Z, Jemal A. Cancer statistics, 2014. CA Cancer J Clin. 2014;64(1):9–29. doi:10.3322/caac.21208.
2. DeSantis CE, Lin CC, Mariotto AB, Siegel RL, Stein KD, Kramer JL, et al. Cancer treatment and survivorship statistics, 2014. CA Cancer J Clin. 2014;64(4):252–71. doi:10.3322/caac.21235.
3. Sutaria D, Grandhi BK, Thakkar A, Wang J, Prabhu S. Chemoprevention of pancreatic cancer using solid-lipid nanoparticulate delivery of a novel aspirin, curcumin and sulforaphane drug combination regimen. Int J Oncol. 2012;41(6):2260–8. doi:10.3892/ijo.2012.1636.
4. Serrano D, Lazzeroni M, Decensi A. Chemoprevention of colorectal cancer: an update. Tech Coloproctol. 2004;8(Suppl 2):s248–52. doi:10.1007/s10151-004-0170-5.
5. Thun MJ, Henley SJ, Patrono C. Nonsteroidal anti-inflammatory drugs as anticancer agents: mechanistic, pharmacologic, and clinical issues. J Natl Cancer Inst. 2002;94(4):252–66.
6. Thakkar A, Sutaria D, Grandhi BK, Wang J, Prabhu S. The molecular mechanism of action of aspirin, curcumin and sulforaphane combinations in the chemoprevention of pancreatic cancer. Oncol Rep. 2013;29(4):1671–7. doi:10.3892/or.2013.2276.
7. Grandhi BK, Thakkar A, Wang J, Prabhu S. A novel combinatorial nanotechnology-based oral chemopreventive regimen demonstrates significant suppression of pancreatic cancer neoplastic lesions. Cancer Prev Res. 2013;6(10):1015–25. doi:10.1158/1940-6207.CAPR-13-0172.
8. Chaudhary A, Sutaria D, Huang Y, Wang J, Prabhu S. Chemoprevention of colon cancer in a rat carcinogenesis model using a novel nanotechnology-based combined treatment system. Cancer Prev Res. 2011;4(10):1655–64. doi:10.1158/1940-6207.CAPR-11-0129.
9. Thakkar A, Chenreddy S, Wang J, Prabhu S. Evaluation of ibuprofen loaded solid lipid nanoparticles and its combination regimens for pancreatic cancer chemoprevention. Int J Oncol. 2015;46(4):1827–34. doi:10.3892/ijo.2015.2879.
10. Frenkel K. Carcinogen-mediated oxidant formation and oxidative DNA damage. Pharmacol Ther. 1992;53(1):127–66.

11. Coussens LM, Werb Z. Inflammatory cells and cancer: think different! J Exp Med. 2001;193(6):F23–6.
12. Farrow B, Evers BM. Inflammation and the development of pancreatic cancer. Surg Oncol. 2002;10(4):153–69.
13. Garcea G, Dennison AR, Steward WP, Berry DP. Role of inflammation in pancreatic carcinogenesis and the implications for future therapy. Pancreatology. 2005;5(6):514–29. doi:10.1159/000087493.
14. Kovacic P, Jacintho JD. Mechanisms of carcinogenesis: focus on oxidative stress and electron transfer. Curr Med Chem. 2001;8(7):773–96.
15. Federico A, Morgillo F, Tuccillo C, Ciardiello F, Loguercio C. Chronic inflammation and oxidative stress in human carcinogenesis. Int J Cancer. 2007;121(11):2381–6. doi:10.1002/ijc.23192.
16. Graf E. Antioxidant potential of ferulic acid. Free Radic Biol Med. 1992;13(4):435–48.
17. Kawabata K, Yamamoto T, Hara A, Shimizu M, Yamada Y, Matsunaga K, et al. Modifying effects of ferulic acid on azoxymethane-induced colon carcinogenesis in F344 rats. Cancer Lett. 2000;157(1):15–21.
18. Mori H, Kawabata K, Yoshimi N, Tanaka T, Murakami T, Okada T, et al. Chemopreventive effects of ferulic acid on oral and rice germ on large bowel carcinogenesis. Anticancer Res. 1999;19(5A):3775–8.
19. Wargovich MJ, Jimenez A, McKee K, Steele VE, Velasco M, Woods J, et al. Efficacy of potential chemopreventive agents on rat colon aberrant crypt formation and progression. Carcinogenesis. 2000;21(6):1149–55.
20. Zhang Z, Rigas B. NF-kappaB, inflammation and pancreatic carcinogenesis: NF-kappaB as a chemoprevention target (review). Int J Oncol. 2006;29(1):185–92.
21. Anderson KE, Johnson TW, Lazovich D, Folsom AR. Association between nonsteroidal anti-inflammatory drug use and the incidence of pancreatic cancer. J Natl Cancer Inst. 2002;94(15):1168–71.
22. Jacobs EJ, Connell CJ, Rodriguez C, Patel AV, Calle EE, Thun MJ. Aspirin use and pancreatic cancer mortality in a large United States cohort. J Natl Cancer Inst. 2004;96(7):524–8.
23. Schernhammer ES, Kang JH, Chan AT, Michaud DS, Skinner HG, Giovannucci E, et al. A prospective study of aspirin use and the risk of pancreatic cancer in women. J Natl Cancer Inst. 2004;96(1):22–8.
24. Roy K, Mao HQ, Huang SK, Leong KW. Oral gene delivery with chitosan–DNA nanoparticles generates immunologic protection in a murine model of peanut allergy. Nat Med. 1999;5(4):387–91. doi:10.1038/7385.
25. Maezaki Y, Tsuji K, Nakagawa Y, Kawai Y, Akimoto M, Tsugita T, et al. Hypocholesterolemic effect of chitosan in adult males. Biosci Biotech Bioch. 1993;57(9):1439–44.
26. Sogias IA, Williams AC, Khutoryanskiy VV. Why is chitosan mucoadhesive? Biomacromolecules. 2008;9(7):1837–42. doi:10.1021/bm800276d.
27. van der Lubben IM, Verhoef JC, Borchard G, Junginger HE. Chitosan and its derivatives in mucosal drug and vaccine delivery. Eur J Pharm Sci. 2001;14(3):201–7.
28. Sakloetsakun D, Perera G, Hombach J, Millotti G, Bernkop-Schnurch A. The impact of vehicles on the mucoadhesive properties of orally administrated nanoparticles: a case study with chitosan-4-thiobutylamidine conjugate. AAPS PharmSciTech. 2010;11(3):1185–92. doi:10.1208/s12249-010-9479-8.
29. Fonte P, Andrade F, Araujo F, Andrade C, Neves J, Sarmento B. Chitosan-coated solid lipid nanoparticles for insulin delivery. Methods Enzymol. 2012;508:295–314. doi:10.1016/B978-0-12-391860-4.00015-X.
30. Hou YZ, Yang J, Zhao GR, Yuan YJ. Ferulic acid inhibits vascular smooth muscle cell proliferation induced by angiotensin II. Eur J Pharmacol. 2004;499(1–2):85–90. doi:10.1016/j.ejphar.2004.07.107.
31. Janicke B, Hegardt C, Krogh M, Onning G, Akesson B, Cirenajwis HM, et al. The antiproliferative effect of dietary fiber phenolic compounds ferulic acid and p-coumaric acid on the cell cycle of Caco-2 cells. Nutr Cancer. 2011;63(4):611–22. doi:10.1080/01635581.2011.538486.
32. Bandugula VR, Prasad R. 2-Deoxy-D-glucose and ferulic acid modulates radiation response signaling in non-small cell lung cancer cells. Tumour Biol. 2013;34(1):251–9. doi:10.1007/s13277-012-0545-6.
33. Hwang ES, Bowen PE. DNA damage, a biomarker of carcinogenesis: its measurement and modulation by diet and environment. Crit Rev Food Sci Nutr. 2007;47(1):27–50. doi:10.1080/10408390600550299.
34. Klaunig JE, Kamendulis LM, Hocevar BA. Oxidative stress and oxidative damage in carcinogenesis. Toxicol Pathol. 2010;38(1):96–109. doi:10.1177/0192623309356453.
35. Seril DN, Liao J, Yang GY, Yang CS. Oxidative stress and ulcerative colitis-associated carcinogenesis: studies in humans and animal models. Carcinogenesis. 2003;24(3):353–62.
36. Konturek PC, Konturek SJ, Brzozowski T. Gastric cancer and *Helicobacter pylori* infection. J Physiol Pharmacol. 2006;57(Suppl 3):51–65.
37. Kumar B, Koul S, Khandrika L, Meacham RB, Koul HK. Oxidative stress is inherent in prostate cancer cells and is required for aggressive phenotype. Cancer Res. 2008;68(6):1777–85. doi:10.1158/0008-5472.CAN-07-5259.
38. Ishikawa K, Takenaga K, Akimoto M, Koshikawa N, Yamaguchi A, Imanishi H, et al. ROS-generating mitochondrial DNA mutations can regulate tumor cell metastasis. Science. 2008;320(5876):661–4. doi:10.1126/science.1156906.
39. Klaunig JE, Kamendulis LM. The role of oxidative stress in carcinogenesis. Annu Rev Pharmacol Toxicol. 2004;44:239–67. doi:10.1146/annurev.pharmtox.44.101802.121851.
40. Ling SS, Magosso E, Khan NA, Yuen KH, Barker SA. Enhanced oral bioavailability and intestinal lymphatic transport of a hydrophilic drug using liposomes. Drug Dev Ind Pharm. 2006;32(3):335–45. doi:10.1080/03639040500519102.
41. Hashida N, Murakami M, Yoshikawa H, Takada K, Muranishi S. Intestinal absorption of carboxyfluorescein entrapped in liposomes in comparison with its administration with lipid-surfactant mixed micelles. J Pharmacobiodyn. 1984;7(3):195–203.
42. Yuan H, Chen J, Du YZ, Hu FQ, Zeng S, Zhao HL. Studies on oral absorption of stearic acid SLN by a novel fluorometric method. Colloids Surf B. 2007;58(2):157–64. doi:10.1016/j.colsurfb.2007.03.002.
43. Sanjula B, Shah FM, Javed A, Alka A. Effect of poloxamer 188 on lymphatic uptake of carvedilol-loaded solid lipid nanoparticles for bioavailability enhancement. J Drug Target. 2009;17(3):249–56. doi:10.1080/10611860902718672.
44. Yuan H, Jiang SP, Du YZ, Miao J, Zhang XG, Hu FQ. Strategic approaches for improving entrapment of hydrophilic peptide drugs by lipid nanoparticles. Colloids Surf B. 2009;70(2):248–53. doi:10.1016/j.colsurfb.2008.12.031.
45. Chen MC, Mi FL, Liao ZX, Hsiao CW, Sonaje K, Chung MF, et al. Recent advances in chitosan-based nanoparticles for oral delivery of macromolecules. Adv Drug Deliv Rev. 2013;65(6):865–79. doi:10.1016/j.addr.2012.10.010.
46. Reagan-Shaw S, Nihal M, Ahmad N. Dose translation from animal to human studies revisited. FASEB J. 2008;22(3):659–61. doi:10.1096/fj.07-9574LSF.
47. Suzuki A, Kagawa D, Fujii A, Ochiai R, Tokimitsu I, Saito I. Short- and long-term effects of ferulic acid on blood pressure in spontaneously hypertensive rats. Am J Hypertens. 2002;15(4 Pt 1):351–7.
48. Huang MT, Smart RC, Wong CQ, Conney AH. Inhibitory effect of curcumin, chlorogenic acid, caffeic acid, and ferulic acid on tumor promotion in mouse skin by 12-*O*-tetradecanoylphorbol-13-acetate. Cancer Res. 1988;48(21):5941–6.
49. Pearson G, Robinson F, Beers Gibson T, Xu BE, Karandikar M, Berman K, et al. Mitogen-activated protein (MAP) kinase pathways: regulation and physiological functions. Endocr Rev. 2001;22(2):153–83. doi:10.1210/edrv.22.2.0428.
50. Adachi T, Kar S, Wang M, Carr BI. Transient and sustained ERK phosphorylation and nuclear translocation in growth control. J Cell Physiol. 2002;192(2):151–9. doi:10.1002/jcp.10124.
51. Im SR, Jang YJ. Aspirin enhances TRAIL-induced apoptosis via regulation of ERK1/2 activation in human cervical cancer cells. Biochem Biophys Res Commun. 2012;424(1):65–70. doi:10.1016/j.bbrc.2012.06.067.
52. Marshall CJ. Specificity of receptor tyrosine kinase signaling: transient versus sustained extracellular signal-regulated kinase activation. Cell. 1995;80(2):179–85.
53. Chen JR, Plotkin LI, Aguirre JI, Han L, Jilka RL, Kousteni S, et al. Transient versus sustained phosphorylation and nuclear accumulation of ERKs underlie anti-versus pro-apoptotic effects of estrogens. J Biol Chem. 2005;280(6):4632–8. doi:10.1074/jbc.M411530200.
54. Sze A, Erickson D, Ren L, Li D. Zeta-potential measurement using the Smoluchowski equation and the slope of the current-time relationship in electroosmotic flow. J Colloid Interface Sci. 2003;261(2):402–10. doi:10.1016/S0021-9797(03)00142-5.

55. Ouyang N, Williams JL, Tsioulias GJ, Gao J, Iatropoulos MJ, Kopelovich L, et al. Nitric oxide-donating aspirin prevents pancreatic cancer in a hamster tumor model. Cancer Res. 2006;66(8):4503–11. doi:10.1158/0008-5472.CAN-05-3118.

56. Detre S, Saclani Jotti g, Dowsett M. A "quickscore" method for immunohistochemical semiquantitation: validation for oestrogen receptor in breast carcinomas. J Clin Pathol. 1995;48(9):876–8.

Characterization of novel carcinoma cell lines for the analysis of therapeutical strategies fighting pancreatic cancer

Dietmar Zechner[1*], Florian Bürtin[1], Jonas Amme[1], Tobias Lindner[2], Tobias Radecke[1], Stefan Hadlich[3], Jens-Peter Kühn[3] and Brigitte Vollmar[1]

Abstract

Background: Preclinical evaluations of chemotherapies depend on clinically relevant animal models for pancreatic cancer. The injection of syngeneic murine adenocarcinoma cells is one efficient option to generate carcinomas in mice with an intact immune system. However, this option is constrained by the paucity of appropriate cell lines.

Results: The murine pancreatic adenocarcinoma cell lines 6606PDA and 7265PDA were compared to the 6606l cell line isolated from a liver metastasis from mice suffering from pancreatic cancer. In tissue culture 6606PDA and 6606l proliferated faster than 7265PDA. 7265PDA cells were, however, significantly more sensitive to gemcitabine as assessed by BrdU-incorporation and trypan blue exclusion assays in vitro. Within 1 week after injection of either one of these three cell lines into the pancreas of C57BL/6J mice, carcinomas were observed by T2 weighted magnetic resonance imaging and histology. Three weeks after injecting 6606PDA or 6606l cells large carcinomas could be characterized, which were surrounded by extensive desmoplastic reaction. After injection of 7265PDA cells, however, remission of cancer was observed between the first and the third week. Compared to 6606PDA cell derived carcinomas a higher apparent diffusion coefficient was quantified by diffusion weighted magnetic resonance imaging in these tumors. This correlated with reduced cancer cell density observed on histological sections.

Conclusion: All three cell lines can be used in vitro for testing combinatorial therapies with gemcitabine. The 6606PDA and 6606l cell lines but not the 7265PDA cell line can be used for evaluating distinct therapies in a syngeneic carcinoma model using C57BL/6J mice. Diffusion-weighted MRI proved to be an appropriate method to predict tumor remission.

Keywords: Syngeneic cancer model, Pancreatic ductal adenocarcinoma, Noninvasive imaging, Cancer remission, Combinatorial therapy, Cancer immunology, Desmoplasia

Background

Although multiple radiation therapies and chemotherapies in addition to surgical intervention have been evaluated over the last decades, the 5-year survival rate of pancreatic cancer patients is still only 7 % [1]. Recently, clinical studies demonstrated prolonged survival of patients after the application of novel combinatorial chemotherapies such as FOLFIRINOX or the combination of gemcitabine with nab-paclitaxel or S-1 [2–4]. However, these novel therapies can prolong the survival of patients only by a few weeks. Since progress in the treatment of pancreatic ductal adenocarcinoma (PDA) has been modest, the evaluation of novel therapies and the investigation of all pathophysiological aspects of PDA continue to be essential.

The evaluation of therapies in tissue culture along with the analysis in an orthotopic cancer model combines the advantages of in vitro studies with the advantages of a clinically relevant animal model [5, 6]. Tissue culture allows the evaluation of combinatorial therapies on isolated cancer cells in a fast and cost efficient way, whereas

*Correspondence: dietmar.zechner@uni-rostock.de
[1] Institute for Experimental Surgery, Rostock University Medical Center, University of Rostock, Schillingallee 69a, 18057 Rostock, Germany
Full list of author information is available at the end of the article

a syngeneic orthotopic cancer model allows the in vivo evaluation of therapies while considering clinically relevant factors such as a desmoplastic reaction, an intact immune system, and pharmacokinetic aspects of applied therapies [7]. It has been suggested that mice with orthotopically implanted syngeneic tumors are clinically more relevant than alternative animal models [7].

However, only few cell lines are available for PDA in a syngeneic orthotopic cancer model. Panc02 cells, derived from C57BL/6 mice after treating the animals with 3-methyl-cholanthrene, were originally characterized more than 30 years ago [8]. These pancreatic adenocarcinoma cells have been used in many studies but have probably accumulated genetic changes over time in distinct laboratories. Recently, the need for additional carcinoma cell lines has been addressed by characterizing cancer cells, which were isolated from genetically modified mice with a C57BL/6 or mixed B6/129 background [9, 10]. However, cells derived from a mixed background require the evaluation of histocompatibility of recipient mice [9]. The 6606PDA cell line, which is syngeneic to the C57BL/6J mouse strain, has first been described in 2011 [11]. This cell line has been reported to generate more differentiated glandular adenocarcinomas than Panc02 cells when injected into the pancreas head [12].

The purpose of this study was to compare the characteristics of two novel cell lines, 7265PDA and 66061, with 6606PDA cells in vitro. In addition, we evaluated these cell lines in a mouse model after orthotopic injection by analyzing tumor growth using magnetic resonance imaging (MRI) at two different time points.

Results and discussion

Characterization of 6606PDA, 6606l, and 7265PDA cells in vitro

When plated on tissue culture dishes, the cells of the murine cell lines, 6606PDA and 6606l, showed a similar morphology. At low cell density these cells had a stretched fibroblast like appearance (Fig. 1a). However,

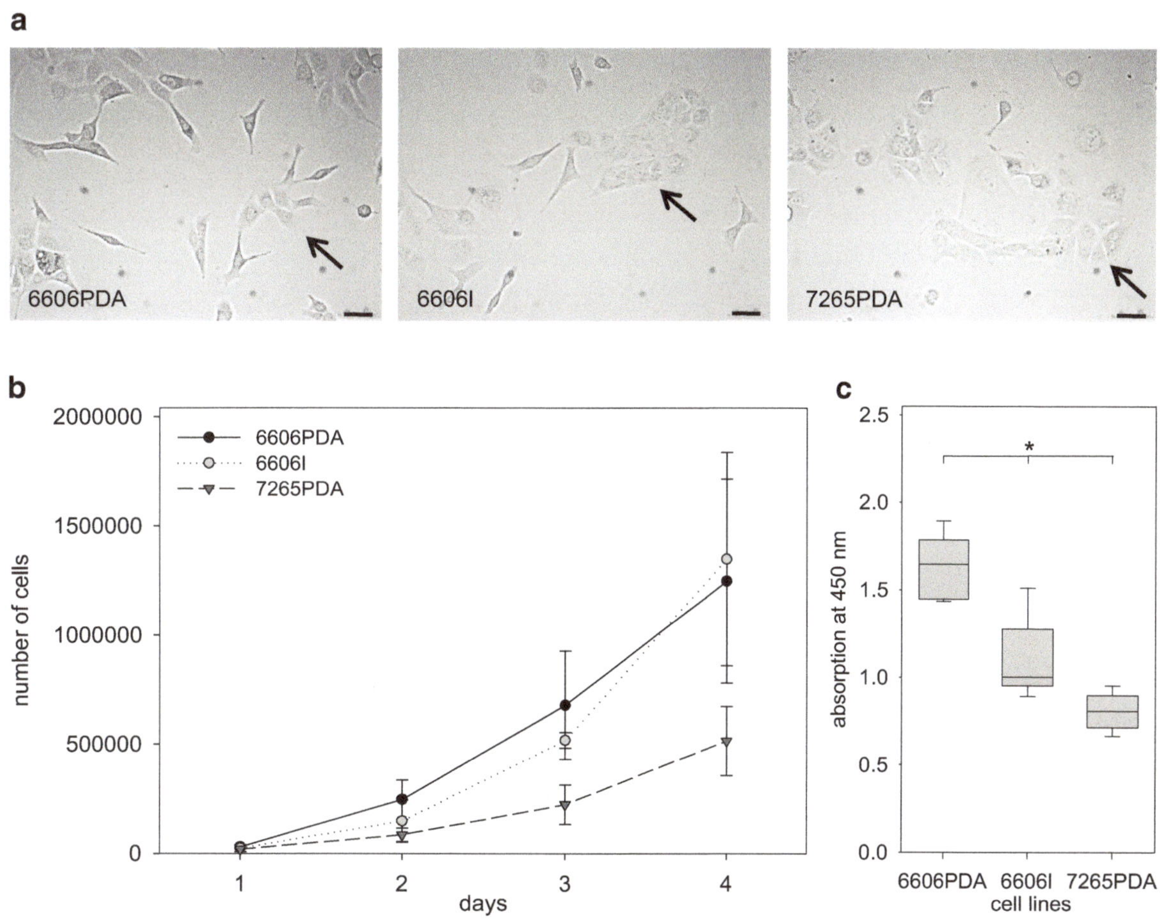

Fig. 1 Characterization of carcinoma cell lines in tissue culture. **a** Characteristic images of 6606PDA, 6606l, and 7265PDA cells grown on tissue culture plates with partial epithelioid morphology (*arrow*). **b** Quantification of cell expansion of indicated cells lines by direct counting of cells (number of independent experiments: 4 for each cell line). **c** Quantification of cell expansion of indicated cells lines by WST-1 assay. Significant differences (*P $\leq$ 0.009) between all three cell lines are indicated in the *box plot* (number of independent experiments: 6 for each cell line). *Bar* 50 μm

when these cells could form intercellular contacts, their appearance changed to a distinct flat epithelioid morphology (Fig. 1a). 7265 PDA cells preferentially showed a flat epithelioid morphology (Fig. 1a). Proliferation of these cells was quantified directly by counting them or indirectly by WST-Assay (Fig. 1b, c). When the cells were subconfluent, 6606PDA cells proliferated faster than 6606l cells, whereas 7265PDA cells were the slowest to divide (Fig. 1b, c).

In order to evaluate if these cell lines are sensitive to gemcitabine, an established drug for chemotherapy, we treated all three cell lines with distinct concentrations of gemcitabine and quantified cell proliferation indirectly by WST-assay (Fig. 2a, b) or directly by measuring

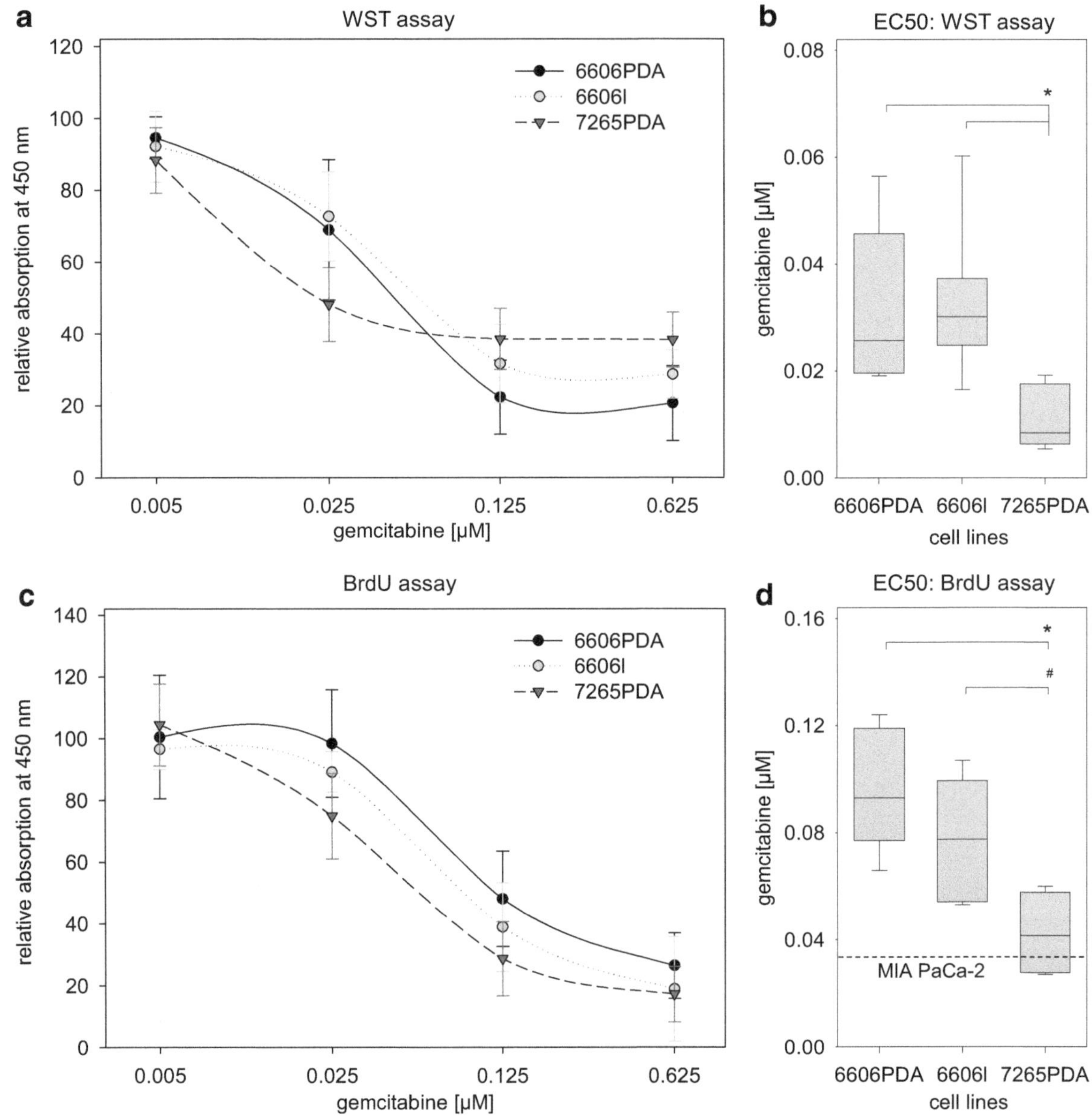

Fig. 2 Inhibition of proliferation by gemcitabine. **a** Quantification of cell proliferation of 6606PDA, 6606l, and 7265PDA cells grown in media containing the indicated gemcitabine concentrations using WST-1 assays. **b** Comparison of EC50 values for each indicated cell line as measured by WST-1 assay. **c** Quantification of gemcitabine dependent cell proliferation of 6606PDA, 6606l, and 7265PDA cells using BrdU incorporation assays. **d** Presentation of EC50 values for each indicated cell line as measured by BrdU incorporation and comparison to published EC50 values from MIA PaCa-2 cells [13]. Significant differences (*P = 0.001) and a tendentious difference (#P = 0.026) are shown in the *box plots* (number of independent experiments: n = 7 for 6606PDA; n = 8 for 6606l, n = 7 for 7265PDA in **a** and **b**; n = 7 for 6606PDA; n = 6 for 6606l, n = 6 in **c** and **d**)

5-bromo-2′-deoxyuridine (BrdU) incorporation (Fig. 2c, d). A concentration dependent inhibition of proliferation was observed with all three cell lines using either assay (Fig. 2a, c). For 7265PDA cells, however, a lower half maximal effective concentration (EC50) of gemcitabine could be defined compared to those of 6606PDA or 6606l cells (Fig. 2b, d). All three cell lines exhibited EC50 values for gemcitabine similar to human cell lines such as MIA PaCa-2 cells [13]. We also quantified cell death of these cell lines after treatment with gemcitabine. Gemcitabine strongly induced cell death in all three cell lines (Fig. 3). Gemcitabine induced a higher percentage of dead cells in 7265PDA cells when compared to gemcitabine treated 6606PDA and 6606l cells (Fig. 3). This confirmed that 7265PDA cells are more sensitive to gemcitabine (Fig. 3). A lower percentage of dead cells was observed after gemcitabine treatment of 6606l cells when compared to 6606PDA cells, although inhibition of proliferation after gemcitabine was similar between 6606PDA and 6606l cells (Figs. 2, 3). Probably mutations, which limit cell death in response to gemcitabine, accumulated in the 6606l cell line. Due to the observed sensitivity to gemcitabine all three cell lines should be especially useful in evaluating additional chemotherapeutical agents in combination with gemcitabine in future. Such preclinical studies have been published for several other cell lines such as AsPC-1, SUIT-2, MIA PaCa-2, or Panc02 cells [14–17].

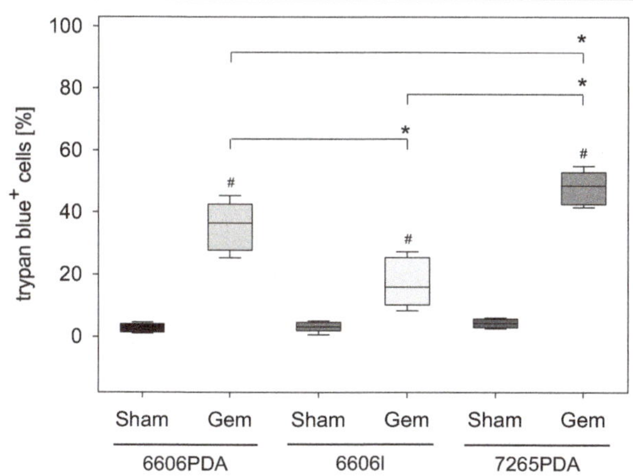

Fig. 3 Induction of cell death by gemcitabine. **a** Quantification of cell death of 6606PDA, 6606l, and 7265PDA cells grown in unsupplemented medium (Sham) or medium supplemented with 625 nM gemcitabine (Gem) using a trypan blue exclusion assay. Significant differences between indicated cohorts (*$P \leq 0.005$); and significant differences between cells of the identical cell line ($^{\#}P \leq 0.001$) grown in gemcitabine versus control medium are shown in the *box plot* (number of independent experiments: n = 10 for 6606PDA; n = 8 for 6606l, n = 7 for 7265PDA)

Characterization of 6606PDA, 6606l, and 7265PDA cells in vivo

In order to evaluate, if these cell lines can be used in a syngeneic orthotopic pancreas carcinoma model, these cells were injected into the pancreas head of C57BL/6J mice on day 0 and the pancreata were analyzed during the early phase (on day 5–7) and during the late phase, on day 20 or 21 (Fig. 4a). After injection of either cell line an insignificant postoperative decline in body weight was observed, but no cachexia developed within 3 weeks (Fig. 4b). The blood glucose concentration was also stable throughout this study (Fig. 4c). These data suggest that within 3 weeks these cell lines cannot be used for examining cachexia or diabetes as paraneoplastic phenomena that have been suggested to occur in patients with pancreatic cancer [18, 19].

To monitor tumors, we assessed the pancreata of mice by 7 T MRI during the early phase (day 5 or 6) and during the late phase of tumor growth (day 20). Carcinomas could be identified during the early phase irrespective of the cell line used (Fig. 5a). Carcinomas could also be identified easily during the late phase when 6606PDA and 6606l cells were injected. However, in most cases carcinomas could not be identified when 7265PDA cells were injected (Fig. 5b). We quantified this observation and noticed that after injecting a total number of 6 animals with 6606PDA cells 6 carcinomas could be identified during the early phase and 6 carcinomas during the late phase of tumor growth (Fig. 5c). When injecting a total number of 6 mice with 6606l cells 5 carcinomas could be identified during the early phase and 4 carcinomas during the late phase (Fig. 5c). The median tumor weight of 6606PDA and 6606l derived tumors on day 21 was 126 mg (interquartile range 101–154 mg) and 145 mg (interquartile range 25–208 mg), respectively (Fig. 5d). Thus, these two cell lines generate carcinomas in immunocompetent C57BL/6J mice and should be particularly valuable in studying various aspects of cancer immunology. When injecting a total number of 11 mice with 7265PDA cells 8 carcinomas could be identified during the early phase of tumor growth and only 1 carcinoma could be observed during the late phase with a tumor weight of 110 mg (Fig. 5c, d). Thus, seven mice have completely lost the tumor within 2 weeks. In this group the number of animals was increased to 11 mice in order to verify the reproducibility of the observed carcinoma remission. Macroscopic inspection of the pancreas after laparotomy of the animals verified that MRI accurately identified the presence or the absence of carcinomas. We also injected a total number of four immunocompromised NMRI-Foxn1$^{nu/nu}$ mice with 7265PDA cells and observed that all mice developed carcinomas

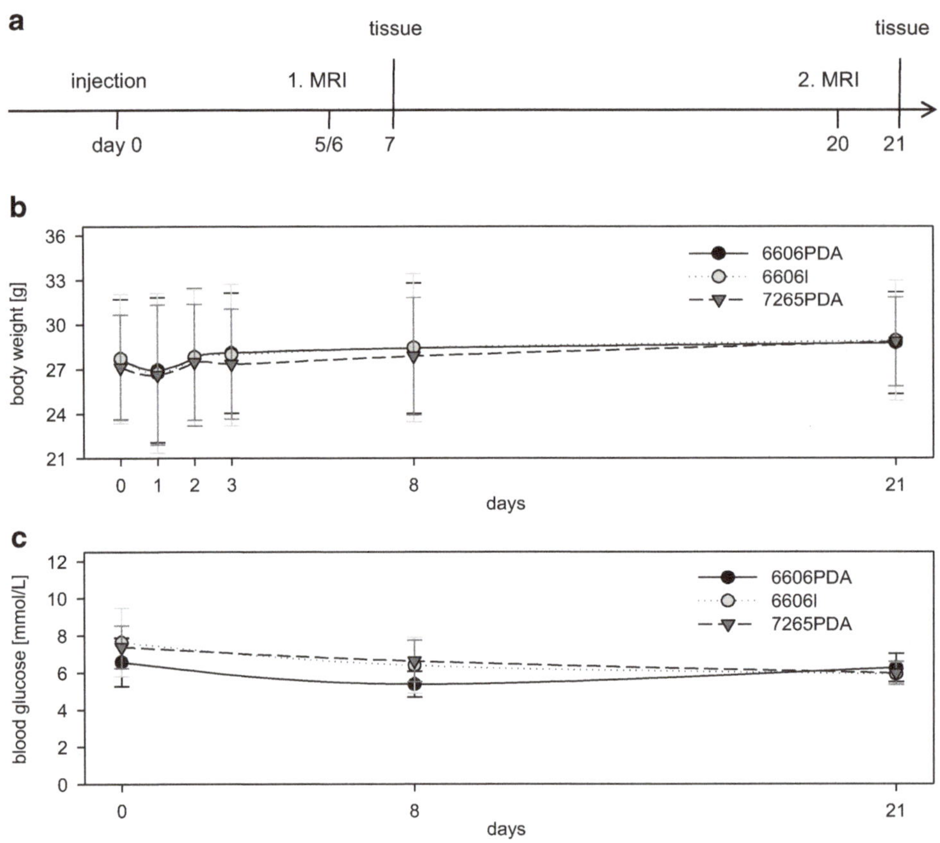

Fig. 4 The Murine carcinoma model. **a** Experimental protocol: injection of carcinoma cells into the pancreas head on day 0, first MRI during early phase (day 5 or 6), second MRI during the late phase of tumor growth (day 20), and analysis of the tissue on day 7 or 21. **b** Mouse body weight at indicated time points after injection of 6606PDA, 6606l, or 7265PDA cells. **c** Blood glucose concentration at indicated time points after injection of 6606PDA, 6606l, or 7265PDA cells. Number of animals analyzed: n = 6 for 6606PDA; n = 6 for 6606l, n = 11 for 7265PDA; 2 independent experiments

within 21 days (median tumor weight: 325 mg; interquartile range 216–563 mg). The remission of carcinomas after injection of 7265PDA cells in C57BL/6J mice suggests that this mouse strain is not syngeneic to this cell line. Indeed, information obtained from the laboratory of David Tuveson (Cambridge, UK) suggests that this cell line was isolated from a mouse with a mixed Bl6/129 background. Thus, for 7265PDA cells the use of immunocompromised mouse strains or mice with matched histocompatibility will be mandatory.

To characterize differences between carcinomas derived from 6606PDA cells and 7265PDA diffusion-weighted MRI was performed during the early phase of tumor growth (Fig. 6a). Interestingly the calculated apparent diffusion coefficient (ADC), measured at the edge of both classes of carcinomas, was higher in carcinomas derived from 7265PDA cells than in carcinomas derived from 6606PDA cells (Fig. 6b). This observation correlated well with the histology of these tumors. 6606PDA cell derived carcinomas were characterized by many densely packed cancer cells (Fig. 6c upper panel). Inflammatory cells surrounded these carcinomas, but only few inflammatory cells were observed within these carcinomas (Fig. 6c upper panel). 7265PDA cell derived carcinomas were characterized by oedema, massive infiltration of inflammatory cells, and few loosely packed cancer cells (Fig. 6c lower panel). These data suggest that less than a week after injection of 7265PDA cells the immune system of C57BL/6J mice prevented the accumulation of densely packed cancer cells. Instead, infiltrating inflammatory cells lead to a local oedema which results in a higher ADC value when diffusion-weighted MRI was performed.

On day 21 cells with epithelial morphology could be observed in carcinomas derived from all three cell lines (Fig. 7a–c). All carcinomas were largely encapsulated by fibroblast like cells (Fig. 7d–f). On individual histological sections of 6606PDA or 6606l derived tumors, the carcinomas lacked complete encapsulation by fibroblast like cells (Fig. 7g–h). This suggests moderate infiltrative

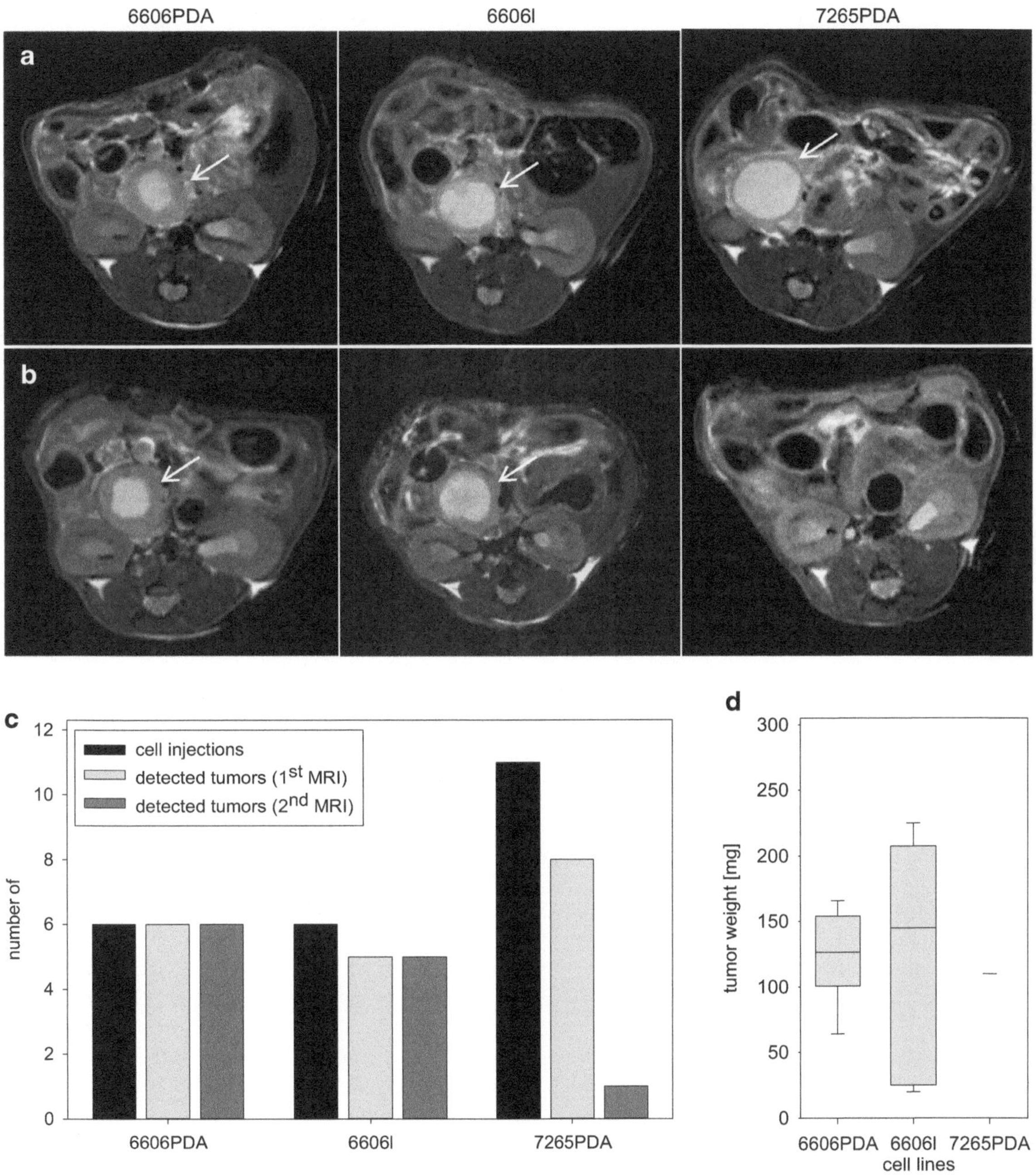

Fig. 5 Characterization of carcinoma cell lines in vivo. **a** Characteristic T2-weighted MRI of 6606PDA, 6606l, and 7265PDA cell derived carcinomas (*arrows*) during early phase of tumor growth (day 5/6). **b** Characteristic T2-weighted MRI of carcinomas (*arrows*) during late phase of tumor growth (day 20). **c** Graphical presentation of the number of cell injections carried out and the number of detected tumors at the first MRI or the second MRI for 6606PDA, 6606l, and 7265PDA cells (number of mice analyzed: n = 6 for 6606PDA; n = 6 for 6606l, n = 11 for 7265PDA). **d** Comparison of tumor weight for indicated cell lines on day 21. Number of tumors analyzed: n = 6 for 6606PDA; n = 5 for 6606l, n = 1 for 7265PDA; 2 independent experiments

growth of the cancer cells (Fig. 7g–h). A deficiency in encapsulation was not observed in the one carcinoma derived from 7265PDA cells (Fig. 7i). Consistent with the observation that infiltrative growth was hardly observed on day 21, we did also not detect any hepatic metastasis by macroscopic evaluation of the liver (data not shown). Since during the early phase (day 5 or day 6) the carcinomas derived from these three cell lines were barely

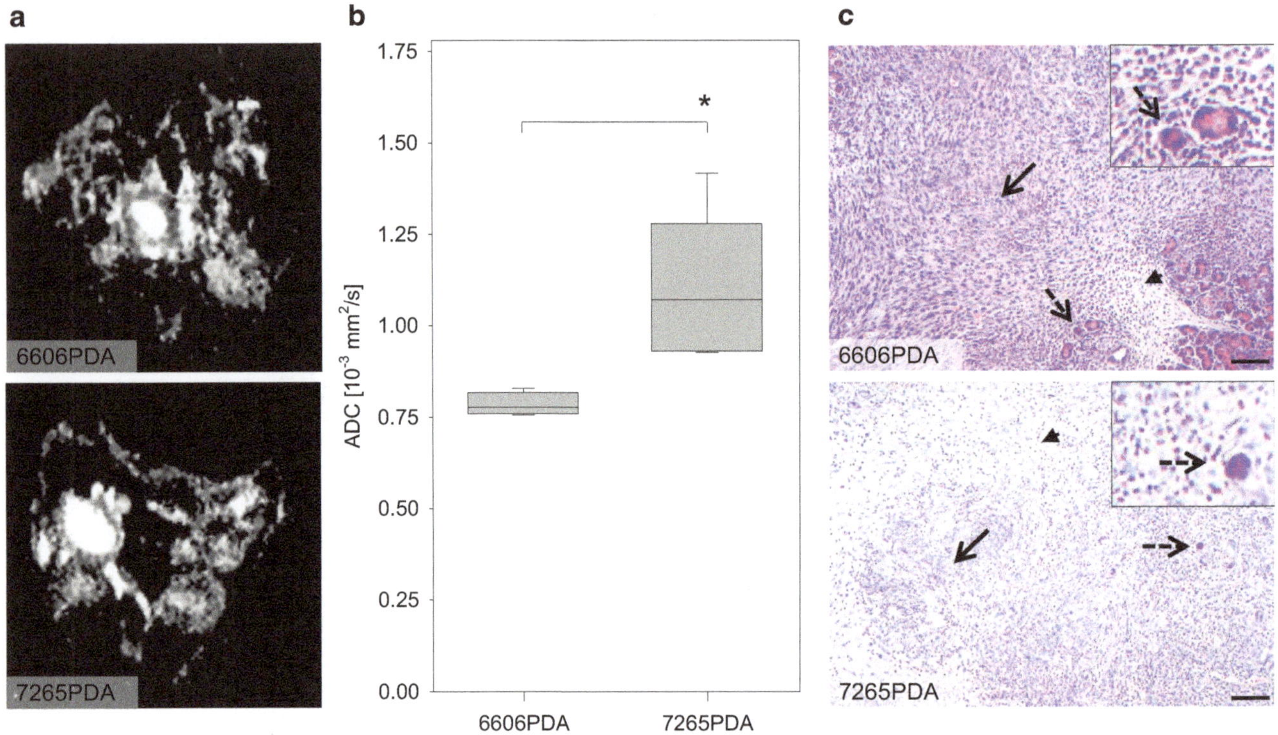

Fig. 6 Characterization of carcinomas by diffusion-weighted MRI and histology during the early phase of tumor growth. **a** Characteristic diffusion-weighted MRI of 6606PDA and 7265PDA cell derived carcinomas (day 5/6). **b** Quantification of water diffusion of 6606PDA and 7265PDA cell derived carcinomas by diffusion-weighted MRI, as given by the ADC value. **c** characteristic haematoxylin/eosin (H/E) staining of histological sections of carcinomas during the early phase of tumor growth (*dotted arrow* pancreatic acinar cells, *arrow* cancer cells, *arrowhead* oedema with infiltrating inflammatory cells). A significant difference between indicated cohorts (*P = 0.01) is shown in the *box plot* (number of tumors analyzed: n = 4 for 6606PDA, n = 6 for 7265PDA; 2 independent experiments). *Bar* 100 μm

encapsulated by fibroblast like cells (Fig. 6c, d, and data not shown), the development of desmoplasia could be studied in this animal model between day 6 and day 21.

Conclusion

The presented experiments describe the applicability of the carcinoma cell lines 6606PDA, 7265PDA, and 6606l for in vitro as well as in vivo studies. The data suggest that (1) all three cell lines will be useful in studying novel combinatorial therapies in vitro using gemcitabine, (2) the 6606PDA and 6606l cells might be very suitable in studying various aspects of cancer immunology in C57BL/6J mice, and that (3) diffusion weighted MRI can be used to define immune mediated cancer rejection.

Methods

Cell culture

The murine cell lines, 6606PDA and 6606l, were isolated from pancreatic carcinoma or a liver metastasis detected in a mouse after p48-cre induced expression of the $KRAS^{G12D}$ oncogene in the pancreas [20]. The 7265PDA cells were derived from a pancreatic carcinoma, which developed after pdx1-creER induced expression of $p53^{R172H}$ and $KRAS^{G12D}$. These three cell lines were a generous gift from Prof. Tuveson (Cambridge, UK) and were isolated in his lab according to Schreiber et al. [21]. Briefly, the tumors were dissected, minced, and digested at 37 °C in a Hank's balanced salt solution containing 2 mg/mL type V collagenase (Sigma, St. Louis, MO, USA). The material was then filtered through nylon mesh and the protease was inactivated by the addition of Dulbecco's modified Eagle medium/F12 (Invitrogen, Carlsbad, CA, USA) supplemented with 10 % fetal bovine serum. For all assays the cells were grown in DMEM high glucose medium (Biochrom GmbH, Berlin, Germany) with 10 % fetal calf serum on uncoated plastic dishes. Expansion of all three cells lines was quantified directly by plating 4×10^3 cells per well in a 12 well plate and counting cells after 24, 48, 72, or 96 h. Expansion of cells was also determined indirectly by WST-assay after plating of 4×10^3 cells per well in a 96 well plate, growing the cells 48 h, and determining cell metabolism with the Cell Proliferation Reagent WST-1 (Roche Diagnostics, Mannheim, Germany). To evaluate inhibition of proliferation

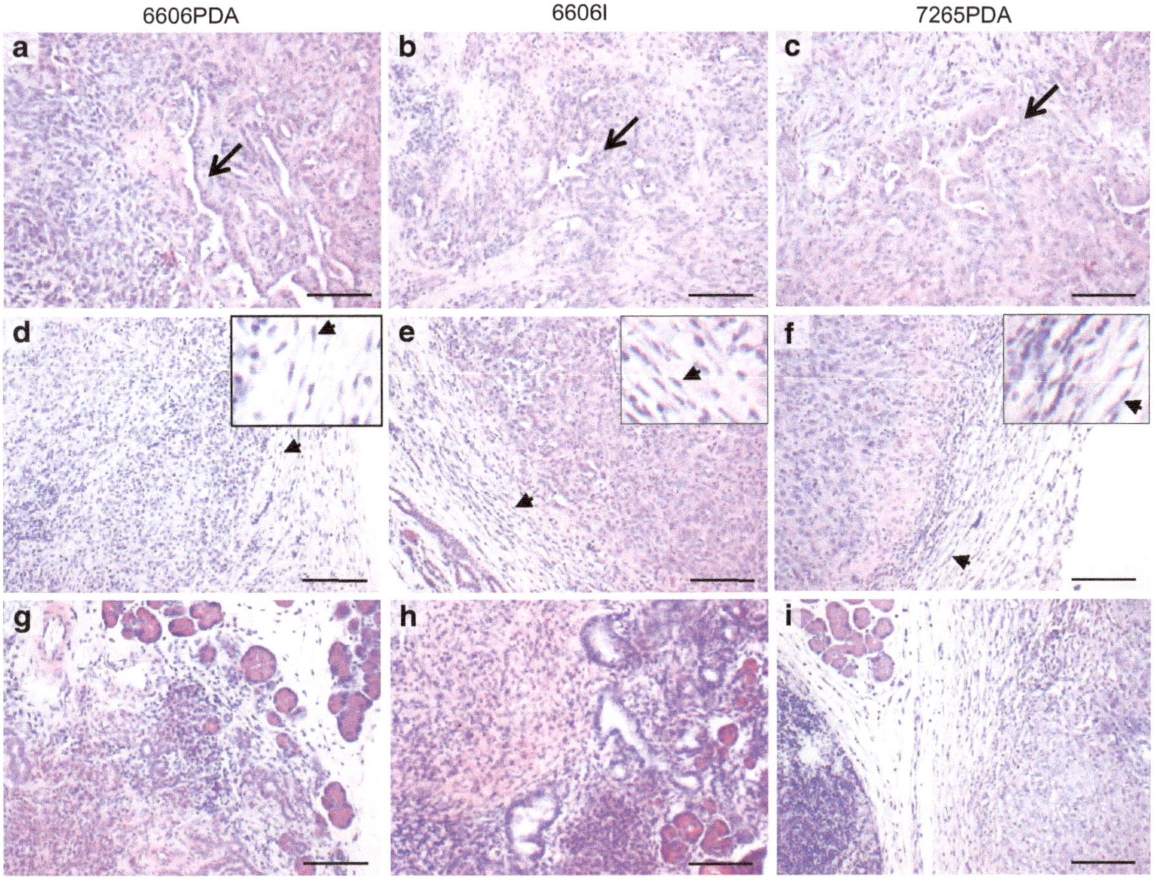

Fig. 7 Characterization of carcinomas by H/E staining during the late phase of tumor growth. **a–c** Histological images of carcinomas, which were derived from 6606PDA, 6606l, or 7265PDA cells, show cells with epithelial morphology on day 21 (*arrows*). **d–f** Representative histological images of carcinomas, which were derived from the indicated cell lines, show that the carcinomas are mostly encapsulated by fibroblast like cells (*arrowheads*). **g–i** In few locations lack of encapsulation was observed in 6606PDA (**g**) or 6606l (**h**) but not in 7265PDA (**i**) derived carcinomas (selected histological images). Number of tumors analyzed: n = 6 for 6606PDA; n = 5 for 6606l, n = 1 for 7265PDA (2 independent experiments). *Bar* 100 μm

by gemcitabine 4×10^3 cells per well were plated in a 96 well plate, grown for 24 h, and treated with the indicated concentration of gemcitabine and the BrdU labeling reagent (Roche Diagnostics, Mannheim, Germany) for additional 24 h. The incorporation of BrdU was then quantified with the colorimetric Cell Proliferation ELISA (Roche Diagnostics). To evaluate induction of cell death by gemcitabine 3×10^4 cells per well were plated in a 24 well plate, incubated for 24 h, and treated with 625 nM gemcitabine or medium lacking gemcitabine for additional 48 h. Cell death was then quantified by trypan blue staining solution (Life Technologies, CA, USA).

Animals and the syngeneic orthotopic carcinoma model

Male C57BL/6J and NMRI-Foxn1$^{nu/nu}$ mice were purchased from The Jackson Laboratory (Bar Harbor, ME) and bred in our local animal facility. Mice were kept on water and standard laboratory chow ad libitum and all experiments were executed in accordance with German legislation and the EU-directive 2010/63/EU. As published previously, laparotomy was performed on anesthetized mice (1.2–2.5 % isoflurane), 2.5×10^5 carcinoma cells were injected (single injection per animal) into the pancreas head, and the abdominal cavity was closed by sutures [22]. For pain relief 5 mg/kg carprofen (Pfizer GmbH, Berlin, Germany) was injected (sc) before surgery and 800 mg/L metamizol (Ratiopharm GmbH, Ulm, Germany) was added to the drinking water until euthanasia of the mice. For sampling blood and tissues animals were anesthetized with 90 mg/kg ketamine (bela-pharm, Vechta, Germany) and 7 mg/kg xylazine (Bayer Health Care, Leverkusen, Germany).

Analysis of the blood and the tissue

Blood glucose concentrations were measured with the blood glucose meter Contour (Bayer Vital, Leverkusen, Germany) and the tissue was sampled on days defined in Fig. 4a. The tissue was processed as described previously

[23]. The histology of carcinomas was evaluated on haematoxylin and eosin (H/E) stained paraffin tissue sections.

Morphological and diffusion-weighted 7 T MRI

MRI was performed on anesthetized (1.2–2.5 % isoflurane) mice at day 5–6 and day 20. Animals were scanned in 7 T small animal MRI (ClinScan, 7.0 T, 290 mT/m gradient strength) with a whole mouse body coil (Bruker, Ettlingen, Germany). The imaging protocol included morphological T2 weighted turbo spin echo (T2w-TSE) and diffusion weighted imaging (DWI). Tumor sizes were assessed in high resolution T2-weighted images of transversal plane images (TR: due to respiratory gating approx. 1900 ms; TE: 45.0 ms; FA: 180°; FoV: 40 mm × 40 mm; matrix: 240 × 320; voxel size: 0.16 × 0.125 × 0.7 mm^3, 24 slices, acquisition time: 9:46 min).

The ADC value was calculated from echo planar imaging DWI-sequence (two b values, $b_1 = 0$, $b_2 = 800$) TR: 9000 ms; TE: 85 ms; FA: 90°; FoV: 35 mm × 35 mm; matrix: 256 × 256; 10 slices of 0.7 mm per slice.

Analysis of MRI data

Images were analyzed employing Slicer3D (National Institutes of Health, Bethesda, Maryland, USA) and ImageJ (National Institutes of Health, Bethesda, Maryland, USA) for ROI placement during ADC evaluation. For evaluation of necrosis and vital tumor tissue T2w images and ADC-maps were superimposed. For each carcinoma the mean ADC of three ROIs, fitted to the outer tumor tissue rim, was calculated.

Statistics

Data presentation and statistics were performed as described previously [22, 23]. The significance of differences was evaluated using a Mann–Whitney rank-sum test followed by the correction for the accumulation of the α error by considering the number of meaningful comparisons. Differences with $P \leq 0.05$, divided by the number of meaningful comparisons, were considered to be significant.

Abbreviations

ADC: Apparent diffusion coefficient; BrdU: 5-Bromo-2′-deoxyuridine; DWI: Diffusion weighted imaging; EC50: Half maximal effective concentration; MRI: Magnetic resonance imaging; H/E: Haematoxylin/eosin.

Authors' contributions

DZ carried out the study design, the interpretation of data, the cell injections into mice, histological evaluations, and drafted the manuscript. All other authors participated in the study (FB: Figs. 2, 3; JA: Figs. 4b–c, 5c–d, 7; TL: Fig. 6a–b; TR: Fig. 1; SH: Figs. 5a–b, 6a–b), carried out the analysis and interpretation of data, and revised the manuscript. JPK and BV made substantial contributions to the design of the study and revision of the manuscript. All authors read and approved the final manuscript.

Author details

[1] Institute for Experimental Surgery, Rostock University Medical Center, University of Rostock, Schillingallee 69a, 18057 Rostock, Germany. [2] Core Facility Small Animal Imaging, Rostock University Medical Center, Schillingallee 69a, 18057, Rostock, Germany. [3] Department of Diagnostic Radiology and Neuroradiology, University Medicine Greifswald, Sauerbruchstr. 1, 17489 Greifswald, Germany.

Acknowledgements

We thank Berit Blendow, Dorothea Frenz, Eva Lorbeer-Rehfeldt, and Maren Nerowski (Institute for Experimental Surgery, University of Rostock) for excellent technical assistance, Marian Loebler for correcting the English text, and Prof. Tuveson (University of Cambridge, UK) for the gift of the 6606PDA, 6606l and 7265PDA cell lines.

Funding

Forschungsförderung der Medizinischen Fakultät der Rostocker Universität (Project 889017).

Compliance with ethical guidelines

Competing interests

The authors declare that they have no competing interests.

References

1. Siegel RL, Miller KD, Jemal A. Cancer statistics, 2015. CA Cancer J Clin. 2015;65(1):5–29.
2. Conroy T, Desseigne F, Ychou M, Bouché O, Guimbaud R, Bécouarn Y, Adenis A, Raoul JL, Gourgou-Bourgade S, de la Fouchardière C, Bennouna J, Bachet JB, Khemissa-Akouz F, Péré-Vergé D, Delbaldo C, Assenat E, Chauffert B, Michel P, Montoto-Grillot C, Ducreux M, Groupe Tumeurs Digestives of Unicancer, PRODIGE Intergroup. FOLFIRINOX versus gemcitabine for metastatic pancreatic cancer. N Engl J Med. 2011;364(19):1817–25.
3. Von Hoff DD, Ervin T, Arena FP, Chiorean EG, Infante J, Moore M, Seay T, Tjulandin SA, Ma WW, Saleh MN, Harris M, Reni M, Dowden S, Laheru D, Bahary N, Ramanathan RK, Tabernero J, Hidalgo M, Goldstein D, Van Cutsem E, Wei X, Iglesias J, Renschler MF. Increased survival in pancreatic cancer with nab-paclitaxel plus gemcitabine. N Engl J Med. 2013;369(18):1691–703.
4. Li Y, Sun J, Jiang Z, Zhang L, Liu G: Gemcitabine and S-1 combination chemotherapy versus gemcitabine alone for locally advanced and metastatic pancreatic cancer: a meta-analysis of randomized controlled trials in Asia. J Chemother. 2015. Epub ahead of print.
5. Ruggeri BA, Camp F, Miknyoczki S. Animal models of disease: pre-clinical animal models of cancer and their applications and utility in drug discovery. Biochem Pharmacol. 2014;87(1):150–61.
6. Kapischke M, Pries A. Animal models of pancreatic cancer for drug research. Expert Opin Drug Discov. 2008;3(10):1177–88.
7. Talmadge JE, Singh RK, Fidler IJ, Raz A. Murine models to evaluate novel and conventional therapeutic strategies for cancer. Am J Pathol. 2007;170(3):793–804.
8. Corbett TH, Roberts BJ, Leopold WR, Peckham JC, Wilkoff LJ, Griswold DP Jr, Schabel FM Jr. Induction and chemotherapeutic response of two transplantable ductal adenocarcinomas of the pancreas in C57BL/6 mice. Cancer Res. 1984;44(2):717–26.
9. Tseng WW, Winer D, Kenkel JA, Choi O, Shain AH, Pollack JR, French R, Lowy AM, Engleman EG. Development of an orthotopic model of invasive pancreatic cancer in an immunocompetent murine host. Clin Cancer Res. 2010;16(14):3684–95.
10. Torres MP, Rachagani S, Souchek JJ, Mallya K, Johansson SL, Batra SK. Novel pancreatic cancer cell lines derived from genetically engineered mouse models of spontaneous pancreatic adenocarcinoma: applications in diagnosis and therapy. PLoS One. 2013;8(11):e80580.

11. Partecke IL, Kaeding A, Sendler M, Albers N, Kühn JP, Speerforck S, Roese S, Seubert F, Diedrich S, Kuehn S, Weiss UF, Mayerle J, Lerch MM, Hadlich S, Hosten N, Heidecke CD, Puls R, von Bernstorff W. In vivo imaging of pancreatic tumours and liver metastases using 7 Tesla MRI in a murine orthotopic pancreatic cancer model and a liver metastases model. BMC Cancer. 2011;11:40.
12. Partecke LI, Sendler M, Kaeding A, Weiss FU, Mayerle J, Dummer A, Nguyen TD, Albers N, Speerforck S, Lerch MM, Heidecke CD, von Bernstorff W, Stier A. A syngeneic orthotopic murine model of pancreatic adenocarcinoma in the C57/BL6 mouse using the Panc02 and 6606PDA cell lines. Eur Surg Res. 2011;47(2):98–107.
13. Shi X, Liu S, Kleeff J, Friess H, Büchler MW. Acquired resistance of pancreatic cancer cells towards 5-fluorouracil and gemcitabine is associated with altered expression of apoptosis-regulating genes. Oncology. 2002;62(4):354–62.
14. Patra CR, Bhattacharya R, Wang E, Katarya A, Lau JS, Dutta S, Muders M, Wang S, Buhrow SA, Safgren SL, Yaszemski MJ, Reid JM, Ames MM, Mukherjee P, Mukhopadhyay D. Targeted delivery of gemcitabine to pancreatic adenocarcinoma using cetuximab as a targeting agent. Cancer Res. 2008;68(6):1970–8.
15. Zhao M, Tominaga Y, Ohuchida K, Mizumoto K, Cui L, Kozono S, Fujita H, Maeyama R, Toma H, Tanaka M. Significance of combination therapy of zoledronic acid and gemcitabine on pancreatic cancer. Cancer Sci. 2012;103(1):58–66.
16. Sun JD, Liu Q, Ahluwalia D, Li W, Meng F, Wang Y, Bhupathi D, Ruprell AS, Hart CP. Efficacy and safety of the hypoxia-activated prodrug TH-302 in combination with gemcitabine and nab-paclitaxel in human tumor xenograft models of pancreatic cancer. Cancer Biol Ther. 2015;16(3):438–49.
17. Brandes F, Schmidt K, Wagner C, Redekopf J, Schlitt HJ, Geissler EK, Lang SA. Targeting cMET with INC280 impairs tumour growth and improves efficacy of gemcitabine in a pancreatic cancer model. BMC Cancer. 2015;15:71.
18. Sah RP, Nagpal SJ, Mukhopadhyay D, Chari ST. New insights into pancreatic cancer-induced paraneoplastic diabetes. Nat Rev Gastroenterol Hepatol. 2013;10(7):423–33.
19. Tan CR, Yaffee PM, Jamil LH, Lo SK, Nissen N, Pandol SJ, Tuli R, Hendifar AE. Pancreatic cancer cachexia: a review of mechanisms and therapeutics. Front Physiol. 2014;5:88.
20. Hingorani SR, Petricoin EF, Maitra A, Rajapakse V, King C, Jacobetz MA, Ross S, Conrads TP, Veenstra TD, Hitt BA, Kawaguchi Y, Johann D, Liotta LA, Crawford HC, Putt ME, Jacks T, Wright CV, Hruban RH, Lowy AM, Tuveson DA. Preinvasive and invasive ductal pancreatic cancer and its early detection in the mouse. Cancer Cell. 2003;4(6):437–50.
21. Schreiber FS, Deramaudt TB, Brunner TB, Boretti MI, Gooch KJ, Stoffers DA, Bernhard EJ, Rustgi AK. Successful growth and characterization of mouse pancreatic ductal cells: functional properties of the Ki-RAS(G12V) oncogene. Gastroenterology. 2004;127(1):250–60.
22. Zechner D, Radecke T, Amme J, Bürtin F, Albert AC, Partecke LI, Vollmar B. Impact of diabetes type II and chronic inflammation on pancreatic cancer. BMC Cancer. 2015;15:51.
23. Bobrowski A, Spitzner M, Bethge S, Mueller-Graf F, Vollmar B, Zechner D. Risk factors for pancreatic ductal adenocarcinoma specifically stimulate pancreatic duct glands in mice. Am J Pathol. 2013;182(3):965–74.

7

PTEN signaling is required for the maintenance of spermatogonial stem cells in mouse, by regulating the expressions of PLZF and UTF1

Wei Zhou[1,2†], Hongfang Shao[3†], Di Zhang[2,4†], Jian Dong[2], Wei Cheng[5], Lu Wang[2], Yincheng Teng[3*] and Zhuo Yu[2*]

Abstract

Background: *Pten* plays a crucial role in the stem cell maintenance in a few organs. *Pten* defect also causes the premature oocytes and ovary aging. We and other groups have found that the phosphatidylinositol-3-OH kinase (PI3K)-Akt signaling regulates the proliferation and differentiation of spermatogonial stem cells (SSCs). PTEN functions as a negative regulator of the PI3K pathway. Thus, we thought that the fate of SSCs might be controlled by *Pten*.

Results: We report that promyelocytic leukaemia zinc finger (PLZF) and undifferentiated embryonic cell transcription factor 1 (UTF1), both of which are germ cell-specific transcriptional factors, are regulated by *Pten*. Conditional deletion of *Pten* leads to reduction in PLZF expression but induction of UTF1, which is associated with SSCs depletion and infertility in males with age.

Conclusion: Our data demonstrate that *Pten* is required for the long-term maintenance of SSCs and precise regulation of spermatogenesis in mouse. The finding of a *Pten*-regulated GFRα1$^+$/PLZF$^-$/UTF1$^+$ progenitor population provides a new insight into the precise mechanisms controlling SSC fate.

Keywords: *Pten* knockout, PLZF, UTF1, Spermatogonial stem cells, PI3K-Akt signaling

Background

Stem cells are capable of renewing themselves to maintain a stem cell pool as a preserved cell source for tissue homeostasis, while they can also differentiate into mature cells to carry out the function of a specific tissue. The precise balance of self-renewal and differentiation of stem cells is critical for the maintenance and function of a tissue or organ throughout life-time. Similar to other stem cells, spermatogonial stem cells (SSCs) renew themselves and meanwhile undergo a dramatic differentiation process-spermatogenesis to generate a large number of sperms consistently. Prior to spermatogenesis, multiple mitotic divisions of SSCs produce subpopulations of SSCs, and the balance of the SSC subpopulations is critical for long-term sperm production. Multiple proteins, such as promyelocytic leukaemia zinc finger (PLZF), GDNF family receptor alpha-1 (GFRα1) and undifferentiated embryonic cell transcription factor 1 (UTF1), are expressed in SSC subpopulations, which plays a crucial role in the maintenance of SSC pool. PLZF and GFRα1 are required in germ cells for stem cell self-renewal [1–3], whereas UTF1 is restricted to a small subset of spermatogonia that make the cells maintain the ability of differentiation [4, 5].

PTEN signaling is critical in governing the stem cell pool not only in the blood system and central neural

*Correspondence: teng_yc@126.com; yuzhuo78@aliyun.com
†Wei Zhou, Hongfang Shaoa and Di Zhang contributed equally to this work
[2] Key Laboratory of Cell Differentiation and Apoptosis of Chinese Ministry of Education, Shanghai Jiao Tong University School of Medicine, Shanghai 200025, China
[3] Centre for Reproductive Medicine, Shanghai Jiao Tong University Affiliated Sixth People Hospital, Shanghai 200233, China
Full list of author information is available at the end of the article

system but also in reproductive system [6–8]. The loss of *Pten* in ovary via conditional knockout triggers premature of oocytes and ovary aging [8]. On the other hand, we and other groups have revealed that the phosphatidylinositol-3-OH kinase(PI3K)/Akt/S6 pathway is a critical signaling in controlling the proliferation and division of SSCs. Disruption of this signaling or *Akt* knockout leads to the loss of spermatogonial cells and infertility in males [9, 10]. PTEN is a major negative regulator of PI3K signaling [11, 12]. To understand the function of *Pten* in regulating SSC fate and fertility in male mouse, we generated conditional *Pten* knockout males using germ cell specific Cre strain, the *Stra8*-Cre mouse. It was turned out that the loss of *Pten* caused reduction of PLZF expression, but induction of UTF1. Thus, conditional *Pten* knockout leads to depletion of SSC pool and infertility with age.

Results

Conditional deletion of *Pten* in spermatogonial cells in mice

STRA8 is a germ-cell-specific protein and is expressed through neonatal spermatogonial cells to meiotic cells [13]. In the *Stra8*-EGFP transgenic mice, spermatogonial stem cells can be labeled by EGFP as characterized by transplantation assay [14]. Therefore, *Stra8*-Cre can be applied to generate SSC-specific gene knockout model. We created SSC-*Pten* null mice by crossing $Pten^{LoxP/LoxP}$ mice with *Stra8*-Cre mice. The *Pten* knockout genotype was identified by examining the genomic allele of *Pten* (Fig. 1a), the *Pten* expression in testis sections of 7 day-old males (Fig. 1b) as well as in whole proteins from adult testes (Fig. 1c). Since *Pten* is also expressed in non-germ cells, we obtained purified haploid spermatids through cell sorting from adult mice to confirm the absence of *Pten* expression in germ cells from crossed mice (Fig. 1d).

Conditional deletion of *Pten* caused overgrowth of testes followed by shrinking and sterility with age

The males with *Pten*-deleted in SSCs were grossly normal through all ages except that the size of testes was of overgrowth within the first 50 days after birth then shrunk afterwards (Fig. 2a). Fertility was found lower in the young *Pten*-deleted males and it was lost progressively after 60 days as measured by mating with wild type females (Fig. 2b). The morphology of testicular tubules cross-section was abnormal as showing larger lumen and

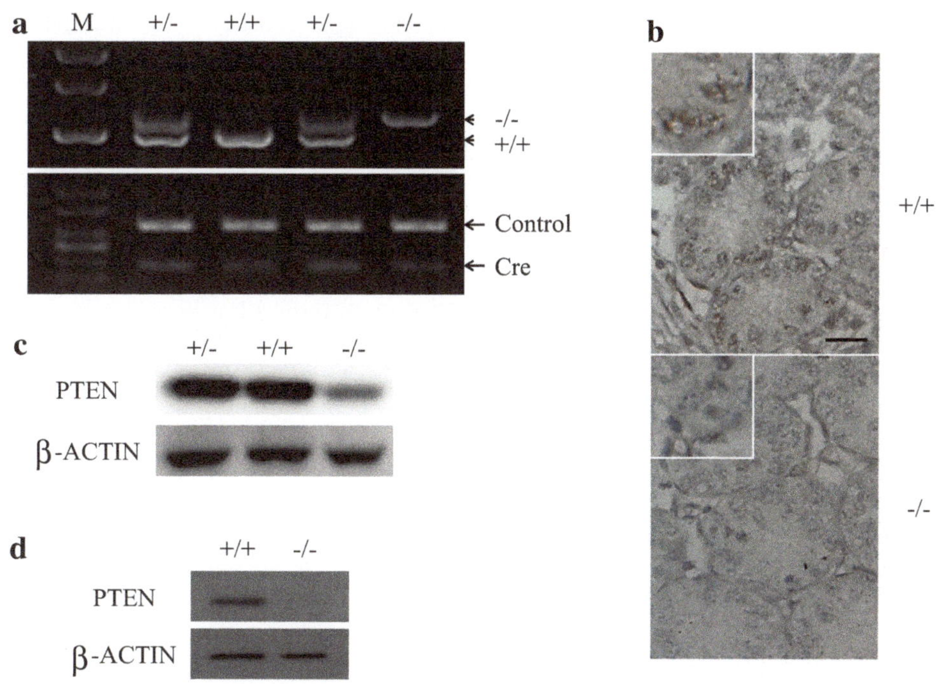

Fig. 1 Cre-recombinase mediated deletion of *Pten* in SSCs. **a** PCR analysis of genotype of *Pten* knockout (KO) mice. *Short arrows* denote the predicted size of *Pten* KO and wild-type (WT) alleles, *long arrows* denote the predicted size of Cre and internal positive control (+/+, wild type; +/−, heterozygote; −/−,homozygote; M, Marker). **b** Immunostaining of PTEN in cross sections of 7 day-old testis. The cytoplasmic staining was observed in spermatogonial cells from $Pten^{+/+}$ section, whereas it was absent in the $Pten^{-/-}$ section (*scale bar* is 20 μm). **c** Western blot analysis of PTEN expression in whole testis of 32 day-old $Pten^{+/+}$, $Pten^{+/-}$, and $Pten^{-/-}$mice. PTEN is also expressed in nongerminal cells, so PTEN expression was detected in $Pten^{-/-}$ testes, but was significantly lower compared with $Pten^{+/+}$ and $Pten^{+/-}$ testes. **d** Absence of PTEN expression in haploid cells from $Pten^{-/-}$ testes. Haploid sperms were isolated from 79 day-old testes of $Pten^{+/+}$ and $Pten^{-/-}$ mice separately by sorting using flow cytometer, then were subjected to Western blotting analysis.

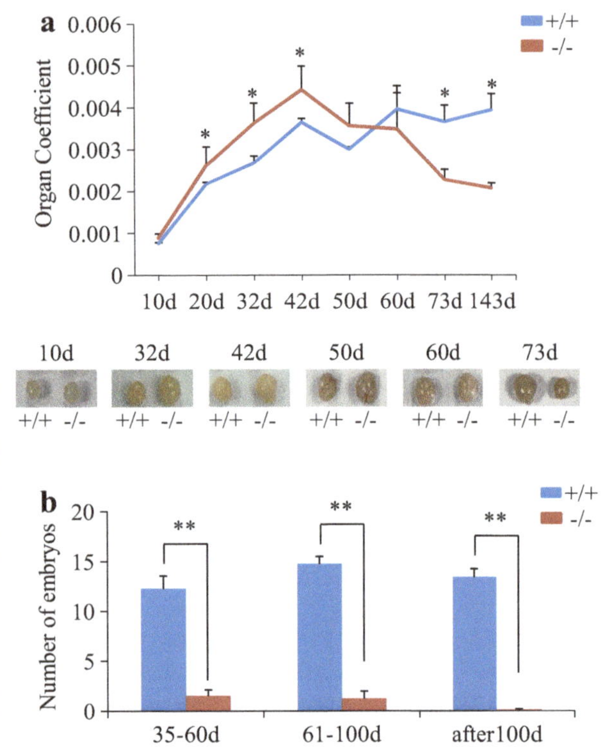

Fig. 2 Overgrowth of testes and fertility loss in $Pten^{-/-}$ mice. **a** Curve of organ coefficient of $Pten^{+/+}$ and $Pten^{-/-}$ testes with age. *Horizontal bars* indicate mean values, n = 3, * $P < 0.05$. **b** In vivo fertility assay of $Pten^{+/+}$ and $Pten^{-/-}$ mice. The mating test was divided into three groups according to the male's age: 35–60 days old, 61–100 days old, and over 100 days old. *Horizontal bars* indicate mean values, n = 22 ** $P < 0.01$.

failure of spermatogenesis with age (Fig. 3a). Furthermore, the rate of spermatogenesis was found very low in the *Pten*-deleted males during young ages, and severe loss of mature sperm production in the adult males epididymis after age of 60 days (Fig. 3b). This overall phenotype is very similar to that of *Pten* knockout in bone marrow stem cells and central neural stem cells as over-expansion of short-term hemeatopoietic stem cell pool and enlarged brain [6–8]. Possibly, the loss of *Pten* might disturb the balance of self-renewal and differentiation and promote excessive differentiation-associated proliferation of SSCs, thereby giving rise to enlarged testes in young mice but causing the depletion of stem cell source and infertility with age.

Loss of *Pten* led to reduction of SSCs in neonatal males

To examine whether the self-renewal of SSCs was influenced by the absence of *Pten*, we used testis cross sections from 7 day-old pups and calculated the number of SSCs. The amount of SSCs expressing both GFRα1 and PLZF was reduced significantly (Fig. 4a, e, f) indicating that *Pten* played a crucial role in SSC self-renewal in the neonatal testis. To further reveal the molecular mechanisms accounting for the phenotype of this *Pten*-knockout testis, we used whole transcriptome sequencing to compare the gene expression profiles between wild type and *Pten*-knockout testes at 32 days old. Interestingly, we found that the expression of UTF1 significantly increased in the *Pten*-knockout testes (Additional file 1: Figure S1B). Next, immunostaining of the cross sections confirmed the increase of UTF1-expressing but PLZF-negative cells in $Pten^{-/-}$ 7 day-old testis (Fig. 4b, g). At the age of day 10, similar to that of day 7, SSCs expressing GFRα1 or PLZF decreased (Fig. 4c, h, i). However, the number of $UTF1^+/PLZF^-$ cells was significantly higher in the *Pten*-knockout testes (Fig. 4d, j). As a chromatin-associated protein, UTF1 is involved in the initiation of ES cell differentiation [15]. In the testis, it has been evidenced that UTF1 is expressed in a subset of spermatogonial cells and germ cell neoplasms, making the SSCs maintain the ability of differentiation [4, 16]. In $Pten^{-/-}$ mouse, we have seldom observed neoplasms in the testes. A number of $UTF1^+/PLZF^-$ cells and few $UTF1^-/PLZF^+$ cells were observed in the cross sections of 32 day-old $Pten^{-/-}$ mouse testis by immunostaining (Additional file 1: Figure S1A), which implied that *Pten*-deletion-induced UTF1 expression might boost SSCs differentiation resulting in testes overgrowth in *Pten* knockout males.

The PTEN signaling regulated the expression of PLZF and UTF1 in SSCs

We further examined the expression of GFRα1, PLZF and UTF1 in *Pten*-deleted testes at day 7 or day 10 using Western blot analysis. Consistent with the data from cross section immunostaining, the expression of GFRα1 and PLZF was reduced at both day 7 and day 10, while UTF1 expression was highly increased at day 10 (Fig. 5a). As the PI3K/AKT/mTOR pathway is an important signaling pathway in regulating the cellular functions, PTEN is a major negative regulator of PI3K signaling. Then, we isolated SSCs from 7 days old pups and cultured them in the presence or absence of PI3K inhibitor or mTOR inhibitor-rapamycin to detect the role of PTEN signaling in SSCs in vitro. We found that PLZF expression was induced by inhibiting the PI3K signaling (Fig. 5b, c). However, in the same cell pool, UTF1 expression was reduced in the presence of PI3K inhibitor or rapamycin (Fig. 5b, c), implying the presence of a reversal relationship between PLZF and UTF1 in the context of the PTEN/PI3K signaling. Furthermore, UTF1 expression was slightly higher with Rapamycin than with PI3K inhibitor, which indicated that other branched pathways, in addition to mTOR signaling, may participate in this regulation. As we all know, PTEN is an inhibitor of PI3K

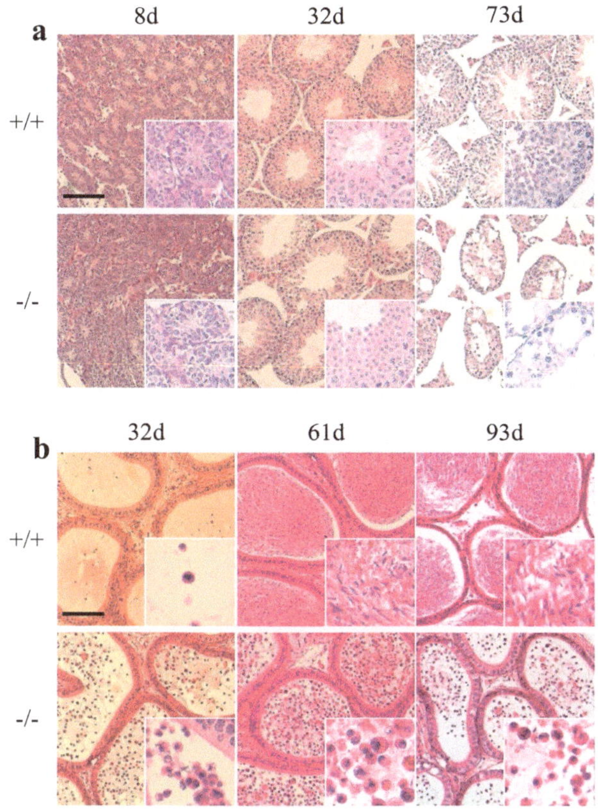

Fig. 3 Abnormal spermatogenesis in *Pten*$^{-/-}$ mice. **a** Hematoxylin and eosin staining of sections from *Pten*$^{+/+}$ and *Pten*$^{-/-}$ testes at 7, 32 and 73 days old (*scale bar* is 100 μm). **b** Hematoxylin and eosin staining of epididymis sections from *Pten*$^{+/+}$ and *Pten*$^{-/-}$ mice at 32, 61, and 93 days old. Massive lack of normal sperm was observed in the epididymis of *Pten*$^{-/-}$ mice (*scale bar* is 100 μm).

signaling. Thus, we proposed that the PLZF and UTF1 expression was regulated by *Pten* in SSCs and *Pten* deletion led to reduction in PLZF expression associated with the increase of UTF1 expression.

A putative model of SSC subpopulation fate controlled by *Pten*

To further identify the properties of UTF1$^+$, PLZF$^+$ and GFRα1$^+$ cells, we performed whole mount staining in 7 day-old tubules to locate their expression in SSC population. As shown in Fig. 6a, although most UTF1 positive cells are positive to both GFRα1 and PLZF, a subpopulation of UTF1$^+$/GFRα1$^+$/PLZF$^-$ SSCs is present. UTF1 protein, which is revealed as a chromatin-associated protein [15], loads on chromosomes in GFRα1$^+$/PLZF$^-$ SSCs (Fig. 6a, upper panel). We observed the dividing spermatogonial cells expressing UTF1 but neither GFRα1 nor PLZF in the 7 day-old testicular tubules of *Pten*$^{-/-}$ males (Fig. 6a, bottom panel). Furthermore, we observed the groups of GFRα1$^-$/PLZF$^-$/UTF1$^+$ cells located adjacent the cells of GFRα1$^+$/PLZF$^-$/UTF1$^+$ in the *Pten*$^{-/-}$ 7 day-old testicular tubules (Fig. 6b). Therefore, we hypothesize a model of SSC fate: A GFRα1$^+$/PLZF$^+$/UTF1$^+$ SSC may undergo asymmetric division, then generate a GFRα1$^+$/PLZF$^+$/UTF1$^+$ cell for self-renewal and another GFRα1$^+$/PLZF$^-$/UTF1$^+$ cell. The latter cell enters cell cycle, loses GFRα1 expression, and later develops into differentiating SSCs (Fig. 6c).

Discussion

Prior to undergoing differentiation of meiosis, spermatogonial stem cells proliferate and form a pool of cells at different division status to meet the dynamics of spermatogenesis. This cell pool is maintained by self-renewal and proliferation of SSCs and exists throughout life time. The transcriptional factor PLZF plays a crucial role in the maintenance of SSC pool in adult males, and PLZF knockout causes a progressive loss of spermatogonia with age [1, 2]. Interestingly, *Pten* knockout male pups have less PLZF positive SSCs even at 7 day-old (Figs. 4a, f). We have reported that PLZF expression is regulated by the PTEN signaling pathway in prostate cells [17]. Similarly, PLZF expression was significantly reduced in the *Pten* knockout SSCs in this study (Fig. 5a), and further experiments in vitro confirmed that in SSCs, PLZF was indeed regulated by the PTEN signaling (Fig. 5b). Thus, in *Pten*$^{-/-}$ males, the loss of SSCs is partly due to the reduction of PLZF expression.

The precise regulation of the balance of self-renewal versus differentiation of stem cells is critical in controlling tissue homeostasis and function. Excessive differentiation-associated proliferation leads to depletion of stem cells and degeneration of tissue with age. In *Pten*$^{-/-}$ males, although the number of SSCs decreased, which occurred as early as 7 days after birth, testes underwent overgrowth or premature of larger size until day 42 but shrank afterward. This phenotype is apparently associated with excessive differentiation-proliferation of SSCs, which disturbs the long-term maintenance of stem cell pool, thereby leading to the exhaustion of spermatogenesis with age. Furthermore, *Pten* knockout induced the expression of UTF1, which is expressed in a subpopulation of spermatogonial cells in the testis [4, 16]. UTF1$^+$ cells were significantly increased in the testis as early as at day 10 in the *Pten*$^{-/-}$ males compared with wild-type males (Fig. 4d). Using immunostaining of a nearly infertile 32 day-old *Pten*$^{-/-}$ testis, many UTF1$^+$/PLZF$^-$ cells and few UTF1$^-$/PLZF$^+$ cells (Additional file 1: Figure S1A) were observed, indicating that *Pten*-deletion-induced UTF1 expression might boost SSCs differentiation associated with the testes overgrowth of *Pten* knockout males. Moreover, it has been reported that UTF1 makes the spermatogonia maintain the ability of differentiation [4] and is involved in the

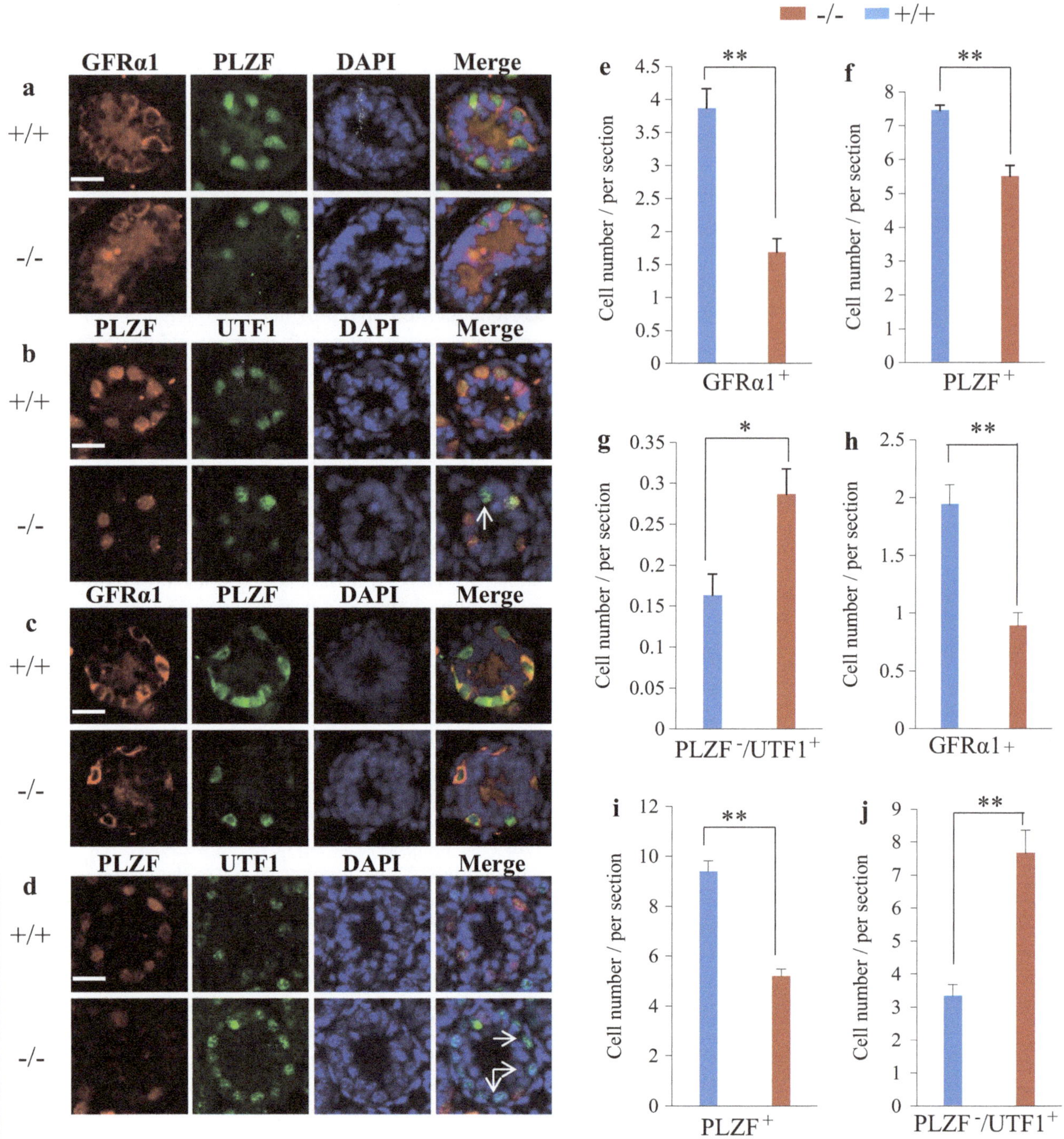

Fig. 4 Reduction of GFRα1 and PLZF positive SSCs and increase of UTF1 positive cells in neonatal *Pten*$^{-/-}$ testes. Staining of 7 day-old testis sections showed the reduction of both GFRα1^{+} SSCs and PLZF^{+} SSCs **a** and the emergence of PLZF^{-}/UTF1^{+} SSCs in the *Pten*$^{-/-}$ testis (**b**, *arrow*). Staining of 10 day-old testis sections showed a significant loss of both GFRα1^{+} SSCs and PLZF^{+} SSCs (**c**) and an increase in the number of PLZF^{-}/UTF1^{+} cells in the *Pten*$^{-/-}$ testis (**d**, *arrows*). Nuclei were counterstained with DAPI (*scale bar* is 20 μm). Based on coimmunofluorescent staining of testicular tubule sections from both *Pten*$^{+/+}$ and *Pten*$^{-/-}$ mice at 7 days old (**e**–**g**) and at 10 day olds (**h**–**j**), the average number ± SEM of GFRα1^{+}, PLZF^{+} and PLZF^{-}/UTF1^{+} cells per tubule cross-section were calculated and presented as *bar graphs*. For the statistical analysis, each five inconsecutive testis sections were counted. *Horizontal bar* indicates mean value, n = 4, *$P < 0.05$, **$P < 0.01$.

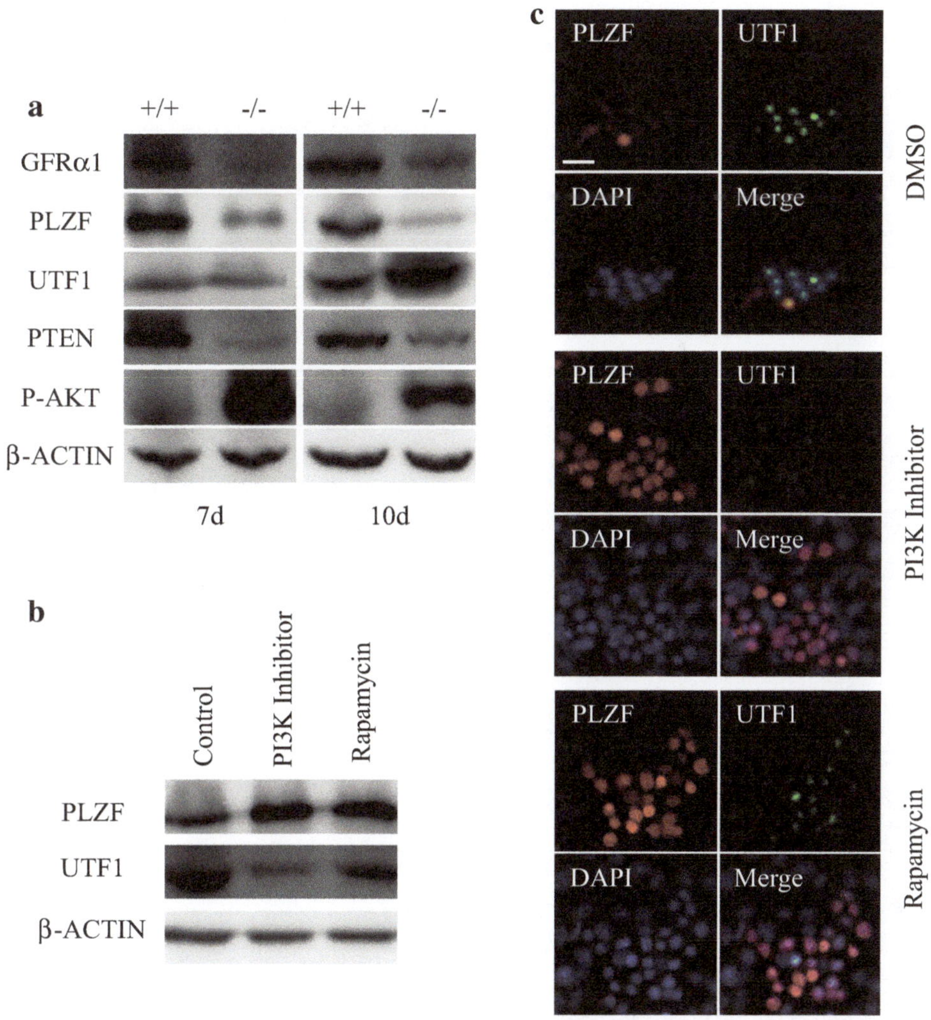

Fig. 5 PLZF and UTF1 are regulated by the PI3K/PTEN signal pathway. **a** Western blot analysis of GFRα1, PLZF, UTF1, PTEN, and P-AKT expression in *Pten*$^{+/+}$ and *Pten*$^{-/-}$ testes at 7 and 10 days old. **b** Western blot analysis of PLZF and UTF1 expression in cultured SSCs isolated from 7 day-old testes. The treatment with PI3K inhibitor or rapamycin lasted for 96 h, DMSO was used as control. **c** Coimmunofluorescent staining of PLZF and UTF1 in SSCs treated with PI3K inhibitor, rapamycin or DMSO, showed that the PI3K signal pathway inhibition induced PLZF but reduced UTF1 expression (*scale bar* is 20 μm).

initiation of ES cell differentiation [15]. All of these results indicate that UTF1^{+} cells are differentiating SSCs. To further identify the properties of UTF1^{+} cells, we performed a three color whole-mount staining of UTF1 with GFRα1 and PLZF of 7 day old tubules to locate UTF1 expression in the SSC population. Notably, a subpopulation of UTF1^{+}/GFRα1^{+}/PLZF^{-} SSC and UTF1^{low}/GFRα1^{+}/PLZF^{+} cell was observed, which seemed to come from the same precursor cell through asymmetric division. Similar subpopulation cells in *Pten*$^{-/-}$ tubule lost both GFRα1 and PLZF expression. Therefore, we hypothesized a model of SSC fate in Fig. 6c. Thus, in this study, *Pten* knockout induced UTF1 expression in addition to causing the loss of PLZF expression. However, further studies should be conducted to address the mechanism how *Pten* regulates PLZF and UTF1 expression.

Although the testes overgrowth in *Pten* knockout males occurred within the first 2 months, the fertility and embryos production were lower compared with wild type males at same ages (Fig. 2b). Apparently, this phenotype is associated with the abnormality of sperms found in the epididymis which lack tails (Fig. 3b). This abnormality may be caused by the differentiation defects before haploid stages or during spermatogenesis because *Pten* is actively expressed in the haploid cells in the testis (Fig. 1d).

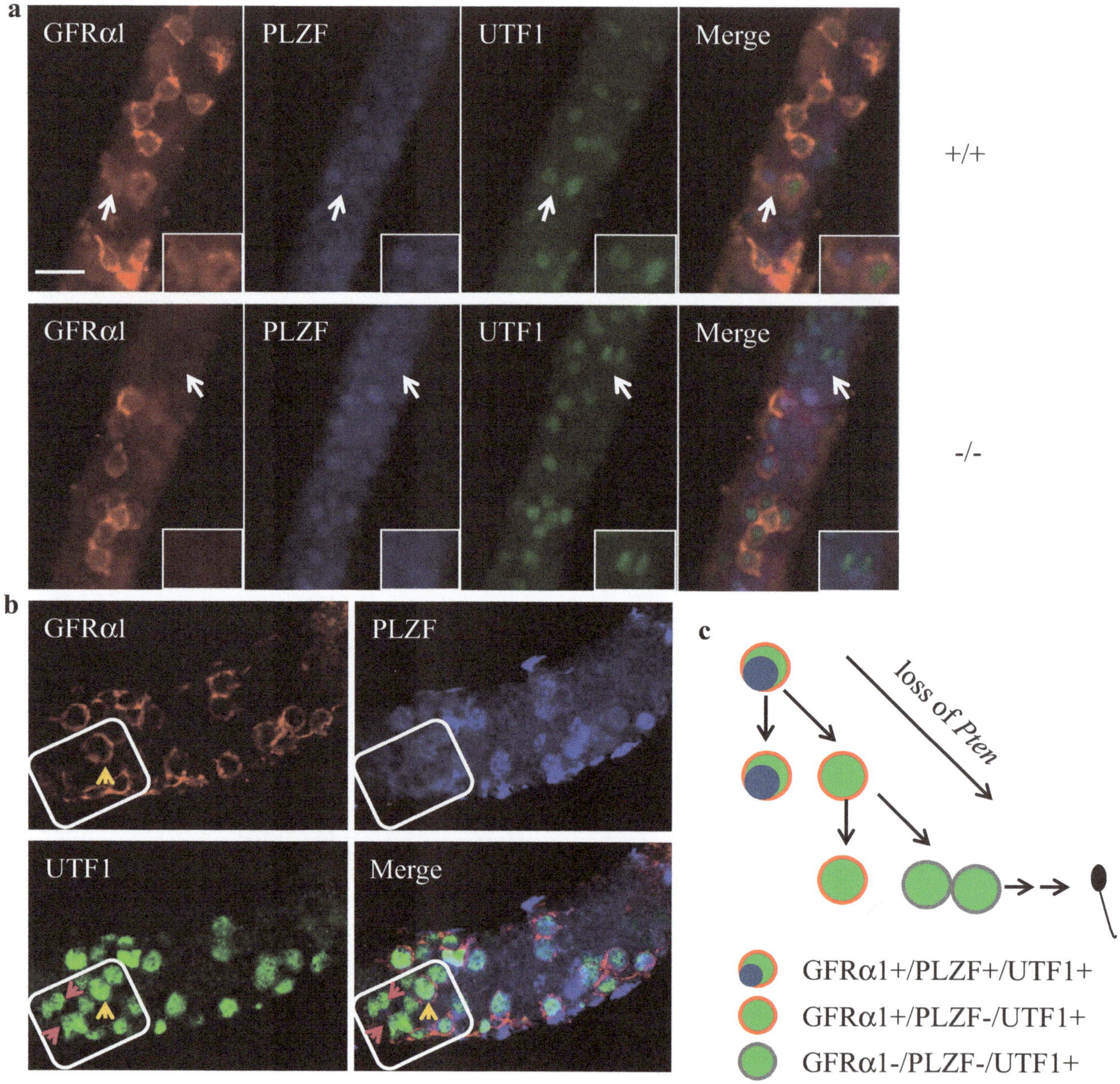

Fig. 6 Loss of *Pten* triggers asymmetric division and increases the differentiation-associated proliferation of SSCs. **a** Whole-mount triple-immunofluorescence of GFRα1, PLZF and UTF1 in seminiferous tubules at 7 days old. In the $Pten^{+/+}$ tubules (*upper panel*), a pair of SSCs (*arrows*) consisting of one GFRα1^{+}/PLZF^{+}/UTF1^{low} cell and the other GFRα1^{+}/PLZF^{-}/UTF1^{+} (with UTF1 on the chromatin, *arrow*) cell was observed, which may undergo an asymmetric division of the stem cell. Meanwhile, a pair of GFRα1^{-}/PLZF^{-}/UTF1^{+} progeny (*arrows*) with UTF1 on chromatin was observed in the completing division in the $Pten^{-/-}$ seminiferous tubules (*lower panel*) (*scale bar* is 20 μm). **b** Whole-mount triple-immunofluorescence of GFRα1, PLZF and UTF1 in $Pten^{-/-}$ seminiferous tubules at 7 days old showing a group (marked in *square*) of GFRα1^{-}/PLZF^{-}/UTF1^{+} cells (*purple arrow*) next to GFRα1^{+}/PLZF^{-}/UTF1^{+} cells (*yellow arrow*) within the context of GFRα1^{+}/PLZF^{+}/UTF1^{+} SSCs. **c** A schematic diagram showing a hypothesis of asymmetric division of SSC in the testis at 7 days old. GFRα1^{+}/PLZF^{+}/UTF1^{+} stem cell underwent a division and gave rise to a GFRα1^{+}/PLZF^{-}/UTF1^{+} progeny, which in turn divided into two GFRα1^{-}/PLZF^{-}/UTF1^{+} cells towards differentiation fate. Loss of *Pten* accelerated this pathway and disturbed the balance of self-renewal versus differentiation of GFRα1^{+}/PLZF^{+}/UTF1^{+} stem cells, thereby causing SSCs depletion and infertility with age.

Collectively, The *Pten*-deletion-induced reduction of PLZF and increased expression of UTF1 apparently disturb the balance of self-renewal and differentiation of SSCs, leading to the depletion of spermatogonial cells and infertility with age.

Conclusion

By studying the model of *Pten* knockout in SSCs, we found that *Pten* is required for the long-term maintenance of SSCs and spermatogenesis. Our study provides a new insight into the precise mechanisms controlling SSC self-renewal versus differentiation to maintain SSC pool and spermatogenesis throughout life time, especially the discovery of a *Pten*-regulated GFRα1$^+$/PLZF$^-$/UTF1$^+$ progenitor population might lead to a new understanding of SSC fate control.

Methods

Animals

Stra8-cre mice (Stock number 008208) and *Pten*$^{LoxP/LoxP}$ mice (Stock number 006440) were purchased from the Jackson Laboratory. *Stra8*-cre males were crossed with *Pten*$^{f/f}$ females to generate *Pten* knockout in SSCs. Genotype of *Stra8*-cre mice and *Pten*$^{f/f}$ mice were determined by PCR analysis using the primers and procedures provided by the Jackson Laboratory or by a previous research [18]. For *Pten* PCR, the *Pten*$^{f/f}$ (1.1 kb) and *Pten* (1 kb) fragments were amplified by using the following primers: 5′-ACTCAAGGCAGGGATGAGC-3′ (forward), 5′-AATCTAGGGCCTCTTGTGCC-3′ (reverse). For *Stra8*-cre PCR, the *Stra8*-cre (179 bp) and *Interleukin 2* (*Il2* internal positive control, 324 bp) fragments were amplified by using primers: 5′-GTGCAAGCTGA ACAACAGGA-3′ (*Stra8*-cre forward), 5′-AGGGACAC AGCATTGGAGTC-3′ (*Stra8*-cre reverse); 5′-CTAGGCC ACAGAATTGAAAGATCT-3′ (*Il2* forward), 5′-GTAGG TGGAAATTCTAGCATCATCC-3′ (*Il2* reverse). Animals used in this study were maintained according to the Guide for the Care and Use of Laboratory Animals (Publication 85-23, revised 1996; National Institutes of Health, Bethesda, MD, USA), and the protocol was approved by Shanghai Jiao Tong University School of Medicine (Shanghai, China)

Histological analysis and immunostaining

Testes and epididymis were fixed in fresh Bouin's fixative, embedded in paraffin and sectioned at 4 μm thickness. After the hematoxylin and eosin staining, the sections were mounted and viewed under a microscope (Carl Zeiss, Maple Grove, MN, USA).

For immunohistochemical staining, testes were fixed in 4% paraformaldehyde, embedded in OCT and sectioned at 8 μm thickness. The endogenous peroxidase activity was blocked by placing the slides in 3% hydrogen peroxidase for 10 min followed by a tap water rinse. After being blocked with 5% BSA, slides were subsequently incubated with the primary antibody against PTEN (1:50 dilution, BOSTER BA1377) at 4°C overnight, slides were then incubated with Biotin conjugated secondary antibody. Following incubation with Streptavidin-Biotin Complex (BOSTER SA1022), visualization was performed with a DAB reaction, thereby resulting in brown staining of structures containing the epitope. Cellular nuclei were counterstained with hematoxylin and slides were permanently mounted and evaluated under a light microscope. For immunofluorescent staining, after blocking with 2% BSA, frozen slides or cell slides were stained with antibodies against PLZF (1:100 dilution, R&D, AF2944), UTF1 (1:1,000 dilution, ABCAM, ab24273) or GFRα1 (1:40 dilution, R&D, AF560). The primary antibodies were revealed with Alexa-555 and Alexa-488 conjugated secondary antibodies together with DAPI to stain the nuclei. The sections were mounted and viewed under a fluorescence microscope. For statistical analysis, five different slides from *Pten*$^{+/+}$ or *Pten*$^{-/-}$ mice were stained and positive cell numbers were calculated and analyzed by one-way ANOVA ($\alpha = 0.05$). For whole-mount staining, with enzymatic dissociation of the testes using 1 mg/ml collagenase for 5 min at 37°C, untangled seminiferous tubules were fixed with 2% paraformaldehyde containing 0.5 mM $CaCl_2$ for 30 min at room temperature. After incubation with 1% Ttriton 100 for 10 min, samples were dehydrated through a series of methanol (25, 50, 75, and 100% in PBS containing 0.5% Triton 100—PBS-T) on ice followed by rehydration in PBS-T. The seminiferous tubules were incubated in a blocking buffer (1% BSA and 4% donkey serum) for 1 h and incubated with the first antibody combination at 4°C overnight. The appropriate second antibodies (Alexa-555, Alexa-488 and Dylight-405 conjugated) were applied onto the samples at room temperature for 2 h. After washing with PBS-T, the samples were mounted and observed under a fluorescence microscope.

Western blot analysis

The proteins were extracted from the cells or testes using the lysis buffer containing 50 mM Tris-HCl (pH7.4), 1 mM EDTA, 150 mM NaCl, 1% sodium deoxycholate, 0.1% SDS, 10 mM sodium fluoride, 1 mM sodium orthavanadate and 1% protease inhibitor cocktail (Sigma-Aldrich Corp, St. Louis, MO, USA). The extracted samples containing 50 μg proteins were subjected to 10%SDS-PAGE and electrophoretically transferred to polyvinylidene difluoride membranes. The filter was probed with PLZF antibody (1:200 dilution, R&D AF2944), UTF1 antibody (1:250 dilution, Chemicon

MAB4337), PTEN antibody (1:1,000 dilution, Millipore 04-035), GFRα1 antibody (1:2,000 dilution, R&D AF560), P-AKT antibody (1:1,000 dilution, Cell Signaling Technology #4058s) and β-actin (Cell Signaling Technology). Appropriate secondary antibodies were used and the antibody-antigen complexes in the membranes were visualized using an enhanced-chemiluminescent detection kit (Millipore). The images were scanned using LAS-4000 mini (FUJIFILM, Minato-ku, Tokyo, Japan).

RNA isolation and RT-PCR analysis

The total RNAs were extracted using TRIzol reagent (Invitrogen) and then the RNAs were reverse transcribed by using a Reverse Transcription kit according to manufacturer's instructions (TaKaRa, DRR037A). The following primers were used for SYBR Green–based real-time PCR (TaKaRa, DRR420A) on a 7900HT Real Time PCR System (Applied Biosystems Inc, USA): *Gapdh* [GenBank: NM_008084.3], 5′-TGCCCCCATGTTTGTGATG-3′ and 5′-TGTGGTCATGAGCCCTTCC-3′; *Pten* [GenBank: NM_008084.3], 5′-TTCATACCAGGACCAGAGGA-3′ and 5′-TTGTCATTATCTGCACGCTCT-3′. Relative gene expression was calculated by the two DDCt method against internal reference gene of glyceraldehyde-3-phosphate dehydrogenase (*Gapdh*).

In vivo fertility assay

To evaluate the effect of $Pten^{-/-}$ on fertility, we carried out in vivo fertility assay. For each experiment, two normal female mice were mated with one $Pten^{+/+}$ or $Pten^{-/-}$ male for 2 weeks and then embryos were counted. This mating test was artificially divided into three groups according to the male's ages as follows: 35–60 days, 61–100 days, and older than 100 days. All statistical analyses were conducted with GraphPAD 5.0.

Isolation of haploid cells

Testes were cut into pieces after removing the tunica albuginea, and testicular fragments in PBS were shocked roughly to wash out the intermediate cells near the lumen. Subsequently, the cells in supernatant were collected and stained with Hoechst 33342 (5 μg/ml). After 90 min of incubation, cells were resuspended in an ice-cold cell solution (PBS with 10% FBS) containing 2 μg/ml of propidium iodide for dead cell discrimination. All the solutions contain verapamil (50 μM/ml) to block the efflux of Hoechst. Finally, sorting was performed on an Influx cell sorter with UV laser (BD Biosciences) [19].

Isolation and culture of spermatogonial stem cells

Testes were removed from pups with fine forceps using sterile procedures and cut into pieces after removing the tunica albuginea. Following a two-step enzymatic digestion at 37°C until the tubules became minimum, supernatants were pipetted and collected quickly. The supernatant was centrifuged to remove the collagenase and the cells were incubated in a dish for 1 h, when the somatic cells had adhered to the bottom of the dish, the supernatants were collected and resuspended in KO-DMEM medium containing 1% FBS and 1,500 units/ml LIF to 6 well plates (for western blotting) or to 12 well plates with covers in each well (for immunofluorescent staining). Recombinant human GDNF and bFGF were added at a final concentration of 20 and 1 ng/ml respectively. Cells were maintained at 34°C in a humidified 5% CO_2 atmosphere [20]. The medium (containing 5 μM PI3K inhibitor or rapamycin 20 nM and growth factors) were changed every other day.

Abbreviations

PTEN: phosphatase and tensin homolog; PLZF: promyelocytic leukaemia zinc finger; UTF1: undifferentiated embryonic cell transcription factor 1; PI(3)K: phosphatidylinositol-3-OH kinase; SSCs: spermatogonial stem cells; Stra8: stimulated by retinoic acid gene 8; EGFP: enhanced green fluorescent protein; GFRα1: GDNF family receptor alpha-1; FOXO3A: forkhead box O3; Il2: interleukin 2; LIF: leukemia inhibitory factor; FBS: fetal bovine serum; GDNF: glial cell-derived neurotrophic factor; bFGF: basic fibroblast growth factor.

Authors' contributions

DZ, JD helped with the mice manipulation, WC and LW did the SSC isolation and culture experiments, WZ performed most of the experiments, HS and YT prepared the manuscript, ZY and WZ designed the research and prepared the manuscript. All authors read and approved the final manuscript.

Author details

[1] Hongqiao International Institute of Medicine, Shanghai Tongren Hospital / Faculty of Basic Medicine, Shanghai Jiao Tong University School of Medicine, Shanghai 200025, China. [2] Key Laboratory of Cell Differentiation and Apoptosis of Chinese Ministry of Education, Shanghai Jiao Tong University School of Medicine, Shanghai 200025, China. [3] Centre for Reproductive Medicine, Shanghai Jiao Tong University Affiliated Sixth People Hospital, Shanghai 200233, China. [4] Institute of Genetics and Developmental Biology, Chinese Academy of Sciences, Beijing 100101, China. [5] College of Public Health, Shanghai Jiao Tong University School of Medicine, Shanghai 200025, China.

Acknowledgements

The other authors wish to dedicate this paper to Dr. Lixin Feng who passed away during the manuscript preparation. This study was supported by Grants from the National Natural Science Foundation of China (31171409, 81000049, 81370654), National Key Basic Research and Development Program of China (2012CB966603), Innovation Program of Shanghai Municipal Education Commission (13G20), and the Program for Professor of Special Appointment (Eastern Scholar) at Shanghai Institutions of Higher Learning.

Compliance with ethical guidelines

Competing interests

The authors declare that they have no competing interests.

References

1. Buaas FW, Kirsh AL, Sharma M, McLean DJ, Morris JL, Griswold MD, et al. Plzf is required in adult male germ cells for stem cell self-renewal. Nat Genet. 2004;36(6):647–52. doi:10.1038/ng1366ng1366.
2. Costoya JA, Hobbs RM, Barna M, Cattoretti G, Manova K, Sukhwani M, et al. Essential role of Plzf in maintenance of spermatogonial stem cells. Nat Genet. 2004;36(6):653–9. doi:10.1038/ng1367ng1367.
3. He Z, Jiang J, Hofmann MC, Dym M. Gfra1 silencing in mouse spermatogonial stem cells results in their differentiation via the inactivation of RET tyrosine kinase. Biol Reprod. 2007;77(4):723–33. doi:10.1095/biolreprod.107.062513.
4. van Bragt MP, Roepers-Gajadien HL, Korver CM, Bogerd J, Okuda A, Eggen BJ, et al. Expression of the pluripotency marker UTF1 is restricted to a subpopulation of early A spermatogonia in rat testis. Reproduction. 2008;136(1):33–40. doi:10.1530/REP-07-0536.
5. Jung H, Roser JF, Yoon M. UTF1, a putative marker for spermatogonial stem cells in stallions. PLoS One. 2014;9(10):e108825. doi:10.1371/journal.pone.0108825.
6. Groszer M, Erickson R, Scripture-Adams DD, Lesche R, Trumpp A, Zack JA, et al. Negative regulation of neural stem/progenitor cell proliferation by the Pten tumor suppressor gene in vivo. Science. 2001;294(5549):2186–9. doi:10.1126/science.1065518.
7. Zhang J, Grindley JC, Yin T, Jayasinghe S, He XC, Ross JT, et al. PTEN maintains haematopoietic stem cells and acts in lineage choice and leukaemia prevention. Nature. 2006;441(7092):518–22. doi:10.1038/nature04747.
8. Reddy P, Liu L, Adhikari D, Jagarlamudi K, Rajareddy S, Shen Y, et al. Oocyte-specific deletion of Pten causes premature activation of the primordial follicle pool. Science. 2008;319(5863):611–3. doi:10.1126/science.1152257.
9. Blume-Jensen P, Jiang G, Hyman R, Lee KF, O'Gorman S, Hunter T. Kit/stem cell factor receptor-induced activation of phosphatidylinositol 3'-kinase is essential for male fertility. Nat Genet. 2000;24(2):157–62. doi:10.1038/72814.
10. Feng LX, Ravindranath N, Dym M. Stem cell factor/c-kit up-regulates cyclin D3 and promotes cell cycle progression via the phosphoinositide 3-kinase/p70 S6 kinase pathway in spermatogonia. J Biol Chem. 2000;275(33):25572–6. doi:10.1074/jbc.M002218200.
11. Maehama T, Dixon JE. The tumor suppressor, PTEN/MMAC1, dephosphorylates the lipid second messenger, phosphatidylinositol 3,4,5-trisphosphate. J Biol Chem. 1998;273(22):13375–8.
12. Stambolic V, Suzuki A, de la Pompa JL, Brothers GM, Mirtsos C, Sasaki T, et al. Negative regulation of PKB/Akt-dependent cell survival by the tumor suppressor PTEN. Cell. 1998;95(1):29–39.
13. Oulad-Abdelghani M, Bouillet P, Decimo D, Gansmuller A, Heyberger S, Dolle P, et al. Characterization of a premeiotic germ cell-specific cytoplasmic protein encoded by Stra8, a novel retinoic acid-responsive gene. J Cell Biol. 1996;135(2):469–77.
14. Giuili G, Tomljenovic A, Labrecque N, Oulad-Abdelghani M, Rassoulzadegan M, Cuzin F. Murine spermatogonial stem cells: targeted transgene expression and purification in an active state. EMBO Rep. 2002;3(8):753–9. doi:10.1093/embo-reports/kvf149.
15. van den Boom V, Kooistra SM, Boesjes M, Geverts B, Houtsmuller AB, Monzen K, et al. UTF1 is a chromatin-associated protein involved in ES cell differentiation. J Cell Biol. 2007;178(6):913–24. doi:10.1083/jcb.200702058.
16. Kristensen DM, Nielsen JE, Skakkebaek NE, Graem N, Jacobsen GK, Rajpert-De Meyts E, et al. Presumed pluripotency markers UTF-1 and REX-1 are expressed in human adult testes and germ cell neoplasms. Hum Reprod. 2008;23(4):775–82. doi:10.1093/humrep/den010.
17. Cao J, Zhu S, Zhou W, Li J, Liu C, Xuan H, et al. PLZF mediates the PTEN/AKT/FOXO3a signaling in suppression of prostate tumorigenesis. PLoS One. 2013;8(12):e77922. doi:10.1371/journal.pone.0077922.
18. Ruan H, Li J, Ren S, Gao J, Li G, Kim R, et al. Inducible and cardiac specific PTEN inactivation protects ischemia/reperfusion injury. J Mol Cell Cardiol. 2009;46(2):193–200. doi:10.1016/j.yjmcc.2008.10.021.
19. Goodell MA. Stem cell identification and sorting using the Hoechst 33342 side population (SP). In: Paul Robinson J et al., editors Current protocols in cytometry/editorial board, Chapter 9:Unit9.18. 2005. doi:10.1002/0471142956.cy0918s34.
20. Wang L, Cao J, Ji P, Zhang D, Ma L, Dym M, et al. Oocyte-like cells induced from mouse spermatogonial stem cells. Cell Biosci. 2012;2(1):27. doi:10.1186/2045-3701-2-27.

Cellular prostatic acid phosphatase (cPAcP) serves as a useful biomarker of histone deacetylase (HDAC) inhibitors in prostate cancer cell growth suppression

Yu-Wei Chou[1,2*], Fen-Fen Lin[2], Sakthivel Muniyan[2], Frank C Lin[2,3], Ching-Shih Chen[4], Jue Wang[5,6], Chao-Cheng Huang[1,7] and Ming-Fong Lin[2,8,9,10*]

Abstract

Background: Prostate cancer (PCa) is the most commonly diagnosed solid tumor and the second leading cancer death in the United States, and also one of the major cancer-related deaths in Chinese. Androgen deprivation therapy (ADT) is the first line treatment for metastatic PCa. PCa ultimately relapses with subsequent ADT treatment failure and becomes castrate-resistant (CR). It is important to develop effective therapies with a surrogate marker towards CR PCa.

Method: Histone deacetylase (HDAC) inhibitors were examined to determine their effects in androgen receptor (AR)/cellular prostatic acid phosphatase (cPAcP)-positive PCa cells, including LNCaP C-33, C-81, C4-2 and C4-2B and MDA PCa2b androgen-sensitive and androgen-independent cells, and AR/cPAcP-negative PCa cells, including PC-3 and DU 145 cells. Cell growth was determined by cell number counting. Western blot analyses were carried out to determine AR, cPAcP and PSA protein levels.

Results: cPAcP protein level was increased by HDAC inhibitor treatment. Valproic acid, a HDAC inhibitor, suppressed the growth of AR/cPAcP-positive PCa cells by over 50% in steroid-reduced conditions, higher than on AR/cPAcP-negative PCa cells. Further, HDAC inhibitor pretreatments increased androgen responsiveness as demonstrated by PSA protein level quantitation.

Conclusion: Our results clearly demonstrate that HDAC inhibitors can induce cPAcP protein level, increase androgen responsiveness, and exhibit higher inhibitory activities on AR/cPAcP-positive PCa cells than on AR/cPAcP-negative PCa cells. Upon HDAC inhibitor pretreatment, PSA level was greatly elevated by androgens. This data indicates the potential clinical importance of cPAcP serving as a useful biomarker in the identification of PCa patient sub-population suitable for HDAC inhibitor treatment.

Keywords: Prostate cancer, Histone deacetylase inhibitor, Cellular prostatic acid phosphatase, Biomarker

Background

Prostate cancer is the most commonly diagnosed solid tumor and the second leading cancer death in United States. While the incidence in Chinese population is lower than in Western countries, it is rising rapidly and becomes one of the major cancer-related deaths in this region [1, 2]. Androgen-deprivation therapy (ADT) is the first line treatment for the advanced metastatic PCa by decreasing the production of androgens or the functions of AR with anti-androgen agents [3–5]. Unfortunately, most PCa will eventually still progress to castration-resistant prostate cancer (CR PCa) which represents an aggressive and incurable phenotype after a certain time period of treatment [4, 6]. Although new FDA approved

*Correspondence: ywchou@cgmh.org.tw; mlin@unmc.edu
[1] Tissue Bank and BioBank, Kaohsiung Chang Gung Memorial Hospital, No. 123, Da-Pi Road, Niao-Song District, Kaohsiung 833, Taiwan, ROC
[2] Department of Biochemistry and Molecular Biology, College of Medicine, 985870 Nebraska Medical Center, University of Nebraska Medical Center, Omaha, NE 68198-5870, USA
Full list of author information is available at the end of the article

therapies demonstrating increased survival benefits for CR PCa treatment exist, there are still no treatment modalities to inhibit the development of CR PCa [3].

Human prostatic acid phosphatase (PAcP), a 100 kDa glycoprotein of two subunits, is a prostate epithelium-specific differentiation antigen: one stays intracellularly, the cellular form (cPAcP), and the other secrets into seminal fluid, the secretory form (sPAcP), both encoded by the same gene [7, 8]. In normal males, circulating sPAcP activity is negligible. Interestingly, the serum activity of sPAcP is significantly elevated in PCa patients, especially in PCa patients with bone metastasis, and also correlated with tumor progression. sPAcP was thus utilized as a surrogate maker for the diagnosis and prognosis of PCa before the availability of prostate-specific antigen (PSA) despite the decreased expression of mRNA levels [9, 10]. sPAcP can also serve as an independent predictor of tumor recurrence following radical prostatectomy [7, 11]. Additionally, several lines of evidence show that cPAcP may serve as an excellent measure to elucidate the molecular mechanism of the relationship between androgens and tyrosine phosphorylation signaling involved in prostate cancer progression [8, 12–15]. cPAcP has been shown to be a negative growth regulator of prostate epithelia through its neutral protein tyrosine phosphatase (PTP) activity by dephosporylating p-Tyr of ErbB-2, which results in regulating androgen sensitivity [5, 12, 15]. Interestingly, cPAcP is involved in the effect of HDAC inhibitors on PCa cell growth suppression via its up-regulation for ErbB-2 dephosphorylation, and knockdown PAcP expression by shRNA reduces the degree of growth suppression by HDAC inhibitor [16]. Collectedly, cPAcP protein serves as a prostate epithelial differentiation marker and functions as a unique prostate-specific tumor suppressor [8].

Histone acetylation is regulated by a dynamic balance between histone acetyl transferases (HATs) and histone deactylases (HDACs), and involved in affecting the chromatin folding during gene expression [17, 18]. HDACs modulate transcriptional activity of hormonal receptors including AR, for example, by altering the stability of the transcriptional pre-initiation complex and/or modifying the chromatin structure. Many lines of evidence demonstrate HDACs over-expression or close association in multiple cancers, including PCa [3, 19]. HDAC inhibitors are epigenetic therapy agents targeting class I and/or class II histone deacetylases which alter not only histone and also non-histone protein function [6, 18]. HDAC inhibitors have been shown to mediate tumor cell differentiation, exhibit a dramatic inhibitory effect on tumor cell proliferation and death [3, 20]. HDAC inhibitors have therefore been considered to be a novel class of cancer treatment agents and a number of inhibitors have been entered into clinical trials for PCa therapy.

A biomarker such as a measurable molecular, cellular, or genetic parameter should indicate the biological or pathological conditions or pharmacological response to the treatments. Drug discovery and development in cancer research is rapidly approaching personalized or mechanism-based targeting therapy. The application of a suitable biomarker in the novel treatment could bring various advantages, such as the increasing potency, specific tumor selectivity, reducing toxicities and side effect profiles, improving the quality of patient's life. HDAC inhibitors may serve as a novel class of anti-cancer agents; to develop a selecting biomarker for patient population who are suitable to HDAC inhibitor treatment requires further identification. In our previous study, we investigated the molecular target by HDAC inhibitors for exploring their potential of CR PCa therapy. We found that cPAcP expression is involved in growth suppression by HDAC inhibitors in AR-positive PCa cells, and HDAC inhibitor pre-treatment could increase androgen responsiveness of those PCa cells [16].

In this study, we tested the hypothesis that cPAcP can serve as a useful biomarker for identifying patients sensitive to HDACi treatments. We analyzed six different HDAC inhibitors which have shown inhibitory activities on tumor cell proliferation and/or viability or entered in various clinical trials, including valproic acid (VPA), sodium butyrate (NaB), suberoylanilide hydroxamic acid (SAHA), PxD 101, MS-275 and AR-42 [6, 16, 20–29] on six AR/cPAcP-positive and four AR/cPAcP-negative PCa cell lines. Our data provide strong evidence for the role of cPAcP expression in various HDAC inhibitors treatment in PCa cells. HDAC inhibitor treatment elevated cPAcP expression level and increased the androgen responsiveness of AR/cPAcP-positive PCa cells as shown by elevated PSA protein levels. Importantly, in steroid-reduced conditions mimicking clinical androgen deprivation therapy, AR/cPAcP-positive PCa cells were more sensitive to inhibitory efficiency of HDAC inhibitors treatment than AR/cPAcP-negative PCa cells. These results have important clinical impacts on identifying a useful biomarker for HDAC inhibitors toward advanced CR PCa treatment and also on predicting clinical treatment outcome.

Results and discussion

Cellular prostatic acid phosphatase (cPAcP) is a unique prostate-specific tumor suppressor and its loss of expression is associated with prostate carcinogenesis [8]. The data also revealed that cPAcP is involved in regulating androgen-stimulated PCa cell growth, and its expression is associated with androgen-sensitive cell proliferation [7, 16]. Previously, we identified that cPAcP is one of molecular targets by HDAC inhibitors in PCa growth suppression. In HDAC inhibitor-treated AR-positive PCa cells, cPAcP is elevated and cell growth is suppressed; conversely, knockdown cPAcP expression by shRNA reduces the degree of growth suppression by HDAC inhibitors [16]. Furthermore, cPAcP in addition to AR plays a critical role in regulating androgen sensitivity of PCa cell proliferation. While AR is essential to androgen sensitivity; the presence of AR alone is not sufficient for androgen responsiveness of growth stimulation. For example, CR PCa cells still express functional AR but are androgen unresponsive. Instead, the expression of cPAcP in those cells is associated with androgen sensitivity. Since cPAcP expression is responsive to but not regulated by androgens, cPAcP level is not consistent with AR level. Importantly, upon VPA pretreatment, the androgen responsiveness of cells was increased, higher than control cells. As a clinical correlation, we selected cPAcP as a surrogate marker and further explored the role of cPAcP expression in PCa cell growth suppression by various HDAC inhibitors and examined whether HDAC inhibitors treatment will indeed alter androgen responsiveness of different PCa cells.

First, we analyzed the basal level of AR, PAcP and PSA proteins in different PCa cell lines. As shown in Figure 1, in regular culture condition, MDA PCa2b AS and AI cells, and LNCaP C-33, C-81, C4-2 and C4-2B cells all express AR protein. Among them, LNCaP cells had an overall higher levels of AR protein than MDA PCa2b cells, and LNCaP C-33 cells expressed the highest AR protein level among these cells examined (Figure 1), correlating with the degree of androgen-stimulated cell growth (data not shown). On the contrary, MDA PCa2b cells express higher levels of cPAcP than LNCaP cells (Figure 1) and have slower cell proliferation [30]. Furthermore, in MDA PCa2b and LNCaP cell models, cPAcP level decreased in AI cells, lower than that in the corresponding AS cells,

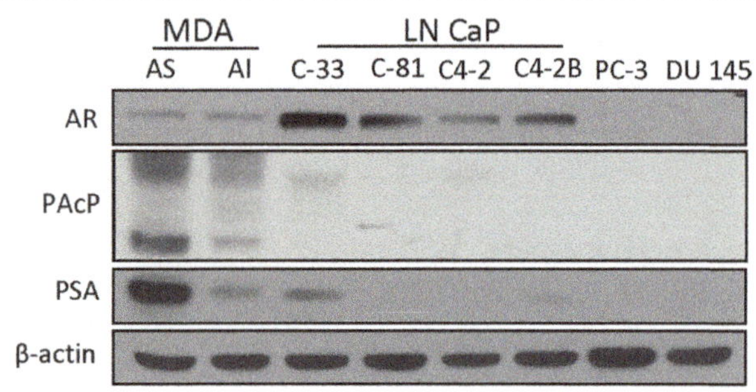

Figure 1 The basal expression levels of AR, cPAcP and PSA were determined in different PCa cell lines. LNCaP C-33/C-81, LNCaP C4-2/C4-2B, MDA PCa2B AS/AI, PC-3 and DU 145 cells that were plated in regular medium for 3 days and then changed with fresh medium for 1 day. The cells were harvested and the total protein was subjected to western blot analyses of functional proteins expression. β-Actin was analyzed and used as a loading control.

respectively. The low PAcP level in AI LNCaP C-81, C4-2 and C4-2B could be seen upon prolonged exposure (data not shown). The PSA protein level is also decreased in AI cells. In comparison, PC-3 and DU 145 cells do not express a detectable level of AR, PAcP and PSA proteins (Figure 1) despite prolonged exposure (data not shown).

We determined the effect of HDAC inhibitor on cPAcP protein level in AR-positive PCa cells and examined their relationship since cPAcP protein functions as a tumor suppressor in PCa cells. We first examined VPA effect on cPAcP protein level. As shown in Figure 2a–c, upon VPA treatment, cPAcP protein levels were greatly elevated in LNCaP C-33 and C4-2B cells, compared with control cells received the solvent alone (Figure 2a, b, Lane #3 vs. #1, right panel), which were decreased by subsequent DHT treatment (Figure 2a, b, Lane #4 vs. #3, right panel). cPAcP protein level had only a slight elevation in VPA-treated MDA PCa2b-AS cells (Figure 2c, Lane #3 vs. #1, right panel), which could be in part due to a very high basal level of cPAcP protein in those cells (Figure 1). Similar phenomenon was observed in LNCaP C-81, C4-2 and MDA PCa2B AI PCa cells (data not shown; [16]). Therefore, the observations on cPAcP protein levels that are increased in all VPA-pretreated PCa cells and then decreased by DHT treatment are inversely correlated with cell growth (Figure 2, Column #1 vs. #3, #3 vs. #4, left panel).

Since androgen sensitivity is an important clinical phenomenon; we examined VPA effect on the androgen responsiveness. Importantly, the PSA level was greatly elevated by 10 nM DHT in VPA-pretreated LNCaP cell lines by over 18-fold, higher than that of control cells without VPA-pretreatment with about fourfold increase (Figure 2a, b, Lane #4 vs. #2, right panel). In VPA-pretreated MDA PCa2b AS cells, PSA protein level was greatly elevated, which is further increased upon DHT treatment (Figure 2c, Lane #4 vs. #3, right panel); despite the fact that DHT alone only had a marginal effect on PSA protein level in the absence of VPA pretreatment, the similar trends were observed in LNCaP C-81, C4-2 and MDA PCa2B AI PCa cell lines (data not shown; [16]). In summary, our data show that VPA pretreatment can increase the degree of androgen sensitivity in cell proliferation by cell number counting and PSA protein level, an androgen-regulated marker, despite that in MDA PCa2b AS cells, VPA pretreatment only greatly enhanced DHT-increased PSA level (Figure 2c, Lane #3 vs. #4, right panel) but not cell growth (Figure 2c, Column #3 vs. #4, left panel). Furthermore, cPAcP protein level was indeed elevated by VPA treatment and then diminished by subsequent DHT treatment (Figure 2, Lane #3 vs. #4, right panels). Since VPA pretreatment greatly enhances DHT-upregulated PSA level, the data indicate that VPA can

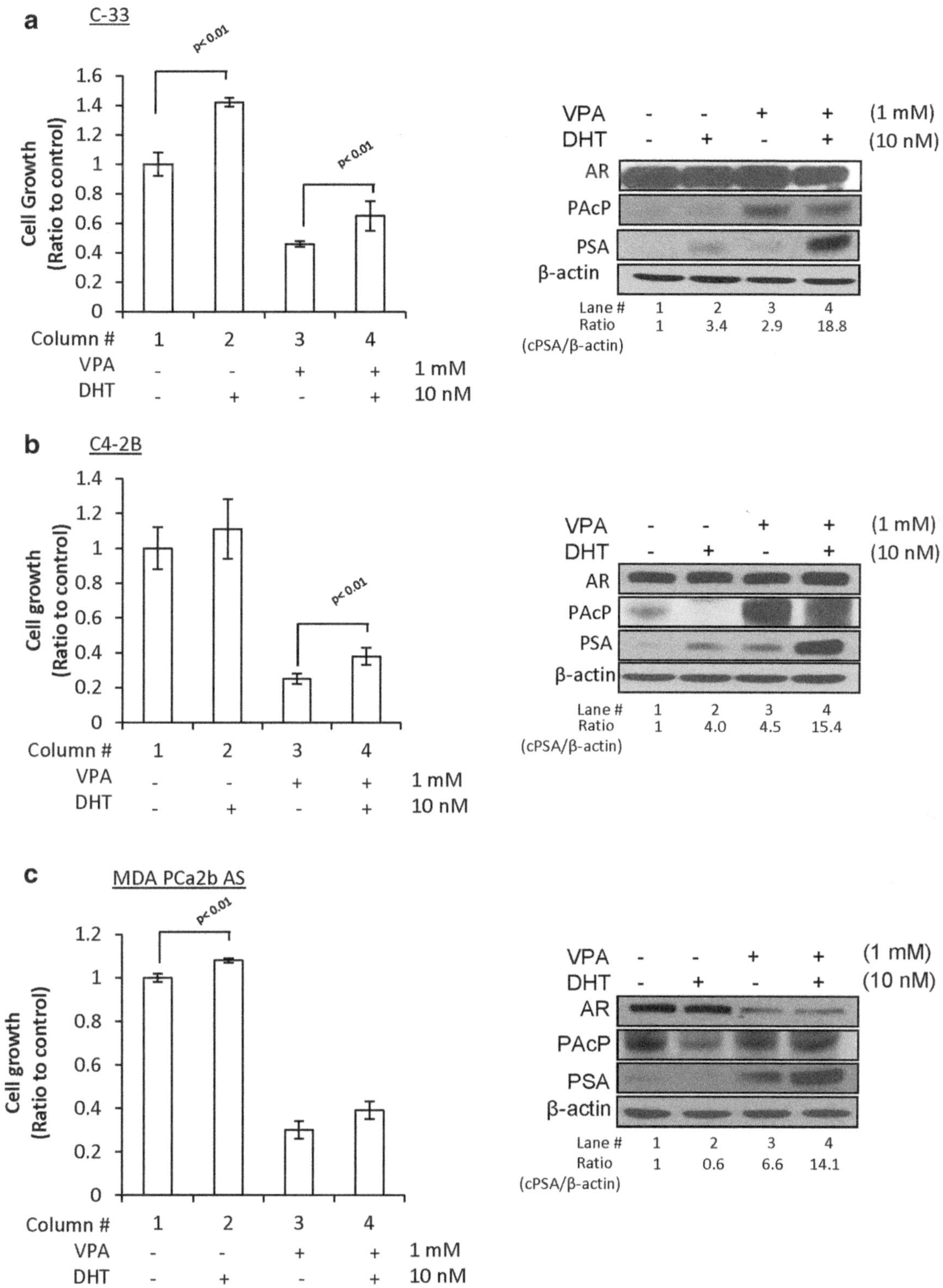

Figure 2 Effect of VPA on androgen responsiveness of PCa cell lines. **a** LNCaP C-33; **b** LNCaP C4-2B; **c** MDA PCa2B AS cells were seeded in 6-wells plate and then treated with 1 mM VPA or solvent for 48 h. Cell were then maintained in a steroid-reduced medium with or without 10 nM DHT for 2 days. Total cell number was counted. The ratio of cell growth was calculated by normalizing the cell number to that of control cells (*column #1*, *left panel*, n = 3×2). Total cell lysate proteins from 3-day DHT treatment were analyzed for cPAcP, PSA, AR protein. β-Actin was analyzed and used as a loading control (*right panel*).

increase androgen responsiveness of AR-positive PCa cells.

We examined whether other HDAC inhibitors could similarly enhance the androgen responsiveness of PCa cells. LNCaP C-81 cells were used as the model for HDAC inhibitors pretreatment since C-81 cells exhibit many biochemical properties of CR PCa cells (16, 31, 32). C-81 cells were treated with HDAC inhibitors including NaB, SAHA, PxD101, MS-275 and AR42. Results of western blot analyses showed that cPAcP protein including the 38 kDa intermediate form and 50 kDa mature form were greatly elevated by all HDAC inhibitor treatments (Figure 3a–e, Lane #3 vs. #1, right panel) and were diminished by subsequently 1 and 10 nM DHT treatments, following the dose-dependent manner (Figure 3a, Lane #4 vs. #3, right panel; Figure 3b–e, Lane #5, 6 vs. Lane #4, right panel). Further analyses on Figures 2 and 3 reveal that the efficacy of HDAC inhibitor's growth suppression is at least in part correlated with the degree of induced expression of cPAcP in addition to cPAcP basal level.

Furthermore, we validated DHT responsiveness by analyzing PSA protein level followed by semi-quantification in HDAC inhibitors-pretreated cells. In absence of DHT, PSA basal levels were greatly elevated by SAHA, PxD 101 and MS-275 treatments, and slightly increased in AR42-treated cells, but not significantly elevated in NaB-treated cells, respectively (Figure 3b–e, Lane #4 vs. #1; Figure 3a, Lane #3 vs. #1, right panel). Importantly, PSA expression levels were greatly elevated by 10 nM DHT in all HDAC inhibitor-pretreated cells by up to 12-fold of that in control cells without HDAC inhibitor pretreatment (Figure 3a, Lane #4 vs. #2; Figure 3b–e, Lane #6 vs. #3 right panel). However, the growth stimulation by DHT was only marginally increased in those HDAC inhibitors-pretreated cells comparing with control cells and only significantly increased in MS-275 and AR42 pretreated cells (Figure 3a, Column #4 vs. #3; Figure 3b–e, Column #5, 6 vs. #4, left panel). The data collectively indicate that HDAC inhibitors exhibit the significant efficacy of growth suppression and can enhance the androgen responsiveness of PSA levels. Nevertheless, the effect of HDAC inhibitors pretreatment on DHT-stimulated cell growth requires further investigation.

Since the expression of cPAcP correlates with growth suppression by HDAC inhibitors, we investigated whether cPAcP protein level can serve as a useful biomarker of identifying the PCa patient sub-population who is potentially responsive to HDAC inhibitors treatment. To mimic the clinical situation of chemotherapy under androgen ablation conditions, cell growth suppression was determined in steroid-reduced (SR) conditions. Six AR/cPAcP-positive PCa cell lines and four AR/cPAcP-negative PCa cell lines including NE 1–3 and NE 1–8 cells, two neuroendocrine prostate cancer cell lines, were examined. After 2 days of VPA treatment, all PCa cells were maintained in SR medium for 72 h. Interestingly, the growth of those AR/cPAcP-positive PCa cells were in general significantly decreased by VPA treatment with more than 50% suppression; while the growth of AR/cPAcP-negative PCa cells was suppressed by less than 50% (Figure 4). The data indicate that cPAcP can potentially serve as a biomarker for HDAC inhibitor treatment with clinical benefits. Those patients can be more sensitive to HDAC inhibitor treatment, i.e., higher growth suppression and enhanced androgen responsiveness.

Conclusion

In summary, the results of our study clearly show that in all HDAC inhibitors-treated AR/cPAcP-positive PCa cells, growth suppression by HDAC inhibitors is associated with elevated cPAcP protein level, and the androgen responsiveness of those PCa cells is also enhanced. PCa cells which exhibit endogenous cPAcP expression are more sensitive to HDAC inhibitors as shown by higher inhibitory efficiency with more than 50% compared with that of PCa without cPAcP expression by HDAC inhibitor treatments (Figure 4). Our data reveal that cPAcP can serve as a biomarker for identifying PCa patients who are sensitive to be treated by HDAC inhibitors. cPAcP can thus serve as a surrogate marker in PCa therapy, predicting clinical outcome to decrease the medical resources waste and improve the treatment efficacy. Furthermore, HDAC inhibitor-treated patients may re-gain their androgen responsiveness and thus are suitable to continue ADT treatment. HDAC inhibitors significantly increase PSA protein level while inhibit PCa cell proliferation, serum PSA cannot serve as a suitable marker for predicating the efficacy of treatments by HDAC inhibitors.

Methods

Materials

RPMI 1640 medium, gentamicin and trypsin/EDTA reagents were purchased from Invitrogen Corporation (Carlsbad, CA, USA). Fetal bovine serum (FBS), charcoal/dextran-treated, certified FBS was from Atlanta Biologicals (Lawrenceville, GA, USA). Acrylamide, protein molecular weight standard markers and Protein Estimation Kit were obtained from Bio-Rad (Hercules, CA, USA). The ECL reagent kit was purchased from Pierce Biotechnology Inc. (Rockford, IL, USA). Histone deacetylase inhibitors including sodium butyrate (NaB), valproic acid (VPA), 5α-dihydrotestosterone (DHT) and anti-β-Actin Ab (AC-15) were from Sigma (St Louis, MO, USA). Other HDAC inhibitors, including suberoylanilide hydroxamic acid (SAHA), AR42 and MS-275, were kindly

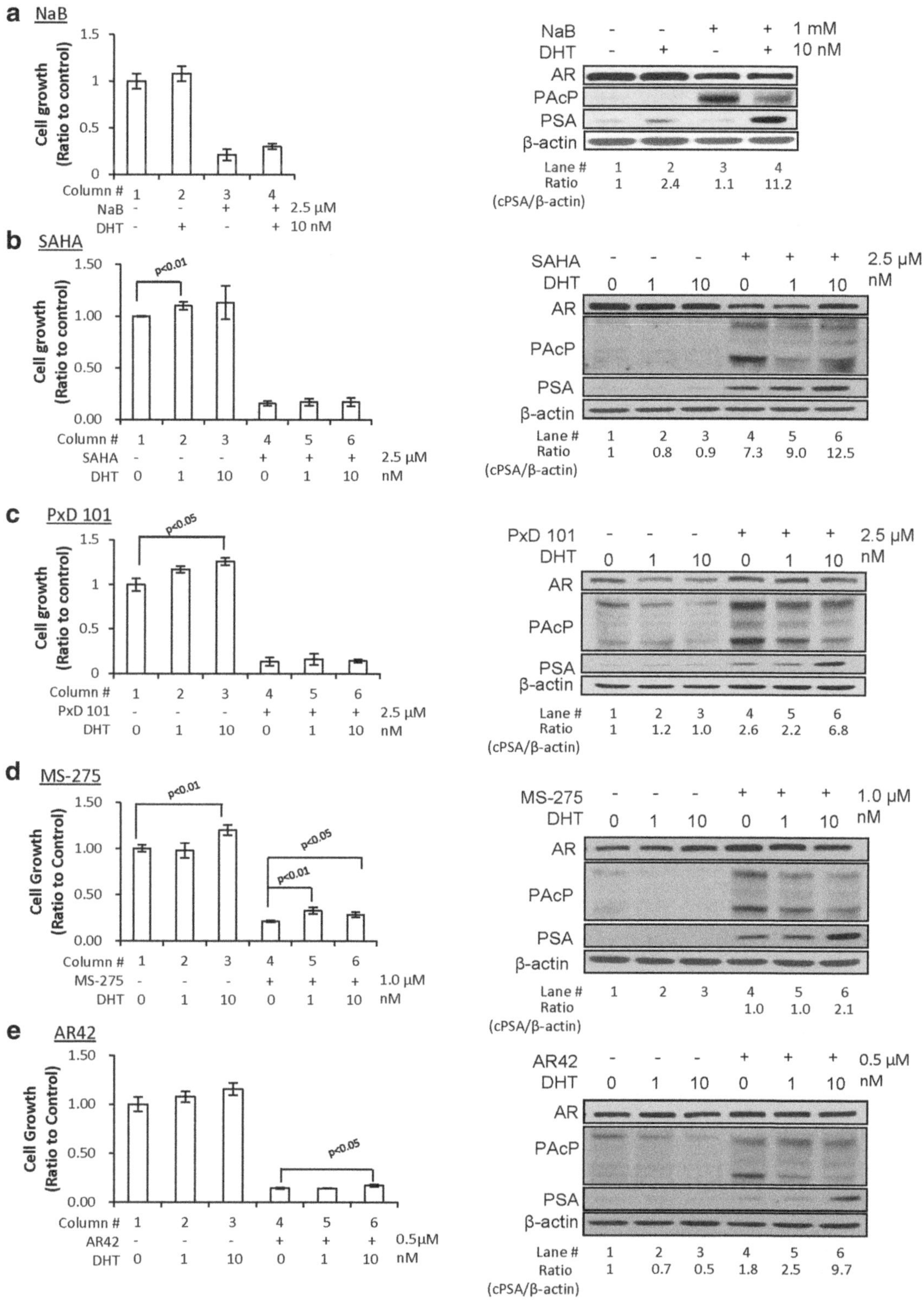

Figure 3 Effects of different HDAC inhibitors on androgen responsiveness of PCa cells. LNCaP C-81 cells were plated in 6-wells plate and then treated with **a** 1 mM NaB; **b** 2.5 μM SAHA; **c** 2.5 μM PxD101; **d** 1.0 μM MS-275; **e** 0.5 μM AR42 or solvent alone for 48 h. Cell were then maintained in a steroid-reduced medium with or without 1 and 10 nM DHT for 3 days. Total cell number was counted. The ratio of cell growth was calculated by normalizing the cell number to that of control cells (*column #1*, *left panel*, n = 3×2). Total cell lysate proteins were analyzed for cPAcP, PSA and AR protein. β-Actin was analyzed and used as a loading control (*right panel*).

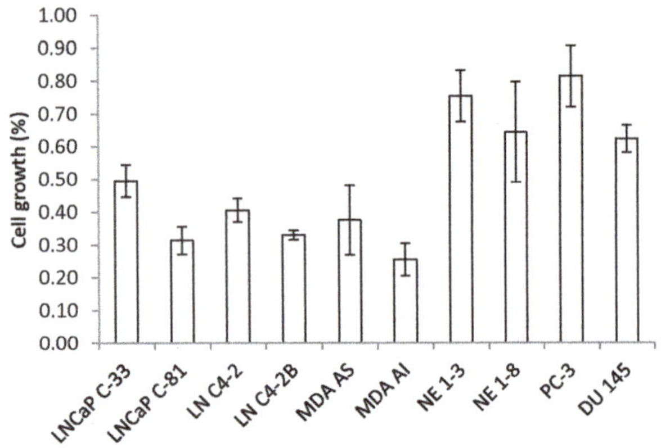

Figure 4 The growth inhibition of VPA treatment on various PCa cells. LNCaP C-33/C-81, LNCaP C4-2/C4-2B, MDA PCa2B AS/AI, NE 1-3/1-8, PC-3 and DU 145 PCa cell lines were plated in 6-wells plates and then treated with 1 mM VPA or solvent for 48 h. Cells were then maintained in a steroid-reduced medium for 3 days. Total cell number was counted. The ratio of cell growth was calculated by normalizing the cell number to that of control cells ($n = 3 \times 2$).

provided by Dr. Ching-Shih Chen at the Ohio State University Comprehensive Cancer Center (Columbus, OH, USA). PxD101 was from Dr. Jue Wang at Medical Oncology section, University of Nebraska Medical Center (Omaha, NE, USA). Rabbit anti-human PAcP Ab (ATM-3) has been described previously [14, 15]. The respective Abs against androgen receptor (AR) and PSA were from Santa Cruz Biotechnology (Santa Cruz, CA, USA).

Cell culture

Human prostate carcinoma cell lines including LNCaP, MDA PCa2b, PC-3 and DU 145 cells were originally purchased from the American Type Culture Collection (Rockville, MD, USA). LNCaP C4-2 and C4-2B cells were purchased from DIANON Company (Oklahoma City, OK, USA). LNCaP C-33/C-81, PC-3 and DU 145 cells were routinely maintained in the regular medium, i.e., phenol red-positive RPMI 1640 medium supplemented with 5% FBS, 2 mM glutamine and 50 μg/ml gentamicin. MDA PCa2b cells were cultured in BRFF-HPC1 medium containing 20% FBS, 2 mM glutamine and 50 μg/ml gentamicin. LNCaP C4-2 and C4-2B cells were grown in DMEM/F12 medium with 10% FBS, 2 mM glutamine, 50 μg/ml gentamicin, 1 mM sodium pyruvate, 2× vitamin C and 1× MEM non-essential amino acid. Cells were split once a week by trypsinization, which was defined as one passage.

The LNCaP PCa cell progression model was originally described by Lin et al. [31] and further characterized by Igawa et al. [32] with passage number less than 35 defined as C-33, passage numbers between 80 and 120 as C-81 cells. LNCaP C-81 cells exhibit many biochemical properties similar to the phenotype of advanced CR PCa, including the intracrine growth regulation, PSA secretion and rapid cell proliferation under steroid-deprived conditions. LNCaP C4-2/C4-2B cells also exhibit androgen independency of growth [33]. Similarly, MDA PCa2b-AI cells, the high passage MDA PCa2b cells, exhibit androgen-independent proliferation as described [12, 34, 35]. In this set of experiments, the passage numbers of MDA PCa2b-AI cells were between about 110 and 125.

Effect of HDAC inhibitor pretreatment on the androgen responsiveness and cell growth suppression of PCa cell lines

Various PCa cell lines, including LNCaP C-33/C-81, LNCaP C4-2/C4-2B and MDA PCa2b AS/AI cells were plated with 3×10^4, 3×10^4 and 1×10^5 cells/well, respectively, in 6-well plates in regular medium for 3 days and then treated with 1 mM VPA or different concentrations of HDAC inhibitors as specified in each experiment for 2 days. Control cells were treated with solvent alone. Subsequently, cells were maintained in a steroid-reduced medium minus or plus 1 and 10 nM DHT for 2 days. Cells were harvested and cell numbers were counted using a Cellometer Auto T4 Image-based cell counter (Nexcelom Bioscience). All experiments were performed in triplicate and repeated at least twice. Results shown were an average or a representative from two or three sets of independent experiments. Cells were lysed for analyzing cPAcP, AR and PSA protein expression. β-Actin was used as a loading control.

To determine the effect of cPAcP on PCa cell growth suppression by HDAC inhibitors, LNCaP (C-33/C-81, C4-2/C4-2B), MDA PCa2B AS/AI, NE1-3/1-8, PC-3 and DU145 PCa cells were plated in 6-well plates in regular medium for 3 days, treated with 1 mM VPA for 2 days and then maintained in steroid-reduced medium for 3 days. Control cells were treated with solvent alone. The cell numbers were counted. The ratio of cell growth was calculated by normalizing the number of experimental cells to that of control cells.

Immunoblotting

For analyzing cellular protein levels, subconfluent cells were harvested by scraping. The cell pellet was rinsed with ice-cold 20 mM HEPES-buffered saline (pH 7.0) and then lysed in ice-cold cell lysis buffer (20 mM Tris–HCl, pH 7.5, 150 mM NaCl, 1 mM EDTA, 1% Nonidet P-40) containing protease and phosphatase inhibitors and the total lysate protein was prepared upon centrifugation. An aliquot of total cellular lysate having 50–120 μg protein was subjected to electrophoresis on SDS–polyacrylamide gels (7.5–12% acrylamide) and then transferred to nitrocellulose membrane for western blot analyses. The membrane filter was blocked by 5% skim milk and subsequently incubated with appropriate primary and secondary Ab. The proteins of interest were visualized by an ECL detection system. For re-probing, the membranes were stripped with a stripping buffer for 30 min at 50°C, blocked and re-hybridized with specific Abs [16].

Statistical analysis

Each experiment was performed in duplicate or triplicates and repeated at least twice as independent experiments, as specified in each figure legend or experiment design, and the mean and standard error values were calculated. The significance of difference (p value) was calculated using independent Student t test and the p value less than 0.05 was considered as significant.

Abbreviations

PCa: prostate cancer; PAcP: prostatic acid phosphatase; HDAC: histone deacetylase.

Authors' contributions

YWC, SM and FCL performed the experiments. YWC wrote the manuscript. FFL provided the technical supports. CSC and JW provided HDAC inhibitors. CCH provided the clinical medical suggestions. MFL conceived and supervised this study, designed the experiments, and revised the manuscript. All authors read and approved the final manuscript.

Author details

[1] Tissue Bank and BioBank, Kaohsiung Chang Gung Memorial Hospital, No. 123, Da-Pi Road, Niao-Song District, Kaohsiung 833, Taiwan, ROC. [2] Department of Biochemistry and Molecular Biology, College of Medicine, 985870 Nebraska Medical Center, University of Nebraska Medical Center, Omaha, NE 68198-5870, USA. [3] Division of Urology, Department of Surgery, University of Arizona Medical Center, Tucson, AZ, USA. [4] Division of Medicinal Chemistry and Pharmacology, College of Pharmacy, The Ohio State University, Columbus, OH, USA. [5] Division of Oncology/Hematology, Department of Internal Medicine, University of Nebraska Medical Center, Omaha, NE, USA. [6] University of Arizona Cancer Center, St. Joseph's Hospital and Medical Center, Phoenix, AZ, USA. [7] Department of Pathology, Kaohsiung Chang Gung Memorial Hospital, and Chang Gung University College of Medicine, Kaohsiung, Taiwan, ROC. [8] Eppley Institute for Research in Cancer and Allied Diseases, University of Nebraska Medical Center, Omaha, NE, USA. [9] Department of Surgery/Urology, University of Nebraska Medical Center, Omaha, NE, USA. [10] School of Pharmacy, Kaohsiung Medical University, Kaohsiung, Taiwan, ROC.

Acknowledgements

This work was supported in part by the National Cancer Institute, National Institute of Health (R01 CA88184); Department of Defense PCa Training Grant (PC094594, PC121645) and the University of Nebraska Medical Center Bridge Fund; Kaohsiung Chang Gung Memorial Hospital, Taiwan (CMRPG8D00631).

Compliance with ethical guidelines

Competing interests

The authors declare that they have no competing interests.

References

1. Ito K. Prostate cancer in Asian men. Nat Rev Urol. 2014;11:197–212.
2. Pu YS. Prostate cancer in Taiwan: epidemiology and risk factors. Int J Androl. 2000;2000(23):34–6.
3. Ellis L, Ku S, Ramakrishnan S, Lasorsa E, Azabdaftari G, Godoy A, et al. Combinatorial antitumor effect of HDACs and the PI3K-Akt-mTOR pathway inhibition in a Pten deficient model of prostate cancer. Oncotarget. 2013;4:2225–36.
4. Muniyan S, Chou YW, Ingersoll MA, Devine A, Morris M, Odero-Marah VA, et al. Antiproliferative activity of novel imidazopyridine derivatives on castration-resistant human prostate cancer cells. Cancer Lett. 2014;353:59–67.
5. Zhang L, Davis JS, Zelivianski S, Lin FF, Schutte R, Davis TL, et al. Suppression of ErbB-2 in androgen-independent human prostate cancer cells enhances cytotoxic effect by gemcitabine in an androgen-reduced environment. Cancer Lett. 2009;285:58–65.
6. Gravina GL, Marampon F, Muzi P, Mancini A, Piccolella M, Negri-Cesi P, et al. PXD101 potentiates hormonal therapy and prevents the onset of castration-resistant phenotype modulating androgen receptor, HSP90, and CRM1 in preclinical models of prostate cancer. Endocr Relat Cancer. 2013;20:321–37.
7. Muniyan S, Chaturvedi NK, Dwyer JG, Lagrange CA, Chaney WG, Lin MF. Human prostatic acid phosphatase: structure, function and regulation. Int J Mol Sci. 2013;14:10438–64.
8. Muniyan S, Ingersoll MA, Batra SK, Lin MF. Cellular prostatic acid phosphatase, a PTEN-functional homologue in prostate epithelia, functions as a prostate-specific tumor suppressor. BBA Rev Cancer. 2014;1846:88–98.
9. Chu TM, Lin MF. PSA and acid phosphatase in the diagnosis of prostate cancer. J Clin Lig Assay. 1998;21:24–34.
10. Papsidero LD, Wojcieszyn JW, Horoszewicz JS, Leong SS, Murphy GP, Chu TM. Isolation of prostatic acid phosphatase-binding immunoglobulin G from human sera and its potential for use as a tumor-localizing reagent. Cancer Res. 1980;40:3032–5.
11. Han M, Partin AW, Pound CR, Epstein JI, Walsh PC. Long-term biochemical disease-free and cancer-specific survival following anatomic radical retropubic prostatectomy: the 15-year Johns Hopkins experience. Urol Clin North Am. 2001;28:555–65.
12. Chuang TD, Chen SJ, Lin FF, Veeramani S, Kumar S, Batra SK, et al. Human prostatic acid phosphatase, an authentic tyrosine phosphatase, dephosphorylates ErbB-2 and regulates prostate cancer cell growth. J Biol Chem. 2010;285:23598–606.
13. Lin MF, Clinton GM. Human prostatic acid phosphatase has phosphotyrosyl protein phosphatase activity. Biochem J. 1986;235:351–7.
14. Lin MF, DaVolio J, Garcia-Arenas R. Expression of human prostatic acid phosphatase activity and the growth of prostate carcinoma cells. Cancer Res. 1992;52:4600–7.
15. Meng TC, Lin MF. Tyrosine phosphorylation of c-ErbB-2 is regulated by the cellular form of prostatic acid phosphatase in human prostate cancer cells. J Biol Chem. 1998;273:22096–104.
16. Chou YW, Chaturvedi NK, Ouyang S, Lin FF, Kaushik D, Wang J, et al. Histone deacetylase inhibitor valproic acid suppresses the growth and increases the androgen responsiveness of prostate cancer cells. Cancer Lett. 2011;311:177–86.
17. Marks PA, Xu WS. Histone deacetylase inhibitors: potential in cancer therapy. J Cell Biochem. 2009;107:600–8.
18. Stimson L, La Thangue NB. Biomarkers for predicting clinical responses to HDAC inhibitors. Cancer Lett. 2009;280:177–83.
19. Makarević J, Tawanaie N, Juengel E, Reiter M, Mani J, Tsaur I, et al. Cross-communication between histone H3 and H4 acetylation and Akt-mTOR signalling in prostate cancer cells. J Cell Mol Med. 2014;18:1460–6.
20. Qian X, Ara G, Mills E, LaRochelle WJ, Lichenstein HS, Jeffers M. Activity of the histone deacetylase inhibitor belinostat (PXD101) in preclinical models of prostate cancer. Int J Cancer. 2008;122:1400–10.
21. Armeanu S, Pathil A, Venturelli S, Mascagni P, Weiss TS, Gottlicher M, et al. Apoptosis on hepatoma cells but not on primary hepatocytes by histone deacetylase inhibitors valproate and ITF2357. J Hepatol. 2005;42:210–7.
22. Fotheringham S, Epping MT, Stimson L, Khan O, Wood V, Pezzella F, et al. Genome-wide loss-of-function screen reveals an important role for the proteasome in HDAC inhibitor-induced apoptosis. Cancer Cell. 2009;15:57–66.
23. Gravina GL, Marampon F, Giusti I, Carosa E, Di Sante S, Ricevuto E, et al. Differential effects of PXD101 (belinostat) on androgen-dependent and androgen-independent prostate cancer models. Int J Oncol. 2012;40:711–20.

24. Huang PH, Chen CH, Chou CC, Sargeant AM, Kulp SK, Teng CM, et al. Histone deacetylase inhibitors stimulate histone H3 lysine 4 methylation in part via transcriptional repression of histone H3 lysine 4 demethylases. Mol Pharmacol. 2011;79:197–206.
25. Huang PH, Plass C, Chen CS. Effects of histone deacetylase inhibitors on modulating H3K4 methylation marks—a novel cross-talk mechanism between histone-modifying enzymes. Mol Cell Pharmacol. 2011;3:39–43.
26. Kang H, Gillespie TW, Goodman M, Brodie SA, Brandes M, Ribeiro M, et al. Long-term use of valproic acid in US veterans is associated with a reduced risk of smoking-related cases of head and neck cancer. Cancer. 2014;120:1394–400.
27. Li J, Xu YH, Lu Y, Ma XP, Chen P, Luo SW, et al. Identifying differentially expressed genes and small molecule drugs for prostate cancer by a bioinformatics strategy. Asian Pac J Cancer Prev. 2013;14:5281–6.
28. Qian DZ, Wei YF, Wang X, Kato Y, Cheng L, Pili R. Antitumor activity of the histone deacetylase inhibitor MS-275 in prostate cancer models. Prostate. 2007;67:1182–93.
29. Wheler JJ, Janku F, Falchook GS, Jackson TL, Fu S, Naing A, et al. Phase I study of anti-VEGF monoclonal antibody bevacizumab and histone deacetylase inhibitor valproic acid in patients with advanced cancers. Cancer Chemother Pharmacol. 2014;73:495–501.
30. Veeramani S, Igawa T, Yuan TC, Lin FF, Lee MS, Lin JS, et al. Expression of p66Shc protein correlates with proliferation of human prostate cancer cells. Oncogene. 2005;24:7203–12.
31. Lin MF, Meng TC, Rao PS, Chang C, Schönthal AH, Lin FF. Expression of human prostatic acid phosphatase correlates with androgen-stimulated cell proliferation in prostate cancer cell lines. J Biol Chem. 1998;273:5939–47.
32. Igawa T, Lin FF, Lee MS, Karan D, Batra SK, Lin MF. Establishment and characterization of androgen-independent human prostate cancer LNCaP cell model. Prostate. 2002;50:222–35.
33. Thalmann GN, Anezinis PE, Chang SM, Zhau HE, Kim EE, Hopwood VL, et al. Androgen-independent cancer progression and bone metastasis in the LNCaP model of human prostate cancer. Cancer Res. 1994;54:2577–81.
34. Chen SJ, Karan D, Johansson SL, Lin FF, Zeckser J, Singh AP, et al. Prostate-derived factor as a paracrine and autocrine factor for the proliferation of androgen receptor-positive human prostate cancer cells. Prostate. 2007;67:557–71.
35. Thalmann GN, Sikes RA, Wu TT, Degeorges A, Chang SM, Ozen M, et al. LNCaP progression model of human prostate cancer: androgen-independence and osseous metastasis. Prostate. 2000;44:91–103.

9

A physical association between the human mutY homolog (hMYH) and DNA topoisomerase II-binding protein 1 (hTopBP1) regulates Chk1-induced cell cycle arrest in HEK293 cells

Se Hee Han[1], Soo-Hyun Hahm[1], An Hue Vy Tran[1], Ji Hyung Chung[2], Myoung-Ki Hong[3], Hyun-Dong Paik[4], Key-Sun Kim[5] and Ye Sun Han[1,6*]

Abstract

Background: Human DNA topoisomerase II-binding protein 1 (hTopBP1) plays an important role in DNA replication and the DNA damage checkpoint pathway. The human mutY homolog (hMYH) is a base excision repair DNA glycosylase that excises adenines or 2-hydroxyadenines that are mispaired with guanine or 7,8-dihydro-8-oxoguanine (8-oxoG). hTopBP1 and hMYH were involved in ATR-mediated Chk1 activation, moreover, both of them were associated with ATR and hRad9 which known as checkpoint-involved proteins. Therefore, we investigated whether hTopBP1 interacted with hMYH, and what the function of their interaction is.

Results: We documented the interaction between hTopBP1 and hMYH and showed that this interaction increased in a hydroxyurea-dependent manner. We also mapped the hMYH-interacting region of hTopBP1 (residues 444–991). In addition, we investigated several cell cycle-related proteins and found that co-knockdown of hTopBP1 and hMYH significantly diminished cell cycle arrest due to compromised checkpoint kinase 1 (Chk1) activation. Moreover, we observed that hMYH was essential for the accumulation of hTopBP1 on damaged DNA, where hTopBP1 interacts with hRad9, a component of the Rad9-Hus1-Rad1 complex. The accumulation of hTopBP1 on chromatin and its subsequent interaction with hRad9 lead to cell cycle arrest, a process mediated by Chk1 phosphorylation and ataxia telangiectasia and Rad3-related protein (ATR) activation.

Conclusions: Our results suggested that hMYH is necessary for the accumulation of hTopBP1 to DNA damage lesion to induce the association of hTopBP1 with 9-1-1 and that the interaction between hMYH and hTopBP1 is essential for Chk1 activation. Therefore, we suggest that the interaction between hMYH and hTopBP1 is crucial for activation of the ATR-mediated cell cycle checkpoint.

Keywords: Human topoisomerase II-binding protein 1 (hTopBP1), Human mutY homolog (hMYH), Human Rad9, Phospho-Chk1, Cell cycle arrest, ATR signaling

*Correspondence: yshan@konkuk.ac.kr
[6] College of Global Integrated Studies, Division of Interdisciplinary Studies, Konkuk University, 120 Neungdong-ro, Gwangjin-gu, Seoul 143-701, Republic of Korea
Full list of author information is available at the end of the article

Background

In response to DNA damage, eukaryotic cells initiate checkpoint control mechanisms that help maintain genome integrity [1, 2]. The ataxia telangiectasia and Rad3-related protein (ATR) signaling cascade is an important pathway involved in the checkpoint control mechanism [3]. During ATR signaling in response to DNA damage, Rad17 forms a complex with 9-1-1 and loads onto stalled replication forks [4–9]. Subsequently, hTopBP1 accumulates on replication protein A (RPA)-coated chromatin and is activated by interacting with hRad9 [4, 8, 10]. Then hTopBP1 interacts with ATR-ATRIP through its ATR-activating domain (AD) and stimulates ATR kinase activity [8, 9]. Activation of ATR phosphorylates a number of downstream proteins that coordinate the cell cycle checkpoint. Chk1 is one of the best-studied substrates of ATR [3]. ATR-activated Chk1 induces a transient cell cycle delay and arrest, which is followed by degradation of cell division cycle 25A (Cdc25A) and inhibition of cyclin-dependent kinase (Cdk) [3, 8]. Consequently, Chk1 activation initiates a reversible cell cycle arrest, a process considered essential for DNA repair [3].

Human DNA topoisomerase II-binding protein 1 (TopBP1) and its orthologs play important roles in DNA replication and checkpoint control [1]. These proteins contain eight BRCA1 C-terminus (BRCT) domains, usually found in proteins that are involved in DNA repair and cell cycle checkpoint mechanisms [3, 11]. Through its interactions with other proteins via its BRCT domains, hTopBP1 performs diverse functions [1]. As part of the DNA damage response, hTopBP1 directly interacts with the ATR-ATRIP complex and activates ATR kinase [1, 12]. hTopBP1 also interacts with the phosphorylated tail of Rad9 [1, 4]. Although binding to the ATR-ATRIP and 9-1-1 complexes occurs independently, both are essential for ATR-mediated Chk1 phosphorylation [1, 4, 12]. Thus, hTopBP1 constitutes an important part of the ATR signaling pathway and acts as a molecular bridge that associates the independently recruited 9-1-1 and ATR-ATRIP complexes, thereby leading to checkpoint activation [4].

One of the oxidative DNA lesions frequently generated upon exposure of cells to reactive oxygen species (ROS) is 7,8-dihydro-8-oxoguanine (8-oxoG) [13]. The presence of 8-oxoG on the replicating strand leads to frequent misincorporation of adenine opposite a lesion, and results in G:C to T:A transversions after replication [13, 14]. Human mutY homolog (MYH) is a DNA glycosylase involved in base excision repair (BER) [5, 13, 14]. This glycosylase initiates BER and reduces G:C to T:A mutations by removing the adenine or 2-hydroxyadenines mispaired with guanine or 8-oxoG that arises through DNA replication errors [5, 13, 15, 16]. hMYH physically and functionally interacts with the 9-1-1 complex [14, 16], and this interaction increases significantly following hydrogen peroxide treatment, implying that the association primarily occurs for DNA repair [6]. In our previous study, we found that depletion of hMYH disrupts ATR and Chk1 activation following hydroxyurea (HU) and ultraviolet treatment [17]. In addition, we also observed endogenous interactions between hTopBP1 and hMYH as well as hRad9 and hMYH [5, 18]. These observations support the claim that hMYH is an important component of the ATR signaling pathway. Importantly, cell cycle checkpoint proteins are recognized as key tumor suppressors, and their direct role in DNA repair, as with hMYH/9-1-1 interaction, can prevent the accumulation of mutations [19]. The connection between DNA repair and cell cycle checkpoints provides an additional mechanism to preserve genomic integrity [19, 20].

Interestingly, a recent report suggested that an unknown factor caused the accumulation of hTopBP1 on damaged DNA, following the interaction between 9-1-1 and hTopBP1 [8]. Based on our finding that hMYH interacts with 9-1-1 and hTopBP1, we identified hMYH as the likely factor involved in ATR-mediated activation of Chk1. We further propose that during the DNA damage response, the association of hMYH with hTopBP1 is necessary for the cell cycle arrest caused by ATR-mediated activation of Chk1. We also conclude that hMYH plays an important role in ATR signaling by interacting with 9-1-1 and hTopBP1.

Results and discussion

hMYH physically interacts with hTopBP1

In our previous study, we observed that endogenous hMYH interacts with hTopBP1 [5]. Here, we examined whether exogenous hMYH interacted with hTopBP1 using a co-IP assay. HEK293 cells were co-transfected with GST/c-Myc-hMYH or GST-hTopBP1/c-Myc-hMYH for 24 h. Then, the cell lysates were immunoprecipitated with an anti-GST antibody, and the precipitated lysates were analyzed by immunoblotting with anti-c-Myc and anti-GST antibodies. c-Myc-tagged hMYH was immunoprecipitated with GST-tagged hTopBP1, but not with GST (Fig. 1a). The association between hMYH and hTopBP1 was confirmed by co-IP with an anti-c-Myc in c-Myc/GST-hTopBP1- or c-Myc-hMYH/GST-hTopBP1-co-transfected cells. We consistently found that GST-tagged hTopBP1 interacted with c-Myc-tagged hMYH, but not with c-Myc (Fig. 1b). Based on our endogenous and exogenous interaction results, we performed GST pull-down assay to determine the physical interaction between hMYH and hTopBP1 (Fig. 1c). We prepared bacterially expressed and purified His-hMYH and GST-hTopBP1. GST or GST-hTopBP1 was immobilized on glutathione Sepharose beads and mixed with purified

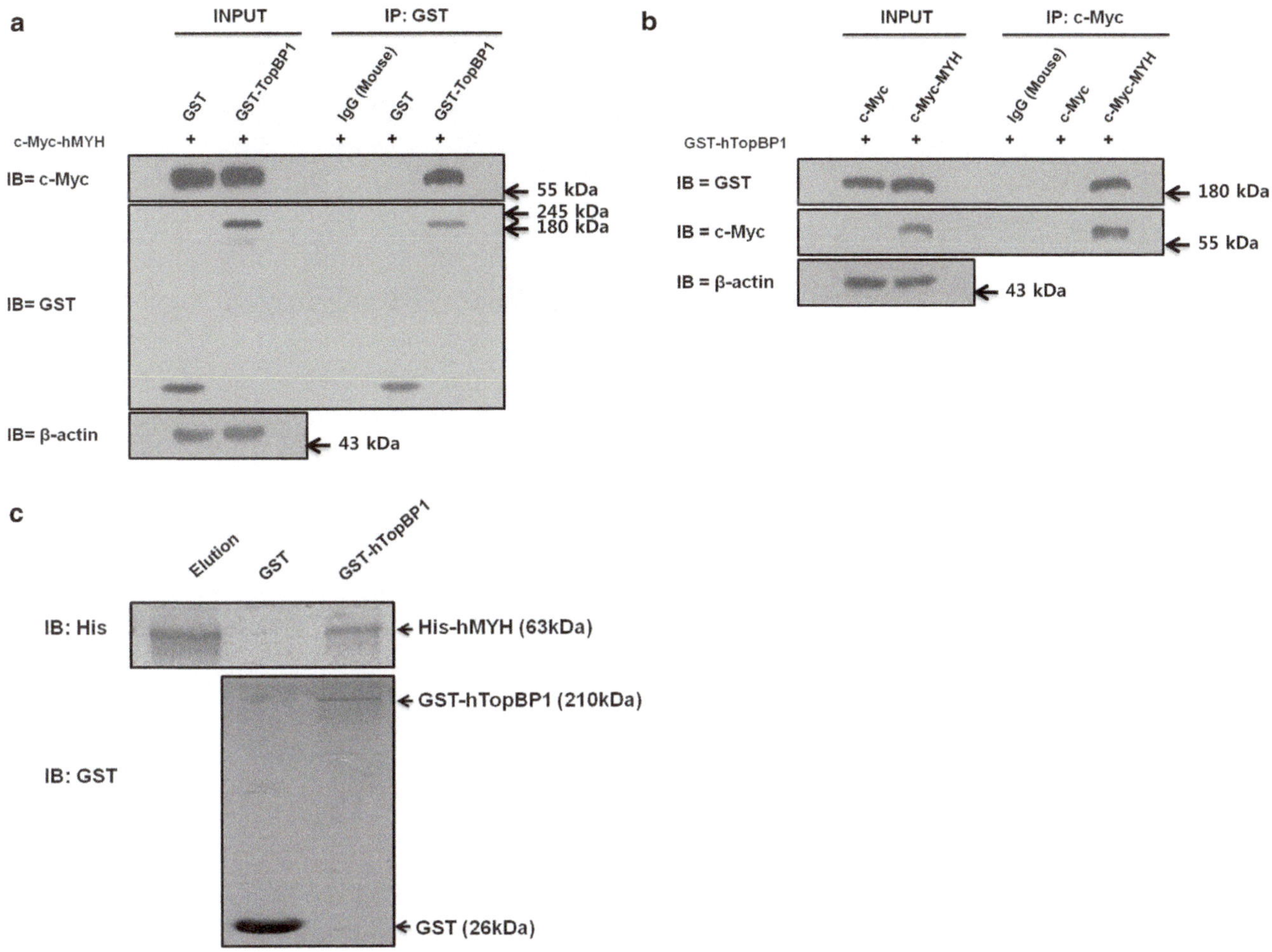

Fig. 1 Interaction between hTopBP1 and hMYH. **a** HEK293 cells were co-transfected with either GST and c-Myc-hMYH or GST-hTopBP1 and c-Myc-hMYH. Cell lysates were subjected to co-immunoprecipitation (IP) and immunoblotting. Co-IP was performed with an anti-GST antibody and protein A/G PLUS-agarose beads. Then, the precipitated proteins were immunoblotted (IB) with anti-GST and anti-c-Myc antibodies. **b** Co-IP was performed using an anti-c-Myc antibody in cells co-transfected with either c-Myc and GST-hTopBP1 or c-Myc-hMYH and GST-hTopBP1. The levels of the precipitated c-Myc- and GST-tagged proteins were assessed by immunoblotting. **c** Equal amount of purified His-hMYH was mixed with GST or GST-hTopBP1 bound glutathione Sepharose beads to pull down. *Lane 1* purified His-hMYH, *lane 2 and 3* pull-downs with GST or GST-hTopBP1, respectively

His-hMYH to pull-down. As we can see in upper panel, His-hMYH was pulled down by GST-hTopBP1, but not by GST alone. This result indicate that a direct interaction between hMYH and hTopBP1. The above results demonstrated that hTopBP1 physically interacts with hMYH.

Effect of HU treatment on the interaction between hMYH and hTopBP1

HU is an inhibitor of ribonucleotide reductase that inhibits DNA replication in cells [18, 21, 22]. HU induces the accumulation of ROS and cell death. It also initiates cell cycle arrest, which in turn facilitates the interaction between hMYH and hTopBP1 [22–24]. Both hMYH and hTopBP1 are involved in DNA repair, and their expression increases following treatment with HU [1]. We examined the effect of HU treatment on the interaction between hTopBP1 and hMYH. HEK293 cells were either treated with HU or left untreated for various durations. After HU treatment, cells were immunoprecipitated with an anti-hTopBP1 antibody for immunoblotting. As shown in Fig. 2a (INPUT), the expression of both hTopBP1 and hMYH were increased by HU treatment. Quantification of their expression (INPUT) confirmed that both hTopBP1 and hMYH were significantly increased by HU treatment (Fig. 2b, left panel). Moreover, the interaction between hTopBP1 and hMYH also increased in HU-treated cells in a time-dependent manner (Fig. 2a).

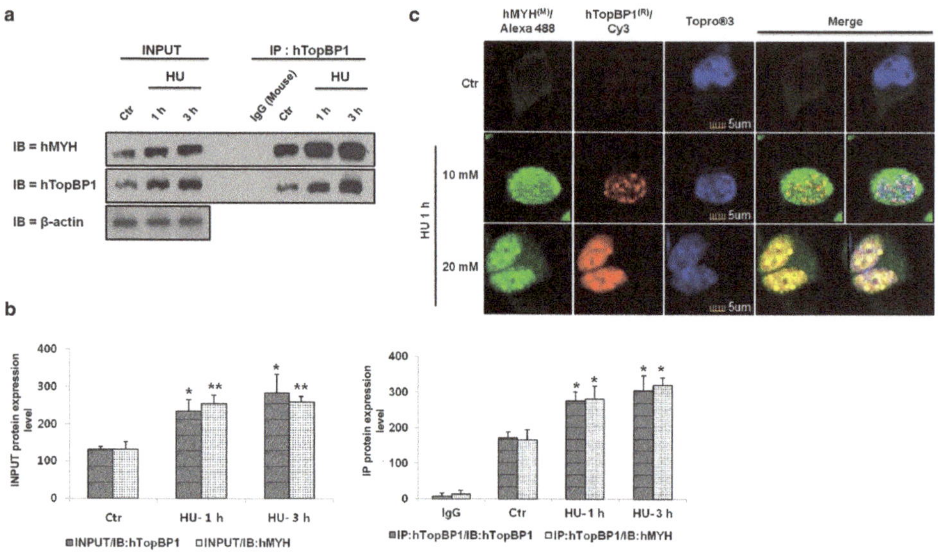

Fig. 2 The interaction between hTopBP1 and hMYH increases following HU treatment. **a** HEK293 cells were incubated with 20 mM HU for 1 or 3 h and then immunoprecipitated with anti-hTopBP1 antibodies. The precipitated proteins were detected using anti-hMYH and anti-hTopBP1 antibodies. β-Actin was used as a loading control. **b** Protein expression levels and their interaction were quantified and are presented as mean ± standard error (of three independent experiments). *P* values were calculated using a paired *t* test. $*p < 0.05$, $**p < 0.01$ compared to the Control (HU-untreated cells). **c** Cells were seeded and grown on coverglass bottom dishes. After 24 h, cells were either untreated or treated with various concentrations of HU for 1 h, fixed with 4 % paraformaldehyde, and permeabilized with 0.1 % Triton X-100 in PBS. Cells were subsequently incubated with anti-hMYH and anti-hTopBP1 antibodies and then stained with Alexa Fluor® 488 (hMYH/*Green*), Cy3 (hTopBP1/*Orange*), and To-pro®-3 (nucleus/*Red*). *Scale bar* 10 μm

Quantification of the co-IP result confirmed that HU treatment significantly increased the interaction between hTopBP1 and hMYH (Fig. 2b, right panel).

We also imaged immunofluorescently stained cells in order to assess hTopBP1 and hMYH co-localization following HU treatment (Fig. 2c). HEK293 cells were prepared in coverglass bottom dishes and were either untreated (control; Ctr) or treated with 10 or 20 mM HU for 1 h. In untreated cells, hMYH was located in the cytoplasm and hTopBP1 was almost exclusively located in the nucleus (Fig. 2c). Therefore, no co-localization was observed. However, when we treated the cells with 10 or 20 mM HU, hMYH expression is increased in nucleus, and we observed co-localization of hTopBP1 and hMYH (yellow in merge). Moreover, their co-localization increased in an HU dose-dependent manner. This result clearly indicated that the interaction between hMYH and hTopBP1 was significantly enhanced by HU in a time- and dose-dependent manner.

The BRCT 4–6 (D2) domain of hTopBP1 interacts with hMYH

To identify the region of hTopBP1 that associates with hMYH, we designed and generated several deletion mutants of hTopBP1 (Fig. 3a). Each deletion mutant was tagged with GST and co-transfected with c-Myc-tagged hMYH. Co-IPs were performed using an anti-c-Myc antibody. We observed that a construct corresponding to the D2 region of hTopBP1 (containing BRCT 4–6, amino acids 444–991) interacted with hMYH (Fig. 3b). This result clearly showed that residues 444–991 of hTopBP1 were necessary for its interaction with hMYH.

Knockdown of hTopBP1 and hMYH affects cell cycle arrest

hTopBP1 and hMYH are required for the phosphorylation of Chk1, which is a checkpoint protein that induces cell cycle arrest following DNA damage [4, 17, 25]. Therefore, we hypothesized that interaction between hTopBP1 and hMYH would trigger the phosphorylation of Chk1. We knocked down the expression of hMYH and hTopBP1, either alone or together in the same cells, using siRNAs as indicated in Fig. 4a. siGFP-transfected cells were used as a control. Cells were treated with HU after transfection, and then protein levels were assessed by immunoblotting, which showed that hTopBP1 and hMYH were successfully knocked down by siRNA treatment (Fig. 4a).

HU induces cell cycle arrest at the G_1/S boundary by inhibiting ribonucleotide diphosphate reductase [24, 26]. Therefore, we decided to investigate Chk1 phosphorylation at Ser 345 by assessing phospho-Chk1 (p-Chk1), an indicator of DNA damage, in HU-treated cells. As expected, a strong signal for p-Chk1 was observed in

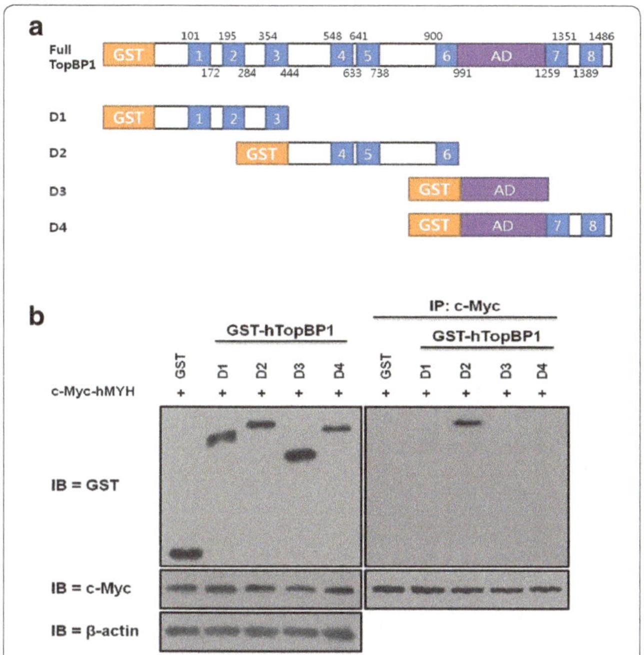

Fig. 3 Identification of the hMYH-interacting domain of hTopBP1. **a** Schematic map of the hTopBP1 deletion mutants to identify the interacting region of hTopBP1. **b** Co-IP and immunoblotting were performed on lysates expressing the various hTopBP1 deletion mutants. For the experiments, HEK293 cells were co-transfected with full-length c-Myc-hMYH and the various GST-hTopBP1 mutants. Co-IP was performed with an anti-c-Myc antibody, and the precipitated proteins were immunoblotted with anti-GST and anti-c-Myc antibodies

HU-treated siGFP-transfected cells (Fig. 4a). However, after knockdown of hTopBP1 or hMYH, Chk1 phosphorylation was significantly reduced in HU-treated cells (lane 5 versus lane 6, $p < 0.01$; lane 5 versus lane 7, $p < 0.05$). Co-knockdown of hTopBP1 and hMYH (siTM) caused a greater reduction in Chk1 phosphorylation than that caused by a similar knockdown of siGFP, siMYH, or siTopBP1 alone (Fig. 4a, lane 5 versus lane 8, $p < 0.01$). Quantification of the Chk1 phosphorylation in Fig. 4a (first panel of Fig. 4c) showed that knockdown of both hTopBP1 and hMYH synergistically reduced Chk1 phosphorylation. Hence, it is possible that the interaction between hMYH and hTopBP1 affects Chk1 phosphorylation.

Next, we examined Cdk2 and Cdc25A to determine the effect of hMYH and hTopBP1 knockdown on substrates downstream of phosphorylated Chk1 signaling. The phosphorylated, inactive form of Cdk2 (p-Cdk2, T14, Y15), which does not promote cell cycle progression, was higher in HU-treated siGFP-transfected cells (Fig. 4b). As expected, we observed a decrease in p-Cdk2 levels in HU-treated siTopBP1-transfected and HU-treated siMYH-transfected cells, compared with that in HU-treated siGFP-transfected cells ($p < 0.05$). Similarly, p-Cdk2 levels in the HU-treated co-knockdown cells were significantly lower than in the HU-treated siGFP-transfected cells (HU-siGFP versus HU-siTM, $p < 0.01$). Additionally, degradation of Cdc25A, which is required for cell cycle arrest, was diminished in HU-treated siTopBP1-transfected and HU-treated siMYH-transfected cells compared to that in the HU-treated siGFP-transfected cells ($p < 0.01$). Moreover, HU-treated co-knockdown (hTopBP1 and hMYH) cells showed a remarkable defect in Cdc25A degradation (HU-siGFP versus HU-siTM, $p < 0.001$). The results shown in Fig. 4b (p-Cdk2 and Cdc25A levels) were quantitatively evaluated (Fig. 4c). The results showed that depletion of both hMYH and hTopBP1 had a synergistic negative effect on cell cycle arrest in HU-treated cells through the diminishment of recovery of DNA damage (Fig. 4; Additional file 1).

hMYH is crucial for the association between hRad9 and hTopBP1

After analyzing our data, we hypothesized that hMYH was likely to affect the activation of ATR signaling [5, 17]. Therefore, we wanted to determine whether hMYH could affect the interaction between hRad9 and hTopBP1, an association that is necessary for inducing ATR activation. To determine the effect of hMYH, we depleted or overexpressed hMYH in HU-treated or untreated HEK293 cells and then conducted an IP assay using an anti-hRad9 antibody (Fig. 5). Figure 5a shows that knockdown of hMYH induced a considerable decrease in the interaction between hRad9 and hTopBP1 compared to that in the control siGFP-transfected cells ($p < 0.05$). We also observed a significant decrease in the interaction between hTopBP1 and hRad9 in HU-treated siMYH-transfected cells compared to that in HU-treated siGFP-transfected cells. Similarly, we also studied the effect of overexpressing hMYH (Fig. 5b). The interaction between hRad9 and hTopBP1 was higher in cells overexpressing hMYH than in cells transfected with an empty expression vector (Fig. 5b, $p < 0.05$). These results suggest that hMYH is a critical factor involved in the interaction between hTopBP1 and hRad9, an important early step in ATR signaling. Moreover, it suggests that hMYH affects the interaction between hRad9 and hTopBP1 through its association with both hRad9 and hTopBP1.

hMYH required for accumulation of hTopBP1 to chromatin

Based on Fig. 5 results, we believed that hMYH affects chromatin association of hTopBP1. Therefore, we have investigated whether hMYH affects hTopBP1 accumulation onto DNA lesion (Fig. 6). To examine whether chromatin association of hTopBP1 is mediated by hMYH,

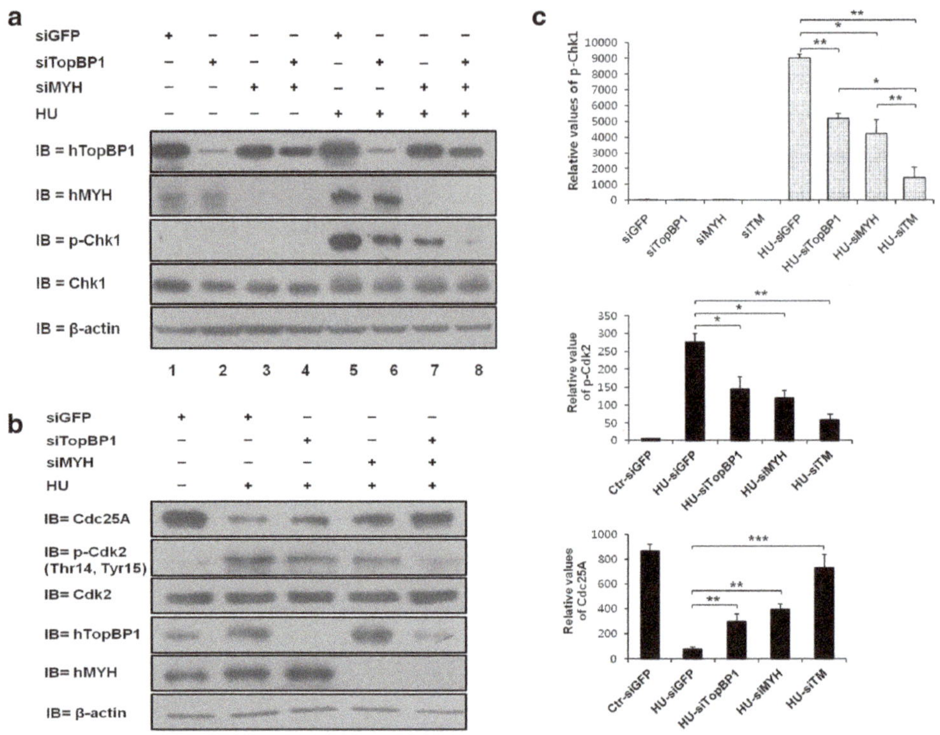

Fig. 4 Knockdown of both hTopBP1 and hMYH affects cell cycle arrest. **a** HEK293 cells were either transfected with individual siRNAs targeted against GFP (siGFP), hMYH (siMYH), and hTopBP1 (siTopBP1) or co-transfected with siTopBP1 and siMYH. Transfected cells were treated with 20 mM HU for 1 h. Total cell lysates were immunoblotted with anti-hTopBP1, anti-hMYH, anti-Chk1, and anti-phospho-Chk1 antibodies. **b** The expression of hTopBP1, hMYH, or both was knocked down, following which the cells were incubated with 20 mM HU for 1 h. The cell lysates were analyzed by immunoblotting with anti-p-Cdk2 (T24, Y15) and anti-Cdc25A antibodies. **c** The relative levels of p-Chk1, Cdc25A, and p-Cdk2 from replicate experiments were quantified and normalized to β-actin, and the normalized data are presented as mean ± standard error (of three independent experiments). *P* values were calculated using a paired *t* test, $^{*}p < 0.05$, $^{**}p < 0.01$, $^{***}p < 0.001$

first we depleted hMYH using siRNA. HEK293 cells were transfected with siGFP or siMYH in HU treated or untreated cells, then chromatin isolation was performed. Chromatin associated proteins were collected and association were examined by western blotting. We observed that association of hMYH onto chromatin was diminished by siMYH treatment. As we expected, association of hTopBP1 onto chromatin was enhanced by HU treatment, however, it was abolished by absence of hMYH. ORC2 was used for loading control of chromatin fractions. This result indicates that hMYH and its interaction with hTopBP1 is important for accumulation of hTopBP1 onto DNA lesion.

Conclusions

DNA damage checkpoints are surveillance mechanisms for preserving genome integrity and ensuring proper cellular responses to stress [3, 14]. The ATR-Chk1 pathway is essential for this DNA damage checkpoint. ATR activation requires several factors, including Rad17-RFC, 9-1-1, hTopBP1, and ATRIP [9, 17, 27]. Based on our studies, we believe that hMYH is a component of the ATR signaling pathway and is required for Chk1 activation [5, 14]. Accordingly, in this study, we sought to elucidate the molecular mechanism underlying the accumulation of hTopBP1 at DNA damage sites. Additionally, we explored the interaction between hTopBP1 and hMYH and delineated its role in DNA damage checkpoint signaling.

We studied the physical interaction between hTopBP1 and hMYH (Fig. 1). Previous observations prompted us to examine whether HU-induced DNA damage could affect the interaction between hTopBP1 and hMYH [5, 17, 28]. Indeed, the expression levels of hMYH and hTopBP1 were increased following HU treatment (Fig. 2a, b). Additionally, the association between endogenous hTopBP1 and hMYH increased in a time-dependent manner following HU treatment (Fig. 2a, b). In addition, hMYH and hTopBP1 co-localization increased in an HU dose-dependent manner (Fig. 2c). These results showed the interplay between hTopBP1 with hMYH related to the DNA damage response pathway. We also demonstrated that the D2 domain of hTopBP1 (residues 444–991) was crucial for its interaction with hMYH (Fig. 3b).

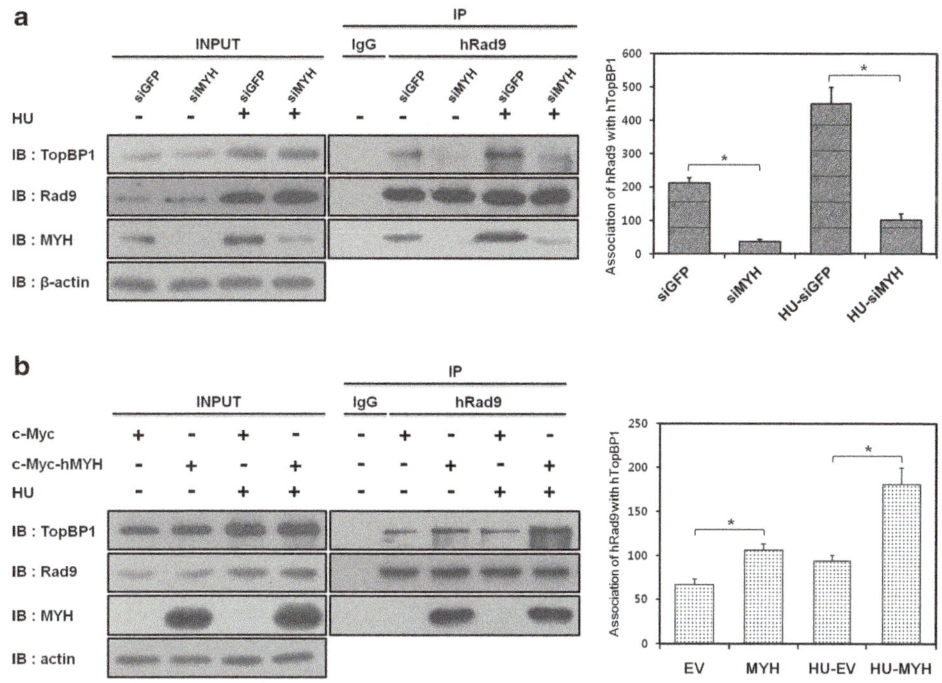

Fig. 5 hMYH is a key factor for the interaction between hTopBP1 and hRad9. **a** HEK293 cells transfected with siGFP or siMYH were either untreated or treated with 20 mM HU for 1 h. The cell lysates were subjected to IP with an anti-hRad9 antibody. Immunoblotting was performed using the indicated antibodies. The bar graph shows the quantification of the interaction between hRad9 and hTopBP1. The values shown represent the mean ± standard error (of three independent experiments). **b** Cells overexpressing c-Myc or c-Myc-hMYH were either untreated or treated 20 mM HU for 1 h. Then, an IP assay was performed with an anti-hRad9 antibody. Immunoblotting was then performed as indicated. Quantification of the association between hRad9 and hTopBP1 is shown as mean ± standard error (of three independent experiments). *P* values were calculated using a paired *t* test, *$p < 0.05$

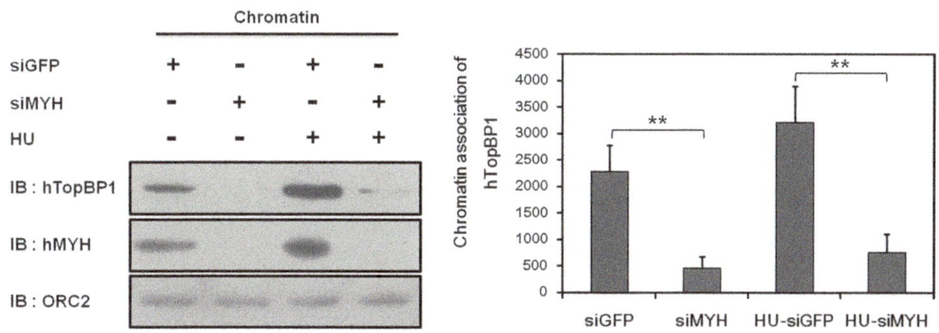

Fig. 6 Knockdown of hMYH affects chromatin association of hTopBP1. siGFP or siMYH transfected HEK293 cells were either untreated or treated with 20 mM HU for 1 h. The cells were lysed and chromatins were collected. Chromatin binding proteins were analyzed by western blotting. ORC2 were used loading control. Quantification of the association of hTopBP1 with chromatin is shown as mean ± standard error (of three independent experiments). *P* values were calculated using a paired *t* test, **$p < 0.01$

Hahm et al., Yan et al., and Liu et al. performed experiments in which either hMYH or hTopBP1 was depleted, and they observed inhibition of Chk1 phosphorylation in these cells [17, 29, 30]. Chk1 phosphorylation is necessary for the progression from cell cycle arrest to DNA repair [25, 31]. Interestingly, we observed that knockdown of both hMYH and hTopBP1 had a synergistic negative effect on cell cycle arrest following HU treatment (Fig. 4). Our observation indicates that the association between hMYH and hTopBP1 is probably required for inducing cell cycle arrest after DNA damage. Therefore, we suggest that this interaction is an important step in checkpoint signaling.

It has been reported that hTopBP1 has a key domain, AD, which is responsible for activating ATR [9, 27].

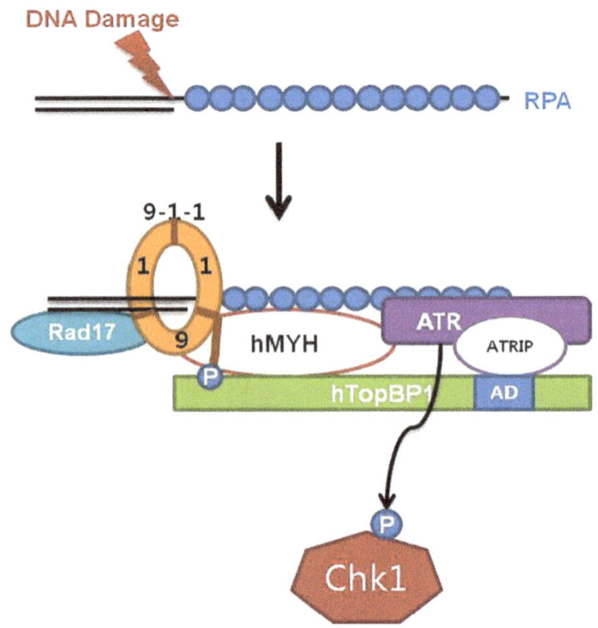

Fig. 7 A model for the involvement of hMYH in ATR-mediated checkpoint signaling. A model for the interaction of hMYH with hRad9 and hTopBP1 at stalled replication forks. See the "Conclusions" section for details

According to Delacroix et al., when hRad9 interacts with hTopBP1, the AD domain of hTopBP1 and the phospho-Ser 387 of hRad9 are involved in Chk1 phosphorylation [4, 8, 32]. Interestingly, we observed that knockdown of hTopBP1 and hMYH affects Chk1 activation (Fig. 4a). Therefore, we decided to determine the role of hMYH in checkpoint signaling. As mentioned above, Lee et al. pointed out that an unknown factor was required for the accumulation of hTopBP1 on the DNA lesion [8]. It was already known that hMYH is involved in the ATR-Chk1 pathway and that it interacts with 9-1-1, RPA, ATR, and hTopBP1, which are components of the ATR-Chk1 pathway [17, 33, 34]. We first proposed that hMYH is the unknown factor involved in accumulation of hTopBP1 onto DNA lesion for inducing the interaction between hRad9 and hTopBP1. Our results clearly demonstrated that chromatin association of hTopBP1 is mediated by hMYH (Fig. 6), therefore, hMYH is indispensable for the interaction between hRad9 and hTopBP1 (Fig. 5).

Based on our findings, we suggested a model (Fig. 7). Following DNA damage, replication is initiated, and RPA binds to ssDNA. Then, hMYH and ATR-ATRIP associate with RPA, which is followed by Rad17/9-1-1 loading on the DNA lesion [8, 35]. hMYH then interacts with hRad9 and ATR and induces the accumulation of hTopBP1 on DNA lesion [5]. Finally, hTopBP1 is activated through its interaction with Ser 387-phosphorylated hRad9 [4]. This association facilitates activation of ATR through the interaction between hTopBP1 and ATR-ATRIP [12, 36]. An important feature of this model is that hMYH is involved in the recruitment of hTopBP1 to damaged DNA after 9-1-1 loading.

Taken together, our results indicated that hMYH is an important factor that recruits and accumulates hTopBP1 on the DNA lesion, where it interacts with hRad9. This is an essential step in the process of Chk1 phosphorylation. In addition, we conclude that hTopBP1 and hMYH are important components of the ATR signaling pathway and suggest that their interaction is necessary for Chk1-mediated cell cycle arrest.

Methods

Cell culture and transfection

Human embryonic kidney (HEK) 293 cells were cultured in Dulbecco's modified Eagle's medium (DMEM; Welgene, Daegu, South Korea), supplemented with 10 % fetal bovine serum (FBS; JR Scientific, Woodland, CA, USA) and 1 % penicillin–streptomycin solution (Welgene) at 37 °C in a 5 % CO_2 incubator. For transfection, cells were seeded (3×10^5–6×10^5 cells/mL) and transiently transfected with Lipofectamine® 2000 (Invitrogen, Carlsbad, CA, USA), according to the manufacturer's protocol. After incubating the cells for 24 h, 20 mM HU was added, and the cells were incubated for an additional 1 h.

siRNA construction

The siRNAs used to knockdown of endogenous hMYH and hTopBP1 were designed and purchased from Santa Cruz Biotechnology, Inc. (Santa Cruz, CA, USA). An siRNA sequence corresponding to nucleotides 415–439 of green fluorescent protein (GFP) was used as a negative control (Santa Cruz). hTopBP1 and hMYH knockdown was performed according to the manufacturer's instructions.

Chromatin fractionation

HEK293 cells were lysed with lysis buffer (10 mM HEPES pH 7.4, 10 mM KCl, 0.05 % NP-40), and nuclear extracts were lysed in Low salt buffer (10 mM Tris–HCl pH 7.4, 0.2 mM $MgCl_2$). Chromatins were collected by centrifugation and chromatin binding proteins were disassociated from chromatin with 0.2 N HCl, and 1 M Tris–HCl pH 8.0 was added. Chromatin binding proteins were quantified using the Bio-Rad DC protein assay kit (Bio-Rad, Hercules, CA, USA).

GST pull-down assay

E. coli BL21 cells (Real Biotech Corporation, Banqiao, Taipei, Taiwan) harboring the expression vectors (pGEX4T1/GST-hTopBP1, pET-28α/His-hMYH) were cultured and induced using isopropylthiogalactoside (IPTG, a final concentration of 0.5 mM) and incubated for 16 h at 18 °C. Cells were harvested and lysed by sonication in lysis buffer [20 mM Tris–Cl (pH 7.5), 500 mM NaCl] together with protease inhibitor cocktail (Sigma-Aldrich, St. Louis, MO, USA). After centrifugation, 5 mg/ml of supernatant were pulled down by glutathione Sepharose 4B beads (GE Healthcare, UK) or Ni–NTA agarose resin (Qiagen, Valencia, CA, USA). Ni–NTA agarose beads bound His-hMYH protein were released from resin by elusion buffer [20 mM Tris–Cl (pH 7.4), 500 mM NaCl] together with various concentration of Imidazole (50–300 mM). Equal concentration of purified His-hMYH (1.95 μg/μl) was then incubated with GST or GST-hTopBP1 in phosphate-buffered saline (PBS; Sigma-Aldrich), and proteins were incubated for 16 h at 4 °C. After incubation, beads was washed with PBS then resuspended with reduced glutathione buffer [50 mM Tris–Cl (pH 8.0), 10 mM reduced glutathione]. Mixture of beads and reduced glutathione buffer were incubated for 15 min and centrifuged, then supernatants were collected and analysed by western blot using His and GST antibody (Santa Cruz).

Western blot analysis

HEK293 cells were harvested and lysed with a lysis buffer [50 mM Tris–HCl (Bio Basic, Markham, Canada), 10 g/mL PMSF, 100 mM NaCl, 5 mM EDTA, 1 % Nonidet P-40, and protease and phosphatase inhibitor cocktail (Sigma-Aldrich)] for 1 h at 4 °C. Protein extracts were collected after centrifugation, and proteins were quantified. Protein samples were separated on an 8 or 12 % SDS-PAGE and transferred to polyvinylidene fluoride (PVDF) membranes (PALL Corporation, NY, USA). The membranes were blocked using 3 % non-fat dry milk (Bio Basic) in Tris-buffered saline with 0.05 % Tween 20 (TBST) for 30 min. The membranes were then incubated with primary antibodies against hMYH (Abnova, Taipei, Taiwan), hTopBP1 (Abcam, Cambridge, UK), hRad9 (Bethyl Laboratories, Montgomery, TX, USA), c-Myc, GST, phospho-Chk1, Chk1, Cdc25A, phospho-Cdk2, Cdk2, and β-actin (Santa Cruz). After incubation with the primary antibodies, the membranes were incubated with the appropriate horseradish peroxidase (HRP)-conjugated secondary antibodies (Santa Cruz). Protein bands were detected with the ECL® Enhanced Chemiluminescence (ECL) analysis system (Thermo Fisher Scientific, Waltham, MA, USA) according to the manufacturer's protocol. The intensity of western blot bands was quantified with Lab Works software (UVP Inc., Upland, CA, USA). Experiments were performed for three times and statistical analysis was conducted using student's t test in Microsoft Excel for measuring the significance between the different values. Data were expressed as means ± standard errors and $p < 0.05$ (paired two-tailed t test, $p < 0.01$, $p < 0.001$) was considered statistically significant.

Immunoprecipitation

Total cell lysates were prepared from cells that were transiently transfected with different sets of expression vectors as described previously. Immunoprecipitation (IP) was conducted by incubating the lysates with anti-c-Myc, anti-GST antibodies (as indicated) for 1 h, and then adding protein A/G PLUS-agarose beads (Santa Cruz). Protein-bead complexes were pelleted by centrifugation and washed with PBS. The immunoprecipitated samples were analyzed by SDS-PAGE, and the immunoblot (IB) analysis was conducted with the indicated antibodies. To assess the endogenous hTopBP1-hMYH and hTopBP1-hRad9 interactions, IPs were conducted using the ImmunoCruz™ IP/WB Optima system (Santa Cruz). Beads were mixed with 1 μg of anti-hTopBP1 or anti-hRad9 antibodies in PBS. Then, the mixture was incubated on a rotator at 4 °C for 3 h. After incubation, the bead-antibody mixture was washed in PBS three times. Cell lysates were quantified, mixed with the bead-antibody mixture, and rotated for 16 h at 4 °C. The mixture was washed with PBS three times and then mixed with 1× loading dye. Samples were boiled, and the supernatant was collected via centrifugation.

Immunofluorescence staining

HEK293 cells were seeded (1×10^5 cells/mL) on coverglass bottom dishes (SPL Life Sciences, Pocheon, South Korea), grown for 24 h, and then treated with various concentrations of HU for 1 h. Cells were fixed with 4 % paraformaldehyde in PBS for 20 min and permeabilized with 0.1 % Triton X-100 in PBS for 10 min. Blocking was performed with 15 % FBS in PBS for 15 min at 37 °C. Cells were incubated with the indicated primary antibodies at 37 °C for 30 min, washed three times with PBS, and then incubated with Alexa Fluor® 488-conjugated anti-mouse IgG (Invitrogen) and Cy3-conjugated anti-rabbit IgG (Sigma-Aldrich) for 30 min at 37 °C. Cells were washed three times with PBS, and the nucleus was counterstained with To-Pro®-3 (Invitrogen). Finally, the cells were analyzed using a confocal fluorescence microscope (Olympus FV-1000; software, Olympus FluoView; Olympus, Center Valley, PA, USA).

Plasmid construction

The hTopBP1 expression vector was constructed as follows: cDNA fragments harboring the D1 (amino acids 1–444; BRCT 1–3), D2 (amino acids 444–991; BRCT 4–6), D3 (amino acids 991–1259; AD), and D4 (amino acids 991–1486; AD and BRCT 7–8) regions of hTopBP1 were generated by PCR. The PCR products were digested with *Bam*H1 and *Not*1 and subsequently ligated into a pEBG vector. The full-length hMYH construct was generated using PCR. The PCR products were cleaved with *Eco*R1 and *Sal*1 and ligated into a pCMV-tag3A vector.

Abbreviations

hMYH: human mutY homolog; hTopBP1: human DNA topoisomerase II-binding protein 1; ATR: ataxia telangiectasia and Rad3-related protein; siRNA: Small interfering RNA; HU: hydroxyurea; Chk1: checkpoint kinase 1; 8-oxoG: 7,8-dihydro-8-oxoguanine; RPA: replication protein A; Cdc25A: cell division cycle 25A; Cdk: cyclin-dependent kinase; BRCT: breast cancer 1 (BRCA1) C-terminus; ROS: reactive oxygen species; GFP: green fluorescent protein.

Authors' contributions

SHH is major contributor in this study. SHH and SH conceived the idea and designed experiment. JHC, HDP, MKH and AHVT contributed to idea. KSK contributed to idea and experiment. SHH and SH performed experiment. SHH and YSH wrote the manuscript. All authors read and approved the final manuscript.

Author details

[1] Department of Advanced Technology Fusion, Konkuk University, 120 Neungdong-ro, Gwangjin-gu, Seoul 143-701, Republic of Korea. [2] Department of Applied Bioscience, College of Life Science, CHA University, 120 Haeryong-ro, Pocheon, Gyeonggi-do 463-836, Republic of Korea. [3] Department of Biological Sciences, Konkuk University, 120 Neungdong-ro, Gwangjin-gu, Seoul 143-701, Republic of Korea. [4] Department of Food Science and Biotechnology of Animal Resources, Konkuk University, 120 Neungdong-ro, Gwangjin-gu, Seoul 143-701, Republic of Korea. [5] Center for Neuroscience, Korea Institute of Science and Technology, 5 Hwarang-ro 14-gil, Seongbuk-gu, Seoul, Republic of Korea. [6] College of Global Integrated Studies, Division of Interdisciplinary Studies, Konkuk University, 120 Neungdong-ro, Gwangjin-gu, Seoul 143-701, Republic of Korea.

Acknowledgements

This work was supported by grants from Konkuk University in 2014.

Compliance with ethical guidelines

Competing interests

The authors declare that they have no competing interests.

References

1. Wang J, Gong Z, Chen J. MDC1 collaborates with TopBP1 in DNA replication checkpoint control. J Cell Biol. 2011;193:267–73.
2. Jeong SY, Kumagai A, Lee J, Dunphy WG. Phosphorylated claspin interacts with a phosphate-binding site in the kinase domain of Chk1 during ATR-mediated activation. J Biol Chem. 2003;278:46782–8.
3. Liu S, Bekker-Jensen S, Mailand N, Lukas C, Bartek J, Lukas J. Claspin operates downstream of TopBP1 to direct ATR signaling towards Chk1 activation. Mol Cell Biol. 2006;26:6056–64.
4. Delacroix S, Wagner JM, Kobayashi M, Yamamoto K, Karnitz LM. The Rad9-Hus1-Rad1 (9-1-1) clamp activates checkpoint signaling via TopBP1. Genes Dev. 2007;21:1472–7.
5. Hahm SH, Chung JH, Agustina L, Han SH, Yoon IS, Park JH, Kang LW, Park JW, Na JJ, Han YS. Human MutY homolog induces apoptosis in etoposide treated HEK293 cells. Oncol Lett. 2012;4:1203–8.
6. Helt CE, Wang W, Keng PC, Bambara RA. Evidence that DNA damage detection machinery participates in DNA repair. Cell Cycle. 2005;4:529–32.
7. Garcia V, Furuya K, Carr AM. Identification and functional analysis of TopBP1 and its homologs. DNA Repair. 2005;4:1227–39.
8. Lee J, Dunphy WG. Rad17 plays a central role in establishment of the interaction between TopBP1 and the Rad9-Hus1-Rad1 complex at stalled replication forks. Mol Biol Cell. 2010;21:926–35.
9. Yan S, Michael WM. TopBP1 and DNA polymerase-α directly recruit the 9-1-1 complex to stalled DNA replication forks. J Cell Biol. 2009;184:793–804.
10. Yan S, Willis J. WD40-repeat protein WDR18 collaborates with TopBP1 to facilitate DNA damage checkpoint signaling. Biochem Biophys Res Commun. 2013;431:466–71.
11. Morishima K, Sakamoto S, Kobayashi J, Izumi H, Suda T, Matsumot Y, Tauchi H, Ide H, Komatsu K, Matsuura S. TopBP1 associates with NBS1 and is involved in homologous recombination repair. Biochem Biophys Res Commun. 2007;362:872–9.
12. Kumagai A, Lee J, Yoo HY, Dunphy WG. TopBP1 activates the ATR-ATRIP complex. Cell. 2006;124:943–55.
13. Van Loon B, Hubscher U. An 8-oxo-guanine repair pathway coordinated by MUTYH glycosylase and DNA polymerase λ. Proc Natl Acad Sci USA. 2009;106:18201–6.
14. Shi G, Chang DY, Cheng CC, Guan X, Venclovas C, Lu AL. Physical and functional interactions between MutY glycosylase homologue (MYH) and checkpoint proteins Rad9-Rad1-Hus1. Biochem J. 2006;400:53–62.
15. Noll DM, Gogos A, Granek JA, Clarke ND. The C-terminal domain of the adenine-DNA glycosylase MutY confers specificity for 8-oxoguanine·adenine mispairs and may have evolved from MutT, an 8-oxo-dGTPase. Biochemistry. 1999;38:6374–9.
16. Kairupan C, Scott RJ. Base excision repair and the role of MUTYH. Hered Cancer Clin Pract. 2007;5:199–209.
17. Hahm SH, Park JH, Ko SI, Lee YR, Chung IS, Chung JH, Kang LW, Han YS. Knock-down of human MutY homolog (hMYH) decreases phosphorylation of checkpoint kinase 1 (Chk1) induced by hudroxyurea and UV treatment. BMB Rep. 2011;44:352–7.
18. Agustina L, Hahm SH, Han SH, Tran AH, Chung JH, Park JH, Han YS. Visualization of the physical and functional interaction between hMYH and hRad9 by Dronpa bimolecular fluorescence complementation. BMC Mol Biol. 2014;15:17.
19. Luncsford PJ, Chang DY, Shi G, Bernstein J, Madabushi A, Patterson DN, Lu AL, Toth EA. A structural hinge in eukaryotic MutY homologues mediates catalytic activity and Rad9-Rad1-Hus1 checkpoint complex interactions. J Mol Biol. 2010;403:351–70.
20. Chang DY, Lu AL. Functional interaction of MutY homolog with proliferating cell nuclear antigen in fission yeast, *Schizosaccharomyces pombe*. J Biol Chem. 2002;277:11853–8.
21. Liu X, Lee YJ, Liou LC, Ren Q, Zhang Z, Wang S, Witt SN. Alpha-synuclein functions in the nucleus to protect against hydroxyurea-induced replication stress in yeast. Hum Mol Genet. 2011;20:3401–14.
22. Davies BW, Kohanski MA, Simmons LA, Winkler JA, Collins JJ, Walker GC. Hydroxyurea induces hydroxyl radical-mediated cell death in *Escherichia coli*. Mol Cell. 2009;36:845–60.

23. Skog S, Tribukait B, Wallström B, Eriksson S. Hydroxyurea-induced cell death as related to cell cycle in mouse and human T-lymphoma cells. Cancer Res. 1987;47:6490–3.
24. Gottifredi V, Shieh S, Taya Y, Prives C. p53 accumulates but is functionally impaired when DNA synthesis is blocked. Proc Natl Acad Sci USA. 2001;98:1036–41.
25. Wagner JM, Karnitz LM. Cisplatin-induced DNA damage activates replication checkpoint signaling components that differentially affect tumor cell survival. Mol Pharmacol. 2009;76:208–14.
26. Borel F, Lacroix FB, Margolis RL. Prolonged arrest of mammalian cells at the G1/S boundary results in permanent S phase stasis. J Cell Sci. 2002;115:2829–38.
27. Yan S, Michael WM. TopBP1 and DNA polymerase α-mediated recruitment of the 9-1-1 complex to stalled replication forks. Cell Cycle. 2009;8:2877–84.
28. Liu K, Bellam N, Lin HY, Wang B, Stockard CR, Grizzle WE, Lin WC. Regulation of p53 by TopBP1: a potential mechanism for p53 inactivation in cancer. Mol Cell Biol. 2009;29:2673–93.
29. Yan S, Lindsay HD, Michael WM. Direct requirement for Xmus101 in ATR-mediated phosphorylation of Claspin bound Chk1 during checkpoint signaling. J Cell Biol. 2006;173:181–6.
30. Liu K, Graves JD, Scott JD, Li R, Lin WC. Akt switches TopBP1 function from checkpoint activation to transcriptional regulation through phosphoserine binding-mediated oligomerization. Mol Cell Biol. 2013;33:4685–700.
31. Tapia-Alveal C, Calonge TM, O'Connell MJ. Regulation of Chk1. Cell Div. 2009;4:8.
32. Mäkiniemi M, Hillukkala T, Tuusa J, Reini K, Vaara M, Huang D, Pospiech H, Majuri I, Westerling T, Mäkelä TP, Syväoja JE. BRCT domain-containing protein TopBP1 functions in DNA replication and damage response. J Biol Chem. 2001;276:30399–406.
33. Parker A, Gu Y, Mahoney W, Lee SH, Singh KK, Lu AL. Human homolog of the MutY repair protein (hMYH) physically interacts with proteins involved in long patch DNA base excision repair. J Biol Chem. 2001;276:5547–55.
34. Lindsey-Boltz LA, Sancar A. Tethering DNA damage checkpoint mediator proteins Topoisomerase IIβ-binding protein 1 (TopBP1) and Claspin to DNA actaxia-telangiectasia mutated and Rad3-related (ATR) phosphorylation of checkpoint kinase1 (Chk1). J Biol Chem. 2011;286:19229–36.
35. Xu YJ, Leffak M. ATRIP from TopBP1 to ATR-in vitro activation of a DNA damage checkpoint. Proc Natl Acad Sci USA. 2010;107:13561–2.
36. Mordes DA, Glick GG, Zhao R, Cortez D. TopBP1 activates ATR through ATRIP and a PIKK regulatory domain. Genes Dev. 2008;22:1478–89.

10

Transplantation of induced pluripotent stem cell-derived renal stem cells improved acute kidney injury

Qing Li[1†], Shou-fu Tian[2,3†], Ye Guo[4], Xin Niu[1], Bin Hu[1], Shang-chun Guo[1], Nian-song Wang[2*] and Yang Wang[1*]

Abstract

Background: Acute kidney injury (AKI) is a severe disease with high morbidity and mortality. Methods that promote repair of the injured kidney have been extensively investigated. Cell-based therapy with mesenchymal stem cells or renal progenitor cells (RPCs) resident in the kidney has appeared to be an effective strategy for the treatment of AKI. Embryonic stem cells or induced pluripotent stem cells (iPSCs) are also utilized for AKI recovery. However, the therapeutic effect of iPSC-derived RPCs for AKI has yet to be determined.

Methods: In this study, we induced iPSCs differentiation into RPCs using a nephrogenic cocktail of factors combined with the renal epithelial cell growth medium. We then established the rat ischemia–reperfusion injury (IR) model and transplanted the iPSC-derived RPCs into the injured rats in combination with the hydrogel. Next, we examined the renal function-related markers and renal histology to assess the therapeutic effect of the injected cells. Moreover, we investigated the mechanism by which iPSC-derived RPCs affect AKI caused by IR.

Results: We showed that the differentiation efficiency of iPSCs to RPCs increased when cultured with renal epithelial cell growth medium after stimulation with a nephrogenic cocktail of factors. The transplantation of iPSC-derived RPCs decreased the levels of biomarkers indicative of renal injury and attenuated the necrosis and apoptosis of renal tissues, but resulted in the up-regulation of renal tubules formation, cell proliferation, and the expression of pro-renal factors.

Conclusion: Our results revealed that iPSC-derived RPCs can protect AKI rat from renal function impairment and severe tubular injury by up-regulating the renal tubules formation, promoting cell proliferation, reducing apoptosis, and regulating the microenvironment in the injured kidney.

Keywords: Acute kidney injury, iPSC-derived RPCs, Renal ischemia–reperfusion injury, Hydrogel

Background

Acute kidney injury (AKI) is characterized by acute tubular injury and a rapid decline in renal function [1]. Renal ischemia is one of the most common causes of AKI. AKI has recently received increasing attention due to the high mortality and morbidity rates of the syndrome [2]. Although pharmacological therapy, modern dialysis techniques, and intermittent or continuous renal replacement therapies exist, the therapeutic approaches for AKI remain very limited. Thus, the establishment of novel therapeutic strategies for ischemic AKI is urgently needed.

In response to acute injury, the adult kidney shows some level of regeneration characterized by the proliferation of the surviving cells and the replacement of the necrotic tubular cells with functional tubular epithelium [3]. The process is hypothesized to involve epithelial cell dedifferentiation, interstitial cell transdifferentiation and/or activation of quiescent stem cells. Over the

*Correspondence: wangniansong2012@163.com; wangy63cn@126.com
†Qing Li and Shou-fu Tian contributed equally to this work
[1] Institute of Microsurgery on Extremities, Shanghai Jiao Tong University Affiliated Sixth People's Hospital, Shanghai 200233, China
[2] Department Nephrology and Rheumatology, Shanghai Jiao Tong University Affiliated Sixth People's Hospital, Shanghai 200233, China
Full list of author information is available at the end of the article

last few years, renal progenitor cells (RPCs) have been isolated from the kidney [4–7]. Several studies have indicated that RPCs appear to play important roles in kidney repair under various pathological conditions [4, 8–10]. However, progenitor cells in the adult kidney are rare, which limits the application of these cells. Therefore, we resorted to other types of stem cells.

Stem cells, including embryonic stem cells (ESCs) and adult stem cells, have the potential of self-renewal and differentiation into multiple cell types and therefore hold great promise in regenerative medicine [11–13]. It was recently reported that stem cells exhibit therapeutic potential for AKI [14–17]. Several studies have demonstrated that the exposure of ESCs to factors required for renal specification, such as retinoic acid, activin A and bone morphogenic proteins (BMPs), does induce their differentiation into renal lineage cells in vitro [18–20]. Vigneau et al. [10] showed that the transplantation of mouse ESCs-derived RPCs can result in the stable integration into proximal tubules with normal morphology and normal polarization injection into developing live newborn mouse kidneys, suggesting the potential of ESCs for application in regenerative therapies. However, the use of ESCs for human therapy raises several safety and ethical concerns.

Induced pluripotent stem cells (iPSCs) are a type of newly defined stem cell with properties similar to those of ESCs in terms of self-renewal and differentiation. These cells were first generated by Yamanaka and colleagues [21]. Since their discovery, iPSCs have shown their advantages in regenerative medicine. iPSCs have also been reported to be effective for AKI. Lee and colleagues [16] showed that the injection of iPSCs into the kidney improves renal function and attenuates renal tubular injury in AKI caused by ischemia–reperfusion injury (IR) and eventually improves the survival rate of rats with AKI. Although iPSCs are an alternative potential cell source for stem cell therapy to protect against AKI, there is also a risk of tumor formation. Therefore, we investigated whether iPSC-derived RPCs have a therapeutic effect on AKI.

In the present study, we examined whether iPSC-derived RPCs can protect against AKI in a rate model of IR. We showed that the differentiation efficiency of iPSCs to RPCs increased when cultured with Renal Epithelial Cell Growth Medium after stimulation with a nephrogenic cocktail of factors. The injection of iPSC-derived RPCs combined with hydrogel, which provides a 3-D structure to the cells, into the kidney of rats with IR could improve renal function and attenuate tubular injury by forming renal tubules in the recipient rat kidney directly, promoting cell proliferation, reducing apoptosis, and regulating the microenvironment in the injured kidney.

Results

Efficient differentiation of RPCs from mouse iPSCs

To investigate whether iPSC-derived RPCs can improve AKI, we first used a nephrogenic cocktail of factors (including retinoic acid, activin A, and BMP7) to induce iPSCs differentiation into RPCs (Additional file 1: Figure S1). The iPS cell line used in this study is tagged with a ubiquitously expressed *gfp* gene. The real-time PCR analysis showed that the expression of the RPC markers PAX2, WT1, Six2 and CD24 increased after RAB treatment (Fig. 1a), indicating that RPCs were successfully induced. As shown by flow cytometry analysis, the PAX2, WT1 and CD24 positive cells were 33.16, 19.56 and 27.82 % respectively (Fig. 1b). Additionally, the mature renal markers AQP1

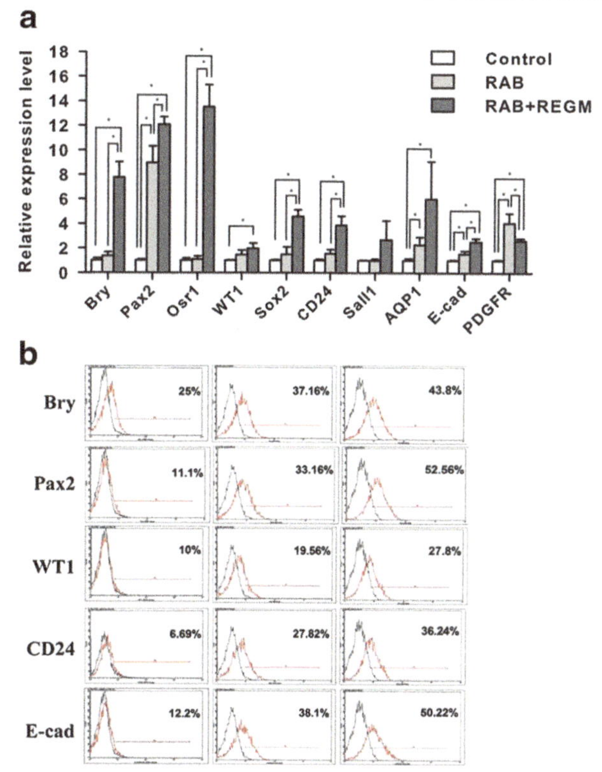

Fig. 1 Efficient differentiation of renal progenitor cells from mouse induced pluripotent stem cells (iPSCs). The renal differentiation of mouse iPSCs was initiated by the formation of embryoid bodies (EBs). After 2 days, retinoic acid, activin A, and BMP7 were added to the differentiation medium, and the cells were exposed to this supplemented media for 5 days (RAB group). After incubation with growth factors for 5 days, the EBs in the RAB + REGM group were cultured in renal epithelial cell growth medium for another 5 days. **a** Real-time PCR analysis of the expression of mesoderm (Bry) and renal lineage genes (Pax2, Osr1, WT1, Six2, CD24, Sal1, AQP1, E-cad and PDGFR). **b** Flow cytometry analysis of the expression of mesoderm renal progenitor-related genes. *Black line*, cells stained with isotype control; *Red line*, cells stained with indicated antibodies. *$P < 0.05$

and E-cadherin were up-regulated upon RAB stimulation (Fig. 1a). To improve the differentiation efficiency of iPSCs into RPCs, the cells were cultured in renal epithelial cell growth medium for another 5 days (Additional file 1: Figure S1). As expected, the expression of the RPCs markers was further up-regulated compared with that of the RAB group, as shown by real-time PCR analysis after 5 days of differentiation in RAB medium (Fig. 1a). Moreover, the PAX2, WT1, and CD24 single-positive cells increased to 52.56, 27.8 and 36.24 % respectively (Fig. 1b), indicating that more RPCs were generated in the RAB + REGM group.

Therapeutic effect of iPSC-derived RPCs in rats with IR-induced AKI

Next, the rat IR model was generated by occlusion of the left renal artery followed by reperfusion and right kidney removal. iPSC-derived RPCs from the RAB + REGM group were injected directly into the renal parenchyma of the injured rats in combination with the hydrogel. The control group (IR-control) was injected with PBS combined with the hydrogel. The levels of BUN and Scr were detected at the indicated times. The plasma levels of BUN and Scr reached their peak levels at day 1 of renal IR in all groups and then decreased gradually (Fig. 2a, b). After RPC transplantation, the plasma levels of BUN and Scr were lower than those of the IR-control group (Fig. 2a, b). To test whether the RPC transplantation has beneficial effects on regeneration after IR, the rats were sacrificed on days 3, 7, 14, and 28, and the renal histology was examined. H&E staining showed that the proximal tubule in the renal cortex in the control group exhibited acute injury and necrosis 3 days after surgery (Fig. 3a):

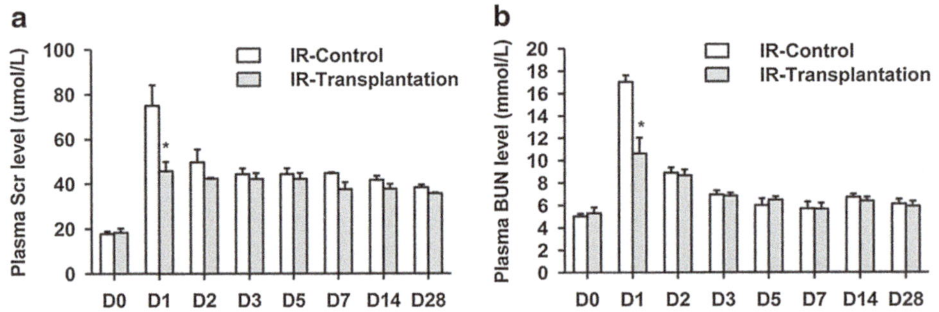

Fig. 2 Generation of rat renal ischemia–reperfusion model. The rat renal ischemia–reperfusion injury (IR) model was generated by occlusion of the left renal artery followed by reperfusion and right kidney removal. iPSC-derived renal progenitor cells were injected into the renal parenchyma of the injured rats in combination with a hydrogel. The Scr (**a**) and BUN (**b**) levels in the plasma were detected at the indicated times. *$P < 0.05$ vs. IR-Control

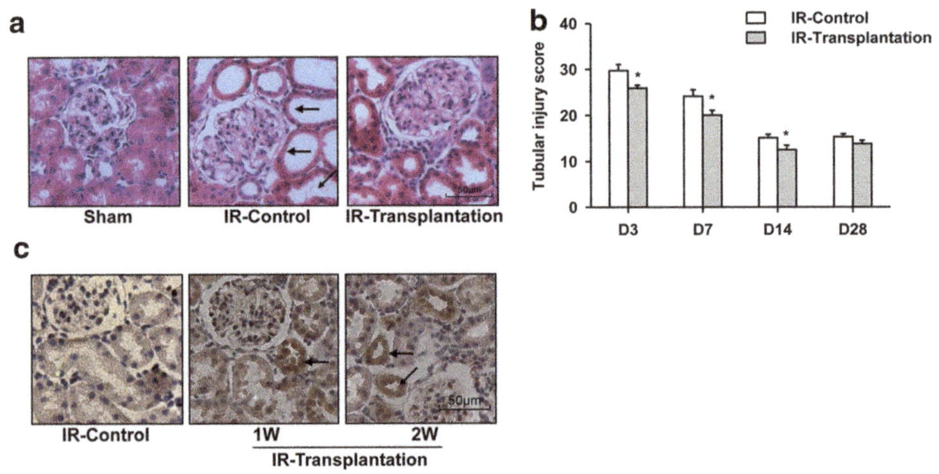

Fig. 3 Transplantation of iPSC-derived renal progenitor cells improved renal tubular damage caused by ischemia–reperfusion. **a** Pathological changes in the kidney on the third day after surgery, as shown by H&E staining. Luminal debris, loss of brush borders and lumen expansion are observed in the injured groups (*black arrow*). **b** The transplantation of iPSC-derived renal progenitor cells reduced the acute tubular necrosis scores. **c** The immunohistochemistry analysis indicated that the injected GFP-positive cells formed a tubular structure (*black arrow*) in the recipient organ at the indicated times after transplantation. *$P < 0.05$ vs. IR-Control. *Scale bar* 50 μm

the brush border of some epithelial cells disappeared; the lumen expanded; some of the tubular epithelial cells detached from the basement membrane; the tubule was obstructed with cellular debris; and the interstitial tubule was infiltrated with inflammatory cells. The histological features of necrotic injury were still severe 7 days after ischemia and began to improve on days 14 and 28. The injury phenotype was decreased in the rat kidney as a result of RPC transplantation. The quantitative analysis of the renal tubular necrosis using the grading scores of Paller et al. [22] is shown in Fig. 3b. These results suggest that the transplantation of iPSC-derived RPCs could improve renal regeneration and function after AKI.

Mechanistic study of the improvement in the renal tubular damage caused by IR as a result of iPSC-derived RPC transplantation

We further investigated the mechanism through which RPCs relieve acute renal injury caused by IR. Previous studies have reported that mouse kidney progenitor cells accelerate renal regeneration after ischemic injury by differentiation into epithelial cells and incorporating into the renal tubule [9, 23–25]. Thus, we first examined the localization of the transplanted iPSC-derived RPCs. Because the iPS cell line used in our study carries a ubiquitously expressed *gfp* gene, it is convenient to trace the injected cells. Using immunohistochemistry, we showed that GFP-positive cells began to form a tubular structure in the recipient kidney 7 days after injection (Fig. 3c). Importantly, no tumor was detected even 3 months after transplantation. Next, the effects of the RPCs on the proliferation and apoptosis of cells in the injured kidney were examined by PCNA staining and TUNEL analyses, respectively. The results showed that the number of PCNA-positive cells increased in the transplanted group compared with that found in the control group on days 7 after injection (Fig. 4a, b), indicating the presence of a greater number of proliferating renal tubular epithelial cells in the kidney after RPC transplantation. In contrast, the cell apoptosis on days 7 was reduced in the RPC-transplanted group, as shown by TUNEL analysis (Fig. 4c, d). Furthermore, we detected the expression levels of the anti-inflammatory factors interleukin-10 (IL-10), basic fibroblast growth factor (bFGF), and transforming growth factor β1 (TGF-β1) and growth factors promoting renal tubular cell repair, namely epidermal growth factor (EGF), hepatocyte growth factor (HGF), and platelet-derived growth factor (PDGF). The real-time PCR analysis showed that the expression of these genes was upregulated to different extents after RPC transplantation (Fig. 5). Altogether, these data indicate that iPSC-derived RPC transplantation improves renal function after IR by directly incorporating into the renal tubule, promoting cell proliferation, reducing apoptosis, and upregulating the expression of pro-renal factors.

Discussion

AKI is an emerging worldwide public health problem with high mortality and morbidity rates and has thus attracted increasing attention. Although traditional therapies show benefits in the treatment of AKI, the therapeutic approaches are still very limited. Recently, stem

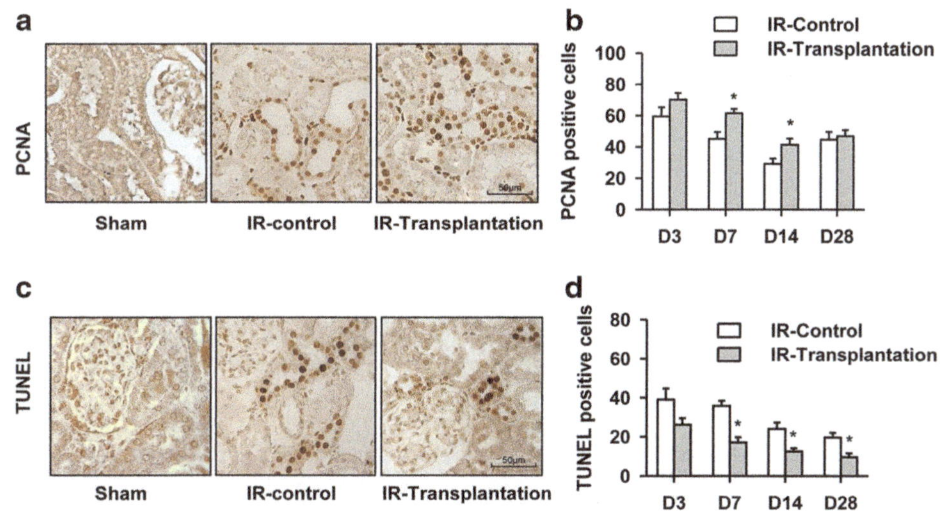

Fig. 4 Cell proliferation was increased and apoptosis was decreased in the transplanted renal parenchyma. **a** The proliferation of renal tubular cells was increased 7 days after cell transplantation, as determined by PCNA staining. **b** Quantitative analysis of PCNA-positive cells in **a**. **c** Renal tubular cell apoptosis was decreased 7 days after cell transplantation, as determined by TUNEL assay. **d** Quantitative analysis of **c**. *$P < 0.05$ vs. IR-Control. *Scale bar* 50 μm

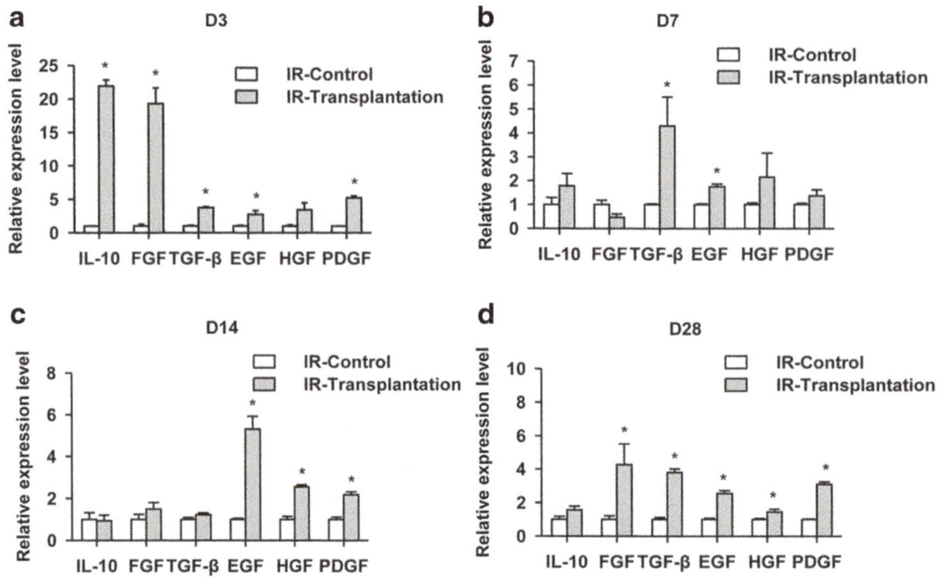

Fig. 5 Anti-inflammatory factors and pro-renal tubular repair factors increased after renal progenitor cell transplantation. Real-time PCR analysis of the expression of anti-inflammatory factors (IL-10, FGF, and TGF-β) and pro-renal tubular repair factors (EGF, HGF, and PDGF) on D3, D7, D14, and D28. The anti-inflammatory factors and pro-renal tubular repair factors in the renal cortex of rats after cell transplantation are up-regulated compared with the levels observed in the control group. *$P < 0.05$ vs. IR-Control

cell-based therapy appeared to be a potential strategy for the prevention of AKI [26]. In the present study, we provide the first demonstration that the transplantation of iPSC-derived RPCs improves renal regeneration and function in a rat model of IR-induced AKI, and the protective effect of the RPCs was mediated by their direct differentiation into renal lineage cells and incorporation into the renal tubule, which resulted in the promotion of cell proliferation and the reduction of apoptosis in the damaged zone. Furthermore, the transplantation of iPSC-derived RPCs promoted the expression of anti-inflammatory factors and pro-renal tubular repair factors, suggesting that RPCs can regulate the microenvironment and facilitate cell survival in the injured kidney.

After ischemic injury, RPCs and mesenchymal stem cells (MSCs) resident in the kidney are activated and show some level of regenerative ability. Several studies have shown the therapeutic potential of isolated primary RPCs or MSCs in experimental AKI models. However, these cells are not available in large volumes. Recent advances demonstrated that iPSCs may be more readily accessible for kidney regeneration [16]. Therefore, in our study, iPSCs were differentiated into renal lineage cells to obtain a sufficient number of RPCs. To the traditional induction medium, we added renal specific growth medium for further induction. Using this modified protocol, the differentiation efficiency of iPSCs into RPCs and mature renal epithelial cells increased. Because kidney regeneration requires many functionally distinct cell types of the nephron, the transplantation of all renal cell types derived from iPSCs may offer the advantage of generating more than one cell type of the adult kidney.

In previous studies, stem cells for the treatment of AKI were mainly injected through the tail vein or the intrarenal artery [9, 16], and the transplanted stem cells in the circulation are mobilized to the injury site in the kidney mediated by chemokines/cytokines and receptor interaction and thereafter enhance renal regeneration. However, the homing efficiency cannot be determined. In our study, RPCs were injected directly into the renal parenchyma in combination with a hydrogel. A hydrogel consists of a network of polymer chains, and the function and structure of a hydrogel are similar to those of a natural extracellular matrix. Therefore, hydrogels are currently widely used as scaffolds in tissue engineering [27–30]. The hydrogel used in our work is composed of polypeptides and can be degraded into natural amino acids in vivo; thus, the hydrogel has no hazardous effect on the injured tissue. After being injected into the renal parenchyma with the RPCs, the liquid hydrogel will quickly transform into a solid structure, which provides a three-dimensional microenvironment for RPC adhesion, migration, proliferation and differentiation. Our results showed that the exogenous cells formed a tubular structure in the injured kidney, indicating that the RPCs could migrate out of the hydrogel and participate in renal regeneration.

The therapeutic mechanisms of primary RPCs for AKI were recently investigated in several studies [9, 23, 31]. It has been reported that the transplanted RPCs can differentiate into renal tubule cells and vessel endothelial cells with the expression of E-cadherin and CD34 [23] and therefore accelerate renal regeneration and prolong survival after AKI. Our result that iPSC-derived RPCs can differentiate into renal tubule cells and form renal tubules in the injured kidney further supports this hypothesis. Moreover, we showed that the transplantation of iPSC-derived RPCs promoted cell proliferation and decreased apoptotic events. The cells also exhibited an anti-inflammatory effect by increasing the expression of anti-inflammatory factors, including TGF-β1. A recent study [32] reported that the presence of TGF-β1 in the homogenate of acute IR-injured renal tissue markedly increases the CXCR4 surface expression of MSCs and promotes the migration of MSCs to SDF-1. Therefore, we hypothesized that the transplantation of RPCs increased the level of TGF-β1 in the injured zone, which in turn regulated the CXCR4 expression of the RPCs, contributing to the migration of the RPCs out of the hydrogel to the injured sites. However, this proposed mechanism requires further investigation.

Collectively, the present study demonstrated that the transplantation of iPSC-derived RPCs is able to protect against kidney injury in an experimental IR rat model. These cells function in both differentiation-dependent and -independent manners by directly forming renal tubules and exerting pro-proliferative, anti-apoptotic, and anti-inflammatory effects. Our data suggest that iPSC-derived RPCs are a potential cellular resource for stem cell-based therapy for IR-induced AKI.

Conclusions

This study reports a modified method for the differentiation of iPSCs into RPCs and provides experimental evidence that iPSC-derived RPCs combined with a hydrogel can improve renal function in AKI and reduce tubular injury in an animal IR model. We believe that iPSC-derived RPCs hold great potential to be used as seed cells for personalized treatment in regenerative medicine.

Methods

IPSCs culture

Undifferentiated iPSCs were routinely cultured and expanded on mitotically inactivated MEFs (50,000 cells/cm^2) in six-well culture plates with mES medium: DMEM supplemented with 15 % FBS, L-glutamine, nonessential amino acids, β-mercaptoethanol (Gibco), and 1000 U/ml LIF (Millipore). The iPS cell line used in the present study was purchased from SiDanSai Biotechnology (Shanghai, China). The sequence of *gfp* gene, for tracing the iPSCs and iPSC-derived cells, was inserted into the chromosome of iPSCs. iPSCs transduced with this sequence showed robust expression of GFP.

Renal differentiation of murine iPSCs

iPSCs were differentiated through embryoid body (EB) formation in EB medium (DMEM supplemented with 15 % FBS, L-glutamine, nonessential amino acids, and β-mercaptoethanol). On day 3 of differentiation, the EBs were transferred to gelatin-coated culture dishes at a density of 10 EBs per 1 ml of medium. The cells in the control group were maintained in EB medium for 5 days, and the medium was changed every 2 days. The cells in the induction group were exposed to a nephrogenic cocktail of factors, including 0.1 μM RA (Sigma), 10 ng/ml activin-A (PeproTech), and 50 ng/ml BMP7 (PeproTech), in the EB medium for 5 days. The induced cells were then cultured in the EB medium alone (RAB group) or in Renal Epithelial Cell Growth Medium (RAB + REGM group) for another 5 days and harvested for further analyses.

Quantitative reverse-transcriptase polymerase chain reaction (RT-PCR)

The total RNA from cells or tissues was extracted using the TRIzol reagent according to the protocol delineated by the manufacturer (Invitrogen-Life Technologies). One microgram of total RNA was reverse transcribed into cDNA with oligo-dT primers and reverse transcriptase (Invitrogen-Life Technologies). Real-time quantitative PCR was performed using SYBR Green (Toyobo Co, Japan). The primers used in the amplification reaction are shown in Table 1.

Flow cytometry

The differentiated cells were detached from the flask using accutase (Invitrogen-Life Technologies). The single cells were fixed with 4 % paraformaldehyde (Sigma) for 15 min, permeabilized with 0.5 % Triton x-100 (Sigma), and blocked with 3 % BSA (Gibco) for 30 min at room temperature. The cells were then incubated with the following primary antibodies for 1 h: Pax2 (1:100; Abcam), Bry (1:100; Abcam), E-cadherin (1:100; Cell Signaling Technology), CD24 (1:200; BD Biosciences), and WT1 (1:50; Santa Cruz Biotechnology Inc). After washing three times, the cells were incubated with the secondary antibody conjugated to Alexa Fluor 594 (1:200; Invitrogen-Life Technologies). The cells were washed to remove any unbound antibody and then analyzed using a flow cytometer (Millipore).

Preparation of hydrogel and cell mixture for injection

Hydrogels belong to a class of biological materials and produce a nanoscale environment similar that of the

Table 1 Primers used for quantitative reverse-transcriptase polymerase chain reaction (RT-PCR)

Genes	Forward primer (5′–3′)	Reverse primer (5′–3′)
m-PAX2	AAGCCCGGAGTGATTGGTG	CAGGCGAACATAGTCGGGTT
m-WT1	CAGTTCCCCAACCATTCCTT	AAGCTGGGAGGTCATTTGGT
m-Brachyury (Bry)	ACCCAGACTCGCCCAATTTT	GGAAAGCAGTGGCTGGTGAT
m-CD24	GTTGCACCGTTTCCCGGTAA	CCCCTCTGGTGGTAGCGTTA
m-Osr1	ATTCACCCTAAGCCAGAGATCA	AGGCCAGGTTAGCGAAATCAA
m-Six2	CTCACCACCACGCAAGTCAG	CTCGGAACTGCCTAGCACC
m-Sall1	CTCAACATTTCCAATCCGACCC	GGCATCCTTGCTCTTAGTGGG
m-E-cad	CTCCAGTCATAGGGAGCTGTC	TCTTCTGAGACCTGGGTACAC
m-AQP1	AGGCTTCAATTACCCACTGGA	GTGAGCACCGCTGATGTGA
m-PDGFR	CCACACCCTTGGGGAATAGT	TTTGAAGGGCAAGGAATGTG
m-GAPDH	ACTTCAACAGCAACTCCCACTC	TAGGCCCCTCCTGTTATTATGG
r-IL-10	TAACTGCACCCACTTCCCAGT	TGGCAACCCAAGTAACCCTTA
r-bFGF	CGACCCACACGTCAAACTAC	CCAGGCGTTCAAAGAAGAAA
r-TGF-β1	GCCCTGGATACCAACTACTGCT	GTTGGTTGTAGAGGGCAAGGAC
r-EGF	CGTCTCAGTGGTCATGGATTT	TCAGAAGAACACGGGAATTGT
r-HGF	CTCTCGTTCCTTGGGATTATTG	GATCCCCCACAGATGTGTTTAT
r-PDGF	ATCGAGCCAAGACACCTCAAAC	ATGGGGGCAGTACAGCAAATAC
r-GAPDH	AGTGCCAGCCTCGTCTCATAG	CGTTGAACTTGCCGTGGGTAG

native extracellular matrix [27–30]. A hydrogel consists of 1 % self-assembling peptides (w/v) and 99 % water (w/v). The detailed constituents and properties and the detailed preparation of the hydrogel used in this study are detailed by the manufacturer (Beaver Nano Technologies, China). Briefly, the hydrogel (1 %) was sonicated for 30 min before use. The cells were suspended with 50 μl of 10 % sucrose solution, and 50 μl of the cell suspension was rapidly and carefully mixed with 50 μl of 1 % hydrogel. Then, 100 μl of PBS (Corning) was carefully added to the top of the cell and hydrogel mixture for instantaneous gelation. The 1 % hydrogel (50 μl) diluted with 150 μl of PBS was used as a control.

Rat renal IR model and injection of RPCs

The renal IR model was generated in 8-week-old male Sprague–Dawley as described previously [16]. Briefly, thirty rats (3–3.5 kg) were anesthetized with chloral hydrate (0.2 mg/g, Sigma), and this step was followed by exposure of the abdomen. For induction of total ischemia in the kidney, the left renal artery was clamped with a small vascular clamp for 45 min. Reperfusion was initiated by removal of the clamp. The right kidney was removed simultaneously. Thirty-four rats survived the IR surgery and no rats died in the following experiments. Then, the hydrogel (200 μl; denoted "IR-control" group) or the suspension of iPSC-derived RPCs (1×10^5 cells in 200 μl of 0.25 % hydrogel per rat; denoted "IR-transplantation" group) was respectively injected into the renal parenchyma of rats (seventeen rats per group). The rats were injected with the immunosuppressant cyclosporine A (Sigma) at a dose of 5 mg/kg per day. Six sham-operated animals underwent similar operative procedures but without clamping of the left renal artery and right kidney nephrectomy. At the indicated time, the blood was collected to measure the levels of blood urea nitrogen (BUN) and serum creatinine (Scr). The rats were killed at the indicated days for the collection of kidney tissue samples. All care and handling of animals was performed with the approval of the Ethical Review Board of Shanghai Six People's Hospital Affiliated to Shanghai Jiaotong University. The animals were raised in a specific pathogen-free (SPF) environment.

Histological analysis and tubular injury score

For the histological analysis, the kidney tissues were fixed with 4 % paraformaldehyde overnight and embedded in paraffin. The paraffin sections (4 μm) were stained with hematoxylin and eosin (H&E, Sigma). The quantitative analysis of the renal tubular injury used the grading scores proposed in a previous study [22]. The sections were evaluated by assessing 10 randomly selected high-power fields (40 × objective), and higher scores represented more severe damage: tubular epithelial cell flattening (1 point), brush border loss (1 point), cell membrane bleb formation (1 or 2 points), interstitial edema (1 point), cytoplasmic vacuolization (1 point), cell necrosis (1 or 2 points), and tubular lumen obstruction (1 or 2 points).

Immunohistochemistry

Immunohistochemical staining was performed with mouse anti-GFP antibody (1:100; Cell Signaling Technology) and mouse anti-proliferating cell nuclear antigen (PCNA, 1:200; Abcam). Briefly, paraffin sections of the kidneys were deparaffinized with xylene and rehydrated in an alcohol series and water. The kidney sections were subjected to antigen retrieval and blocked with a peroxidase-blocking reagent. The sections were incubated with the primary antibody overnight at 4 °C. After washing, the kidney sections were incubated with horseradish peroxidase-conjugated secondary antibody (ZSJQ-BIO, China) for 1 h at room temperature. The sections were visualized with 3,3′-diaminobenzidine (DAB, ZSGQ-BIO) and counterstained with hematoxylin. The number of positive cells was evaluated by counting the stained cells per high-power field in at least 20 randomly selected fields. The apoptotic cells in the kidney were detected by terminal deoxynucleotidyl transferase (TdT)-mediated digoxigenin deoxyuridine nick-end labeling (TUNEL, Promega) staining according to the protocol delineated by the manufacturer. The TUNEL-negative controls were stained without TdT enzyme.

Statistical analysis

All of the experiments were performed at least three times. The data are shown as the mean ± SEM. Differences were analyzed using one-way analysis of variance (ANOVA). Values of $P < 0.05$ were considered statistically significant.

Authors' contributions

YW and NSW conceived the idea, designed the experiments, and provided their funds to the study. SFT, YG and SCG participated in the experiments of Cell-culture and animal experiments. XN and BH were responsible for Data collection and analysis. QL and SFT contributed to Manuscript writing. All authors read and approved the final manuscript.

Author details

[1] Institute of Microsurgery on Extremities, Shanghai Jiao Tong University Affiliated Sixth People's Hospital, Shanghai 200233, China. [2] Department Nephrology and Rheumatology, Shanghai Jiao Tong University Affiliated Sixth People's Hospital, Shanghai 200233, China. [3] Department of Integration of Traditional Chinese and Western Medicine, The First Affiliated Hospital of Soochow University, Suzhou 215006, China. [4] Department of Neurosurgery, Shandong Jining No. 1 People's Hospital, Jining 272011, China.

Acknowledgements

This work was financially supported by the National Natural Science Foundation of China (No: 81170640, 30960385).

Compliance with ethical guidelines

Competing interests

The authors declare that they have no competing interests.

References

1. Thodani R, Pascual M, Bonventre J. Medical progress: acute renal failure. N Engl J Med. 1996;334:1448–60.
2. Lameire NH, Bagga A, Cruz D, De Maeseneer J, Endre Z, Kellum JA, et al. Acute kidney injury: an increasing global concern. Lancet. 2013;382(9887):170–9.
3. Sharfuddin AA, Molitoris BA. Pathophysiology of ischemic acute kidney injury. Nat Rev Nephrol. 2011;7(4):189–200.
4. Bussolati B, Bruno S, Grange C, Buttiglieri S, Deregibus MC, Cantino D, et al. Isolation of renal progenitor cells from adult human kidney. Am J Pathol. 2005;166(2):545–55.
5. Lazzeri E, Mazzinghi B, Romagnani P. Regeneration and the kidney. Curr Opin Nephrol Hypertens. 2010;19(3):248–53.
6. Sagrinati C, Netti GS, Mazzinghi B, Lazzeri E, Liotta F, Frosali F, et al. Isolation and characterization of multipotent progenitor cells from the Bowman's capsule of adult human kidneys. J Am Soc Nephrol. 2006;17(9):2443–56.
7. Smeets B, Boor P, Dijkman H, Sharma SV, Jirak P, Mooren F, et al. Proximal tubular cells contain a phenotypically distinct, scattered cell population involved in tubular regeneration. J Pathol. 2013;229(5):645–59.
8. Angelotti ML, Ronconi E, Ballerini L, Peired A, Mazzinghi B, Sagrinati C, et al. Characterization of renal progenitors committed toward tubular lineage and their regenerative potential in renal tubular injury. Stem Cells. 2012;30(8):1714–25.
9. Han X, Zhao L, Lu G, Ge J, Zhao Y, Zu S, et al. Improving outcomes of acute kidney injury using mouse renal progenitor cells alone or in combination with erythropoietin or suramin. Stem Cell Res Ther. 2013;4(3):74.
10. Vigneau C, Polgar K, Striker G, Elliott J, Hyink D, Weber O, et al. Mouse embryonic stem cell–derived embryoid bodies generate progenitors that integrate long term into renal proximal tubules in vivo. J Am Soc Nephrol. 2007;18(6):1709–20.
11. Cherry AB, Daley GQ. Reprogrammed cells for disease modeling and regenerative medicine. Annu Rev Med. 2013;64:277.
12. Singec I, Jandial R, Crain A, Nikkhah G, Snyder EY. The leading edge of stem cell therapeutics. Annu Rev Med. 2007;58:313–28.
13. Tabar V, Studer L. Pluripotent stem cells in regenerative medicine: challenges and recent progress. Nat Rev Genet. 2014;15(2):82–92.
14. Bi B, Schmitt R, Israilova M, Nishio H, Cantley LG. Stromal cells protect against acute tubular injury via an endocrine effect. J Am Soc Nephrol. 2007;18(9):2486–96.
15. Humphreys BD. Kidney injury, stem cells and regeneration. Curr Opin Nephrol Hypertens. 2014;23(1):25.
16. Lee P-Y, Chien Y, Chiou G-Y, Lin C-H, Chiou C-H, Tarng D-C. Induced pluripotent stem cells without c-Myc attenuate acute kidney injury via downregulating the signaling of oxidative stress and inflammation in ischemia-reperfusion rats. Cell Transplant. 2012;21(12):2569–85.
17. Morigi M, Introna M, Imberti B, Corna D, Abbate M, Rota C, et al. Human bone marrow mesenchymal stem cells accelerate recovery of acute renal injury and prolong survival in mice. Stem Cells. 2008;26(8):2075–82.
18. Kim D, Dressler GR. Nephrogenic factors promote differentiation of mouse embryonic stem cells into renal epithelia. J Am Soc Nephrol. 2005;16(12):3527–34.
19. Morizane R, Monkawa T, Itoh H. Differentiation of murine embryonic stem and induced pluripotent stem cells to renal lineage in vitro. Biochem Biophys Res Commun. 2009;390(4):1334–9.
20. Xia Y, Nivet E, Sancho-Martinez I, Gallegos T, Suzuki K, Okamura D, et al. Directed differentiation of human pluripotent cells to ureteric bud kidney progenitor-like cells. Nat Cell Biol. 2013;15(12):1507–15.

21. Takahashi K, Yamanaka S. Induction of pluripotent stem cells from mouse embryonic and adult fibroblast cultures by defined factors. Cell. 2006;126(4):663–76.
22. Paller MS, Hoidal J, Ferris TF. Oxygen free radicals in ischemic acute renal failure in the rat. J Clin Investig. 1984;74(4):1156.
23. Lee PT, Lin HH, Jiang ST, Lu PJ, Chou KJ, Fang HC, et al. Mouse kidney progenitor cells accelerate renal regeneration and prolong survival after ischemic injury. Stem Cells. 2010;28(3):573–84.
24. Maeshima A, Sakurai H, Nigam SK. Adult kidney tubular cell population showing phenotypic plasticity, tubulogenic capacity, and integration capability into developing kidney. J Am Soc Nephrol. 2006;17(1):188–98.
25. Minuth WW, Denk L, Castrop H. Generation of tubular superstructures by piling of renal stem/progenitor cells. Tissue Eng Part C Methods. 2008;14(1):3–13.
26. Osafune K. In vitro regeneration of kidney from pluripotent stem cells. Exp Cell Res. 2010;316(16):2571–7.
27. Farnebo S, Woon CY, Schmitt T, Joubert L-M, Kim M, Pham H, et al. Design and characterization of an injectable tendon hydrogel: a novel scaffold for guided tissue regeneration in the musculoskeletal system. Tissue Eng Part A. 2014;20(9–10):1550–61.
28. Lei Y, Schaffer DV. A fully defined and scalable 3D culture system for human pluripotent stem cell expansion and differentiation. Proc Natl Acad Sci. 2013;110(52):E5039–48.
29. Sargeant TD, Desai AP, Banerjee S, Agawu A, Stopek JB. An in situ forming collagen–PEG hydrogel for tissue regeneration. Acta Biomater. 2012;8(1):124–32.
30. Sun J, Wei D, Zhu Y, Zhong M, Zuo Y, Fan H, et al. A spatial patternable macroporous hydrogel with cell-affinity domains to enhance cell spreading and differentiation. Biomaterials. 2014;35(17):4759–68.
31. Sallustio F, Costantino V, Cox SN, Loverre A, Divella C, Rizzi M, et al. Human renal stem/progenitor cells repair tubular epithelial cell injury through TLR2-driven inhibin-A and microvesicle-shuttled decorin. Kidney Int. 2013;83(3):392–403.
32. Si XY, Li JJ, Yao T, Wu XY. Transforming growth factor-β1 in the microenvironment of ischemia reperfusion-injured kidney enhances the chemotaxis of mesenchymal stem cells to stromal cell-derived factor-1 through upregulation of surface chemokine (C-X-C motif) receptor 4. Mol Med Rep. 2014;9(5):1794–8.

11

The biological role of actinin-4 (*ACTN4*) in malignant phenotypes of cancer

Kazufumi Honda[1,2*]

Abstract

Invasion and metastasis are malignant phenotypes in cancer that lead to patient death. Cell motility is involved in these processes. In 1998, we identified overexpression of the actin-bundling protein actinin-4 in several types of cancer. Protein expression of actinin-4 is closely associated with the invasive phenotypes of cancers. Actinin-4 is predominantly expressed in the cellular protrusions that stimulate the invasive phenotype in cancer cells and is essential for formation of cellular protrusions such as filopodia and lamellipodia. *ACTN4* (gene name encoding actinin-4 protein) is located on human chromosome 19q. *ACTN4* amplification is frequently observed in patients with carcinomas of the pancreas, ovary, lung, and salivary gland, and patients with *ACTN4* amplifications have worse outcomes than patients without amplification. In addition, nuclear distribution of actinin-4 is frequently observed in small cell lung, breast, and ovarian cancer. Actinin-4, when expressed in cancer cell nuclei, functions as a transcriptional co-activator. In this review, we summarize recent developments regarding the biological roles of actinin-4 in cancer invasion.

Keywords: Cancer invasion, Metastasis, Actinin-4 (ACTN4), Actin-bundling protein, Biomarker

Background

Despite successful complete resection at the primary cancer site, poor outcomes are occasionally observed in patients due to failure to control distant metastasis. Controlling metastasis is expected to improve the survival rate of patients with cancer [1, 2]. The mechanisms of cancer metastasis, which occurs in a multistep process, have been investigated to identify new therapeutic strategies for patients with cancer. During formation of metastatic lesions, carcinoma cells destroy the basement membrane, invade the surrounding extracellular matrix, intravasate through the endothelium into the circulation, extravasate again though the capillary vessels, and finally establish secondary tumors at distant sites [1, 3, 4]. The dynamic assembly of the actin cytoskeleton is important in this multistep process of forming metastatic lesions. In particular, the actin cytoskeleton plays important roles in the formation of cellular protrusions known as filopodia, lamellipodia, and invadopodia [5–10].

Alpha-actinin is an actin cross-linking protein that belongs to the spectrin superfamily. Four isoforms of alpha-actinin have been identified: alpha-actinin-1 (gene name; *ACTN1*) [11], actinin-2 (*ACTN2*) [12], actinin-3 (*ACTN3*) [12], and actinin-4 (*ACTN4*) [13]. These isoforms are classified into two groups: muscle (*ACTN2* and *ACTN3*) and non-muscle isoforms (*ACTN1* and *ACTN4*) [14]. Muscle-type isoforms of actinins are only expressed in skeletal and smooth muscle, where they mediate actin filament bundling and interactions with the Z-disk. On the other hand, non-muscle type isoforms are only expressed in non-muscle cells, where they also mediate actin filament bundling and interact with cell membranes. Non-muscle types in particular are associated with cell adhesion and cell migration. We originally identified *ACTN4* as a metastasis-related gene in cancer in 1998 [13] and have investigated the biological mechanisms and clinical implications of actinin-4 in cancer metastasis.

In this review, I mainly describe the involvement of actinin-4 in cancer metastasis and review recent studies of the biological function of actinin-4 in cancer and human diseases.

*Correspondence: khonda@ncc.go.jp
[1] Department of Chemotherapy and Clinical Research, National Cancer Center Research Institute, 5-1-1 Tsukiji Chuoku, Tokyo 104-0045, Japan
Full list of author information is available at the end of the article

Isolation of *ACTN4*, a metastasis-related gene

We generated a mouse monoclonal antibody that strongly reacts to the highly invasive phenotype of breast carcinoma, and we identified the full-length cDNA for the protein that was recognized by this antibody. This cDNA encodes a fourth novel isoform of alpha-actinin and was named actinin-4. Human actinin-4 is composed of 911 amino acids, and the amino acid homology with actinin-1 is 86% [13]. Alpha-actinin family members form an anti-parallel dimer with an actin-binding domain (ABD), which is composed of two calponin homology (CH) domains at the N-terminus of each monomer. Adjacent to the ABD, four spectrin repeats are followed by a C-terminal calmodulin (CaM)-like domain consisting of two EF-hand repeats (Fig. 1a) [14]. This molecular architecture results in the formation of a rod-shaped molecule with ABD and CaM domains at both ends, allowing cross-linking of bundles of actin filaments (Fig. 1b). Moreover, non-muscle alpha-actinins interact with actin filaments to connect with the plasma membrane through beta 1–3 integrins, vinculin, and alpha-catenin (Fig. 1c) [14–16].

Immunohistochemical analysis with the anti-actinin-4-specific antibody revealed significant overexpression of actinin-4 in histological subtypes of breast cancer with high invasive ability. Patients with overexpression of actinin-4 in invasive ductal adenocarcinoma of the breast show worse prognosis for overall survival than patients without overexpression. Immunocytochemistry following the wound healing assay to evaluate the invasiveness of cancer cells revealed that actinin-4 predominantly accumulates at artificial invasive fronts [13].

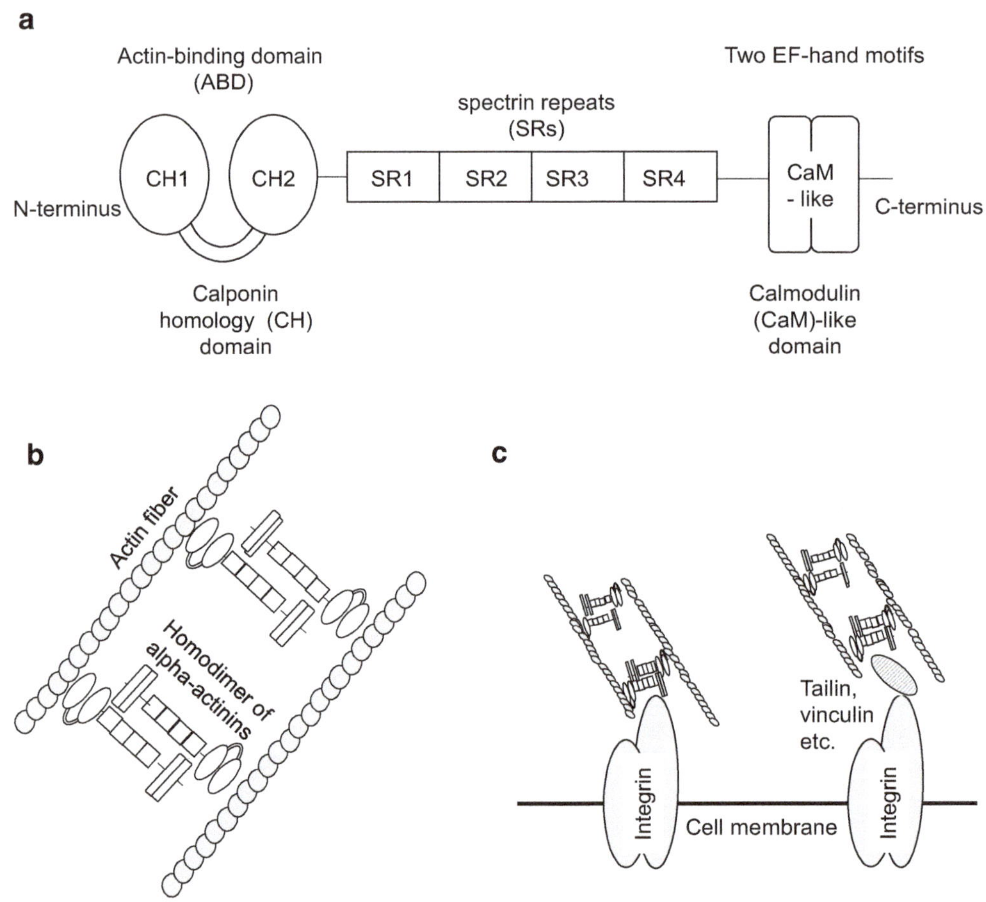

Fig. 1 Schematic of the domain structure of alpha-actinins (**a**). Alpha-actinins are composed of an actin-binding domain (ABD), four spectrin repeats (SRs), and a calmodulin (CaM)-like domain. ABDs are composed of two calponin homology (CHs) domains (CH1 and CH2). CaM-like domains are composed of two EF-hand motifs. Schematic of actin bundling with alpha-actinins (**b**). Actinins form an anti-parallel dimer, and homodimers of actinins bundle actin fibers by interacting with the ABD. Schematic of interactions between actin fibers and cell membranes (**c**). Actin fibers bundled with actinins directly or indirectly interact with the cell membrane through integrins.

The correlation between protein overexpression of actinin-4 and metastatic ability of cancer cells

Cancer cells, which are at the invasive front of cancer tissues, show an increased ability to migrate and metastasize, and show loss of epithelial integrity and specialization, a phenotype known as epithelial to mesenchymal transition (EMT) [10, 17]. Cells at the invasive fronts of colorectal cancer show reduced expression of E-cadherin, lose their cell–cell adhesions, and aggressively invade the stroma [18–21]. In colorectal cancer, overexpression of actinin-4 and EMT are observed in cells at the invasive front. We generated colorectal cancer cells (DLD1-TetOff-*ACTN4*) that express N-terminal HA-tagged actinin-4 under control of the tetracycline regulatory system and confirmed the distribution of exogenous actinin-4 with immunocytochemistry. When exogenous actinin-4 was overexpressed in DLD1-TetOff-*ACTN4* cells, filopodia and lamellipodia, which are involved in cell migration, were predominantly observed on the cell surface compared with before overexpression. DLD1-TetOff-*ACTN4* cells are highly motile in a cell motility assay, and animal experiments to confirm the metastatic ability revealed a significant increase in lymph node metastases compared with control cells [22]. On the other hand, an siRNA-mediated decreased in actinin-4 protein in a colon cancer cell line (SW480) reduces the cellular protrusions that are associated with cancer invasion [23].

Similar phenomena are observed in pancreatic cancer. Overexpression of actinin-4 is observed in invasive ductal adenocarcinoma of the pancreas, and such patients have a worse prognosis for overall survival than patients with weak actinin-4 expression [24]. In addition, actinin-4 is mainly observed at the invadepodia of cells from a pancreatic cancer cell line [25]. When actinin-4 is reduced in the pancreatic cancer cell line, BxPC3-KD-ACTN4, with *ACTN4* siRNA, the invasive ability in the invasion assay is decreased [23]. Transplantation of pancreatic cancer cells with siRNA-mediated reduction of *ACTN4* expression into the pancreas of mice revealed no destructive invasion into the pancreas compared with control cells. Patients with ovarian cancer with overexpression of actinin-4 show similar results, including a worse outcome than patients without overexpression [26].

Interestingly, Angrwal et al. recently showed that actinin-4 interacts with murine double minute 2 homolog (MDM2) binding protein (MTBP) [27, 28]. MDM2 is a major negative regulator of the tumor suppressor, p53, but also has p53-independent roles in tumorigenesis [29]. Iwakuma et al. reported that MTBP suppresses tumor metastasis and revealed an endogenous protein–protein interaction between actinin-4 and MTBP [28]. They showed that constitutive overexpression of actinin-4 in two different osteosarcoma cell lines, SaO2-LM7 (p53 null) and U2OS (p53 wild-type), increases the migration potential in both cell lines as expected. However, concomitant overexpression of MTBP significantly decreases the potential for cell migration that is mediated by overexpression of actinin-4 in both cell lines [27, 28]. Thus, MTBP inhibits cell migration that is mediated by overexpression of actinin-4 independent of p53.

In addition, actinin-4 is overexpressed in colorectal cancer [22, 23], pancreatic cancer [24, 25], ovarian cancer [26], osteosarcoma [27, 28], lung cancer [30–33], oral squamous cell carcinoma [34], salivary gland carcinoma [35], bladder cancer, breast cancer [36, 37], and esophageal cancer [38]. Reports describing overexpression of actinin-4 in association with metastasis and malignant phenotypes in cancers are summarized in Table 1. The biological function and binding partners of actinin-4 that are associated with cell invasion are shown in Fig. 2.

Amplification of *ACTN4* in cancer and clinical utility as a biomarker for decisions regarding the therapeutic strategy

Although overexpression of actinin-4 protein has been reported in several types of cancers, the cause of overexpression is not clearly understood. If overexpression is due to a genetic alteration in *ACTN4*, an oncogene may be actively associated with cancer invasion and metastasis. *ACTN4* is located on chromosome 19q13, and amplification of the 19q13.1 locus has been reported frequently in several cancers including pancreatic and ovarian cancers [39–47]. We used specific fluorescence in situ hybridization (FISH) of *ACTN4* to investigate *ACTN4* amplifications in patients with pancreatic cancer [24]. *ACTN4* amplifications occurred in 38% of patients with invasive ductal adenocarcinoma of the pancreas with protein overexpression of actinin-4 [24]. Patients with ovarian cancer and *ACTN4* amplification have been observed, and patients with stage III and IV disease with gene amplification show significantly worse overall survival than patients without gene amplification [48]. The status of gene amplification may more accurately predict the outcome of patients with stage III and IV ovarian cancer than immunohistochemical analysis with the anti-actinin-4 antibody. In addition, positive statistical significance between *ACTN4* amplification and the efficacy of post-operative chemotherapy was seen in patients with stage III and IV ovarian cancer [48, 49].

The clinical benefits of *ACTN4* amplification as a prognostic factor are also observed in stage I adenocarcinoma of the lung and salivary gland carcinoma, and *ACTN4* amplification is a stricter prognostic biomarker

Table 1 Representative reports describing the importance of actinin-4 in malignant tumors

Type of malignant tumor	Observations
Brain tumors	1. Correlation between histological grade and protein expression of actinin-4 in gliomas [81] 2. Association of actinin-4 with cell migration in gliomas [82] 3. Overexpression of actinin-4 in high-grade astrocytomas [83]
Head and neck cancer	4. Positive correlation between *ACTN4* amplification and the histological grade of salivary gland carcinomas. The importance of *ACTN4* amplification as a prognostic biomarker in salivary gland carcinomas [35] 5. Positive correlation between invasive classification of oral squamous cell carcinoma and protein expression of actinin-4 [34] 6. Correlation between histological grade and protein expression in thyroid cancer [84]
Lung cancer	7. Utility of *ACTN4* amplification as a prognostic biomarker for stage I adenocarcinoma of the lung [50] 8. Overexpression of actinin-4 mRNA in NSCLC [31] 9. Identification of a splice variant of actinin-4 in SCLC as a cancer testis antigen [30]. Utility of a splice variant of actinin-4 in the lung as a prognostic biomarker for high-grade malignant neuroendocrine tumors [33] 10. Expression of actinin-4 in blood samples of patients with NSCLC and utility as a diagnostic biomarker for NSCLC [85]
Breast cancer	11. Identification of actinin-4 as a novel actin-bundling protein, and utility of actinin-4 as a prognostic biomarker for invasive ductal breast cancer [13] 12. Summary of actinin-4 as a translational coactivator in breast cancer [15, 65] 13. Identification of protein–protein interactions between estrogen receptors and actinin-4 [70]
Esophageal cancer	14. Overexpression of actinin-4 according to clinical stage in esophageal cancer [74]
Pancreatic cancer	15. First evidence of *ACTN4* amplification in cancer. Identification of actinin-4 overexpression in patients with invasive ductal adenocarcinoma of the pancreas with poor prognosis [24] 16. Clinical utility of *ACTN4* amplification as a predictive biomarker for chemoradiotherapy in LAPC [57] 17. Association of actinin-4 with invadopodia in pancreatic cancer [25]
Colorectal cancer	18. Identification of overexpression of actinin-4 in areas of EMT in colorectal cancer [22] 19. Involvement of actinin-4 in the formation of cellular protrusions that are associated with invasion and migration [23]
Ovarian cancer	20. Identification of actinin-4 overexpression in ovarian cancer, and correlation between actinin-4 overexpression and overall survival in patients with ovarian cancer [26] 21. Utility of *ACTN4* amplification as a prognostic biomarker in ovarian cancer [48] 22. Accumulation of *ACTN4* amplification in high-grade clear cell carcinoma of ovarian cancer [49] 23. Identification of *ACTN4* amplification in fallopian tube carcinomas [86]
Bladder cancer	24. Reduced invasive ability with *ACTN4* siRNA in bladder cancer cell lines [36] 25. Correlation between histological grade in bladder cancer and actinin-4 protein expression [37]
Prostate cancer	26. Protein complex that includes actinin-4 and androgen receptor in the nucleus. Actinin-4 protein expression is reduced in the nucleus of high-grade prostate cancer [80]
Melanoma	27. Association of actinin-4 with amoeboid-type invasiveness of melanoma cells [87]
Leukemia	28. Identification of the fusion gene *MLL-ACTN4* in adult CD10-negative B-cell precursor acute lymphoblastic leukemia [88, 89]
Osteosarcoma	29. Protein–protein interactions between MTBP and actinin-4 in osteosarcoma [27, 28]

than immunohistochemistry for overall survival in these patients.

Although the clinical benefit of adjuvant chemotherapy in patients with non-small cell lung cancer (NSCLC) who have undergone complete surgical resection has been observed in stage II–IIIA in some prospective clinical trials, the benefit has not been seen in stage I NSCLC [50–52]. If patients with stage I adenocarcinoma of the lung with potential metastasis can be identified with *ACTN4* amplification of surgical specimens, adjuvant chemotherapy for such patients may have a clinical benefit in terms of patient selection.

Compared to prognostic biomarkers, predictive biomarkers to select a specific treatment strategy by evaluating the metastasis ability are urgently needed. For example, local treatment such as surgery and radiotherapy could be effective in patients without distant metastases. However, local therapies are not sufficiently effective for metastatic lesions. Patients with micrometastasis, which cannot be detected with imaging, should not undergo local therapy. Treatment options for locally advanced pancreatic cancer (LAPC) include chemotherapy alone, induction chemotherapy followed by chemoradiotherapy (CRT), or definitive CRT. Numerous randomized trials have been performed to compare the survival benefit of chemotherapy alone and CRT for LAPC [53, 54]. Results have been contradictory, and the most effective treatment has not been defined for patients with LAPC [55, 56]. Radiotherapy involving the primary site does not have sufficiently high impact for patients

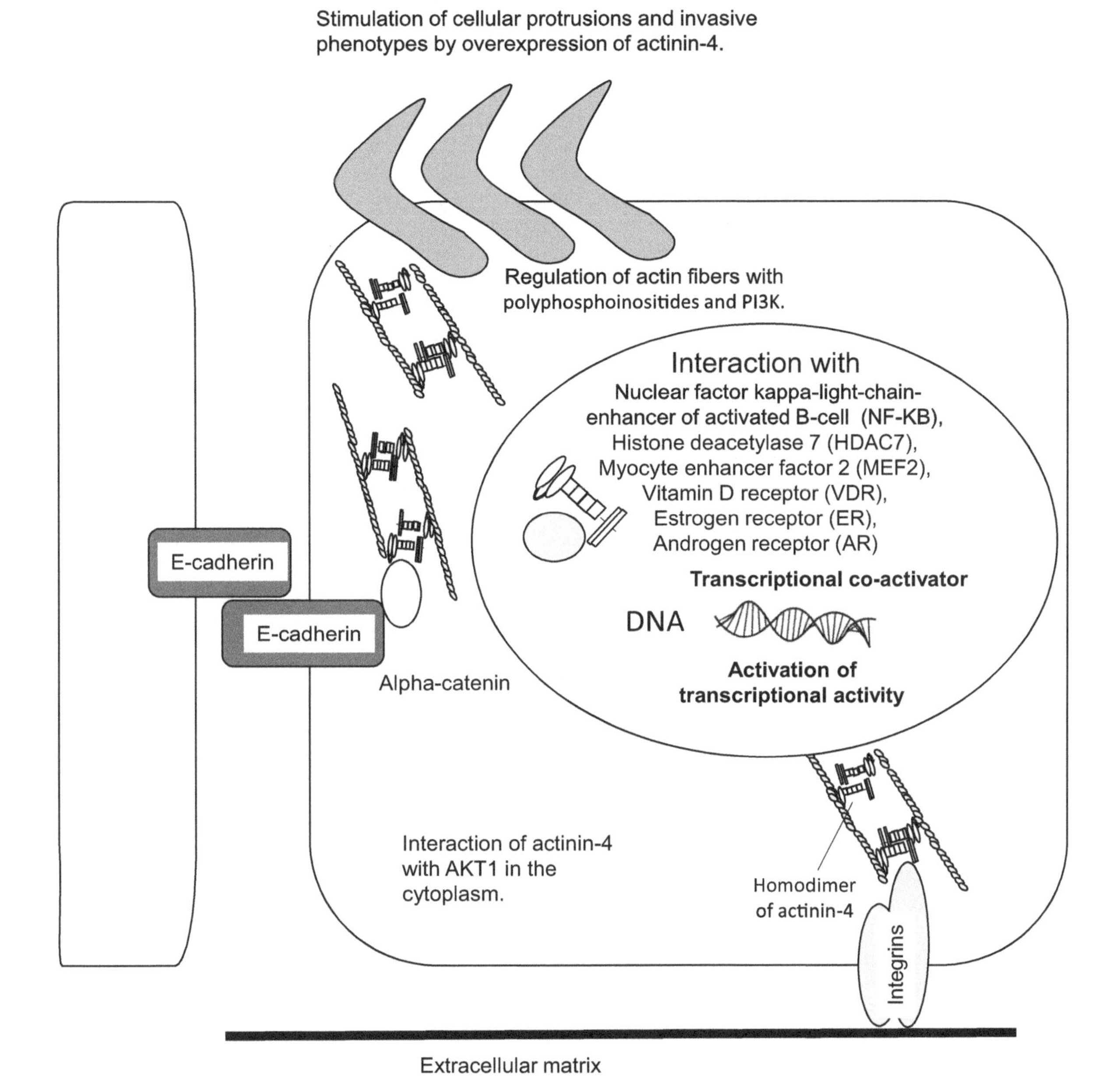

Fig. 2 Cellular distribution of protein complexes that include actinin-4. The protein complexes that include actinin-4 and some binding partners are located in the cytoplasm and nucleus, and include integrins [14], alpha catenins [14], polyphosphoinositides [76], phosphoinositide 3-kinase (PI3K) [77], v-akt murine thymoma viral oncogene homolog 1 (AKT1) [78], nuclear factor kappa-light-chain-enhancer of activated B-cell (NF-κB) [75], histone deacetylase 7 (HDAC7) [65, 70], myocyte enhancer factor 2 (MEF2) [65, 79], vitamin D receptor (VDR) [15, 70], estrogen receptor (ER) [79], and androgen receptor [80] (AR).

with occult distant metastasis, because radiotherapy does not treat distant metastatic lesions. However, imaging technology to accurately detect extremely small micrometastatic lesions has not been developed. Therefore, identification of biomarkers that can accurately evaluate the metastatic potential of biopsy samples from patients with LAPC will be very important for deciding the best personalized therapeutic strategy.

We used biopsy specimens and FISH analysis to retrospectively investigate the *ACTN4* copy number in patients with LAPC who underwent chemotherapy or CRT [57]. In such patients who underwent CRT, those with a normal *ACTN4* copy number showed a better prognosis for overall survival than patients with an increased *ACTN4* copy number. However, in patients who underwent chemotherapy, no statistically significant difference was observed between increased and normal *ACTN4* copy numbers. Thus, *ACTN4* may be a potential biomarker for metastatic ability and for predicting the effectiveness of CRT in LAPC [57].

Specific expression of an alternative splice variant of *ACTN4* in small cell lung cancer (SCLC) and mutation in focal segmental glomerular sclerosis (FSGS)

A tumor-specific alternative splice variant of *ACTN4* was found in SCLC [30]. Exon 8 of *ACTN4* is skipped in this variant, and another exon is inserted in its place (ACTN4-SpEx8), resulting in the changes N249G, A251L, and S264C in exon 8 [30]. Among normal tissues and various cancer cell lines, we observed expression of ACTN4-SpEx8 only in a SCLC cell line and normal testis. Thus, ACTN4-SpEx8 is considered a cancer testis antigen. We established a specific antibody against ACTN4-SpEx8 and observed protein expression in SCLC and large cell neuroendocrine carcinoma (LCNEC) with immunohistochemistry among pathological samples of adenocarcinoma, squamous cell carcinoma, LCNEC, carcinoid, and SCLC. Patients with SCLC and LCNEC and ACTN4-SpEx8 protein expression have a worse outcome for overall survival than patients without such expression [33]. The altered amino acids, N249G, A251L, and S264C, are very close to the mutations that are observed in familial FSGS [58, 59], which occur in exon 8 of *ACTN4* and result in the changed amino acids K255E and T259I. The three-dimensional structure of ACTN2 has been studied in detail [60], and the mutated sites are located on the surface of the separation between the CH1 and CH2 domains. For actinin to bind to actin, the three-dimensional structure of the CH1 and CH2 domains of actinin changes from a closed to an open conformation [61–63]. The substitution of amino acids in ACTN4-SpEx8 and the *ACTN4* mutation in familial FSGS may affect the conformation of these domains.

Moreover, alteration of the affinity of actinin-4 for binding to actin filaments may be an important factor in the poor prognosis of SCLC and the effacement of foot processes in the podocytes of the glomerulus in FSGS. Recently, Ehrlicher and Pollak et al. demonstrated that in FSGS, a K255E mutation in *ACTN4* changes the cellular biological properties in which increasing the affinity for actin increases cellular forces and work and decreases cellular movement. This type of mutation in this part in *ACTN4* affects actinin binding kinetics to modulate cellular dynamics and force generation, and suggests the mechanisms by which such physical defects lead to human diseases [64].

The role of actinin-4 as a transcriptional coactivator in cancer

Aberrant transcripts that fail to regulate the expression of mRNA are a cause of cancer development. Transcription of mRNA is strictly regulated in normal cells. Nuclear localization of actinin-4 is frequently observed in breast cancer [13], ovarian cancer [26], and SCLC [30] cells. However, the biological role of this nuclear localization is not clear, although a novel function other than cancer invasion is likely.

Early observation of actinin-4 as a transcriptional coactivator began with a report of protein–protein interactions among actinin-4, class II histone deacetylases, and myocyte enhancer factor 2s (MEF2s). A protein complex containing these three proteins increases the transcriptional activity of MEF2s. Chakraborty and Kao's group provided the first evidence that actinin-4 plays a role as a transcriptional coactivator [65]. Moreover, they reported the important roles of actinin-4 in breast cancer cell nuclei. Nuclear hormone receptors including the vitamin D receptor and steroid hormone receptors such as the estrogen receptor (ER) are ligand-activated transcription factors that control homeostasis, cell differentiation, proliferation, and development [66–68]. In particular, the ER plays a very important role in the development of breast cancer, and Tamoxifen, a competitive inhibitor of ERs, is used as a molecular targeted drug in ER-positive patients [69]. Recently, Kao's group also reported that estradiol (E2) promotes recruitment of actinin-4 to the promoter of *pS2*, an ER target gene in the ER-positive breast cancer cell line, MCF7 [70, 71]. The fact that actinin-4 regulates ER-alpha-mediated transcriptional activation suggests that actinin-4 may play a role in E2-mediated regulation of breast cancer cell proliferation. In fact, decreased actinin-4 protein expression due to siRNA in MCF7 cells significantly reduces E2-mediated induction of ER-alpha target genes and abolishes estrogen-mediated proliferation of cancer cells [70]. In addition, actinin-4 and ER interact [71], suggesting that actinin-4 functions as a transcriptional co-activator with ER-alpha in some subtypes of breast cancer [15].

Nuclear factor-kappa B (NF-κB) is a transcription factor that regulates cell proliferation, the immune response, cell differentiation, and apoptosis by controlling the expression of mRNA for genes encoding inflammatory cytokines, chemokines, and adhesion molecules [72, 73]. Babakov et al. reported that actinin-4 and NF-κB change their cellular localization from the cytoplasm to the nucleus when actin fibers are disrupted by cytochalasin D. The interaction between actinin-4 and NF-κB was demonstrated with immunoprecipitation following epidermal growth factor or tumor necrosis factor-alpha

(TNF-alpha) stimulation [74]. Zaho et al. also clearly demonstrated that actinin-4 expression is essential for the transcriptional activity of NF-κB in the presence of TNF-alpha [75]. The NF-κB and TNF-alpha pathway is important for cancer development, during which actinin-4 may play an important role in regulating transcription events through the NF-κB pathway. The biological functions of actinin-4 as a transcriptional co-activator are summarized in Fig. 2.

Although the nuclear localization of actinin-4 was reported in breast cancer, ovarian cancer, prostate cancer, and SCLC, a correlation between the localization of actinin-4 and clinical findings of patients with cancer is not clearly understood. The biological mechanisms of the translocation of actinin-4 to the nucleus from the cytoplasm should be clarified for innovative drug development for actinin-4.

Conclusion and future perspective

Here we described the biological roles of actinin-4, which is closely associated with cancer invasion and cell motility. Overexpression of actinin-4 protein and *ACTN4* amplification are biomarkers for evaluating the potential metastatic ability in an individual patient with cancer, and actinin-4 expression may be useful for selecting the optimal therapy for patients. In particular, predicting late metastasis after surgery is an important clinical issue. To utilize actinin-4 as a biomarker in the clinical setting, prospective clinical trials should be done.

Recent studies of actinin-4 demonstrated not only a role in cancer invasion, but also its biological role as a transcriptional co-activator. Actinin-4 is aggressively involved in the tumorigenesis of breast cancer, and this concept is attracting a lot of attention. The localization of actinin-4 in the nucleus is very interesting in terms of tumorigenesis.

Targeted therapy for actinin-4 has not been developed. Recently, the three-dimensional structure of actinin-2 has been reported [60]. Using this information, we hope that a drug for molecular targeted therapy for actinin-4 will be developed. Although these proteins have distinct physiological and cellular functions, actinin-2 and actinin-4 share 80% similarity in amino acid sequence. Basic studies of the biology of actinin-4 have the potential to overcome human diseases.

Abbreviations

ABD: actin-binding domain; ACTNs: alpha-actinins; CaM: calmodulin; CH: calponin homology; CRT: chemoradiotherapy; EMT: epithelial to mesenchymal transition; ER: estrogen receptor; FISH: fluorescence in situ hybridization; FSGS: focal segmental glomerular sclerosis; LCNEC: large cell neuroendocrine carcinoma; LAPC: locally advanced pancreatic cancer; MDM2: murine double minute 2 homolog; MTBP: murine double minute binding protein; MEF2: myocyte enhancer factor 2; NSCLC: non-small cell lung cancer; NF-κB: nuclear factor-kappa B; SCLC: small cell lung cancer; ACTN4-SpEx8: splice variant of ACTN4; TNF-alpha: tumor necrosis factor-alpha.

Author details

[1] Department of Chemotherapy and Clinical Research, National Cancer Center Research Institute, 5-1-1 Tsukiji Chuoku, Tokyo 104-0045, Japan. [2] AMED-CREST AMED, Japan Agency for Medical Research and Development, 1-7-1 Otemachi, Chiyoda, Tokyo 100-0004, Japan.

Acknowledgements

This work was supported by an Applied Research for Innovative Treatment of Cancer Grant from the Ministry of Health, Labor and Welfare of Japan [to KH]; Japan Agency for Medical Research and Development (AMED) Practical Research for Innovation Cancer Control (15ck0106101h0002, to K. H.); P-direct [to KH]; AMED-CREST AMED, [to KH]; a Grant-in Aid for Scientific Research (B), and a Challenging Exploratory Research grant from the Ministry of Education, Culture, Sports, Science and Technology (MEXT) of Japan [to KH]; and the National Cancer Center Research and Development Fund [23-A-38, 23-A-11] [to KH].

Compliance with ethical guidelines

Competing interests

The author declares that he has no competing interests.

References

1. Palmer TD, Ashby WJ, Lewis JD, Zijlstra A. Targeting tumor cell motility to prevent metastasis. Adv Drug Deliv Rev. 2011;63(8):568–81.
2. Yano T, Okamoto T, Fukuyama S, Maehara Y. Therapeutic strategy for postoperative recurrence in patients with non-small cell lung cancer. World J Clin Oncol. 2014;5(5):1048–54.
3. Fidler IJ. The pathogenesis of cancer metastasis: the 'seed and soil' hypothesis revisited. Nat Rev Cancer. 2003;3(6):453–8.
4. Kedrin D, van Rheenen J, Hernandez L, Condeelis J, Segall JE. Cell motility and cytoskeletal regulation in invasion and metastasis. J Mammary Gland Biol Neoplasia. 2007;12(2–3):143–52.
5. Yamaguchi H, Miki H, Takenawa T. Neural Wiskott-Aldrich syndrome protein is involved in hepatocyte growth factor-induced migration, invasion, and tubulogenesis of epithelial cells. Cancer Res. 2002;62(9):2503–9.
6. Parsons JT, Horwitz AR, Schwartz MA. Cell adhesion: integrating cytoskeletal dynamics and cellular tension. Nat Rev Mol Cell Biol. 2010;11(9):633–43.
7. Mattila PK, Lappalainen P. Filopodia: molecular architecture and cellular functions. Nat Rev Mol Cell Biol. 2008;9(6):446–54.
8. Paz H, Pathak N, Yang J. Invading one step at a time: the role of invadopodia in tumor metastasis. Oncogene. 2014;33(33):4193–202.
9. Machesky LM. Lamellipodia and filopodia in metastasis and invasion. FEBS Lett. 2008;582(14):2102–11.
10. Morris HT, Machesky LM. Actin cytoskeletal control during epithelial to mesenchymal transition: focus on the pancreas and intestinal tract. Br J Cancer. 2015;112(4):613–20.
11. Youssoufian H, McAfee M, Kwiatkowski DJ. Cloning and chromosomal localization of the human cytoskeletal alpha-actinin gene reveals linkage to the beta-spectrin gene. Am J Hum Genet. 1990;47(1):62–72.
12. Beggs AH, Byers TJ, Knoll JH, Boyce FM, Bruns GA, Kunkel LM. Cloning and characterization of two human skeletal muscle alpha-actinin genes located on chromosomes 1 and 11. J Biol Chem. 1992;267(13):9281–8.
13. Honda K, Yamada T, Endo R, Ino Y, Gotoh M, Tsuda H, et al. Actinin-4, a novel actin-bundling protein associated with cell motility and cancer invasion. J Cell Biol. 1998;140(6):1383–93.
14. Otey CA, Carpen O. Alpha-actinin revisited: a fresh look at an old player. Cell Motil Cytoskelet. 2004;58(2):104–11.
15. Hsu KS, Kao HY. Alpha-actinin 4 and tumorigenesis of breast cancer. Vitam Horm. 2013;93:323–51.
16. Sjoblom B, Salmazo A, Djinovic-Carugo K. Alpha-actinin structure and regulation. Cell Mol Life Sci CMLS. 2008;65(17):2688–701.
17. Lopez-Novoa JM, Nieto MA. Inflammation and EMT: an alliance towards organ fibrosis and cancer progression. EMBO Mol Med. 2009;1(6–7):303–14.

18. Ono M, Sakamoto M, Ino Y, Moriya Y, Sugihara K, Muto T, et al. Cancer cell morphology at the invasive front and expression of cell adhesion-related carbohydrate in the primary lesion of patients with colorectal carcinoma with liver metastasis. Cancer. 1996;78(6):1179–86.
19. Hirohashi S. Inactivation of the E-cadherin-mediated cell adhesion system in human cancers. Am J Pathol. 1998;153(2):333–9.
20. Hirohashi S, Kanai Y. Cell adhesion system and human cancer morphogenesis. Cancer Sci. 2003;94(7):575–81.
21. Ino Y, Gotoh M, Sakamoto M, Tsukagoshi K, Hirohashi S. Dysadherin, a cancer-associated cell membrane glycoprotein, down-regulates E-cadherin and promotes metastasis. Proc Natl Acad Sci USA. 2002;99(1):365–70.
22. Honda K, Yamada T, Hayashida Y, Idogawa M, Sato S, Hasegawa F, et al. Actinin-4 increases cell motility and promotes lymph node metastasis of colorectal cancer. Gastroenterology. 2005;128(1):51–62.
23. Hayashida Y, Honda K, Idogawa M, Ino Y, Ono M, Tsuchida A, et al. E-cadherin regulates the association between beta-catenin and actinin-4. Cancer Res. 2005;65(19):8836–45.
24. Kikuchi S, Honda K, Tsuda H, Hiraoka N, Imoto I, Kosuge T, et al. Expression and gene amplification of actinin-4 in invasive ductal carcinoma of the pancreas. Clin Cancer Res Off J Am Assoc Cancer Res. 2008;14(17):5348–56.
25. Welsch T, Keleg S, Bergmann F, Bauer S, Hinz U, Schmidt J. Actinin-4 expression in primary and metastasized pancreatic ductal adenocarcinoma. Pancreas. 2009;38(8):968–76.
26. Yamamoto S, Tsuda H, Honda K, Kita T, Takano M, Tamai S, et al. Actinin-4 expression in ovarian cancer: a novel prognostic indicator independent of clinical stage and histological type. Mod Pathol Off J US Can Acad Pathol Inc. 2007;20(12):1278–85.
27. Agarwal N, Adhikari AS, Iyer SV, Hekmatdoost K, Welch DR, Iwakuma T. MTBP suppresses cell migration and filopodia formation by inhibiting ACTN4. Oncogene. 2013;32(4):462–70.
28. Iwakuma T, Agarwal N. MDM2 binding protein, a novel metastasis suppressor. Cancer Metastasis Rev. 2012;31(3–4):633–40.
29. Iwakuma T, Lozano G. MDM2, an introduction. Mol Cancer Res MCR. 2003;1(14):993–1000.
30. Honda K, Yamada T, Seike M, Hayashida Y, Idogawa M, Kondo T, et al. Alternative splice variant of actinin-4 in small cell lung cancer. Oncogene. 2004;23(30):5257–62.
31. Yamagata N, Shyr Y, Yanagisawa K, Edgerton M, Dang TP, Gonzalez A, et al. A training-testing approach to the molecular classification of resected non-small cell lung cancer. Clin Cancer Res Off J Am Assoc Cancer Res. 2003;9(13):4695–704.
32. Noro R, Honda K, Tsuta K, Ishii G, Maeshima AM, Miura N, et al. Distinct outcome of stage I lung adenocarcinoma with ACTN4 cell motility gene amplification. Ann Oncol Off J Eur Soc Med Oncol ESMO. 2013;24(10):2594–600.
33. Miyanaga A, Honda K, Tsuta K, Masuda M, Yamaguchi U, Fujii G, et al. Diagnostic and prognostic significance of the alternatively spliced ACTN4 variant in high-grade neuroendocrine pulmonary tumours. Ann Oncol Off J Eur Soc Med Oncol ESMO. 2013;24(1):84–90.
34. Yamada S, Yanamoto S, Yoshida H, Yoshitomi I, Kawasaki G, Mizuno A, et al. RNAi-mediated down-regulation of alpha-actinin-4 decreases invasion potential in oral squamous cell carcinoma. Int J Oral Maxillofac Surg. 2010;39(1):61–7.
35. Watabe Y, Mori T, Yoshimoto S, Nomura T, Shibahara T, Yamada T, et al. Copy number increase of ACTN4 is a prognostic indicator in salivary gland carcinoma. Cancer Med. 2014;3(3):613–22.
36. Koizumi T, Nakatsuji H, Fukawa T, Avirmed S, Fukumori T, Takahashi M, et al. The role of actinin-4 in bladder cancer invasion. Urology. 2010;75(2):357–64.
37. Yoshii H, Ito K, Asano T, Horiguchi A, Hayakawa M, Asano T. Increased expression of alpha-actinin-4 is associated with unfavorable pathological features and invasiveness of bladder cancer. Oncol Rep. 2013;30(3):1073–80.
38. Fu L, Qin YR, Xie D, Chow HY, Ngai SM, Kwong DL, et al. Identification of alpha-actinin 4 and 67 kDa laminin receptor as stage-specific markers in esophageal cancer via proteomic approaches. Cancer. 2007;110(12):2672–81.
39. Bellacosa A, de Feo D, Godwin AK, Bell DW, Cheng JQ, Altomare DA, et al. Molecular alterations of the AKT2 oncogene in ovarian and breast carcinomas. Int J Cancer. 1995;64(4):280–5.
40. Cheng JQ, Godwin AK, Bellacosa A, Taguchi T, Franke TF, Hamilton TC, et al. AKT2, a putative oncogene encoding a member of a subfamily of protein-serine/threonine kinases, is amplified in human ovarian carcinomas. Proc Natl Acad Sci USA. 1992;89(19):9267–71.
41. Kallioniemi A, Kallioniemi OP, Piper J, Tanner M, Stokke T, Chen L, et al. Detection and mapping of amplified DNA sequences in breast cancer by comparative genomic hybridization. Proc Natl Acad Sci USA. 1994;91(6):2156–60.
42. Kim TM, Yim SH, Lee JS, Kwon MS, Ryu JW, Kang HM, et al. Genome-wide screening of genomic alterations and their clinicopathologic implications in non-small cell lung cancers. Clin Cancer Res Off J Am Assoc Cancer Res. 2005;11(23):8235–42.
43. Rao PH, Arias-Pulido H, Lu XY, Harris CP, Vargas H, Zhang FF, et al. Chromosomal amplifications, 3q gain and deletions of 2q33-q37 are the frequent genetic changes in cervical carcinoma. BMC Cancer. 2004;4:5.
44. Ried T, Petersen I, Holtgreve-Grez H, Speicher MR, Schrock E, du Manoir S, et al. Mapping of multiple DNA gains and losses in primary small cell lung carcinomas by comparative genomic hybridization. Cancer Res. 1994;54(7):1801–6.
45. Staal SP. Molecular cloning of the akt oncogene and its human homologues AKT1 and AKT2: amplification of AKT1 in a primary human gastric adenocarcinoma. Proc Natl Acad Sci USA. 1987;84(14):5034–7.
46. Tang TC, Sham JS, Xie D, Fang Y, Huo KK, Wu QL, et al. Identification of a candidate oncogene SEI-1 within a minimal amplified region at 19q13.1 in ovarian cancer cell lines. Cancer Res. 2002;62(24):7157–61.
47. Thompson FH, Nelson MA, Trent JM, Guan XY, Liu Y, Yang JM, et al. Amplification of 19q13.1-q13.2 sequences in ovarian cancer. G-band, FISH, and molecular studies. Cancer Genet Cytogenet. 1996;87(1):55–62.
48. Yamamoto S, Tsuda H, Honda K, Onozato K, Takano M, Tamai S, et al. Actinin-4 gene amplification in ovarian cancer: a candidate oncogene associated with poor patient prognosis and tumor chemoresistance. Mod Pathol Off J US Can Acad Pathol Inc. 2009;22(4):499–507.
49. Yamamoto S, Tsuda H, Honda K, Takano M, Tamai S, Imoto I, et al. ACTN4 gene amplification and actinin-4 protein overexpression drive tumour development and histological progression in a high-grade subset of ovarian clear-cell adenocarcinomas. Histopathology. 2012;60(7):1073–83.
50. Strauss GM, Herndon JE 2nd, Maddaus MA, Johnstone DW, Johnson EA, Harpole DH, et al. Adjuvant paclitaxel plus carboplatin compared with observation in stage IB non-small-cell lung cancer: CALGB 9633 with the Cancer and Leukemia Group B, Radiation Therapy Oncology Group, and North Central Cancer Treatment Group Study Groups. J Clin Oncol Off J Am Soc Clin Oncol. 2008;26(31):5043–51.
51. Pisters KM, Evans WK, Azzoli CG, Kris MG, Smith CA, Desch CE, et al. Cancer Care Ontario and American Society of Clinical Oncology adjuvant chemotherapy and adjuvant radiation therapy for stages I-IIIA resectable non small-cell lung cancer guideline. J Clin Oncol Off J Am Soc Clin Oncol. 2007;25(34):5506–18.
52. Pignon JP, Tribodet H, Scagliotti GV, Douillard JY, Shepherd FA, Stephens RJ, et al. Lung adjuvant cisplatin evaluation: a pooled analysis by the LACE Collaborative Group. J Clin Oncol Off J Am Soc Clin Oncol. 2008;26(21):3552–9.
53. Chauffert B, Mornex F, Bonnetain F, Rougier P, Mariette C, Bouche O, et al. Phase III trial comparing intensive induction chemoradiotherapy (60 Gy, infusional 5-FU and intermittent cisplatin) followed by maintenance gemcitabine with gemcitabine alone for locally advanced unresectable pancreatic cancer. Definitive results of the 2000-01 FFCD/SFRO study. Ann Oncol Off J Eur Soc Med Oncol ESMO. 2008;19(9):1592–9.
54. Loehrer PJ Sr, Feng Y, Cardenes H, Wagner L, Brell JM, Cella D, et al. Gemcitabine alone versus gemcitabine plus radiotherapy in patients with locally advanced pancreatic cancer: an Eastern Cooperative Oncology Group trial. J Clin Oncol Off J Am Soc Clin Oncol. 2011;29(31):4105–12.
55. Savir G, Huber KE, Saif MW. Locally advanced pancreatic cancer. Looking beyond traditional chemotherapy and radiation. JOP J Pancreas. 2013;14(4):337–9.
56. Mian OY, Ram AN, Tuli R, Herman JM. Management options in locally advanced pancreatic cancer. Curr Oncol Rep. 2014;16(6):388.

57. Watanabe T, Ueno H, Watabe Y, Hiraoka N, Morizane C, Itami J, et al. ACTN4 copy number increase as a predictive biomarker for chemoradiotherapy of locally advanced pancreatic cancer. Br J Cancer. 2015;112(4):704–13.
58. Kaplan J, Pollak MR. Familial focal segmental glomerulosclerosis. Curr Opin Nephrol Hypertens. 2001;10(2):183–7.
59. Kaplan JM, Kim SH, North KN, Rennke H, Correia LA, Tong HQ, et al. Mutations in ACTN4, encoding alpha-actinin-4, cause familial focal segmental glomerulosclerosis. Nat Genet. 2000;24(3):251–6.
60. Ribeiro Ede A, N Pinotsis Jr, Ghisleni A, Salmazo A, Konarev PV, Kostan J, et al. The structure and regulation of human muscle alpha-actinin. Cell. 2014;159(6):1447–60.
61. Lee SH, Weins A, Hayes DB, Pollak MR, Dominguez R. Crystal structure of the actin-binding domain of alpha-actinin-4 Lys255Glu mutant implicated in focal segmental glomerulosclerosis. J Mol Biol. 2008;376(2):317–24.
62. Liu J, Taylor DW, Taylor KA. A 3-D reconstruction of smooth muscle alpha-actinin by CryoEm reveals two different conformations at the actin-binding region. J Mol Biol. 2004;338(1):115–25.
63. Galkin VE, Orlova A, Salmazo A, Djinovic-Carugo K, Egelman EH. Opening of tandem calponin homology domains regulates their affinity for F-actin. Nat Struct Mol Biol. 2010;17(5):614–6.
64. Ehrlicher AJ, Krishnan R, Guo M, Bidan CM, Weitz DA, Pollak MR. Alpha-actinin binding kinetics modulate cellular dynamics and force generation. In: Proceedings of the National Academy of Sciences of the United States of America. 2015 Apr 27. pii: 201505652. [Epub ahead of print].
65. Chakraborty S, Reineke EL, Lam M, Li X, Liu Y, Gao C, et al. Alpha-actinin 4 potentiates myocyte enhancer factor-2 transcription activity by antagonizing histone deacetylase 7. J Biol Chem. 2006;281(46):35070–80.
66. Mangelsdorf DJ, Evans RM. The RXR heterodimers and orphan receptors. Cell. 1995;83(6):841–50.
67. Mangelsdorf DJ, Thummel C, Beato M, Herrlich P, Schutz G, Umesono K, et al. The nuclear receptor superfamily: the second decade. Cell. 1995;83(6):835–9.
68. Francis GA, Fayard E, Picard F, Auwerx J. Nuclear receptors and the control of metabolism. Annu Rev Physiol. 2003;65:261–311.
69. Jordan VC, Brodie AM. Development and evolution of therapies targeted to the estrogen receptor for the treatment and prevention of breast cancer. Steroids. 2007;72(1):7–25.
70. Khurana S, Chakraborty S, Cheng X, Su YT, Kao HY. The actin-binding protein, actinin alpha 4 (ACTN4), is a nuclear receptor coactivator that promotes proliferation of MCF-7 breast cancer cells. J Biol Chem. 2011;286(3):1850–9.
71. Khurana S, Chakraborty S, Zhao X, Liu Y, Guan D, Lam M, et al. Identification of a novel LXXLL motif in alpha-actinin 4-spliced isoform that is critical for its interaction with estrogen receptor alpha and co-activators. J Biol Chem. 2012;287(42):35418–29.
72. DiDonato JA, Mercurio F, Karin M. NF-kappaB and the link between inflammation and cancer. Immunol Rev. 2012;246(1):379–400.
73. Tornatore L, Thotakura AK, Bennett J, Moretti M, Franzoso G. The nuclear factor kappa B signaling pathway: integrating metabolism with inflammation. Trends Cell Biol. 2012;22(11):557–66.
74. Babakov VN, Petukhova OA, Turoverova LV, Kropacheva IV, Tentler DG, Bolshakova AV, et al. RelA/NF-kappaB transcription factor associates with alpha-actinin-4. Exp Cell Res. 2008;314(5):1030–8.
75. Zhao X, Hsu KS, Lim JH, Bruggeman LA, Kao HY. Alpha-Actinin 4 potentiates nuclear factor kappa-light-chain-enhancer of activated B-cell (NF-kappaB) activity in podocytes independent of its cytoplasmic actin binding function. J Biol Chem. 2015;290(1):338–49.
76. Fukami K, Sawada N, Endo T, Takenawa T. Identification of a phosphatidylinositol 4,5-bisphosphate-binding site in chicken skeletal muscle alpha-actinin. J Biol Chem. 1996;271(5):2646–50.
77. Shibasaki F, Fukami K, Fukui Y, Takenawa T. Phosphatidylinositol 3-kinase binds to alpha-actinin through the p85 subunit. Biochem J. 1994;302(Pt 2):551–7.
78. Ding Z, Liang J, Lu Y, Yu Q, Songyang Z, Lin SY, et al. A retrovirus-based protein complementation assay screen reveals functional AKT1-binding partners. Proc Natl Acad Sci USA. 2006;103(41):15014–9.
79. Khurana S, Chakraborty S, Lam M, Liu Y, Su YT, Zhao X, et al. Familial focal segmental glomerulosclerosis (FSGS)-linked alpha-actinin 4 (ACTN4) protein mutants lose ability to activate transcription by nuclear hormone receptors. J Biol Chem. 2012;287(15):12027–35.
80. Jasavala R, Martinez H, Thumar J, Andaya A, Gingras AC, Eng JK, et al. Identification of putative androgen receptor interaction protein modules: cytoskeleton and endosomes modulate androgen receptor signaling in prostate cancer cells. Mol Cell Proteomics : MCP. 2007;6(2):252–71.
81. Fukushima S, Yoshida A, Honda K, Maeshima AM, Narita Y, Yamada T, et al. Immunohistochemical actinin-4 expression in infiltrating gliomas: association with WHO grade and differentiation. Brain Tumor Pathol. 2014;31(1):11–6.
82. Henry WI, Dubois J, Quick QA. The microtubule inhibiting agent epothilone B antagonizes glioma cell motility associated with reorganization of the actin-binding protein alpha-actinin 4. Oncol Rep. 2011;25(3):887–93.
83. Quick Q, Skalli O. Alpha-actinin 1 and alpha-actinin 4: contrasting roles in the survival, motility, and RhoA signaling of astrocytoma cells. Exp Cell Res. 2010;316(7):1137–47.
84. Tanaka N, Yamashita T, Yamamoto S, Matsunobu T, Tsuda H, Honda K, et al. Histological growth pattern of and alpha-actinin-4 expression in thyroid cancer. Anticancer Res. 2014;34(6):3157–63.
85. Wang MC, Chang YH, Wu CC, Tyan YC, Chang HC, Goan YG, et al. Alpha-actinin 4 is associated with cancer cell motility and is a potential biomarker in non-small cell lung cancer. J Thorac Oncol Off Publ Int Assoc Study Lung Cancer. 2015;10(2):286–301.
86. Nowee ME, Snijders AM, Rockx DA, de Wit RM, Kosma VM, Hamalainen K, et al. DNA profiling of primary serous ovarian and fallopian tube carcinomas with array comparative genomic hybridization and multiplex ligation-dependent probe amplification. J Pathol. 2007;213(1):46–55.
87. Shao H, Li S, Watkins SC, Wells A. Alpha-Actinin-4 is required for amoeboid-type invasiveness of melanoma cells. J Biol Chem. 2014;289(47):32717–28.
88. Burmeister T, Meyer C, Schwartz S, Hofmann J, Molkentin M, Kowarz E, et al. The MLL recombinome of adult CD10-negative B-cell precursor acute lymphoblastic leukemia: results from the GMALL study group. Blood. 2009;113(17):4011–5.
89. Yang JJ, Park TS, Lee ST, Seo JY, Oh SH, Cho EH, et al. Molecular characterization and clinical course of MLL-ACTN4 rearrangement in therapy-related hematologic malignancies. Haematologica. 2014;99(4):e49–51.

12

A review on hepatocyte nuclear factor-1beta and tumor

Dan-Dan Yu[†], Shi-Wei Guo[†], Ying-Ying Jing[†], Yu-Long Dong and Li-Xin Wei[*]

Abstract

Hepatocyte nuclear factor-1beta (HNF1β) was initially identified as a liver-specific transcription factor. It is a homeobox transcription factor that functions as a homodimer or heterodimer with HNF1α. HNF1β plays an important role in organogenesis during embryonic stage, especially of the liver, kidney, and pancreas. Mutations in the HNF1β gene cause maturity-onset diabetes of the young type 5 (MODY5), renal cysts, genital malformations, and pancreas atrophy. Recently, it has been shown that the expression of HNF1β is associated with cancer risk in several tumors, including hepatocellular carcinoma, pancreatic carcinoma, renal cancer, ovarian cancer, endometrial cancer, and prostate cancer. HNF1β also regulates the expression of genes associated with stem/progenitor cells, which indicates that HNF1β may play an important role in stem cell regulation. In this review, we discuss some of the current developments about HNF1β and tumor, the relationship between HNF1β and stem/progenitor cells, and the potential pathogenesis of HNF1β in various tumors.

Keywords: Hepatocyte nuclear factor-1beta (HNF1β), Cancer, Stem/progenitor cells, Pathogenesis

Background

Hepatocyte nuclear factors (HNFs) are a group of transcription factors that play important roles in regulating transcription of the liver specific genes. HNFs are expressed predominately in the liver and form a complicated network regulating liver development and hepatocyte differentiation. However, these transcription factors are not restricted to hepatocytes, they are also expressed in many other tissues. Nevertheless, the liver is the only tissue in which a significant number of different HNFs are expressed at the same time [1]. Four major families of HNFs have been described. HNF1α and HNF1β, members of the HNF1 family contain a POU-homeodomain and bind to DNA as homodimers [2]. The HNF3 proteins (HNF3α, β and γ) belong to the forkhead transcription factors and contain a 110 amino acid DNA binding domain [3]. HNF4 is a member of the nuclear hormone receptor family and binds DNA as a homodimer [4]. There are two isoforms of HNF4, HNF4α and HNF4γ, encoded by two separate genes HNF4A and HNF4G in humans [1]. HNF6 contains a bipartite onecut-homeodomain sequence and binds to specific DNA sequences of numerous target gene promoters [5]. Among these HNFs, HNF1β is one of the most important during development and tumorigenesis. In this review, we will focus on HNF1β, which regulates the expression of genes that are expressed in the liver, kidney, and pancreas, and has been identified to cause various human diseases.

The HNF1β gene (TCF2) is located on chromosome 17q12 [6]. The first description of HNF1β mutations associated with disease was in 1997. In humans, heterozygous germline mutations in HNF1β cause maturity-onset diabetes of the young, subtype 5 (MODY5), which is associated with congenital abnormalities, including polycystic kidneys, an abnormal genital tract, and severe pancreatic hypoplasia [7]. HNF1β, also called variant HNF1 (vHNF1) or LFB3, is a homeodomain protein that plays an essential role in the liver-specific expression of many genes during differentiation and development [8]. HNF1β binds to DNA as a homodimer or heterodimer with the related protein HNF1α [9]. The expression ratio of HNF1β is different in each organ. At the adult stage,

*Correspondence: weilixin_smmu@163.com
†Dan-Dan Yu, Shi-Wei Guo and Ying-Ying Jing contributed equally to this work
Tumor Immunology and Gene Therapy Center, Eastern Hepatobiliary Surgery Hospital, The Second Military Medical University, 225 Changhai Road, 200438 Shanghai, China

HNF1β is strongly expressed throughout the biliary system, and in several epithelia organized in tubules, such as the pancreatic exocrine ducts and the kidney tubules [10]. Expression of HNF1β is also seen in the periportal hepatocytes, thymus, genital tract, lung and gut [9, 10]. HNF1β is involved in embryonic development and metabolism of the kidney, pancreas, liver and biliary system. Recent studies have shown that expression of HNF1β is associated with cancer risk in several tumors, and HNF1β plays an important role in tumorigenesis.

HNF1β status in various tumors

Hepatobiliary malignancies

HNF1β has been demonstrated to be associated with the risk of hepatocellular carcinoma (HCC). The HNF1 family plays a dominant role in liver-specific transcription. Hepatocyte differentiation is linked to the expression of liver-specific proteins and that the expression patterns are controlled primarily at their transcription levels. It is suggested that HNF1α and HNF1β may play distinct roles in regulating gene expression in differentiation and maturity of hepatocytes. Studies showed that cultured cells derived from differentiated hepatoma cells express HNF1α, whereas cultured dedifferentiated hepatoma cells express HNF1β instead of HNF1α. Analysis of the expression of HNF1α and HNF1β mRNA HCC tissues by RT-PCR assay showed that the ratio of HNF1α/HNF1β mRNA is closely linked to histological differentiation of HCC [11]. The ratio of HNF1α/HNF1β mRNA is higher in well-differentiated cases than in poorly-differentiated and undifferentiated cases. There were more HNF1α than HNF1β transcripts in well-differentiated HCC, but fewer HNF1α than HNF1β transcripts in poorly differentiated HCC. Western blot revealed that the levels of HNF1β protein were similar in well and poorly differentiated HCC, but higher than in the surrounding non-cancerous portions [12]. HNF1β is expressed in hepatic endoderm of foregut during embryonic development and precedes HNF1α expression. In the process of hepatic development and carcinogenesis, members of the HNF1 family regulates the activity of the AFP promoter. Shim et al. examined the expression of alphafetoprotein (AFP), HNF1α, and HNF1β with immunohistochemistry in HCC tumor [13]. The results showed that expression of HNF1β was related to a serum AFP level and AFP expression. Upstream regulation of AFP expression by HNF1β at the transcriptional level may operate specifically during the course of HCC progression following recurrence. The expression of HNF1β in tumor tissue could predict recurrence and HCC-specific death after transplantation [13]. HNF1β also plays an important role in the regulatory network in mouse liver cells. When HNF1β is suppressed by siRNA, the expression level of HNF4α, HNF1α, HNF3 (HNF3α, β and γ), and HNF6 are significantly downregulated [14]. In mouse hepatoma cells, HNF1β regulated many genes. Albumin, α-fetoprotein, insulin-like growth factor binding protein 1 and HNF1 genes were downregulated by RNAi of HNF1β, while alcohol dehydrogenase 2, α1-antitrypsin, α-fibrinogen and apolipo-protein AII genes were upregulated [14]. However, the study of HNF1β and HCC is limited. Thus, further study is still needed to understand the role of HNF1β in hepatocarcinogenesis in HCC and clinical use of HNF1β expression.

HNF1β is expressed in biliary precursor cells and plays a crucial role in extrahepatic biliary development [10]. Biliary tract cancer (BTC) originates from epithelial cells of the hepatic biliary duct system and the gallbladder. Study shows expression of HNF1β is relatively low in BTC, and HNF1β is nonessential in the biliary tract cancers differentiation and maintenance [15].

Pancreatic cancer

Pancreatic carcinoma is the fourth most common cause of death among cancers. In pancreas, HNF1β is a useful marker to identify clear cell carcinomas, and its overexpression may predict worse survival. Kim et al. [16] found that HNF1β was overexpressed in clear cell carcinomas and in the clear cell components of ductal carcinomas with clear cell features. High expression of HNF1β showed worse survival regardless of morphologic subtype.

Colorectal cancer

Colorectal cancer (CRC) is the third and fourth most common cancer in females and males. Studies have indicated that the accumulation of genetic and epigenetic alterations could result in the transformation of normal colonic epithelial cells to adenocarcinomas [17]. SILVA et al. investigated the epigenetic changes (DNA methylation) in 24 candidate genes in CRC tumors, and identified five candidate hypermethylated (HM) genes as CRC biomarkers. These genes include RUNX3, PCDH10, SFRP5, IGF2 and HNF1β [17]. Thus, HNF1β may be used as a biomarker for the detection of early-stage of CRC.

Renal and urinary tract cancer

Several studies suggest a role of HNF1β in tumor formation and various kinds of renal disease. Renal cell carcinoma (RCC) accounts for more than 80 % of kidney tumors. Studies found that HNF1β expression was reduced in tumor tissue compared with normal kidney tissue. HNF1β is essential for the maintenance of well-ordered renal tissue growth, and downregulation or loss of expression is correlated with malignant transformation and dedifferentiation. HNF1β is a prognostic factor and a potential tumor suppressor, and could be a potential therapeutic target for RCC [18]. Chromophobe renal cell carcinoma (ChRCC) is a rare type of kidney cancer and accounts for 5 % of all kidney cancer. Lack of HNF1β expression plays an important role in the pathogenesis of ChRCC, and may serve as a good diagnostic maker [19]. Rebouissou et al. screened for HNF1β inactivation in 35 renal neoplasms and found biallelic HNF1β inactivation in 2 chromophobe renal carcinomas by association of a germline mutation and a somatic gene deletion. This finding suggested that germline mutations of HNF1β may predispose to renal tumors and proposed that HNF1β may functions as a tumor suppressor gene in ChRCC through a PKHD1 expression control [20]. Gad et al. studied 46 cases of ChRCC, but no mutations were identified in all coding exons of the HNF1β gene. They found that mutations in BHD and TP53 genes but not in HNF1β gene were detected in a large series of sporadic ChRCC [21]. Papillary renal cell carcinomas make up about 15 % of renal cell tumors in surgical series. The HNF1β protein is expressed only in differentiating tubules of fetal kidney and overexpressed in adult tumors of embryonal origin, such as papillary RCCs. The gain and overexpression of the HNF1β gene is associated with the delayed tubular differentiation in precursor lesions [22]. Clear cell adenocarcinoma (CCA) of the urinary tract is a rare tumor that is histologically similar to CCA of the female genital tract [23]. Brimo et al. reported that HNF1β was a useful marker in differentiating clear cell adenocarcinomas of the bladder/urethra from invasive high-grade transitional/urothelial carcinoma and other types of bladder adenocarcinomas and to a lesser extent from nephrogenic adenomas [8].

Prostate cancer

Prostate cancer is one of the most common male malignancies. Recently, a large study has shown that an HNF1β sequence variant confers an increased prostate cancer risk. The first report of HNF1β associated with prostate cancer risk was in a genome-wide association study (GWAS) searching for sequence variants in 1501 Icelandic men with prostate cancer and 11,290 controls, and the variant, rs4430796, in HNF1β at chromosome 17q12 was the earliest loci to be discovered for prostate cancer [6]. It was later replicated in two GWAS in the UK and the United States [24, 25]. Then a second independent variant, rs11649743, located at chromosome 17q12 and separated by a recombination hotspot from the first variant, was subsequently found to be associated with risk [26]. A large-scale fine mapping study of a region on 17q12 associated with prostate cancer confirmed the previously established signals and found evidence that additional variants contribute to the risk of prostate cancer [27]. In this study, the best model for prostate cancer risk in the HNF1β region included five SNPs, rs4430796, rs7405696, rs4794758, rs1016990 and rs3094509, and these SNPs together capture more of the risk associated with this region. Zhang et al. explored the loci associated with prostate risk in a Northern Chinese population and indicated that AG on HNF1β (rs4430796, A) could be associated with PSA increase [28]. Hu et al. identified 12 prostate cancer risk genes potentially connected and related to HNF1β. Six of them, BAG1, ERBB4, ESR1, HSPD1, NR4A1, and PIK3CG, were found to participate in the KEGG pathways. The results indicated that the prostate cancer risk role of HNF1β could possibly be associated with modulating the relationships between androgenic hormone and prostate cancer [29].

Ovarian and endometrial cancer

HNF1β was identified from large-scale gene expression studies as being a useful marker of ovarian and uterine clear cell carcinomas. Clear cell carcinoma (CCC) of the ovary has the worst prognosis of all of the epithelial ovarian cancers. A study has demonstrated that the expression of HNF1β is significantly upregulated in ovarian CCC cell lines, while non-CCC ovarian cancer cell lines rarely express this protein, also, reduction of HNF1β induced apoptotic cell death in ovarian CCC cell lines [30]. HNF1β would be not only an excellent CCC-specific molecular marker but also a molecular target for the therapy of ovarian CCC. Yamamoto et al. found that the incidence of HNF1β immunoreactivity differed significantly between CCCs and other histology in both the ovary and the endometrium, which suggested that HNF1β would be an excellent marker for distinguishing CCCs from other lesions in both the ovary and the endometrium [31]. It was demonstrated by Kao et al. that the overexpression of HNF1β is specific for ovarian CCC among ovarian carcinomas [32]. The HNF1β gene plays an important role in the biology of ovarian CCC. Knockdown of HNF1β in ovarian CCC cells resulted in a significant increase in proliferation, while overexpression of HNF1β in the serous ovarian cancer cell line caused cell growth to be significantly decreased [33]. Downregulation of HNF1β could contribute to drug resistance in ovarian cancer and that HNF1β may perform its drug resistance-related functions through four pathways including ErbB signaling, focal adhesion, apoptosis and p53 signaling [34]. Terasawa et al. observed for the first time that HNF1β gene is a target for epigenetic inactivation in ovarian cancer. HNF1β was methylated in 53 % of ovarian cancer cell lines and in 26 % of primary ovarian cancers (especially in the non-clear cell types), resulting in loss of the gene's expression. Restoration of HNF1β expression induced expression of HNF4α, a transcriptional target of HNF1β, indicating that epigenetic silencing of HNF1β leads to alteration of the hepatocyte nuclear factor network in tumours [35]. Shen et al. found a differential effect of HNF1β on the serous and clear cell subtypes of ovarian cancer, a loss-of-function role in serous and a gain-of function role in clear cell ovarian cancers, and variants in this gene differentially affect genetic susceptibility to these subtypes [36].

Endometrial cancer is the most common gynecological cancer in developed countries. A genome-wide association study identified single nucleotide polymorphisms in HNF1β associated with endometrial cancer risk in women of European background [37]. SNP rs4430796 was identified as an endometrial cancer susceptibility locus close to HNF1β on chromosome 17q. Setiawan et al. provided additional evidence that HNF1β is involved in endometrial cancer etiology [38]. The HNF1β SNPs (rs4430796 and rs7501939) were associated with endometrial cancer risk in two independent studies and that the associations were observed across multiple racial/ethnic groups [38]. A recent genome-wide association study replicated previously identified associations with genetic markers near the HNF1β locus in a multiethnic population from nine studies, but no novel variants reached genome-wide significance [39]. In endometrial cancer, different from ovarian clear cell carcinoma, HNF1β should be used with caution as a diagnostic marker because of its lack of specificity [40].

The potential pathogenic mechanisms of HNF1β in cancer

Epigenetic processes and epigenetic changes

The aberrant expression of HNF1β in tumors is associated with epigenetic processes and epigenetic changes. In humans, one of the epigenetic mechanisms that regulate expression of genes is methylation of the clusters of CpG dinucleotides, called CpG islands. A probable mechanism of aberrant up-regulation of HNF1β in ovarian clear cell carcinoma is hypomethylation of the HNF1β CpG island [35]. Terasawa et al. reported that methylation of the HNF1β CpG island was rare in ovarian CCC, but common in non-CCC ovarian cancers or various cancer cell lines [35]. Hypomethylation of the HNF1β CpG island probably participates in the up-regulation of HNF1β in ovarian CCC. Epigenetic inactivation of HNF1β is also seen in colorectal, gastric, and pancreatic cancer cell lines, suggesting involvement of epigenetic inactivation of HNF1β in tumorigenesis [41]. HNF1β mutations are known to affect expression of downstream genes such as HNF4α, PKHD1 and UMOD [20]. HNF4α is upregulated by inducing HNF1β expression, which suggests alterations in the hepatocyte nuclear factor network can be reversed by inducing HNF1β through demethylation of the gene [35]. Another potential contributors to the HNF1β overexpression are histone acetylation and gene amplification. Methylation was associated with histone deacetylation, and when treating cells with histone deacetylase inhibitor combined with methyltransferase inhibitor, HNF1β expression was synergistically induced [35]. Studies showed that homeobox genes, such as the TLX1, HOXB13, and HNF1B genes methylation play a critical role in the insurgence and/or progression of breast cancer [42]. In Sporadic colorectal cancer (CRC), hypermethylated gene HNF1β was identified, which may be a useful epigenetic marker for non-invasive CRC screening [17].

The HNF1β target genes

The pathway with which HNF1β is involved in cancer is less understood. HNF1β has been identified as one of the most highly overexpressed genes in ovarian CCC. In ovarian CCC cell lines, one of the most markedly up-regulated genes was osteopontin (OPN), which is probably a direct target gene of HNF1β, since OPN contains functional HNF1β binding sites in the promoter region [43]. It was reported that OPN expression is elevated in ovarian CCC and is closely associated with HNF1β over-expression. HNF1β is likely to participate in OPN up-regulation in CCC [44]. OPN has been recognized to play important roles in the process of tumorigenesis. OPN binds to several cell surface receptors and induces several signal transduction pathways, which contribute to tumorigenesis by the inhibition of apoptosis or the activation of matrix-degrading proteases [45]. The reduction of HNF1β might have caused a reduction of OPN, followed by an increase in apoptotic activity. Data showed that checkpoint kinase (Chk) 1 protein is persistently activated in the HNF1β-overexpressing CCC cells [46]. Chk1 might function in the cellular survival pathways that enhance DNA damage repair, thereby granting chemoresistance. Inhibition of Chk1 selectively abrogates the repair of damaged DNA, sensitizes cancer cells to radiotherapy, or increases cancer cell death in the presence of p53 mutations [47]. The Chk1 inhibitor might be a novel target for developing cancer therapeutics in the HNF1β positive cells [46]. Pathway enrichment analysis of 36 genes which co-occurred with HNF1β, ovarian cancer and drug resistance was performed by Li et al. [34]. Four pathways including ErbB signaling, focal adhesion, apoptosis and p53 signaling were enriched, suggesting that HNF1β may contribute to drug resistance in ovarian cancer via those pathways. HNF1β may also play a critical role in a cytoprotective effect against forthcoming oxidative stress. HNF1β may upregulate OGG1 gene expression to counteract ROS mediated mitochondrial dysfunction [48]. OGG1 also known as 8-oxoguanine glycosylase is a DNA glycosylase enzyme involved in base excision repair. Senkel et al. established a human embryonic kidney cell line (HEK293) expressing HNF1β and identified 25 HNF1β-regulated genes. Eight of the 25 genes were significantly up-regulated in ovarian CCC compared to the other ovarian cancer types. The genes SPP1, DPP4, SAH, RBPMS, CD24, NID2, LAMB1, RHOB and SOX9 are deregulated in ovary CCC due to the overexpression of HNF1β [43]. The genes dipeptidyl peptidase 4 (DPP4), and osteopontin (SPP1) are most likely direct target genes, as they contain functional HNF1 binding sites in their promoter region. DPP4 plays a major role in glucose metabolism and appears to work as a suppressor in the development of cancer [49]. RBPMS (RNA binding protein multiple splicing) may be an HNF1β target involved in kidney formation. CD24 is a cell adhesion molecule that is identified as a progenitor marker. NID2 encodes a member of basement membrane proteins that control a large number of cellular activities [50]. LAMB1 (Laminin, beta 1) is a member of noncollagenous constituent of basement members. Sox9 [sex-determining region Y (SRY)-box 9 protein] plays critical roles during embryogenesis. Sox9 is required for development, differentiation, and lineage commitment in various tissues. Studies showed that 22 of 54 genes highly up-regulated in ovarian CCC were involved in downstream targets of HNF1β. These genes include GLRX, GPx3, TST, SOD2, NNMT, ANXA4, UGT1A1, DPPIV, ACE2, Collectrin, TFPI2, MAP3K5/ASK1, Octamer4, PAX8, G6Pase, GK, GLUT2, ALDOB, OPN, and FXYD2 [51]. Genes reported to be upregulated by HNF1β include NNMT, ANXA4, UGT1A1, FXYD2, TFPI2, MAP3K5/ASK1, G6Pase, GK, GLUT2, and mTOR [51]. GLRX (Glutaredoxin), GPx3 (glutathione peroxidase 3), TST (thiosulfate sulfurtransferase), SOD2 (superoxide dismutase2), NNMT (Nicotinamide N-methyltransferase), ANXA4 (Annexin A4), and UGT1A1 (UDP-glycosyltransferase 1 family polypeptide A1) are responsible for drug metabolism and liver detoxification. DPPIV (Dipeptidyl peptidase IV), ACE2 (Angiotensin converting enzyme2), Collectrin, and TFPI2 (Tissue factor pathway inhibitor 2) are proteases involved in oxidative stress. MAP3K5/ASK1 and mTOR are related to signal transduction pathways. Octamer4 (Octamer-binding transcription factor 4) and PAX8 (Paired box gene 8) are transcription factors involved in oxidative stress. G6Pase (Glucose-6-phosphatase), GK (Glucokinase), GLUT2 (Glucose transporter type 2), and ALDOB (Aldolase B) are related to metabolism. FXYD2 (domain-containing ion transport regulator 2) is known as the gamma subunit of the Na, K-ATPase. HNF1β also regulates the expression of CD44v9, which binds several target molecules and specifically regulates cell functions, including migration, growth, survival, anti-apoptosis, immune response and redox status [52]. In human hepatoma cells, HNF4α has been suggested to be directly regulated by HNF1β [53]. The HNF1β-dependent pathway might provide new insights into regulation of glycogen synthesis, detoxification and resistance to anticancer agents.

The signaling related to stem cells

HNF1β has been described as a key regulator of biliary development and is partially regulated by Notch signaling [54]. The Notch pathway has been implicated in the regulation of self-renewal of adult stem cells and differentiation of precursors along a specific cell lineage, in normal embryonic development and organogenesis [15]. Studies showed that HNF1β expression is regulated by Notch2 [54]. Notch2 is a member of the notch family, and it is used to isolate, identify and localise pancreatic cancer stem-like cells. Studies showed that $Notch2^{+}$ cells in human pancreatic cancer Bxpc-3 and Panc-1 cells have the properties of cancer stem cells, with strong tumourigenic ability [55]. Gene expression microarray data demonstrated that Notch2 is one of the most upregulated genes in a cancer stem cell-like population [56]. Moreover, aberrant Notch2 signaling induces the formation of human liver cancers with HpSC features [57].

HNF1β and stem/progenitor cells

Genes and pathways regulating stem and progenitor cells are increasingly recognized in tumorigenesis. Tumors may often originate from the transformation of normal stem cells, since similar signalling pathways may regulate self-renewal in stem cells and cancer cells. According to the cancer stem cell (CSC) hypothesis, a few CSC with self-renewal and multipotentiality differentiation exist in tumors, and these cells can create heterogeneity in a tumor through abnormal proliferation and differentiation. In HEK293 cells and ovary CCC, HNF1β activates the CD24 gene, a cell surface protein that has recently been identified as a marker of the renal progenitor population in the uninduced metanephric mesenchyme [43]. CD24 is highly expressed in many human cancers [58], and is often used to identify and enrich CSCs in cancers such as ovarian and pancreatic cancer. High expression of CD24 is involved in tumor progression and metastasis. SOX9 was down-regulated upon HNF1β overexpression in HEK293 cells. SOX9 is overexpressed in a wide range of human cancers, particularly, in tissues where it plays critical roles in their development and in stem/progenitor cells [59]. SOX9 might contribute to carcinogenesis through effects on stem cells. The HNF1β target gene osteopontin is also shown to be expressed in progenitor cells. OPN is overexpressed by liver progenitors in humans and mice. OPN upregulation during liver injury is a conserved repair response, and influences liver progenitor cell function [60]. A high OPN expression level is associated with poor prognosis and metastasis in several cancer patients. The expression of CD44 variant forms is regulated by several molecules including OPN. CD44 interacts with osteopontin and regulates its cellular functions leading to tumor progression. HNF1β also regulates the expression of CD44v9. CD44 is a multifunctional class I transmembrane glycoprotein with a variety of functions including participation in cell adhesion and migration as well as modulation of cell–matrix interactions [61]. The majority of cancer cell lines express high levels of CD44. CD44 is one of the cell surface markers associated with cancer stem cells in several types of tumor, including breast, prostate, pancreas, ovarian, and colorectal cancers [52, 58]. Overexpression of CD44 indicated bad clinical features and poor prognosis.

In liver development, HNF1β is involved in the hepatobiliary specification of hepatoblasts to cholangiocytes, and it is strongly expressed throughout the embryonic and adult biliary epithelium. Immunostaining of patients with advanced alcoholic liver disease showed that ductular reaction cells were positive for HNF1β, whereas HNF1β was not expressed in mature hepatocytes [62]. It is demonstrate that HNF1β is expressed in liver progenitor cells (LPC), and may also play a role in the maintenance of the hepatobiliary cell phenotype. Lineage tracing demonstrated that HNF1β+ cells give rise to the expansion of cells with a LPC phenotype and to periportal hepatocytes after liver injury [62]. Yu et al. reported that the induced hepatic stem cells (iHepSCs) can be directly induced from mouse embryonic fibroblasts by overexpressing two key transcription factors, HNF1β and Foxa3 [63]. HNF1β has a critical role in the induction of iHepSCs. Pancreatic multipotent progenitor cells (MPCs) produce acinar, endocrine and duct cells during organogenesis [64]. HNF1β has been identified in these pancreatic progenitor cells before differentiation into endocrine or exocrine cells [65, 66]. Study showed that Sox9 directly bound to three genes, including HNF1β, HNF6, Foxa2, in vitro and in intact cells, and regulated their expression. In turn, both Foxa2 and HNF1β regulated Sox9 expression, demonstrating feedback circuits between these genes. Foxa2 (forkhead box protein A2), also known as HNF3β, is a member of the forkhead class of DNA-binding proteins. Foxa2 play an important role in the regulation of metabolism and in the differentiation of the pancreas and liver. HNF6 is correlated to cell proliferation, differentiation and organogenesis, hepatic metabolism [5]. HNF1β, HNF6, and Foxa2 are simultaneously expressed in several regions in the early endoderm, including the developing gut and liver, and persist in the duct cells of the adult pancreas [65]. Transient knockdown of Sox9 levels by nearly 50 % resulted in a 50 % increase in the expression of HNF1β [65]. HNF1β which is expressed before HNF6 in the endoderm, was found to be critical for HNF6 expression. HNF6 controls the initiation of the expression of pancreatic and duodenal homeobox 1 (Pdx1), the earliest marker of pancreatic precursor cells [67]. Therefore, the sequential activation of HNF1β, HNF6, and Pdx1 in the endoderm appears to control the generation of pancreatic precursors. Studies showed that Pdx1 contributed to the specification of pancreatic endocrine progenitors by participating in the Hnf6, Sox9, Hnf1β, Foxa2 transcription factor cross-regulatory network and by regulating Ngn3 directly [68]. Ngn3 (neurogenin3) plays an important role in pancreatic development and the differentiation of endocrine cells. Ngn3 is also one of the pancreatic progenitor markers. Because HNF1β is required for Ptf1a expression in the developing pancreatic bud, Ptf1a may also be downstream of HNF1β when generating pancreatic precursors in the endoderm [67]. Ptf1a (pancreas transcription factor 1a) is expressed in early bud pancreatic multipotent progenitor cells, with an instructive role in distinguishing pancreatic fate from the adjacent organs [64]. All these studies showed that HNF1β is closely related to stem/progenitor cells.

Conclusions

HNF1β plays an important role in tumorigenesis of various organs. High expression of HNF1β showed worse survival in both pancreatic carcinoma and hepatocellular carcinoma. HNF1β expression is reduced in renal cell carcinoma compared with normal kidney tissue. HNF1β may functions as a tumor suppressor gene in renal cell carcinoma. In prostate cancer, the studies of HNF1β focus mainly on the single nucleotide polymorphisms. Genome-wide association studies have discovered at least 30 susceptibility loci for prostate cancer. It is demonstrated that HNF1β would be an excellent marker for distinguishing CCCs from other lesions in both the ovary and the endometrium. In ovarian cancer, down-regulation of HNF1β may contribute to drug resistance, thus estoration of HNF1β function could be a therapeutic approach. Many genetic and epigenetic alterations of HNF1β gene as well as several genetic networks and signaling pathways that are considered to be involved in the development and progression of tumor. The details of the regulatory pathways and their mechanisms are still under investigation. Studies also showed that HNF1β is closely associated with stem/progenitor cells. However, the potential pathogenic mechanisms of HNF1β in cancer and regulatory mechanisms in stem cells are still less understood. Thus, further study for HNF1β with tumor and stem cell is still needed.

Authors' contributions
DDY, SWG, YYJ, YLD and LX W planned the manuscript outline. DDY, SWG and YYJ wrote the draft manuscript, YLD revised the manuscript, LXW finalized the manuscript. All authors read and approved the final manuscript.

Acknowledgements
This project was supported by Key Basic Research Project of China (Grant No. 2011CB966200, 2012CBA01303); National Natural Science Foundation of China (Grant No. 31171321, 81201584,81372312, 81372330); Special Funds for National key Sci-Tech Special Project of China (Grant No. 2012ZX10002-016, 2012ZX10002011-011); Shanghai Science and Technology Committee (Grant No. 12431900802, 12ZR1439800, 12ZR1454200); Shanghai municipal education commission (Grant No. 14ZZ086) and Science Fund for Creative Research Groups, NSFC, China (Grant No. 81221061).

Competing interests
The authors declare that they have no competing interests.

References
1. Azmi AS, Bao GW, Gao J, Mohammad RM, Sarkar FH. Network insights into the genes regulated by hepatocyte nuclear factor 4 in response to drug induced perturbations: a review. Curr Drug Discov Technol. 2013;10(2):147–54.
2. Mendel DB, Hansen LP, Graves MK, Conley PB, Crabtree GR. HNF-1 alpha and HNF-1 beta (vHNF-1) share dimerization and homeo domains, but not activation domains, and form heterodimers in vitro. Genes Dev. 1991;5(6):1042–56.
3. Yang JY, Hung MC. Deciphering the role of forkhead transcription factors in cancer therapy. Curr Drug Targets. 2011;12(9):1284–90.
4. Watt AJ, Garrison WD, Duncan SA. HNF4: a central regulator of hepatocyte differentiation and function. Hepatology. 2003;37(6):1249–53.
5. Wang K, Holterman AX. Pathophysiologic role of hepatocyte nuclear factor 6. Cell Signal. 2012;24(1):9–16.
6. Gudmundsson J, Sulem P, Steinthorsdottir V, Bergthorsson JT, Thorleifsson G, Manolescu A, Rafnar T, Gudbjartsson D, Agnarsson BA, Baker A, et al. Two variants on chromosome 17 confer prostate cancer risk, and the one in TCF2 protects against type 2 diabetes. Nat Genet. 2007;39(8):977–83.
7. Horikawa Y, Iwasaki N, Hara M, Furuta H, Hinokio Y, Cockburn BN, Lindner T, Yamagata K, Ogata M, Tomonaga O, et al. Mutation in hepatocyte nuclear factor-1 beta gene (TCF2) associated with MODY. Nat Genet. 1997;17(4):384–5.
8. Brimo F, Herawi M, Sharma R, Netto GJ, Epstein JI, Illei PB. Hepatocyte nuclear factor-1beta expression in clear cell adenocarcinomas of the bladder and urethra: diagnostic utility and implications for histogenesis. Hum Pathol. 2011;42(11):1613–9.
9. Edghill EL, Bingham C, Ellard S, Hattersley AT. Mutations in hepatocyte nuclear factor-1beta and their related phenotypes. J Med Genet. 2006;43(1):84–90.
10. Coffinier C, Gresh L, Fiette L, Tronche F, Schutz G, Babinet C, Pontoglio M, Yaniv M, Barra J. Bile system morphogenesis defects and liver dysfunction upon targeted deletion of HNF1beta. Development. 2002;129(8):1829–38.
11. Ninomiya T, Hayashi Y, Saijoh K, Ohta K, Yoon S, Nakabayashi H, Tamaoki T, Kasuga M, Itoh H. Expression ratio of hepatocyte nuclear factor-1 to variant hepatocyte nuclear factor-1 in differentiation of hepatocellular carcinoma and hepatoblastoma. J Hepatol. 1996;25(4):445–53.
12. Wang W, Hayashi Y, Ninomiya T, Ohta K, Nakabayashi H, Tamaoki T, Itoh H. Expression of HNF-1 alpha and HNF-1 beta in various histological differentiations of hepatocellular carcinoma. J Pathol. 1998;184(3):272–8.
13. Shim JH, Lee HC, Han S, Kang HJ, Yu E, Lee SG. Hepatocyte nuclear factor 1beta is a novel prognostic marker independent of the Milan criteria in transplantable hepatocellular carcinoma: a retrospective analysis based on tissue microarrays. Liver transplant Off Publ Am Assoc Study Liver Dis Int Liver Transplant Soc. 2013;19(3):336–45.
14. Tanaka T, Tomaru Y, Nomura Y, Miura H, Suzuki M, Hayashizaki Y. Comprehensive search for HNF-1beta-regulated genes in mouse hepatoma cells perturbed by transcription regulatory factor-targeted RNAi. Nucleic Acids Res. 2004;32(9):2740–50.
15. Mazur PK, Riener MO, Jochum W, Kristiansen G, Weber A, Schmid RM, Siveke JT. Expression and clinicopathological significance of notch signaling and cell-fate genes in biliary tract cancer. Am J Gastroenterol. 2012;107(1):126–35.
16. Kim L, Liao J, Zhang M, Talamonti M, Bentrem D, Rao S, Yang GY. Clear cell carcinoma of the pancreas: histopathologic features and a unique biomarker: hepatocyte nuclear factor-1beta. Mod Pathol Off J US Can Acad Pathol Inc. 2008;21(9):1075–83.
17. Silva TD, Vidigal VM, Felipe AV, De Lima JM, Neto RA, Saad SS, Forones NM. DNA methylation as an epigenetic biomarker in colorectal cancer. Oncol Lett. 2013;6(6):1687–92.
18. Buchner A, Castro M, Hennig A, Popp T, Assmann G, Stief CG, Zimmermann W. Downregulation of HNF-1B in renal cell carcinoma is associated with tumor progression and poor prognosis. Urology. 2010;76(2):507 (e506–511).
19. Wang CC, Mao TL, Yang WC, Jeng YM. Underexpression of hepatocyte nuclear factor-1beta in chromophobe renal cell carcinoma. Histopathology. 2013;62(4):589–94.
20. Rebouissou S, Vasiliu V, Thomas C, Bellanne-Chantelot C, Bui H, Chretien Y, Timsit J, Rosty C, Laurent-Puig P, Chauveau D, et al. Germline hepatocyte nuclear factor 1alpha and 1beta mutations in renal cell carcinomas. Hum Mol Genet. 2005;14(5):603–14.
21. Gad S, Lefevre SH, Khoo SK, Giraud S, Vieillefond A, Vasiliu V, Ferlicot S, Molinie V, Denoux Y, Thiounn N, et al. Mutations in BHD and TP53 genes, but not in HNF1beta gene, in a large series of sporadic chromophobe renal cell carcinoma. Br J Cancer. 2007;96(2):336–40.
22. Szponar A, Yusenko MV, Kuiper R, van Kessel AG, Kovacs G. Genomic profiling of papillary renal cell tumours identifies small regions of DNA alterations: a possible role of HNF1B in tumour development. Histopathology. 2011;58(6):934–43.
23. Young RH, Scully RE. Clear cell adenocarcinoma of the bladder and urethra. A report of three cases and review of the literature. Am J Surg Pathol. 1985;9(11):816–26.
24. Eeles RA, Kote-Jarai Z, Giles GG, Olama AA, Guy M, Jugurnauth SK, Mulholland S, Leongamornlert DA, Edwards SM, Morrison J, et al. Multiple newly identified loci associated with prostate cancer susceptibility. Nat Genet. 2008;40(3):316–21.
25. Thomas G, Jacobs KB, Yeager M, Kraft P, Wacholder S, Orr N, Yu K, Chatterjee N, Welch R, Hutchinson A, et al. Multiple loci identified in a genome-wide association study of prostate cancer. Nat Genet. 2008;40(3):310–5.
26. Sun J, Zheng SL, Wiklund F, Isaacs SD, Purcell LD, Gao Z, Hsu FC, Kim ST, Liu W, Zhu Y, et al. Evidence for two independent prostate cancer risk-associated loci in the HNF1B gene at 17q12. Nat Genet. 2008;40(10):1153–5.
27. Berndt SI, Sampson J, Yeager M, Jacobs KB, Wang Z, Hutchinson A, Chung C, Orr N, Wacholder S, Chatterjee N, et al. Large-scale fine mapping of the HNF1B locus and prostate cancer risk. Hum Mol Genet. 2011;20(16):3322–9.
28. Zhang YR, Xu Y, Yang K, Liu M, Wei D, Zhang YG, Shi XH, Wang JY, Yang F, Wang X, et al. Association of six susceptibility Loci with prostate cancer in northern chinese men. Asian Pac J Cancer Prev APJCP. 2012;13(12):6273–6.
29. Hu YL, Zhong D, Pang F, Ning QY, Zhang YY, Li G, Wu JZ, Mo ZN. HNF1b is involved in prostate cancer risk via modulating androgenic hormone effects and coordination with other genes. Genet Mol Res GMR. 2013;12(2):1327–35.
30. Tsuchiya A, Sakamoto M, Yasuda J, Chuma M, Ohta T, Ohki M, Yasugi T, Taketani Y, Hirohashi S. Expression profiling in ovarian clear cell carcinoma: identification of hepatocyte nuclear factor-1 beta as a molecular marker and a possible molecular target for therapy of ovarian clear cell carcinoma. Am J Pathol. 2003;163(6):2503–12.
31. Yamamoto S, Tsuda H, Aida S, Shimazaki H, Tamai S, Matsubara O. Immunohistochemical detection of hepatocyte nuclear factor 1beta in ovarian and endometrial clear-cell adenocarcinomas and nonneoplastic endometrium. Hum Pathol. 2007;38(7):1074–80.

32. Kao YC, Lin MC, Lin WC, Jeng YM, Mao TL. Utility of hepatocyte nuclear factor-1beta as a diagnostic marker in ovarian carcinomas with clear cells. Histopathology. 2012;61(5):760–8.
33. Okamoto T, Mandai M, Matsumura N, Yamaguchi K, Kondoh H, Amano Y, Baba T, Hamanishi J, Abiko K, Kosaka K, et al. Hepatocyte nuclear factor-1beta (HNF-1beta) promotes glucose uptake and glycolytic activity in ovarian clear cell carcinoma. Mol Carcinog. 2015;54(1):35–49.
34. Li J, Zhang Y, Gao Y, Cui Y, Liu H, Li M, Tian Y. Downregulation of HNF1 homeobox B is associated with drug resistance in ovarian cancer. Oncol Rep. 2014;32:979–88.
35. Terasawa K, Toyota M, Sagae S, Ogi K, Suzuki H, Sonoda T, Akino K, Maruyama R, Nishikawa N, Imai K, et al. Epigenetic inactivation of TCF2 in ovarian cancer and various cancer cell lines. Br J Cancer. 2006;94(6):914–21.
36. Shen H, Fridley BL, Song H, Lawrenson K, Cunningham JM, Ramus SJ, Cicek MS, Tyrer J, Stram D, Larson MC, et al. Epigenetic analysis leads to identification of HNF1B as a subtype-specific susceptibility gene for ovarian cancer. Nat Commun. 2013;4:1628.
37. Spurdle AB, Thompson DJ, Ahmed S, Ferguson K, Healey CS, O'Mara T, Walker LC, Montgomery SB, Dermitzakis ET, Australian National Endometrial Cancer Study G, et al. Genome-wide association study identifies a common variant associated with risk of endometrial cancer. Nat Genet. 2011;43(5):451–4.
38. Setiawan VW, Haessler J, Schumacher F, Cote ML, Deelman E, Fesinmeyer MD, Henderson BE, Jackson RD, Vockler JS, Wilkens LR, et al. HNF1B and endometrial cancer risk: results from the PAGE study. PLoS One. 2012;7(1):e30390.
39. De Vivo I, Prescott J, Setiawan VW, Olson SH, Wentzensen N, Australian National Endometrial Cancer Study G, Attia J, Black A, Brinton L, Chen C et al. Genome-wide association study of endometrial cancer in E2C2. Hum Genet. 2014;133(2):211–24.
40. Fadare O, Liang SX. Diagnostic utility of hepatocyte nuclear factor 1-beta immunoreactivity in endometrial carcinomas: lack of specificity for endometrial clear cell carcinoma. Appl Immunohistochem Mol Morphol AIMM/Off Publ Soc Appl Immunohistochem. 2012;20(6):580–7.
41. Kato N, Tamura G, Motoyama T. Hypomethylation of hepatocyte nuclear factor-1beta (HNF-1beta) CpG island in clear cell carcinoma of the ovary. Virchows Arch Int J Pathol. 2008;452(2):175–80.
42. Tommasi S, Karm DL, Wu X, Yen Y, Pfeifer GP. Methylation of homeobox genes is a frequent and early epigenetic event in breast cancer. Breast Cancer Res BCR. 2009;11(1):R14.
43. Senkel S, Lucas B, Klein-Hitpass L, Ryffel GU. Identification of target genes of the transcription factor HNF1beta and HNF1alpha in a human embryonic kidney cell line. Biochim Biophys Acta. 2005;1731(3):179–90.
44. Kato N, Motoyama T. Overexpression of osteopontin in clear cell carcinoma of the ovary: close association with HNF-1beta expression. Histopathology. 2008;52(6):682–8.
45. Rangaswami H, Bulbule A, Kundu GC. Osteopontin: role in cell signaling and cancer progression. Trends Cell Biol. 2006;16(2):79–87.
46. Shigetomi H, Higashiura Y, Kajihara H, Kobayashi H. Targeted molecular therapies for ovarian cancer: an update and future perspectives (Review). Oncol Rep. 2012;28(2):395–408.
47. Morgan MA, Parsels LA, Zhao L, Parsels JD, Davis MA, Hassan MC, Arumugarajah S, Hylander-Gans L, Morosini D, Simeone DM, et al. Mechanism of radiosensitization by the Chk1/2 inhibitor AZD7762 involves abrogation of the G2 checkpoint and inhibition of homologous recombinational DNA repair. Cancer Res. 2010;70(12):4972–81.
48. Yamada Y, Shigetomi H, Onogi A, Haruta S, Kawaguchi R, Yoshida S, Furukawa N, Nagai A, Tanase Y, Tsunemi T, et al. Redox-active iron-induced oxidative stress in the pathogenesis of clear cell carcinoma of the ovary. Int J Gynecol Cancer Off J Int Gynecol Cancer Soc. 2011;21(7):1200–7.
49. Masur K, Schwartz F, Entschladen F, Niggemann B, Zaenker KS. DPPIV inhibitors extend GLP-2 mediated tumour promoting effects on intestinal cancer cells. Regul Pept. 2006;137(3):147–55.
50. Kuk C, Gunawardana CG, Soosaipillai A, Kobayashi H, Li L, Zheng Y, Diamandis EP. Nidogen-2: a new serum biomarker for ovarian cancer. Clin Biochem. 2010;43(4–5):355–61.
51. Kajihara H, Yamada Y, Kanayama S, Furukawa N, Noguchi T, Haruta S, Yoshida S, Sado T, Oi H, Kobayashi H. Clear cell carcinoma of the ovary: potential pathogenic mechanisms (Review). Oncol Rep. 2010;23(5):1193–203.
52. Akasaka J, Uekuri C, Shigetomi H, Koike M, Kobayashi H. Hepatocyte nuclear factor (HNF)-1beta and its physiological importance in endometriosis. Biomed Rep. 2013;1(1):13–7.
53. Hatzis P, Talianidis I. Regulatory mechanisms controlling human hepatocyte nuclear factor 4 alpha gene expression. Mol Cell Biol. 2001;21(21):7320–30.
54. Fabris L, Cadamuro M, Guido M, Spirli C, Fiorotto R, Colledan M, Torre G, Alberti D, Sonzogni A, Okolicsanyi L, et al. Analysis of liver repair mechanisms in Alagille syndrome and biliary atresia reveals a role for notch signaling. Am J Pathol. 2007;171(2):641–53.
55. Zhou ZC, Dong QG, Fu DL, Gong YY, Ni QX. Characteristics of Notch2(+) pancreatic cancer stem-like cells and the relationship with centroacinar cells. Cell Biol Int. 2013;37(8):805–11.
56. Charafe-Jauffret E, Ginestier C, Iovino F, Wicinski J, Cervera N, Finetti P, Hur MH, Diebel ME, Monville F, Dutcher J, et al. Breast cancer cell lines contain functional cancer stem cells with metastatic capacity and a distinct molecular signature. Cancer Res. 2009;69(4):1302–13.
57. Strazzabosco M, Fabris L. Notch signaling in hepatocellular carcinoma: guilty in association! Gastroenterology. 2012;143(6):1430–4.
58. Jaggupilli A, Elkord E. Significance of CD44 and CD24 as cancer stem cell markers: an enduring ambiguity. Clin Dev Immunol. 2012;2012:708036.
59. Matheu A, Collado M, Wise C, Manterola L, Cekaite L, Tye AJ, Canamero M, Bujanda L, Schedl A, Cheah KS, et al. Oncogenicity of the developmental transcription factor Sox9. Cancer Res. 2012;72(5):1301–15.
60. Coombes JD, Swiderska-Syn M, Dolle L, Reid D, Eksteen B, Claridge L, Briones-Orta MA, Shetty S, Oo YH, Riva A, et al. Osteopontin neutralisation abrogates the liver progenitor cell response and fibrogenesis in mice. Gut. 2015;64(7):1120–31.
61. Luo Z, Wu RR, Lv L, Li P, Zhang LY, Hao QL, Li W. Prognostic value of CD44 expression in non-small cell lung cancer: a systematic review. Int J Clin Exp Pathol. 2014;7(7):3632–46.
62. Rodrigo-Torres D, Affo S, Coll M, Morales-Ibanez O, Millan C, Blaya D, Alvarez-Guaita A, Rentero C, Lozano JJ, Maestro MA, et al. The biliary epithelium gives rise to liver progenitor cells. Hepatology. 2014;60(4):1367–77.
63. Yu B, He ZY, You P, Han QW, Xiang D, Chen F, Wang MJ, Liu CC, Lin XW, Borjigin U, et al. Reprogramming fibroblasts into bipotential hepatic stem cells by defined factors. Cell Stem Cell. 2013;13(3):328–40.
64. Pan FC, Bankaitis ED, Boyer D, Xu X, Van de Casteele M, Magnuson MA, Heimberg H, Wright CV. Spatiotemporal patterns of multipotentiality in Ptf1a-expressing cells during pancreas organogenesis and injury-induced facultative restoration. Development. 2013;140(4):751–64.
65. Lynn FC, Smith SB, Wilson ME, Yang KY, Nekrep N, German MS. Sox9 coordinates a transcriptional network in pancreatic progenitor cells. Proc Natl Acad Sci USA. 2007;104(25):10500–5.
66. Hattersley AT, Pearson ER. Minireview: pharmacogenetics and beyond: the interaction of therapeutic response, beta-cell physiology, and genetics in diabetes. Endocrinology. 2006;147(6):2657–63.
67. Poll AV, Pierreux CE, Lokmane L, Haumaitre C, Achouri Y, Jacquemin P, Rousseau GG, Cereghini S, Lemaigre FP. A vHNF1/TCF2-HNF6 cascade regulates the transcription factor network that controls generation of pancreatic precursor cells. Diabetes. 2006;55(1):61–9.
68. Oliver-Krasinski JM, Kasner MT, Yang J, Crutchlow MF, Rustgi AK, Kaestner KH, Stoffers DA. The diabetes gene Pdx1 regulates the transcriptional network of pancreatic endocrine progenitor cells in mice. J Clin Investig. 2009;119(7):1888–98.

13

Zinc ferrite nanoparticle-induced cytotoxicity and oxidative stress in different human cells

Hisham A. Alhadlaq[1], Mohd Javed Akhtar[2] and Maqusood Ahamed[2*]

Abstract

Background: Zinc ferrite nanoparticles (NPs) have shown potential to be used in biomedical field such as magnetic resonance imaging and hyperthermia. However, there is limited information concerning the biological response of zinc ferrite NPs. This study was designed to evaluate the cytotoxicity of zinc ferrite NPs in three widely used in vitro cell culture models: human lung epithelial (A549), skin epithelial (A431) and liver (HepG2) cells. Zinc ferrite NPs were characterized by electron microscopy and dynamic light scattering. Cell viability, cell membrane damage, reactive oxygen species (ROS), glutathione (GSH), mitochondrial membrane potential (MMP), transcriptional level of apoptotic genes were determined in zinc ferrite NPs exposed cells.

Results: Zinc ferrite NPs were almost spherical shaped with an average size of 44 nm. Zinc ferrite NPs induced dose-dependent cytotoxicity (MTT and LDH) and oxidative stress (ROS and GSH) in all three types of cells in the dosage range of 10–40 μg/ml. Transcriptional level of tumor suppressor gene p53 and apoptotic genes (bax, caspase-3 and caspase-9) were up-regulated while the anti-apoptotic gene bcl-2 was down-regulated in cells after zinc ferrite NPs exposure. Furthermore, higher activity of caspase-3 and caspase-9 enzymes was also observed in zinc ferrite NPs treated cells. ROS generation, MMP loss and cell death in all three types of cells were abrogated by *N*-acetyl cysteine (ROS scavenger), which suggests that oxidative stress might be one of the plausible mechanisms of zinc ferrite NPs cytotoxicity. It is worth mentioning that there was marginally difference in the sensitivity of three cell lines against zinc ferrite NPs exposure. Cytotoxicity of zinc ferrite NPs were in following order; A549 > HepG2 > A431.

Conclusion: Altogether, zinc ferrite NPs induced cytotoxicity and oxidative stress in A549, A431 and HepG2 cells, which is likely to be mediated through ROS generation. This study warrants further investigation to explore the potential mechanisms of toxicity of zinc ferrite NPs in normal cells as well as in animal models.

Keywords: Zinc ferrite nanoparticles, A549, A431, HepG2, Human health, Cytotoxicity, Reactive oxygen species

Background

Magnetic nanoparticles (NPs) hold great promise in biomedical applications including hyperthermia, biosensor, magnetic resonance imaging (MRI) and drug delivery [1–3]. Over the years, magnetite (Fe_3O_4) was the most studied magnetic NPs. In the last decade, it became easier to develop new and more effective types of magnetic NPs [4]. Spinel ferrite NPs with the general formula MFe_2O_4 (where M is A is divalent cation of Zn, Ni, Mn, Mg or Co) are very important materials because of their interesting magnetic and electrical properties with good chemical and thermal stabilities [5]. However, their biomedical application may ultimately be limited, because of the limited knowledge on biological response of these NPs [6, 7]. Therefore, it is necessary to explore the biological fate and possible toxic response of magnetic NPs for their successful implications in biomedical field.

Zinc ferrite ($ZnFe_2O_4$) NPs, a lesser investigated class of spinel ferrites, frequently utilized as a contrasting agent in MRI and spintronics devices [8]. Despite the

*Correspondence: maqusood@gmail.com
[2] King Abdullah Institute for Nanotechnology, King Saud University, Riyadh 11451, Saudi Arabia
Full list of author information is available at the end of the article

potential application of zinc ferrite NPs, there is a serious lack of information concerning the toxicity of this material both at in vitro and in vivo level. Some significant studies demonstrated the toxic effects of zinc ferrite NPs. Recently, Saquib et al. [9] suggested that zinc ferrite NPs trigger apoptosis and/or necrosis in human amnion epithelial (WISH) cells through mitochondria dependent intrinsic apoptotic pathway. Zinc ferrite NPs have also been reported to induce chromosomal aberration in the meristematic root cells of sunflower [10].

Toxicological investigations using animal models are both expensive and time taking. Therefore, a search for suitable alternative in vitro models to precisely predict the in vivo toxicity is indispensable. Human cell lines have been shown to be good in vitro models and sensitive tools for high-throughput toxicity screening and have the potential to reduce the use of animals in toxicity studies. Cell lines can be utilized for the generation of mechanistic data that could potentially be used for toxicity assessments. Therefore, we have chosen three widely used in vitro cell culture models; human lung epithelial (A549), skin epithelial (A431) and liver (HepG2) cells as tools to explore the cytotoxicity of zinc ferrite NPs.

Exposure to NPs could occur through the air, skin, food and the use of medical devices [11]. The respiratory tract and skin represents the main route of NPs exposure for workers employed in the manufacturing and handling. The NPs have high possibility to deposit in the respiratory system and can retain in the lungs for a long time where they provoke oxidative stress and an inflammatory burden with respect to their fine-sized equivalents [12, 13]. On the other hand, liver is a primary site of NPs accumulation after they get entry to circulatory system [14]. Studies suggest that NPs get absorbed as they pass through the gastrointestinal tract and distributed different vital organs including liver via the circulatory system [15, 16]. Therefore, we have selected human lung (A549), skin (A431) and liver (HepG2) cell lines to explore cytotoxic response of zinc ferrite NPs. These cell lines have been widely used in nanotoxicity research [17–20].

The underlying mechanisms of toxicity of NPs are not fully explored. One mechanism more often argued is the induction of oxidative damage of cell macromolecules, either due to the reactive oxygen species (ROS) generation or by inactivation of antioxidant defense system [21, 22]. ROS generation is a crucial factor not only in apoptotic pathway, but also in genetic damage, inflammation and several other cellular processes [23, 24]. Our earlier studies have shown that magnetic NPs have potential to induce ROS mediated cytotoxicity in different human cells [20, 25, 26]. In the present study, we investigated the cytotoxicity and oxidative stress response of zinc ferrite NPs in three different types of human cells (A549, A431 and HepG2). To achieve this goal, we determined the cell viability, cell membrane damage, ROS, glutathione (GSH), mitochondrial membrane potential (MMP) and transcriptional level of some apoptotic genes in zinc ferrite NPs exposed cells.

Methods

Chemicals and reagents

Dulbecco's modified eagle's medium (DMEM), penicillin–streptomycin and fetal bovine serum were purchased from Invitrogen (Carlsbad, CA, USA). The 3-(4,5-dimethylthiazol-2-yl)-2, 5-diphenyltetrazoliumbromide (MTT), 3-amino-7-dimethylamino-2-methyl-phenazine hydrochloride (neutral red), *N*-acetylcysteine (NAC), rhodamine-123 (Rh123) and 2,7-dichlorofluorescin diacetate (DCFH-DA) were bought from Sigma-Aldrich (St. Louis, MO, USA). Kits for lactate dehydrogenase (LDH) and caspase assays were obtained from Bio-Vision Inc. (Milpitas, CA, USA). Other chemicals were of analytical grade and bought from available commercial sources.

Zinc ferrite nanoparticles

Dry nanopowder of zinc ferrite ($ZnFe_2O_4$) [Product No. 633844, <100 nm particle size (BET), >99 % trace metals basis] was obtained from Sigma-Aldrich (St. Louis, MO, USA). Zinc ferrite NPs were further characterized in our laboratory.

Zinc ferrite nanoparticle characterization

Structural characterization of zinc ferrite NPs was done by field emission scanning electron microscope (FESEM, JSM-7600F, JEOL Inc., Japan) and field emission transmission electron microscopy (FETEM, JEM-2100F, JEOL Inc., Japan) at an accelerating voltage of 15 and 200 kV, respectively. In FETEM study, 1 mg/ml suspension of zinc ferrite NPs was prepared in de-ionized water. Then suspension was sonicated at room temperature for 15 min at 40 W to avoid NPs agglomeration. To determine the size of NPs, stock suspension was diluted to appropriate working solutions. Further, a drop of aqueous suspension of zinc ferrite NPs was poured onto a carbon-coated copper grid, air-dried and FETEM measurements were performed.

Behavior of zinc ferrite NPs in aqueous state (e.g. water and culture medium) was evaluated by dynamic light scattering (DLS) (Nano-ZetaSizer-HT, Malvern, UK) as reported elsewhere [27]. Briefly, zinc ferrite nano-powder were suspended in de-ionized water and culture medium at the concentration of 40 μg/ml. This suspension was further sonicated at room temperature for 15 min at 40 W and performed the DLS measurements. We have utilized concentration of 40 μg/ml for DLS study because this was the highest dosage level employed in cytotoxicity studies.

Cell culture and exposure of zinc ferrite nanoparticles

A549, A431 and HepG2 cells were obtained from American Type Culture Collection (ATCC) (Manassas, VA, USA). Cells were cultured in DMEM medium supplemented with 10 % FBS and 100 U/ml penicillin–streptomycin at 5 % CO_2 and 37 °C. At 85 % confluence, cells were harvested using 0.25 % trypsin and were sub-cultured for further experiments. Cells were allowed to attach on the surface of culture flask for 24 h before NP exposure. Dry powder of zinc ferrite NPs was suspended in DMEM medium at a concentration of 1 mg/ml and diluted to appropriate dosages (10–40 µg/ml). The different concentrations of NPs were then sonicated at room temperature for 15 min at 40 W to avoid agglomeration of NPs before exposure to cell. In some experiments, cells were pre-exposed for 1 h with 10 mM of NAC before 24 h co-exposure with or without zinc ferrite NPs. Cells not exposed to zinc ferrite NPs served as controls in each experiment. Selection of 10–40 µg/ml dosage range of zinc ferrite NPs was based on preliminary dose–response experiments (data not shown).

Cell viability assay

Cell viability assay was done following the method as described by Mossman [28] with few changes [25]. This assay evaluates the mitochondrial function by determining the ability of living cells to reduce MTT into blue formazon product. Briefly, 10,000 cells/well were seeded in 96-well plates and exposed to different concentrations of zinc ferrite NPs (10–40 µg/ml) for 24 h. After the treatment time completed, culture medium was taken out from each well to avoid interference of NPs and replaced with new medium containing MTT solution in an amount equal to 10 % of culture volume and incubated for 3 h at 37 °C until a purple-colored formazan product developed. The resulting formazan product was dissolved in acidified isopropanol. Then, 96-well plate was centrifuged at 2300*g* for 5 min to settle down the remaining NPs. Further, 100 µl supernatant was transferred to new 96-well plate, and the absorbance was taken at 570 nm utilizing a microplate reader (Synergy-HT, BioTek, USA).

Lactate dehydrogenase leakage assay

Lactate dehydrogenase (LDH) assay was carried out using a BioVision LDH-cytotoxicity colorimetric assay kit as per the manufacturer's instruction. Briefly, 10,000 cells/well were seeded in 96-well plates and treated to different concentrations of zinc ferrite NPs (10–40 µg/ml) for 24 h. At the end of the exposure time, 96-well plate was centrifuged at 2300*g* for 5 min to settle down the NPs. Then, 100 µl of the supernatant was transferred to a new 96-well plate that already contained 100 µl of the reaction mixture from the BioVision kit and incubated for 30 min at room temperature. After the incubation time completed, absorbance of the solution was determined at 340 nm with help of a microplate reader (Synergy-HT, BioTek, USA). The LDH levels in the culture medium versus those present within cells were measured and compared with the control values according to the manufacturer's protocol.

Reactive oxygen species assay

Intracellular reactive oxygen species (ROS) generation after the treatment of zinc ferrite NPs was evaluated using 2,7-dichlorofluorescin diacetate (DCFH-DA) as reported by Wang and Joseph [29] with few changes described in our previous publication [30]. The ROS level was measured by two methods; fluorometric quantitative assay by micro-plate reader and cell imaging by fluorescence microscopy. For fluorometric assay, 10,000 cells/well were seeded in 96-well black-bottomed culture plates and allowed to attach on the surface for 24 h in a CO_2 incubator at 37 °C. Further, cells were treated with zinc ferrite NPs (10–40 µg/ml) for 24 h. After the exposure completed, were washed twice with HBSS before being incubated in 1 ml of working solution of DCFH-DA for 30 min at 37 °C. After this, cells were lysed in alkaline solution and centrifuged at 2300*g* for 10 min. A 200 µl supernatant was transferred to a new 96-well plate, and fluorescence was measured at 485 nm excitation and 520 nm emission utilizing the microplate reader (Synergy-HT, BioTek, USA). The values were presented as a percent of fluorescence intensity relative to the controls.

A parallel set of cells (5×10^4 cells/well in a 24-well transparent plate) were assayed for intracellular fluorescence using a fluorescence microscope (OLYMPUS CKX 41), with images captured at the magnification of 20×.

Cell extract preparation

Crude cell extract were prepared according to the protocol described in our earlier work [31]. Cell extract were used for glutathione (GSH), caspase-3 and caapase-9 enzymes assays. In brief, cells were cultured in 75-cm^2 culture flask and treated with zinc ferrite NPs (10–80 µg/ml) for 24 h. After the exposure completed, cells were harvested in ice-cold phosphate buffer saline by scraping and washed with phosphate buffer saline at 4 °C. The cell pellets were then lysed in cell lysis buffer [1 × 20 mM Tris–HCl (pH 7.5), 150 mM NaCl, 1 mM Na_2EDTA, 1 % Triton, 2.5 mM sodium pyrophosphate]. Following centrifugation (15,000*g* for 10 min at 4 °C) the cell extract (supernatant) was stored in ice for biochemical assays.

Glutathione assay

Intracellular glutathione (GSH) content was estimated utilizing Ellman's method [32]. In brief, a mixture of 0.1 ml of crude cell extract and 0.9 ml of 5 % TCA was centrifuged at 2300*g* for 15 min. After that 0.5 ml of the supernatant was added into 1.5 ml of 0.01 % DTNB and the reaction was monitored at 412 nm. The content of GSH was presented in terms of nmole/mg protein.

Mitochondrial membrane potential assay

Mitochondrial membrane potential (MMP) was estimated using the method of Zhang et al. [33] with few changes [34]. Briefly, cells (5×10^4 cells/well) were exposed to different concentrations (10–40 µg/ml) of zinc ferrite NPs for 24 h. After the completion of exposure time, cells were harvested and washed twice with PBS. Then, cells were treated with 10 µg/ml of Rh-123 fluorescent dye for 1 h at 37 °C in dark. Furthermore, cells were washed twice with PBS then the fluorescence intensity of Rh-123 dye was determined using upright fluorescence microscope (OLYMPUS CKX 41) by grabbing the images at 20× magnification.

A parallel set of cells (1×10^4 cells/well) in 96-well plate were analyzed for quantification of Rh-123 using the microplate reader (Synergy-HT, BioTek, USA).

Quantitative assay of apoptotic genes by real-time PCR

Cells were cultured in 6-well plates and treated with zinc ferrite NPs at a dosage of 20 µg/ml for 24 h. After the completion of exposure time, total RNA was extracted by Qiagen RNeasy mini Kit (Valencia, CA, USA) according to the manufacturer's protocol. The RNA content was estimated using Nanodrop 8000 spectrophotometer (Thermo-Scientific, Wilmington, DE, USA), and the integrity of RNA was visualized on a 1 % agarose gel using the gel documentation system (Universal Hood II, BioRad, Hercules, CA, USA). The first strand of cDNA was synthesized from 1 µg of total RNA by the reverse transcriptase using M-MLV (Promega, Madison, WI, USA) and oligo (dT) primers (Promega) according to the manufacturer's instructions. Quantitative real-time PCR was performed by QuantiTect SYBR Green PCR kit (Qiagen) using the ABI PRISM 7900HT Sequence Detection System (Applied Biosystems, Foster City, CA, USA). Two microliters of template cDNA was added to the final volume of 20 µl of reaction mixture. Real-time PCR cycle parameters included 10 min at 95 °C followed by 40 cycles involving denaturation at 95 °C for 15 s, annealing at 60 °C for 20 s, and elongation at 72 °C for 20 s. The sequences of the specific sets of primer for p53, bax, bcl-2, caspase-3, caspase-9 and β-actin utilized in the present investigation are given in our previous study [25]. Expressions of selected genes were normalized to the β-actin gene, which was used as controls.

Determination of caspase-3 and caspase-9 enzymes activity

Caspase-3 and caspase-9 enzymes activity was evaluated in exposed and control cells using Bio-Vision colorimetric assay kits. Preparation of cell extract is reported above. This assay is based on the principle that activated caspases in apoptotic cells cleave the synthetic substrates to release free chromophore *p*-nitroanilide (pNA), which is measured at 405 nm. The pNA was generated after specific action of caspase-3 and caspase-9 on tertrapeptide substrates DEVD-pNA and LEHD-pNA, respectively [25, 35]. In brief, reaction mixture consisted of 50 µl of cell extract protein (as prepared above), 50 µl of 2× reaction buffer (containing 10 mM dithiothreitol) and 5 µl of 4 mM DEVD-pNA (for caspase-3) or LEHD-pNA (for caspase-9) substrate in a total volume of 105 µl. The reaction mixture was incubated at 37 °C for 1 h and absorbance of the final product was estimated utilizing the microplate reader (Synergy-HT, BioTek, USA) at 405 nm according to kit's instruction.

Protein assay

Protein content was estimated by the Bradford method [36] using bovine serum albumin as the standard.

Statistical analysis

Statistical significance was measured by one-way analysis of variance followed by Dunnett's multiple comparison tests. Significance was ascribed at $p < 0.05$.

Results

Zinc ferrite nanoparticle characterization

Techniques such as FETEM, FESEM and DLS was used to characterize the zinc ferrite NPs. FESEM image depicts the surface morphology zinc ferrite NPs (Fig. 1a). Figure 1b shows the typical TEM image of zinc ferrite NPs. As we can see in Fig. 1c the high resolution TEM indicated the crystalline behavior of zinc ferrite NPs. TEM and SEM images have shown that particles were almost spherical with smooth surfaces. The average size of NPs was calculated from estimating over 120 particles in random fields of TEM view. The average size of zinc NPs was approximately 44.3 nm. Figure 1d shows the size distribution frequency of zinc ferrite NPs.

Characterization of zinc ferrite NPs in aqueous state by DLS technique is given in Table 1. Secondary particle size (hydrodynamic size) of zinc ferrite NPs in de-ionized water and cell culture medium was 312 and 289 nm, respectively. Further, zeta-potential of zinc ferrite NPs in water and culture medium was −18 and −23 mV, respectively.

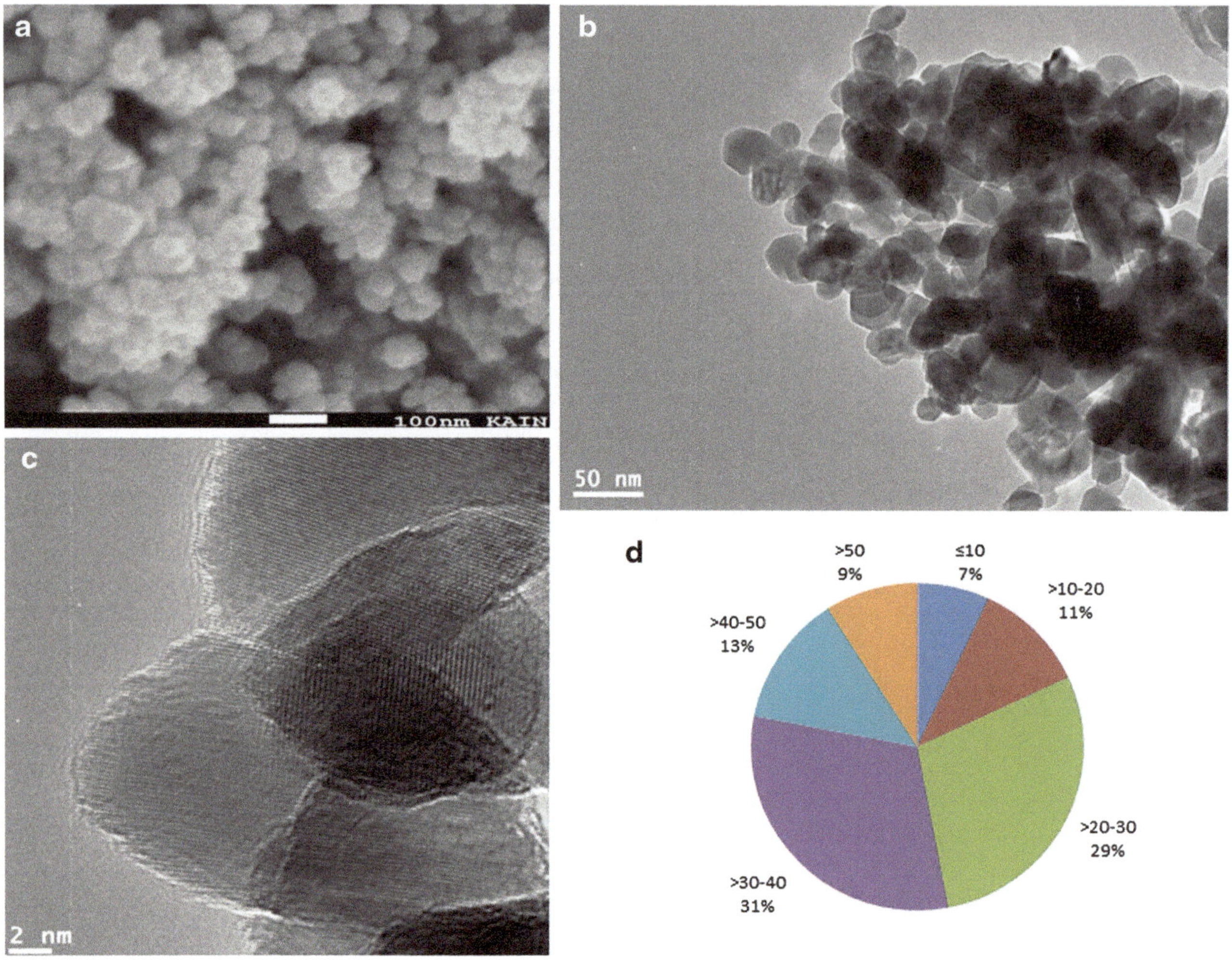

Fig. 1 Electron microscopy characterization of zinc ferrite NPs. **a** FESEM image, **b** FETEM image, **c** FETEM image with high resolution and **d** frequency of particle size distribution

Table 1 Dynamic light scattering characterization of zinc ferrite NPs

	De-ionized water (mean ± SD)	Culture media (mean ± SD)
DLS characterization of zinc ferrite NPs		
Hydrodynamic size (nm)	312 ± 67	289 ± 55
Zeta potential (−mV)	18 ± 8	23 ± 7

Zinc ferrite nanoparticles reduced the cell viability

A431, A549 and HepG2 cells were treated with zinc ferrite NPs (10–40 μg/ml) for 24 h and cell viability was determined by MTT assay. Results have shown that zinc ferrite NPs significantly decreased the viability of all three types of cells in a dose-dependent manner. We also observed that zinc ferrite NPs induced cytotoxicity in following order A549 cells > HepG2 cells > A431 cells. Cell viability was decreased to 81, 63 and 38 % for A431 and 74, 57 and 31 % for HepG2, while 67, 48 and 25 % for A549 cells, at the concentrations of 10, 20, and 40 μg/ml, respectively ($p < 0.05$ for each) (Fig. 2).

Zinc ferrite nanoparticle-induced membrane damage

LDH is an enzyme widely found in the cytosol that converts lactate to pyruvate. When the integrity of plasma membrane is disrupted, LDH leaks into media and its extracellular content increases depending upon the extent of NPs cytotoxicity. Therefore, higher level of LDH in culture medium indicates higher cytotoxic response of NPs. We also observed that zinc ferrite NPs induced LDH leakage dose-dependently in all three types of cells (Fig. 3). Effects of zinc ferrite NPs on A549 cells was higher than those of HepG2 and A431 cells. LDH leakage in A431 cells was increased to 119, 130 and 143 %, and 125, 149 and 163 % for HepG2, while 129, 155 and 172 % were A549 cells for the dosages of 10, 20 and 40 μg/ml, respectively ($p < 0.05$ for each) (Fig. 3).

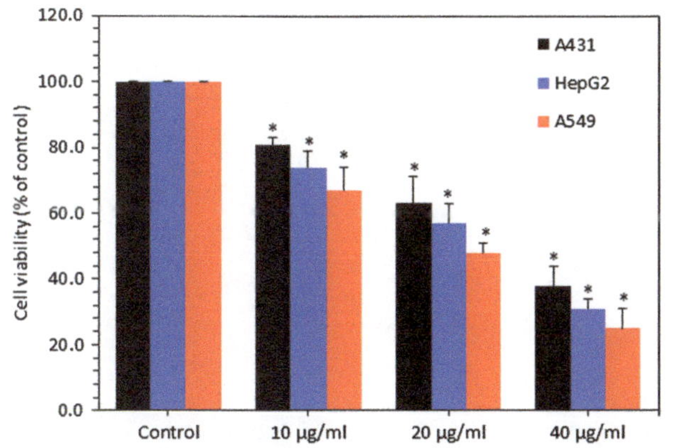

Fig. 2 Zinc ferrite NPs reduced the viability of A431, HepG2 and A549 cells. Data represented are mean ± SD of three identical experiments made in three replicate. *Significant difference as compared to the controls ($p < 0.05$ for each)

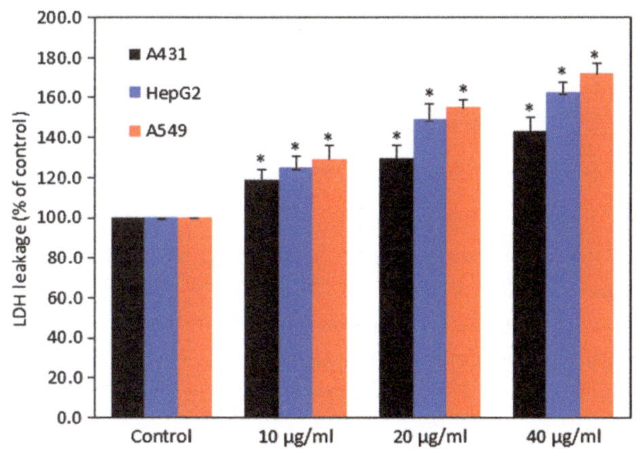

Fig. 3 Zinc ferrite NPs induced membrane damage in A431, HepG2 and A549 cells. Data represented are mean ± SD of three identical experiments made in three replicate. *Significant difference as compared to the controls ($p < 0.05$ for each)

Zinc ferrite nanoparticle-induced reactive oxygen species generation

ROS generation has been suggested to be involved in several cellular events including inflammation, senescence mutation, DNA damage and apoptosis. We evaluated the potential of zinc NPs to induce intracellular ROS generation in A431, HepG2 and A549 cells. Quantitative results indicated that zinc ferrite NPs induced ROS generation dose-dependently in all three types of cells ($p < 0.05$ for each) (Fig. 4a). Fluorescent microscopy results also suggested that zinc ferrite NPs treated cells show higher intensity of green fluoresce of DCF dye (ROS generation marker) than those of the control cells (Fig. 4b).

Zinc ferrite nanoparticle-reduced glutathione level

Antioxidant GSH depletion and changes in the activity of various antioxidant enzymes indicative of lipid peroxidation have been implicated in oxidative damage of cellular macromolecules [37]. Therefore, we further examined the GSH level in A431, HepG2 and A549 cells exposed to zinc ferrite NPs at the concentrations of 10, 20 and 40 µg/ml for 24 h. Results showed that zinc ferrite NPs reduced the level of GSH in all three types of cell in a dose-dependent manner (Fig. 5).

Zinc ferrite nanoparticle-reduced mitochondrial membrane potential

Earlier studies have shown that MMP loss during the process of apoptosis [23]. We studied the effect of zinc ferrite NPs on MMP in A431, HepG2 and A549 cells. Quantitative data showed that zinc ferrite NPs induced MMP loss in a dose-dependent manner in all three types of cells ($p < 0.05$ for each) (Fig. 6a). Fluorescence microscopy results were also according to the quantitative data. The brightness of the fluorescent intensity was decreased in cells treated with zinc ferrite NPs that shows a significant loss MMP (Fig. 6b).

Zinc ferrite nanoparticle-altered the expression of apoptotic genes

Quantitative real-time PCR was used to analyze the expression of mRNA level of various genes involved in apoptosis (p53, bax, bcl-2, caspase-3 and caspase-9) in A431, HepG2 and A549 cells exposed to zinc ferrite NPs at a concentration of 20 µg/ml for 24 h. We noticed that zinc ferrite NPs altered the expression of these genes in all three types of cells ($p < 0.05$ for each) (Fig. 7a). Transcription expression level of tumor suppressor gene p53 and pro-apoptotic gene bax were up-regulated while the expression of anti-apoptotic gene bcl-2 was down-regulated in cells treated with zinc ferrite NPs. We also observed the higher expression of caspase-3 and caspase-9 genes in NPs treated cells as compared to the control.

Zinc ferrite nanoparticle-induced the activity of caspase-3 and caspase-9 enzymes

In support of real-time PCR results, we further determined the activity of caspase-3 and caspase-9 enzymes in A431, HepG2 and A549 cells treated with zinc ferrite NPs at a concentration of 20 µg/ml for 24 h. Results have shown that zinc ferrite NPs increased the activity of both apoptotic enzymes (caspas-3 and caspase-9) in all three types of cells ($p < 0.05$ for each) (Fig. 7b).

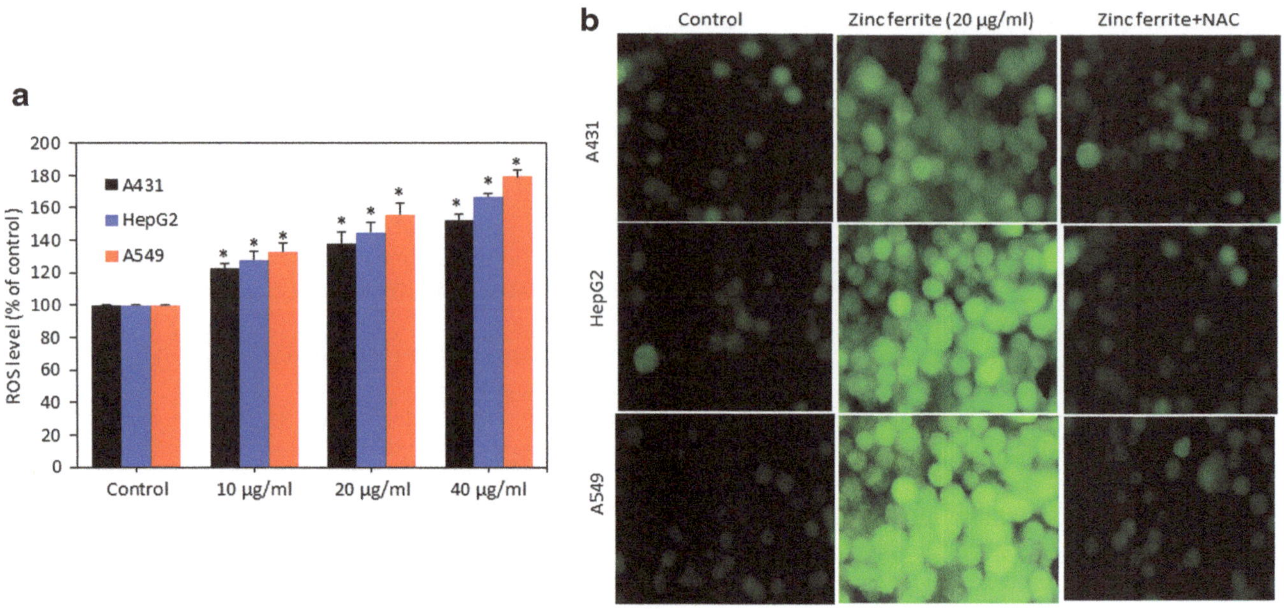

Fig. 4 Zinc ferrite NPs induced ROS generation in A431, HepG2 and A549 cells. **a** Percentage change in ROS generation in all three cells after zinc ferrite NPs exposure at the concentrations of 0, 10, 20 and 40 µg/ml for 24 h. **b** Representative microphotographs showing ROS generation in A431, HepG2 and A549 cells after zinc ferrite NPs exposure at a concentration of 20 µg/ml for 24 h. Images were captured with a fluorescence microscope (OLYMPUS CKX 41). Data represented are mean ± SD of three identical experiments made in three replicate. *Significant difference as compared to the controls ($p < 0.05$ for each)

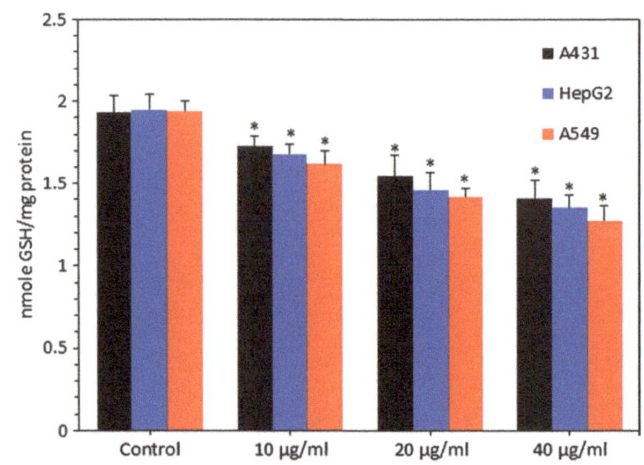

Fig. 5 Zinc ferrite NPs induced GSH depletion in A431, HepG2 and A549 cells. Data represented are mean ± SD of three identical experiments made in three replicate. *Significant difference as compared to the controls ($p < 0.05$ for each)

Zinc ferrite nanoparticle- induced cytotoxicity through ROS generation

In order to investigate whether ROS generation might plays a critical role in cytotoxicity of zinc ferrite NPs, cells were exposed to zinc ferrite NPs in the presence of NAC (ROS scavenger). Results showed that NAC abolished almost fully the cytotoxic effect of zinc ferrite NPs in all three types of cells (A431, HepG2 and A549) (Fig. 8).

Taken together, there was marginally difference in the sensitivity of three cells against zinc ferrite NPs exposure. Cytotoxic response of zinc ferrite NPs were in following order; A549 cells > HepG2 cells > A431cells. However, the modes of action of cytotoxicity of zinc ferrite NPs in all three cells were look similar.

Discussion

Despite many advantages in using spinel ferrite NPs, evidences are increasing to indicate that spinet ferrite NPs may cause toxic effects to human cells [9, 20, 25, 38]. Although the beneficial effects of zinc ferrite ($ZnFe_2O_4$) have attracted considerable attention in biomedical application, their human and environmental hazards should also be considered. Therefore, in this study, we have examined the toxicological effects of zinc ferrite NPs in three different cell lines of human body. The NPs may pose toxic effects due to their tiny size and unique physiochemical properties [27]. Therefore, it is essential to characterize the NPs before their toxicological investigations. The principal parameters of NPs are their size, shape, crystallanity, purity/impurity, hydrodynamic size and agglomeration/dispersion that influence the biological interaction of NPs [21, 27, 39]. We have employed

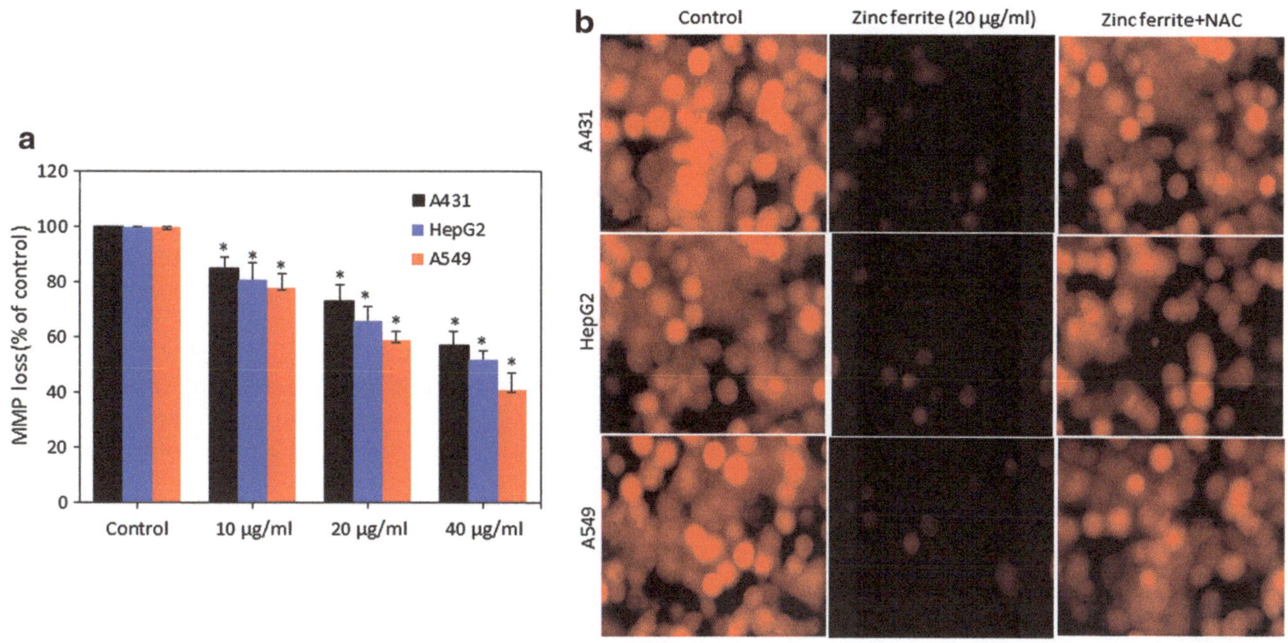

Fig. 6 Zinc ferrite NPs induced MMP loss in A431, HepG2 and A549 cells. **a** Percentage change in MMP in all three cells after zinc ferrite NPs exposure at the concentrations of 0, 10, 20 and 40 µg/ml for 24 h. **b** Representative microphotographs showing MMP loss in A431, HepG2 and A549 cells after zinc ferrite NPs exposure at a concentration of 20 µg/ml for 24 h. Images were captured with a fluorescence microscope (OLYMPUS CKX 41). Data represented are mean ± SD of three identical experiments made in three replicate. *Statistically significant difference as compared to control ($p < 0.05$)

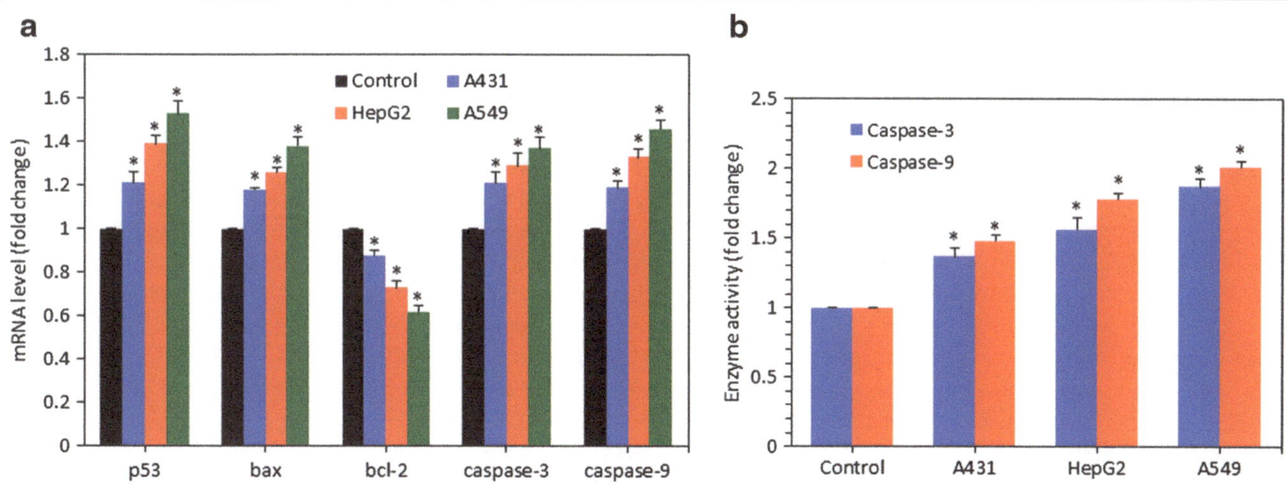

Fig. 7 Zinc ferrite NPs induced apoptotic response in A431, HepG2 and A549 cells. **a** Regulation of mRNA levels of apoptotic genes in all the cells after exposure to zinc ferrite NPs at a concentration of 20 µg/ml for 24 h. The mRNA levels were determined by quantitative real-time PCR as described in "Methods" section. **b** Activity of caspase-3 and caspase-9 enzymes in A431, HepG2 and A549 cells after exposure to zinc ferrite NPs at a concentration of 20 µg/ml for 24 h. Data represented are mean ± SD of three identical experiments made in three replicate. *Significant difference as compared to the controls ($p < 0.05$ for each)

SEM, TEM and DLS techniques to characterize the NPs. The SEM image suggested the smooth surfaces of NPs. The primary particle size of zinc ferrite measured by TEM was approximately 44 nm. High-resolution TEM images represented the crystalline behavior of this material. Secondary particle size (aqueous suspension) of the NPs is also regarded as an important parameter for in vitro assays. Therefore, extent of aggregation and

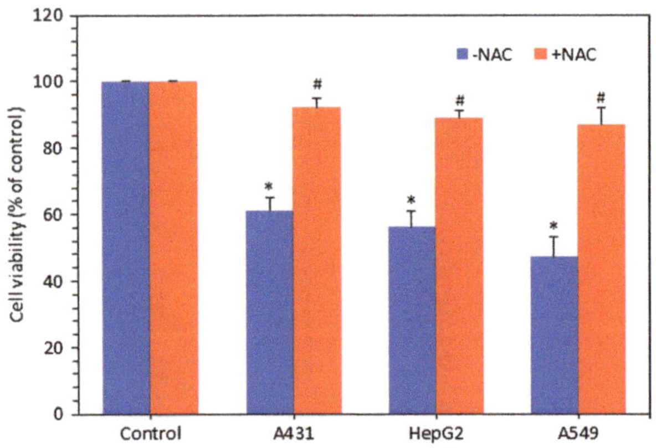

Fig. 8 Zinc ferrite NPs induced cytotoxicity in A431, HepG2 and A549 cells through ROS generation. Cells were exposed to zinc ferrite NPs at a concentration of 20 μg/ml in the presence of 10 mM *N*-acetyl-cystein (NAC) for 24 h. At the end of the exposure time, cell viability was determined. We observed that NAC significantly preserved the viability of all three cells induced by zinc ferrite NPs. Data represented are mean ± SD of three identical experiments made in three replicate. *Significant difference as compared to the controls ($p < 0.05$ for each). #Significant inhibitory effect of NAC on cell viability reduction ($p < 0.05$ for each)

secondary size of zinc ferrite NPs in water and cell culture medium was evaluated through dynamic light scattering (DLS). The DLS is widely used to determine the size of Brownian NPs in colloidal suspensions in the nano and submicron ranges [44]. We observed that the secondary particle size (hydrodynamic diameter) of zinc ferrite NPs was several times higher as compared with the primary size measured by TEM. The greater size of NPs in liquid medium than the primary size could be due to tendency of NPs to aggregate in aqueous state. This finding is supported by other studies, [40, 41] and has been briefly discussed in our earlier work [42]. The average hydrodynamic size of NPs in cell culture medium were slightly smaller (289 nm) as compared to de-ionized water (312 nm), which indicates the possible interaction of zinc ferrite NPs with the protein of culture media, which has been widely reported with different NPs that leads to the formation of 'protein corona' [43, 44]. The tendency of particles to form aggregates depends on the surface modification and charge. The surface charge of zinc ferrite NPs measured as zeta potential was around −18 and −23 mV for water and culture medium, respectively.

After characterization of zinc ferrite NPs, we performed a series of tests to determine the cytotoxic potential of zinc ferrite NPs in in vitro systems. Because of the limited metabolic capacity of the in vitro models, the biotransformation of a chemical in vitro may be minimal compared with that in in vivo systems. However, despite their known limited metabolic capacity, in vitro cell lines still represent promising tools for the development of high-throughput, predictive and mechanism-based assays to evaluate the potential toxicity of agents such as NPs [26]. As demonstrated in Fig. 2, it is evident that A549, A431 and HepG2 cells responded differently to zinc ferrite NPs exposure. The viability values indicate that A549 cells were more sensitive to the NPs exposure than A431 and HepG2 cells after 24 h. Decrease in cell viability after zinc ferrite NPs treatment were in following order; A549 cells > HepG2 cells > A431 cells. LDH leakage from cells is also an evidence of cell membrane damage. Studies have shown that LDH level was elevated in cells culture medium after exposure of cells to the magnetic NPs [20, 45]. Our results also demonstrated that LDH leakage was higher in a dose-dependent manner in all three types of cells treated with zinc ferrite NPs.

Normally, NPs enter into cells through endocytosis and localize in the vacuoles and cell cytoplasm of the cells [46, 47]. During internalization by endocytosis, magnetic NPs may undergo dissolution or degradation due to acidic pH of endosomes, [48] and release iron (Fe) ions that most likely promotes the generation of ROS via Haber–Weiss and/or Fenton reactions, and consequently cause oxidative damage to cell macromolecules [49]. Fe ions can also potentially escape into the cytoplasm and become a part of accessible Fe ions called the labile iron pool, which has also been shown to exist in the nucleus [50, 51]. Moreover, the tiny size with large surface area makes NPs more compatible for generation of ROS in the cell. Cancer cells as compared to normal cells are under greater intrinsic oxidative stress due to alterations in metabolism and higher accumulation of ROS due to an imbalance between ROS generation and elimination [52]. Higher sensitivity of cancer cells toward ROS generation due to NPs exposure as compared to normal cells makes them more suitable to explore the potential mechanisms of ROS mediated toxicity of NPs. We also observed ROS level was significantly higher whereas the antioxidant GSH level was significantly lower in all three A549, A431 and HepG2 cells exposed to zinc ferrite NPs. Moreover, induction ROS generation as well as reduction in cell viability due to zinc ferrite NPs exposure was efficiently prevented by antioxidant NAC treatment. These findings suggest that ROS generation might be the primarily responsible for the cytotoxicity of zinc ferrite NPs. This observation was according to the earlier findings in various human cell lines that indicate ROS generation and oxidative stress due to magnetic NPs [9, 53].

We further observed MMP loss against zinc ferrite NPs exposure in all three human cells. Changes in mitochondrial activity was based on cationic fluorescent probe Rh123, indicated the role of oxidative stress in toxicity of zinc ferrite NPs. We assume that lesser fluorescence intensity of Rh123 indicates perturbation of inner mitochondrial membranes, and consequently mitochondrial dysfunction as a result of ROS. Because ROS scavenger NAC significantly prevents the loss of MMP in zinc ferrite NPs treated cells. The transcriptional data on modulation of p53 and bax/bcl-2 ratio and release of caspases have strengthened the role of zinc ferrite in inducing mitochondrial dependent apoptotic pathway. In general, the caspases are crucial for the activation and execution of apoptosis. The main intrinsic pathway is characterized by mitochondrial dysfunction, with the release of cytochrome c, activation of caspase 9, and subsequently of caspase 3 enzyme [54]. Typically, p53 is activated when DNA damage occurs or cells are stressed and p53 is translocated to the nucleus, where it can induce pro-apoptotic gene expression on the mitochondrial membrane and activate the effector caspases and accelerate cell death [9, 55].

Conclusion

Our results have shown that zinc ferrite NPs induced cytotoxicity (MTT and LDH) in human lung (A549), skin (A431) and (HepG2) cells in a dose-dependent manner. Zinc ferrite NPs were also found to induce oxidative stress dose-dependently, indicated by ROS generation and glutathione depletion. Cytotoxicity of zinc ferrite NPs was effectively abolished *N*-acetyl-cysteine (ROS scavenger) indicating that oxidative stress might be one of the possible causes of zinc ferrite NPs toxicity. Zinc ferrite NPs also showed apoptotic response in all three cells evident by loss of MMP and alteration in the regulation of the apoptotic genes (p53, bax, bcl-2, caspase-3, and caspase-9). The sensitivity of these three cells against zinc ferrite NPs exposure was marginally different. Cytotoxic response of zinc ferrite NPs were in following order; A549 cells > HepG2 cells > A431 cells. Overall, present investigation suggests that zinc ferrite NPs induced cytotoxicity was mediated through ROS generation. Further studies are underway to explore the toxic potential of zinc ferrite NPs at in vivo level.

Authors' contributions

HAA, MJA, and MA performed the experiments and analyzed the data. MA conceived of the study, and participated in its design and coordination and helped to draft the manuscript. All authors read and approved the final manuscript.

Author details

[1] Department of Physics and Astronomy, College of Science, King Saud University, Riyadh 11451, Saudi Arabia. [2] King Abdullah Institute for Nanotechnology, King Saud University, Riyadh 11451, Saudi Arabia.

Acknowledgements

The authors would like to extend their sincere appreciation to the Deanship of Scientific Research at King Saud University for its funding through research group no RG-1435-308.

Compliance with ethical guidelines

Competing interests

The authors declare that they have no competing interests.

References

1. Sun C, Lee JSH, Zhang M. Magnetic nanoparticles in MR imaging and drug delivery. Adv Drug Deliv Rev. 2008;60:1252–65.
2. Taylor EN, Webster TJ. The use of superparamagnetic nanoparticles for prosthetic biofilm prevention. Int J Nanomedicine. 2009;4:145–52.
3. Klostergaard J, Seeney CE. Magnetic nanovectors for drug delivery. Nanomedicine. 2012;8(Suppl 1):S37–50.
4. Song Q, Zhang ZJ. Correlation between spin-orbital coupling and the superparamagnetic properties in magnetite and cobalt ferrite spinel nanocrystals. J Phys Chem B. 2006;110:11205–9.
5. Willard MA, Kurihara LK, Carpenter EE, Calvin S, Harris VG. Chemically prepared magnetic nanoparticles. Int Mat Rev. 2004;49:125–70.
6. Hafeli UO, Riffle JS, Harris-Shekhawat L, Carmichael-Baranauskas A, Mark F, Dailey JP, et al. Cell uptake and in vitro toxicity of magnetic nanoparticles suitable for drug delivery. Mol Pharm. 2009;6(5):1417–28.
7. Lartigue L, Wilhelm C, Servais J, Factor C, Dencausse A, Bacri J-C, et al. Nanomagnetic sensing of blood plasma protein interactions with iron oxide nanoparticles: impact on macrophage uptake. ACS Nano. 2012;6(3):2665–78.
8. Barcena C, Sra AK, Chaubey GS, Khemtong C, Liu JP, Gao J. Zinc ferrite nanoparticles as MRI contrast agents. Chem Commun. 2008;19:2224–6.
9. Saquib Q, Al-Khedhairy AA, Ahmad J, Siddiqui MA, Dwivedi S, Khan ST, Musarrat J. Zinc ferrite nanoparticles activate IL-1b, NFKB1, CCL21 and NOS2 signaling to induce mitochondrial dependent intrinsic apoptotic pathway in WISH cells. Toxicol Appl Pharmacol. 2013;273(2):289–97.
10. Vochita G, Creanga D, Focanici-Ciurlica EL. Magnetic nanoparticle genetic impact on root tip cells of sunflower seedlings. Water Air Soil Pollut. 2012;223:2541–9.
11. Oberdorster G, Oberdorster E, Oberdorster J. Nanotoxicology: an emerging discipline evolving from studies of ultrafine particles. Environ Health Perspect. 2005;113:823–39.
12. Madl AK, Pinkerton KE. Health effects of inhaled engineered and incidental nanoparticles. Crit Rev Toxicol. 2009;39:629–58.
13. Ursini CL, Cavallo D, Fresegna AM, Ciervo A, Maiello R, Tassone P, Buresti G, Casciardi S, Iavicoli S. Evaluation of cytotoxic, genotoxic and inflammatory response in human alveolar and bronchial epithelial cells exposed to titanium dioxide nanoparticles. J Appl Toxicol. 2014;34(11):1209–19.
14. Johnston HJ, Hutchison GR, Christensen FM, Peters S, Hankin S, Stone V. Identification of the mechanisms that drive the toxicity of TiO_2 particulates: the contribution of physicochemical characteristics. Part Fibre Toxicol. 2009;6:33.
15. Chen Z, Meng H, Yuan H, Xing G, Chen C, Zhao F, et al. Identification of target organs of copper nanoparticles with ICPMS technique. J Radioanal Nucl Chem. 2007;272:599–603.
16. Wang B, Feng W, Wang M, Wang T, Gu T, Zhu M, et al. Acute toxicological impact of nano- and submicro-scaled zinc oxide powder on healthy adult mice. J Nanopart Res. 2008;2008(10):263–76.
17. Barillet S, Jugan ML, Laye M, Leconte Y, Herlin-Boime N, Reynaud C, et al. In vitro evaluation of SiC nanoparticles impact on A549 pulmonary cells: cyto-, genotoxicity and oxidative stress. Toxicol Lett. 2010;198:324–30.
18. Shukla RK, Sharma V, Pandey AK, Singh S, Sultana S, Dhawan A. ROS-mediated genotoxicity induced by titanium dioxide nanoparticles in human epidermal cells. Toxicol In Vitro. 2011;25:231–41.
19. Piret JP, Jacques D, Audinot JN, Mejia J, Boilan E. Copper (II) oxide nanoparticles penetrate into HepG2 cells, exert cytotoxicity via oxidative stress and induce pro-inflammatory response. Nanoscale. 2012;2012(4):7168–84.
20. Ahamed M, Alhadlaq HA, Alam J, Khan MA, Ali D, Alarafi S. Iron oxide nanoparticle-induced oxidative stress and genotoxicity in human skin epithelial and lung epithelial cell lines. Curr Pharm Des. 2013;19(37):6681–90.

21. Nel A, Xia T, Madler L, Li N. Toxic potential of materials at the nanolevel. Science. 2006;311:622–7.
22. Kumar A, Pandey AK, Singh SS, Shanker R, Dhawan A. Engineered ZnO and TiO(2) nanoparticles induce oxidative stress and DNA damage leading to reduced viability of *Escherichia coli*. Free Radic Biol Med. 2011;51(10):1872–81.
23. Sharma V, Anderson D, Dhawan A. Zinc oxide nanoparticles induce oxidative DNA damage and ROS-triggered mitochondria mediated apoptosis in human liver cells (HepG2). Apoptosis. 2012;17(8):852–70.
24. Magdolenova Z, Collins A, Kumar A, Dhawan A, Stone V, Dusinska M. Mechanisms of genotoxicity. A review of in vitro and in vivo studies with engineered nanoparticles. Nanotoxicology. 2014;8(3):233–78.
25. Ahamed M, Akhtar MJ, Siddiqui MA, Ahmad J, Musarrat J, Al-Khedhairy AA, Alrokayan SA. Oxidative stress mediated apoptosis induced by nickel ferrite nanoparticles in cultured A549 cells. Toxicology. 2011;2011(283):101–8.
26. Ahamed M, Akhtar MJ, Alhadlaq HA, Khan MAM, Alrokayan SA. Comparative cytotoxic response of nickel ferrite nanoparticles in human liver HepG2 and breast MFC-7 cancer cells. Chemosphere. 2015;135:278–88.
27. Murdock RC, Braydich-Stolle L, Schrand AM, Schlager JJ, Hussain SM. Characterization of nanomaterial dispersion in solution prior to in vitro exposure using dynamic light scattering technique. Toxicol Sci. 2008;101:239–53.
28. Mossman T. Rapid colorimetric assay for cellular growth and survival: application to proliferation and cytotoxicity assays. J Immunol Methods. 1983;65:55–63.
29. Wang H, Joseph JA. Quantifying cellular oxidative stress by dichlorofluorescin assay using microplate reader. Free Radic Biol Med. 1999;27:612–6.
30. Siddiqui MA, Alhadlaq HA, Ahmad J, Al-Khedhairy AA, Musarrat J, Ahamed M. Copper oxide nanoparticles induced mitochondria mediated apoptosis in human hepatocarcinoma cells. PLoS One. 2013;8:e69534.
31. Ahmad J, Ahamed M, Akhtar MJ, Alrokayan SA, Siddiqui MA, Musarrat J, Al-Khedhairy AA. Apoptosis induction by amorphous silica nanoparticles mediated through reactive oxygen species generation in human liver cell line HepG2. Toxicol Appl Pharmacol. 2012;259:160–8.
32. Ellman GI. Tissue sulfhydryl groups. Arch Biochem Biophys. 1959;82:70–7.
33. Zhang Y, Jiang L, Jiang L, Geng C, Li L, Shao J, Zhong L. Possible involvement of oxidative stress in potassium bromateinduced genotoxicity in human HepG2 cells. Chem Biol Int. 2011;189:186–91.
34. Ahamed M, Alhadlaq HA. Nickel nanoparticle-induced dose-dependent cyto-genotoxicity in human breast carcinoma MCF-7cells. Onco Targets Ther. 2014;7:269–80.
35. Berasain C, Garcia-Trevijano ER, Castillo J, Erroba E, Santamaria M, Lee DC. Novel role for amphiregulin in protection from liver injury. J Biol Chem. 2005;280:19012–20.
36. Bradford MM. A rapid and sensitive method for the quantitation of microgram quantities of protein utilizing the principle of protein-dye binding. Anal Biochem. 1976;72:248–54.
37. Ahamed M, AlSalhi MS, Siddiqui MKJ. Silver nanoparticle applications and human health. Clin Chim Acta. 2010;411:1841–8.
38. Horev-Azaria L, Baldi G, Beno D, Bonacchi D, Golla-Schindler U, Kirkpatrick JC, et al. Predictive toxicology of cobalt ferrite nanoparticles: comparative in vitro study of different cellular models using methods of knowledge discovery from data. Part Fibre Toxicol. 2013;10:32.
39. Yu KO, Grabinski CM, Schrand AM, Murdock RC, Wang W, Gu B, et al. Toxicity of amorphous silica nanoparticles in mouse keratinocytes. J Nanopart Res. 2009;11:15–24.
40. Sharma V, Shukla RK, Saxena N, Parmar D, Das M, Dhawan A. DNA damaging potential of zinc oxide nanoparticles in human epidermal cells. Toxicol Lett. 2009;185:211–8.
41. Bai W, Zhang Z, Tian W, He X, Ma Y, Zhao Y, Chai Z. Toxicity of zinc oxide nanoparticles to zebrafish embryo: a physicochemical study of toxicity mechanism. J Nanopart Res. 2009;12:1645–54.
42. Ahamed M, Posgai R, Gorey TJ, Nielsen M, Hussain S, Rowe J. Silver nanoparticles induced heat shock protein 70, oxidative stress and apoptosis in *Drosophila melanogaster*. Toxicol Appl Pharmacol. 2010;242:263–9.
43. Lundqvist M, Stigler J, Elia G, Lynch I, Cerdevall T, Dawson K. Nanoparticle size and surface properties determine the protein corona with possible implications for biological impacts. Proc Natl Acad Sci USA. 2008;105:14265–70.
44. Lynch I, Dawson K. Protein–nanoparticle interactions. Nanotoday. 2008;3:40–7.
45. Mahmoudi M, Laurent S, Shokrgozar MA, Hosseinkhani M. Toxicity evaluations of superparamagnetic iron oxide nanoparticles: cell "vision" versus physicochemical properties of nanoparticles. ACS Nano. 2011;5:7263–6.
46. Hussain S, Thomassen L, Ferecatu I, Borot MC, Andreau K, Martens J, et al. Carbon black and titanium dioxide nanoparticles elicit distinct apoptotic pathways in bronchial epithelial cells. Part Fibre Toxicol. 2010;7:10.
47. Saquib Q, Al-Khedhairy AA, Siddiqui MA, Abou-Tarboush FM, Azam A, Musarrat J. Titanium dioxide nanoparticles induced cytotoxicity, oxidative stress and DNA damage in human amnion epithelial (WISH) cells. Toxicol In Vitro. 2012;2012(26):351–61.
48. Singh N, Jenkins GJS, Nelson BC, Marquis BJ, Maffeis TGG, Brown AP, et al. The role of iron redox state in the genotoxicity of ultrafine superparamagnetic iron oxide nanoparticles. Biomaterials. 2012;33:163–70.
49. Soenen SJH, Himmelreich U, Nuytten N, Pisanic TR, Ferrari A, De Cuyper M. Intracellular nanoparticle coating stability determines nanoparticle diagnostics efficacy and cell functionality. Small. 2010;6:2136–45.
50. Kruszewski M, Iwaneńko T. Labile iron pool correlates with iron content in the nucleus and the formation of oxidative DNA damage in mouse lymphoma L5178Y cell lines. Acta Biochim Pol. 2003;50:211–5.
51. Petrat F, de Groot H, Rauen U. Subcellular distribution of chelatable iron: a laser scanning microscopic study in isolated hepatocytes and liver endothelial cells. Biochem J. 2001;356:61–9.
52. Cairns RA, Harris IS, Mak TW. Regulation of cancer cell metabolism. Nat Rev Cancer. 2011;11(2):85–95.
53. Al-Qubaisi MS, Rasedee A, Flaifel MH, Ahmad SH, Hussein-Al-Ali S, Hussein MZ, et al. Cytotoxicity of nickel zinc ferrite nanoparticles on cancer cells of epithelial origin. Int J Nanomedicine. 2013;8:2497–508.
54. Porter AG, Jänicke RU. Emerging roles of caspase-3 in apoptosis. Cell Death Differ. 1999;6:99–104.
55. Farnebo M, Bykov VN, Wiman KG. The p53 tumor suppressor: a master regulator of diverse cellular processes and therapeutic target in cancer. Biochem Biophys Res Commun. 2010;396:85–9.

14

The expansion of autologous adipose-derived stem cells in vitro for the functional reconstruction of nasal mucosal tissue

Xiao Xu, Liang Li, Cheng Wang, Yang Liu, Chong Chen, Junling Yan, Hong Ding and Su-yang Tang*

Abstract

Background: It is established that adipose-derived stem cells (ADSCs) produce and secrete cytokines/growth factors that antagonize mucosal injury. However, the exact molecular basis underlying the treatment effects exerted by ADSCs is ill understood, and whether ADSCs cooperate with adipose tissue particles to improve mucosal function in patients with empty nose syndrome (ENS) has not been explored. We investigated the impact of ADSCs on nasal mucosa, the associated mechanisms, and their use in the treatment of patients with ENS.

Results: The nasal endoscope and mucociliary clearance assessments were significantly improved ($P < 0.05$) in patients with ($n = 28$) and without ($n = 2$) a rudimentary turbinate that received ADSCs combined with fat granules transplantation. Patients experienced a significant improvement in nasal obstruction and nasal mucociliary clearance after nasal turbinate angioplasty ($P < 0.05$). H&E staining, Masson's staining, and AB-PAS staining confirmed that inflammation was significantly reduced, collagenous fibers became aligned, fewer deposits were observed, and the mucosal proteins generated from caliciform cells increased following treatment. After a 14-day incubation period, ADSCs developed a polygonal cobblestone shape characteristic of human epithelial cells. Furthermore, immunohistochemical analysis revealed the presence of epithelial markers such as cytokeratin-7, and cytokeratin-19. Western blot analysis showed the presence of specific epithelial cell markers including cytokeratin-7, cytokeratin-14 and cytokeratin-19 in these epithelial like cells (ELC); these markers had low expression levels of ADSCs.

Conclusions: The reconstruction of mucosal function by nasal turbinate angioplasty combined with ADSCs and autologous adipose tissue particle transplantation significantly improved the symptoms of patients with ENS. This is a new procedure that will improve mucosal restoration treatment options in patients with ENS. Furthermore, we undertook preliminary explorations of the underlying mechanisms involved, and found that transplantation of ADSCs could induce epithelial cells to improve mucosa function in patients with ENS in the micro-environment of injection areas.

Keywords: Adipose derived stem cells, Empty nose syndrome, Turbinate reconstruction, Nasal mucosa

Background

In recent years, rapid developments in regenerative medicine have identified seed cells and applicable cell stroma for tissue engineering to restore tissue damage. Adipose-derived stem cells (ADSCs) are excellent tissue engineering seed cells with several advantages compared to other stem cells: they are abundant in source, easy to find and culture, not rejected, safe, will undergo translayer multiple differentiation, and proliferate rapidly [1–4]. Empty nose syndrome (ENS) is an iatrogenic disorder most often recognized by the presence of paradoxical nasal obstruction despite an objectively wide, patent nasal fossa. The term 'empty nose syndrome' was initially used to describe certain symptoms associated with tissue

*Correspondence: 2278645614@qq.com
Skin and Reconstructive Medicine Department, The General Hospital of Chinese People's Armed Police Forces, Beijing, People's Republic of China

loss and radiographic findings of a paucity of normal anatomic structures within the nasal cavities. After the removal of the inferior nasal concha, 20 % of patients will develop ENS [5, 6]. The severity of the subjective sensation caused by ENS does not correlate with the findings of objective examinations and can cause conflict between patients and doctors. There is no established treatment for the nasal symptoms experienced by patients with ENS; developing such treatments is an important clinical priority.

Results

ADSC transplantation improved nasal mucosal clinical symptoms

Flow cytometric analysis demonstrated that ADSCs were positive for CD73, CD90, and CD105, and negative for CD19, CD34, CD45, and HLA-DR (Fig. 1). The ADSCs were also capable of osteogenic and adipogenic differentiation when cultured in the appropriate inducing media. Assessment of the degree of osteogenic and adipogenic diffentiation via Alizarin Red S and Oil Red O staining, respectively, revealed good results (Fig. 2). Following the transplantation of ADSCs and fat particles into the areas of nasal damage to form turbinates, 30 ENS patients displayed no signs of infection or allergy. Of these patients, symptoms improved in 28, including increased moistening of the nasal mucosa, decreased tension of the mucosa and of nasal cavity pain when breathing, and improved quality of sleep. Two patients experienced improvement of nasal cavity dryness. However, excessive breathing remained an issue.

ADSCs transplantation improved the function of the nasal mucosa in patients with ENS

Nasal endoscopy was conducted 3 months after treatment, and the nasal cavities of patients were visibly more erythematous, secreted more mucus and had fewer scabs (Fig. 3).

Mucociliary clearance (MCC) assessments

Saccharine clearance times were 1526.23 $\pm$ 1000.43 s preoperatively, 1457.13 $\pm$ 1078.23 s at 3 months follow-up, 1232.03 $\pm$ 499.45 s at 6 months follow-up, and 1501.00 $\pm$ 1159.85 s at 9 months follow-up. Mucociliary clearance assessments showed improvement of saccharine clearance times in the study group at 3 and 6 months postoperatively (Fig. 4).

Acoustic rhinometry assessments: ADSCs improved nasal resistance and mucociliary clearance assessments, and reduced the nasal volumes and the cross-sectional areas of the nasal cavities of patients with ENS

Acoustic rhinometry assessments showed improvements in nasal resistance (NAR), mucociliary clearance assessments (MCCs), nasal volumes (NVs), and in the minimum cross-sectional areas (MCAs) of the nasal cavities of patients at 3, 6, and 9 months postoperatively. The improvements in NAR and in MCAs were not statistically significant at 3 and 6 months after surgery, but where so, when compared to the initial visit, 9 months after surgery ($^*P < 0.05$). The values of NV reduced after the implantation surgery and the change of NV average overall scores were statistically significant between the initial visit versus those of 3 and 9 months after treatment ($^*P < 0.05$). One patient has been observed over a period of 18 months. The symptoms of nasal crusting and difficulty with nasal breathing improved further (data not shown). The acoustic rhinometry and endoscopic imaging findings were not significantly different 9 months after surgery. However, the saccharine clearance time was greatly improved at 18 months compared to that at 12 months after surgery (data not shown) (Fig. 4).

ADSC transplantation treatment improved the histological appearance of the nasal mucosa of patients with ENS

Lymphocytes and neutrophils infiltrated the nasal mucosa prior to ADSCs injection (Fig. 5a). After ADSCs injection, the nasal mucosa section had fewer infiltrated lymphocytes and neutrophils 30 days following treatment (Fig. 5b). Deposits of thickened and disorganized collagenous fibers were seen using Mason's staining between the glands in the nasal mucosa prior to ADSC injection (Fig. 5c). Thirty days later, the collagenous fibers were aligned in the nasal mucosa, and collagenous fiber deposition was decreased in the glands (Fig. 5d). As revealed by AB-PAS staining of mucosa tissue, mucosal proteins generated from cyathiform cells were limited and the submucosal glands showed compensatory hyperplasia (Fig. 5e). Thirty days later the mucosal proteins generated from cyathiform cells were evenly distributed throughout the nasal mucosa (Fig. 5f).

Differentiated human ADSCs expressed epithelial markers

After 14 days of ADSC culture in a differentiating medium containing 20–30 ng/ml EGF, 20–30 % of the cells acquired a rounded/polygonal shape. They proliferated, and formed an adherent monolayer, organized in cobblestone-pattern clusters (Fig. 6). While pure populations of ADSCs downregulated the expression of cytokeratin 19 (CK19), immunohistochemical analysis revealed that the differentiated cells from the dark blue cobblestone-pattern clusters were positive for CK19 (Fig. 6). Microscopic analysis using Lucia software (Nikon Corporation Co., Kanagawa, Japan), showed that these constituted approximately 60 % of the total cells.

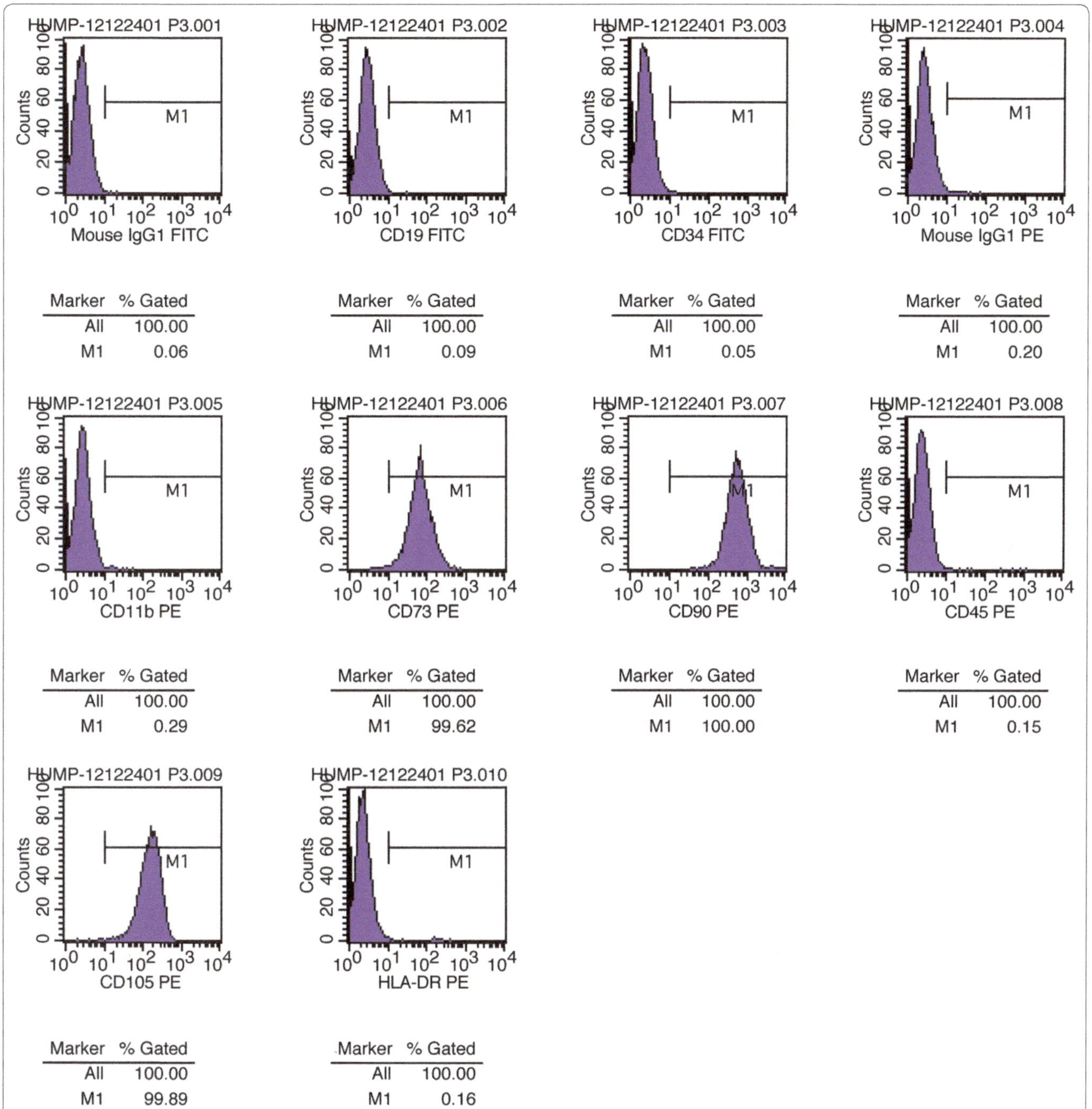

Fig. 1 Flow cytometric analysis. ADSCs are positive for CD73, CD90, and CD105, and negative for CD19, CD34, CD45, and HLA-DR

Sustained upregulation of CK7, CK14 and CK19 in ADSCs leads to an increase in and the activation of epithelial-like cells revealed by western blotting

To demonstrate the progressive epithelial determination of ADSCs, multiple markers specific for epithelial cells were selected and evaluated using western blot analysis. As shown in Fig. 7, cytokeratin-7 (CK7), cytokeratin-14 (CK14), and cytokeratin-19 (CK19) were mainly expressed in epithelial-like cells (ELC), but rarely in ADSCs.

Discussion

ENS often occurs several months or years following nasal cavity surgery, and the diagnosis mainly relies on objective symptoms, signs, and the clinical history. Researchers have hypothesized that decreased nasal

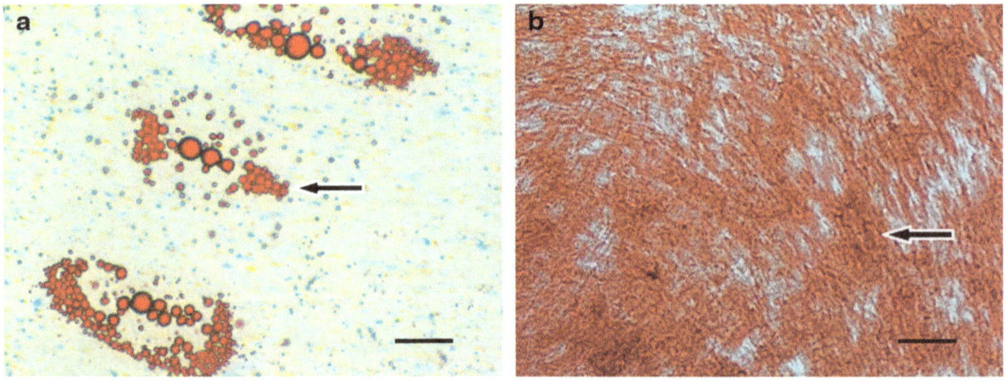

Fig. 2 Characterization of ADSCs. Adipogenic differentiation of ADSCs was assessed by Oil Red O staining. The *arrow* indicates a lipid droplet. The osteogenic ability of the ADSCs was assessed using Alizarin *red* staining. The *arrow* shows a calcium nodule. Magnification: ×400 (**a**) and ×400 (**b**)

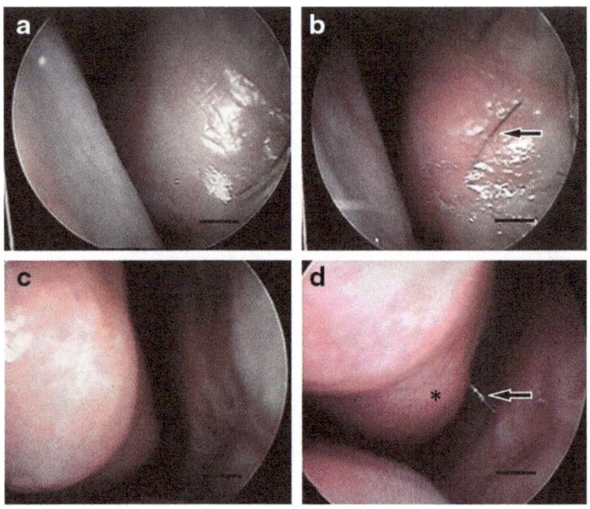

Fig. 3 Nasal endoscopy. Prior to the injection of fat tissue combined with ADSCs (**a**, **c**). Recovery of the nasal turbinate morphology (*Asterisk* was shown). The nasal mucosa rhinothrix has grown (**b**, indicated by the *arrow*). The nasal cavity became more erythematous, and secreted more mucus (**d**, indicated by the *arrow*)

mucosa and changes in nasal resistance participate in the occurrence of ENS [7]. The nasal mucosa has glands and receptors to heat, humidify, and clean the inspired air, as well as immune functions. The specific anatomical structure of the nose adjusts the nasal cavity airflow and laminar conditions. Patients with ENS complain of reduced quality of life as a result of reduced nasal functions.

The protection of the nasal mucosa and prevention of ENS following nasal cavity surgeries are a major concern among otolaryngologists. Surgeons use hydroxyapatite, autogenous cartilage [8], Medpor, Gore-Tex, or acellular dermal tissue to support the nasal mucosa of patients with ENS and improve nasal resistance and ventilation. These treatments are effective, but their effect on the recovery of ENS mucosa function is unclear.

This study identified that the injection of ADSCs combined with fat particles during intranasal minimal invasive-turbinate shaping surgery to treat ENS is an effective treatment option. ADSCs possess many advantages, including a wide range of sources, easy access, minor tissue damage after injections, rapid proliferation, a stable phenotype and heredity, low immunogenicity, and the potential to differentiate into mesoblastic adipose cells, osteoblasts, chondrocyte, vADSCsular endothelial cells, and epidermal cells, among others. The expansion of ADSCs in vitro will increase the rate of survival of transplanted cells, and improve the revADSCsularization of transplanted cells, decrease the rate of absorption, liquefaction, and fat cell infection for a successful single transplant shaping effect [8–10]. Patients given this treatment experience an improvement of symptoms associated with dryness of the nasal cavity and contradictory nasal resistance [11]. Although contradictory nasal resistance indicates that patients feel a subjective nasal obstruction, it is not consistent with nasal examinations that find substantially widened nasal cavity volumes [12]. Following surgery, the heating and humidifying functions of nasal cavity patients were greatly improved, and the pain in the face and nasal cavity disappear when breathing, which resulted in improved quality of sleep. Therefore, ADSCs and fat particles used in intranasal minimal invasive-turbinate shaping surgery, rebuild the ENS nasal mucosa of patients, enhance the area of turbinate mucosa, and improve nasal cavity physiological functioning.

All body surfaces and cavities, including the skin, gastrointestinal tract, urogenital system and breast ducts are lined by epithelial tissue. This provides a protective barrier. Cell loss from it must be precisely balanced by cell

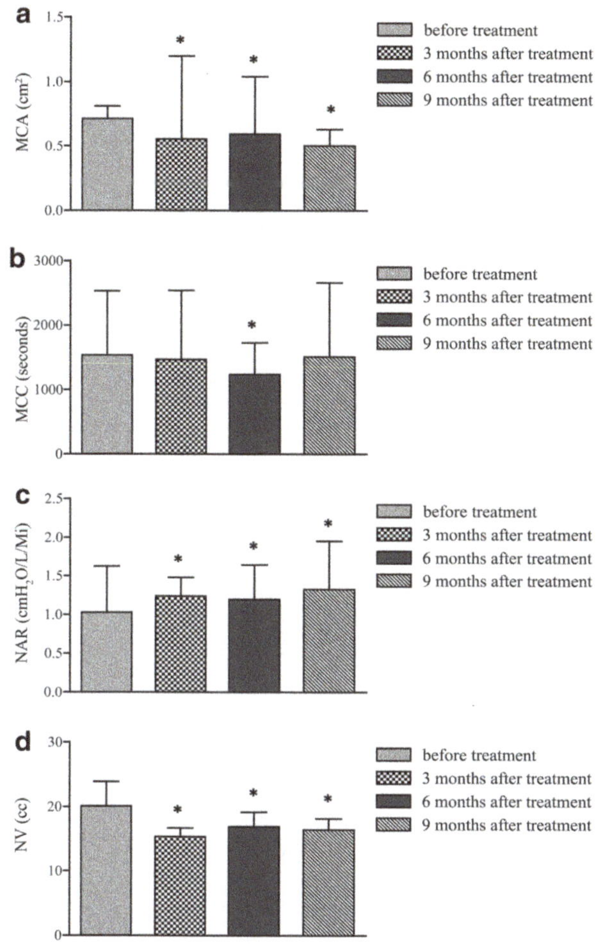

Fig. 4 Values of nasal resistance, Nasal volume, Minimum cross-sectional area, and mucociliary clearance before and after surgery. **a** After ADSC injection, the MCA of the nasal cavity is decreased. **b** After ADSCs injection, the MCC of the nasal cilium is decreased. **c** After ADSC injection, the NAR of the nasal cavity is increased. **d** After ADSC injection, the NV of the nasal cavity is increased. All values are presented as mean ± SD, n = 28, *P < 0.05

production, in order to maintain epithelial homeostasis. The source of the cells involved in tissue repair after injury is largely unknown and is controversial. One possible source is stem-like progenitor cells. These are probably the most important, but are rare components of the proliferative compartment of epithelial tissues. They have been identified in a variety of tissues including neural [13], vADSCsular [14], hepatic [15], pancreatic [16] and epidermal [17]. Several studies have shown that MSCs, HSCs and unfractionated bone-marrow derived cells can give rise, in vivo, to epithelial cell types in lung and other tissues [18–21].

The nasal epithelial coils have two important functions; they act as a protective barrier and are involved in the transport of ions and water. Epithelial ion and water transportation is the basis of mucociliary transport [22–26].

Nasal mucosa epithelial cells are mainly composed of four types of cells: ciliated columnar cells, Non-ciliated columnar epithelium (75 %), basal cells (5 %) and mucous cells [27, 28]. Basal cells are located in the deepest parts of the epithelial layer, and are anchored to the basilar membrane by hemidesmosomes [29], were not exposed to the cavosurface of cells layer. CK 14 is expressed on their surface. Basal cells have the ability to differentiate into the mucus cilium, and they have important roles in epithelial injury repair [28, 30]. CK7 and CK19 are amongst the most basic cell keratin groups in nasal epithelial cells [31]. We concluded that the increase of cytokine 7, 14 and 19 secretion from ELC enhanced the number of basal cells in the transplantation area available for differentiating into mucus cilium, and that this improved the nasal mucosa function in patients with ENS. In addition, undoubtedly, ADSC transplantation also increased the survival of transplanted adipocytes. Both mechanisms may play a part in shaping the turbinate and increasing the area of the nasal mucosa.

This study used fat particles combined with ADSCs during intranasal minimally invasive, turbinate shaping surgery in 30 patients with ENS. The results indicate that the treatment was effective. However, further research will be needed to verify the clinical effect and mechanism of action of ADSC injections.

Conclusion

We found evidence that ADSC transplantation treatment improved the nasal mucosa function of patients with ENS, and that combined use of both treatments synergistically reconstructed the turbinate morphology of patients with ENS. Mechanistically, ADSC transplantation improved the function of epithelial cell by up-regulating the expression of CK7, 14, 19 caused by the nasal mucosa injury micro-environment. However, ENS nasal mucosa reconstruction is complex, involving a multitude of signaling pathways and a variety of molecules. Consequently, other molecular mechanisms may also contribute to the beneficial effects seen with ADSC transplantation, and deserve to be the focus of future investigations.

Methods

Clinical data

Patients with ENS treated in the Skin Regeneration Department and Otolaryngological Department of the General Hospital of the Armed Police Forces between August 2014 and January 2015 were studied. The SCL-90 physiological Methods Symptom Check List (250 below), Self-Rating Anxiety Scale (SAS, medium below), and

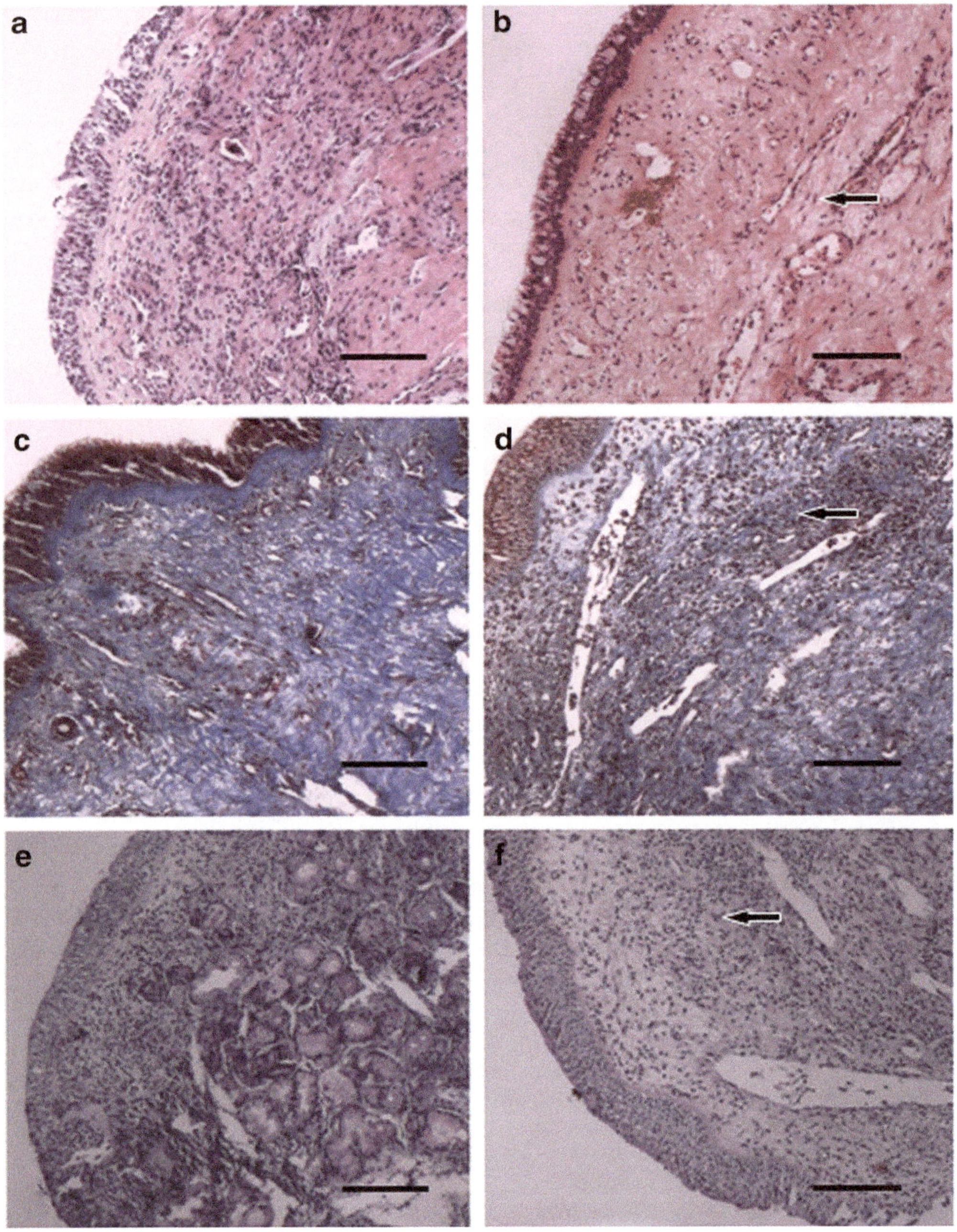

Fig. 5 H&E staining, Masson's staining and AB-PAS staining. Prior to the injection of ADSCs (**a**, **c**) compared to the findings 30 days after the injection of ADSCs (**b**, **d**), the nasal mucosa was infiltrated with lymphocytes and neutrophils (**b**). Furthermore, the collagenous fibers became aligned and collagenous fiber deposition (*arrow*) decreased after treatment (**d**). After AB-PAS staining for mucosa tissue, each group of mucosa shows as followed figures **e** and **f**. Mucosal proteins generated from cyathiform cell were discontinued, and the gland under mucosa experience compensatory hyperplasia (**e**); 30 days after ADSC injections (**f**), mucosal proteins generated from the cyathiform cell were evenly distributed throughout the nasal mucosa

Self-Rating Depression Scale (SDS, medium below) were used to identify participants. We chose 30 patients, 20 men and 10 women, aged between 22 and 30 years (average 26), with secondary ENS caused by a bilateral nasal cavity operation. All patients were in good health without any systemic diseases. The symptoms of the subjects were described as aridity of the nasal mucosa, excessive ventilator function, dry and cold inspiration, and poor sleep

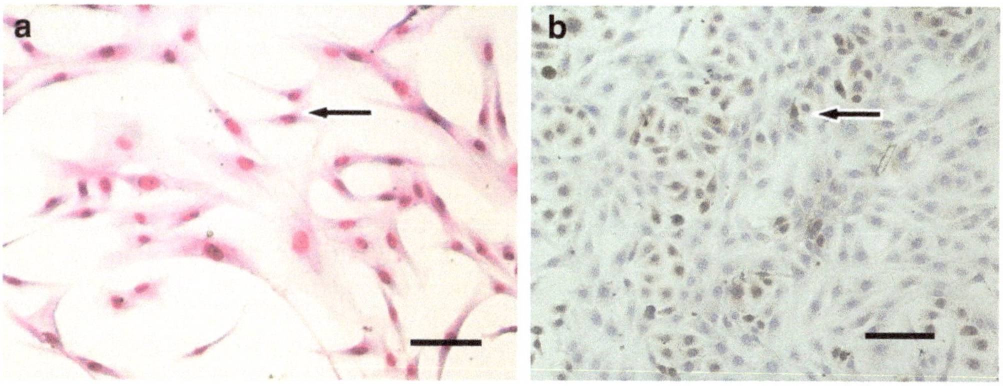

Fig. 6 Epithelial-like morphology. The ADSCs with a fusiform shape after Giemsa's staining were used as negative controls. Immunocytochemical analysis of the differentiated cells from cobblestone-pattern clusters (*arrow*) showed that they were positive for CK-19. Magnification: ×40 (**a**) and ×400 (**b**). *Scale bars* are 100 μm

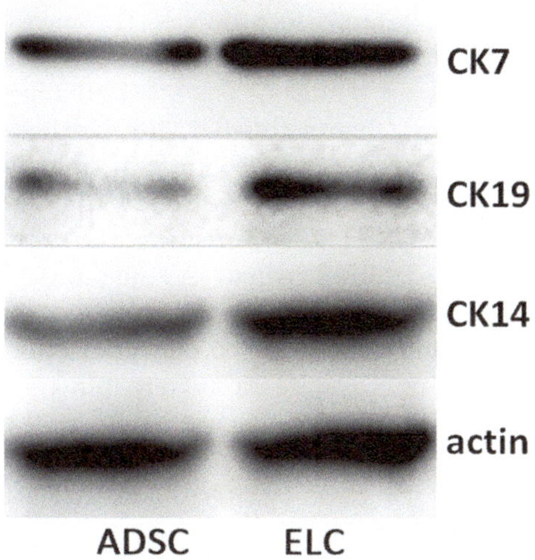

Fig. 7 ELC expression of epithelial markers. We evaluated ADSC trans-differentiation into ELC using several epithelial markers, including CK7, CK14 and CK19. Western blot analysis ELC showed high expression of CK7, CK14 and CK19 proteins. However, a small number of bands were detected in ADSCs

quality. Each patient was inspected by nasal endoscopy using the Sino-Nasal Outcome Test 20 (SNOT-20) [32], nasal sound resistance, and nasal mucociliary clearance investigations prior to surgery. All patients gave written informed consent. The study was approved by the Board of Ethics of the General Hospital of the Chinese Armed Police Forces.

Isolation and preparation of ADSCs

Each individual was tested for communicable diseases by regular antigen-specific antibody examinations (including for hepatitis, syphilis, and AIDS), to ensure that they were in good health. Approximately 15–20 ml of fat particles was extracted from the lower abdomen and thigh by liposuction. The samples were treated with 0.1 % collagenase, trypsin digestion, and centrifuged to remove fat. The cells were re-suspended and filtered through a 200-mesh sieve, and the samples were centrifuged again in order to split red blood cells. The cells were then washed twice in PBS, and the extracted cells were re-suspended in high glucose DMEM containing 15 % fetal bovine serum at an appropriate density in a sterile culture dish. After 4–5 days, media was added to the cells and they were passaged every subsequent 3 days by 0.05 % trypsin digestion when the cells reached a density of 85 %. At the third generation (P3), all cells were examined and free of mycoplasma, human originated particular virus, and endotoxin in accordance with the People's Republic of China pharmacopoeia 2010 (edition 3, Appendix A). Tests to confirm cell form and activity, karyotype, and ADSC immunophenotype were also all normal.

Immunophenotyping by flow cytometry

ADSC surface marker analysis using flow cytometry was performed on a FACS Calibur unit (Becton–Dickinson Biosciences, San Jose, CA, USA). Cells were stained with phycoerythrin-conjugated antibodies for CD19, CD34, CD11b, CD105, CD73, CD90, CD45 and HLA-DR (Becton–Dickinson Biosciences). For osteogenic and adipogenic differentiation, ADSCs were incubated with MesenCult Osteogenic or Adipogenic Stimulatory Medium (STEMCELL Technologies, Vancouver, Canada) for 2–3 weeks. Osteogenic and adipogenic differentiation was evaluated using Alizarin Red S and Oil Red O (Sigma-Aldrich, St. Louis, MO, USA) staining, respectively.

Adipogenic and Osteogenic differentiation

ADSCs were further tested for their ability to differentiate into adipogenic lineages [33]. To achieve this, ADSCs were seeded in 12-well plates at a concentration of 46104 cells/ml and cultured in adipogenic differentiation medium (StemPro, Gibco, and Grand Island, NY). After 7 days in culture, cells were fixed in 4 % paraformaldehyde and the intracellular lipid content were visualized using Oil Red O. Briefly, cells were fixed with 10 % formalin for 1 h at room temperature. Then, they were washed with DI water and prepared by adding 60 % isopropanol for 5 min at room temperature. After 5 min, the isopropanol was discarded and the cells were incubated with Oil Red O working solution (Fisher Scientific) for 5 min at room temperature. The Cells were then washed with tap water. Hematoxilin was used as counterstaining. For osteogenic differentiation, ADSCs were incubated with MesenCult Osteogenic Stimulatory Medium (STEMCELL Technologies, Vancouver, Canada)for 2–3 weeks. Osteogenic differentiation was evaluated using Alizarin Red S and (Sigma-Aldrich St. Louis, MO, USA) staining, respectively.

Transplantation of ADSCs and fat particles to form a turbinate plasty

We treated 30 patients with ENS; some had residual turbinates. ADSC injection into areas of nasal mucosa damage were conducted every 10 days for a total of four injections. For the two ENS patients without residual turbinate tissues, the injection of ADSCs to areas of nasal mucosal damage were conducted every 10 days for three injections; furthermore, 1–5 ml autogenous fat particles were extracted, and then mixed with 1×10^7–5×10^7 ADSCs (third to sixth generation), under the inferior or middle turbinate. Nasal endoscopy, nasal sound resistance, and nasal mucociliary clearance examinations were conducted at 3, 6, and 9 months after treatment.

Outcome measurements

The data of symptom scores, endoscopy, mucociliary clearance (MCC), and acoustic rhinometry (Danish Rhinomanometer RhinoScan 2000, Interacostics A/S, Assens, Denmark) were gathered before and 3, 6, and 9 months after surgery. We also evaluated the mean value of nasal resistance (NAR), nasal volume (NV), and nasal minimum cross-sectional area (MCA) through an acoustic rhinometry examination. NAR is calculated according to Ohm's law: $1/R = 1/Rr + 1/Rl$ (R = total nasal resistance, Rr = right nasal cavity resistance, Rl = left nasal cavity resistance). NV is calculated according to the following formula: $NV = Vr + Vl$ (NV = total nasal volume, Vr = volume of the right nasal cavity, Vl = volume of the left nasal cavity). MCA is the average cross-sectional area of the bilateral nasal cavities. The assessment of MCC was determined with the saccharine method [34].

Tissue histological analysis

Nasal mucosa (0.1×0.1 cm^2) were resected before and 30 days after the injections began and fixed in 10 % formalin neutral buffered solution, embedded in polyester wax and sectioned into 6-mm slices on polylysine-coated glass slides. The sections were subjected to hematoxylin & eosin (H&E), Masson's trichrome, immunohistochemistry, and Alcian blue-periodic acid-Schiff (AB-PAS) staining.

Masson's trichome staining was performed with a kit from Sigma (St. Louis, MO, USA) according to the manufacturer's protocol. The collagen fibers were stained blue and myocardium was stained red. Immunohistochemistry for collagen I was performed using the SABC kit (Maxim, Fuzhou, China) according to the manufacturer's instructions. The tissue sections were incubated with primary antibodies against collagen I (1:50 dilution) overnight at 4 °C, and then incubated with biotinylated secondary antibody for 30 min at room temperature followed by 30 min of incubation with streptavidin peroxidase (Dako LSAB + HRP kit). After rinsing the samples, the sections were visualized using DAB and the slides were counterstained with hematoxylin. All fields was taken under a light microscope at 200× magnification.

For AB-PAS staining, tissue sections were immersed in a solution of alcian blue and 3 % acetic acid for 30 min. Samples were then immersed in Schiff's reagent for 15 min to promote oxidation before undergoing a final counterstain in hematoxylin.

Differentiation of ADSCs to epithelial-like cells

Human ADSCs obtained as described above were plated in uncoated flasks and entered into the differentiation process at the second passage (usually 35–42 days from the initial isolation). The culture medium was DMEM low-glucose (1 g/l) with 10 % FBS, initially supplemented with 8 μg/l epidermal growth factor (EGF, Peprotech Inc., Rocky Hill, USA), and 30 % conditioned medium [35]. After 7–14 days from the initial plating, when the cells acquired a rounded or polygonal shape, the expression of the epithelial marker, cytokeratin 19, was assessed.

Western blot analysis

Briefly, human ADSC samples and epithelial-like cells were selected using the same method, lysed in RIPA buffer and protein lysates and were separated on 8 % SDS polyacryamide gel by electrophoresis. The proteins were transferred to PVDF membranes, which were incubated with CK7 antibody (Abcam, USA), CK19 antibody (Abcam, USA), CK14 antibody (Abcam, USA), and actin (BOSTER, Wuhan, China). The membranes were washed and incubated with horseradish peroxidase-conjugated anti-goat IgG antibody (BOSTER, Wuhan, China). The blots were visualized with chemiluminescence.

Statistical analysis

SPSS 19.0 software (SPSS Inc., Chicago, IL, USA) was used to conduct statistical analysis and results are shown as the mean ± SD. One-way analysis of variance was used to compare groups, and we further compared groups of two by a one-way analysis of variance analysis. Statistical significance was set at $P < 0.05$.

Authors' contributions

XX carried out most of the experiments and drafted the manuscript; LL carried out the in vivo studies; CC and CW assisted in the in vitro and vivo studies; LY participated in the design of the studies; JLW and LY participated in the design of the studies; YZ participated in the design of the studies; SYT conceived the studies, coordinated the experiments and was involved in the drafting the manuscript and revising it. All authors read and approved the final manuscript.

Acknowledgements

We would like to express our gratitude to Minghui Li, who is from Liao Ning Medical College, for his contribution to patient work, and we would also like to thank Xiaobing Wu, who is from Military Medical Sciences, for her contribution to analysis and interpretation of ADSCs with flow cytometry.

Compliance with ethical guidelines

Competing interests

The authors declare that they have no competing interests.

References

1. Zuk PA, Zhu M, Mizuno H, et al. Multilineage cells from human adipose tissue: implications for cell-based therapies. Tissue Eng. 2001;7(2):211–28.
2. Gimble JM, Katz AJ, Bunnell BA. Adipose-derived stem cells for regenerative medicine. Circ Res. 2007;100(9):1249–60.
3. Fraser JK, Wulur I, Alfonso Z, Hedrick MH. Fat tissue: an under appreciated source of stem cells for biotechnology. Trends Biotechnol. 2006;24(4):150–4.
4. Zavan B, Michelotto L, Lancerotto L, et al. Neural potential of a stem cell Feb. 32(1):47–54.
5. Chhabra N, Houser SM. The diagnosis and management of empty nose syndrome. Otolaryngol Clin North Am. 2009;42(2):311–30.
6. Bhandarkar ND, Smith TL. Outcomes of surgery for inferiorturbinate hypertrophy. Curr Opin Otolaryngol Head Neck Surg. 2010;18(1):49–53.
7. Naftali S, Rosenfeld M, Wolf M, et al. The air-conditioning capacity of the human nose. Ann Biomed Eng. 2005;33(4):545–53.
8. Tang SY, Li Y, Yan JL, et al. Clinical studies in vitro amplification of autologous fat stem cells mediated by autologous fat transplantation. Chin Med Biotechnol. 2013;8(6):433–8.
9. Yan JL, Di GH, Ding H, et al. Auto-adipose stem cells facilitate autologous fat transfer for breast augmentation. Chin J Tissue Eng. 2013;17(5):878–85.
10. Xu YW, Liu LP, Xu YF. Effects of adipose tissues derived stem cells compounding with type I collagen on growth of transplanted tissue in nude mice. J Zhengzhou Univ (Med Sci). 2014;49(2):255–7.
11. Dipak S, Prepageran N, Haslinda S, et al. The role of sensation in subjective and objective evaluation of nasal patency. Indian J Otolaryngol Head Neck Surg. 2011;63(1):10–4.
12. Houser SM. Surgical treatment for empty nose syndrome. Arch Otolaryngol Head Neck Surg. 2007;133(9):858–63.
13. Gage HH, et al. Mammalian neural stem cells. Science. 2000;287:1433–8.
14. Kuznetsov SA, Mankani MH, Gronthos S, Satomura K, Bianco P, Robey PG. Circulating skeletal stem cells. J Cell Biol. 2001;153:1133–9.
15. Alison MR, Poulsom R, Forbes SJ. Update on hepatic stem cells. Liver. 2001;21:367–73.
16. Bonner-Weir S, Sharma A. Pancreatic stem cells. J Pathol. 2002;197:519–26.
17. Janes SM, Lowell S, Hutter C. Epidermal stem cells. J Pathol. 2002;197:479–91.
18. Krause DS, Theise ND, Collector MI, Henegariu O, Hwang S, Gardner R, Neutzel S, Sharkis SJ. Multiorgan, multi-lineage engraftment by a single bone marrow-derived stem cell. Cell. 2001;105:369–77.
19. Kotton DN, Ma BY, Cardoso WV, Sanderson EA, Summer RS, Williams MC, Fine A. Bone marrow derived cells as progenitors of lung alveolar epithelium. Development. 2001;128:5181–8.
20. Petersen BE, Bowen WC, Patrene KD, Mars WM, Sullivan AK, Murase N, Boggs SS, Greenberger JS, Goff JP. Bone marrow as a potential source of hepatic oval cells. Science. 1999;284:1168–70.
21. Pereira RF, Halford KW, O'Hara MD, Leeper DB, Sokolov BP, Pollard MD, Bagasra O, Prockop DJ. Marrow stromal cells from marrow can serve as long-lasting precursor cells for bone, cartilage, and lung in irradiated mice. Proc Natl Acad Sci. 1995;92:4857–61.
22. Matsui H, Davis CW, Tarran R, Boucher RC. Osmotic water permeabilities of cultured, well-differentiated normal and cytic fibrosis airway epithelia. J Clin Invest. 2000;105:1419–27.
23. Knowles MR, Boucher RC. Mucus clearance as a primary innate defense mechanism for mammalian airways. J Clin Investig. 2002;109:571–7.
24. Tarran Robert, Button Brian, et al. Normal and cystic fibrosis airway surface liquid homeostasis. J Biol Chem. 2005;280(42):35751–9.
25. Wine JJ. The genesis of cystic fibrosis lung disease. J Clin Investig. 1999;103:309–12.
26. Guggino WB. Cystic fibrosis salt/fluid controversy:in the thick of it. Nat Med. 2001;7:888–9.
27. Schmidt MC, Peter H, et al. In vitro cell models to study nasal mucosal permeability and metabolism. Adv Drug Deliv Rev. 1998;29(1–2):51–79.
28. Crystal RG, Randell SH, et al. Airway epithelial cells: current concepts and challenges. Proc Am Thorac Soc. 2008;5(7):772–7.
29. Zhen Dong GM, Guan WL, Chang, et al. The expression and significance of gene protein related to cell cycle and apoptosis in nasal polyp tissue. Zhonghua Otolaryngol Dep J. 2000;35(6):l29–431.
30. Rock JR, Onaitis MW, et al. Basal cells as stem cells of the mouse trachea and human airway epithelium. Proc Natl Acad Sci. 2009;106(31):12771–5.
31. Mygind N, Dahl R. Anatomy, physiology and function of the nasal cavities in health and disease. Adv Drug Deliv Rev. 1998;29(1–2):3–12.
32. Piccirillo JF, Merritt MG Jr, Richards ML. Psychometric and clinimetric validity of the 20-item sino-nasal outcome test (SNOT-20). Otolaryngol Head Neck Surg. 2002;126:41–7.
33. Zuk P, Zhu M, Ashjian P, et al. Human adipose tissue is a source of multipotent stem cells. Mol Biol Cell. 2002;13:4279–95.
34. Rutland J, Cole PJ. Nasal mucociliary clearance and ciliary beat frequency in cystic fibrosis compared with sinusitis and bronchiectasis. Thorax. 1981;36:654–8 **(grade B)**.
35. JFL, XBF, ZYS et al. The isolation and culture of epidermal stem cell. J Mil Med. 2000;386–387.

MicroRNA-720 promotes in vitro cell migration by targeting Rab35 expression in cervical cancer cells

Yunlan Tang[1], Yi Lin[1], Chuang Li[1], Xunwu Hu[1], Yi Liu[1], Mingyang He[1], Jun Luo[2], Guihong Sun[3], Tao Wang[4], Wenxin Li[1] and Mingxiong Guo[1*]

Abstract

Background: MicroRNA-720 (miR-720), a nonclassical miRNA, is involved in the initiation and progression of several tumors. In our previous studies, miR-720 was shown to be significantly upregulated in cervical cancer tissues compared with normal cervical tissues. However, the precise biological functions of miR-720, and its molecular mechanisms of action, are still unknown.

Results: Microarray expression profiles, luciferase reporter assays, and western blot assays were used to validate *Rab35* as a target gene of miR-720 in HEK293T and HeLa cells. The regulation of Rab35 expression by miR-720 was assessed using qRT-PCR and western blot assays, and the effects of exogenous miR-720 and Rab35 on cell migration were evaluated in vitro using Transwell® assay, wound healing assay, and real-time analyses in HeLa cells. The influences of exogenous miR-720 on cell proliferation were evaluated in vitro by the MTT assay in HeLa cells. In addition, expression of E-cadherin and vimentin associated with epithelial-mesenchymal transition were also assessed using western blot analyses after transfection of miR-720 mimics and Rab35 expression vectors. The results showed that the small GTPase, Rab35, is a direct functional target of miR-720 in cervical cancer HeLa cells. By targeting Rab35, overexpression of miR-720 resulted in a decrease in E-cadherin expression and an increase in vimentin expression and finally led to promotion of HeLa cell migration. Furthermore, reintroduction of Rab35 3′-UTR(−) markedly reversed the induction of cell migration in miR-720-expressing HeLa cells.

Conclusions: The miR-720 promotes cell migration of HeLa cells by downregulating Rab35. The results show that miR-720 is a novel cell migration-associated gene in cervical cancer cells.

Keywords: miR-720, Cervical cancer cells, Rab35, Cell migration

Background

Discovered in 1993, microRNAs (miRNAs) are a class of short, non-coding RNAs that are highly efficient gene expression regulators in various cellular processes [1–5]. They modulate gene expression predominantly through an interaction with the 3′-UTR of their target mRNAs [6, 7]. Increasing evidence suggests that dysfunctions of miRNAs are involved in the initiation and progression of cancer [8, 9], as well as in animal developmental processes [10]. It has been reported that miR-720 is not a classic miRNA, but is probably a fragment of tRNA [11]. Hara et al. identified miR-720 as a novel miRNA regulator in the differentiation of dental pulp cells [12]. Other studies suggested that circulating miR-720 was a novel serum biomarker in some tumors, such as colorectal cancers [13] and myelomas [14]. Furthermore, miR-720 could act as a colorectal cancer-promoting factor, and could be a marker for the prognosis of colorectal cancer [15]. Previous results have reported that miR-720 is also frequently decreased in breast cancer and functions as an anti-metastatic gene by downregulating TWIST1 [16]. Our previous studies suggested that miR-720 expression

*Correspondence: guomx@whu.edu.cn
[1] College of Life Sciences and State Key Laboratory of Virology, Wuhan University, 430072 Wuhan, People's Republic of China
Full list of author information is available at the end of the article

is significantly upregulated in cervix uteri squamous cell carcinoma tissues, when compared with normal cervix uteri tissues [17]. Cervical cancer is the third most commonly diagnosed cancer, and the fourth most common type of cancer among women, worldwide [18]. However, the roles of miR-720 in the initiation and progression of cervical cancer are still largely unknown.

The small GTPase, Rab35, is a member of the RAS oncogene family. It regulates many essential cellular processes, such as recycling from endosomes for neurite outgrowth [19–25], exosome release [26], cytokinesis [27], and actin cytoskeleton organization [28–31] by cycling between a GTP-bound active form and a GDP-bound inactive form [32]. In addition, Rab35 is involved in the early stage of FcγR-mediated phagocytosis in macrophages [33] and also acts as a regulator of vesicle transport required specifically for phagocytosis [34]. Although Rab35 has been shown to regulate various cellular processes, its precise roles in these processes are not fully understood. Moreover, several recent studies have reported that dysfunctions of Rab35 also exert vital functions, such as regulation of myoblast fusion and cadherin-dependent adherens junction formation [35]. Some studies showed that Wnt5a promotes breast cancer cell migration via the Dvl2/Rab35/Rac1 signaling pathway [36], and Rab35 maintains cadherins at the cell surface to promote cell–cell adhesion [37].

In the present study, we therefore sought to determine the role of miR-720 in cervical cancer cells. We first defined miR-720 as a new, in vitro cell migration-associated miRNA in HeLa cells. And overexpression or inhibition of miR-720 did not significantly affect HeLa cell proliferation. Moreover, we identified Rab35, a key regulator of endosomal membrane trafficking, as a direct and functional target of miR-720. The newly identified miR-720/Rab35 axis provides a molecular mechanism for abnormal cell migration in cervical cancer cells via its effects on the expression of an epithelial marker, E-cadherin, and a mesenchymal marker, vimentin.

Results

miR-720 promotes cell migration but does not affect cell proliferation in HeLa cells

In our previous study, we found the expression level of miR-720 was significantly upregulated in cervical cancer tissues compared to normal adjacent tissues [17]. To further explore its functions in the development and progression of cervical cancer, we assessed the influence of miR-720 on cell migration and cell proliferation in HeLa cells, by gain- and loss-of-function analyses. First, we showed that miR-720 mimics could lead to a significant increase in miR-720 expression (Fig. 1a). Then, cell migration assays were performed after HeLa cells were

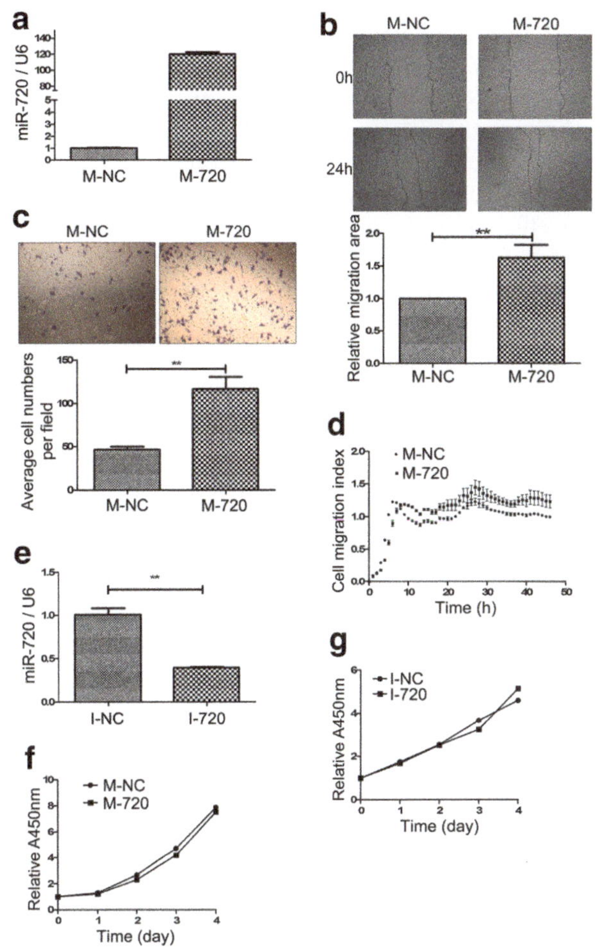

Fig. 1 MiR-720 promotes cell migration but does not affect cell proliferation in HeLa cells. **a** The qRT-PCR analysis of miR-720 expression indicated that HeLa cells transfected with miR-720 mimics (M-720) showed a significant increase in miR-720 expression compared with cells transfected with the microRNA mimic negative control (M-NC). **b** Representative photographs of wound healing assays (100×) show that HeLa cells transfected with miR-720 mimics result in a significant improvement in wound healing ability. The statistical results of cell migration area measured by Image J software demonstrate a significant difference in cell migration ability caused by overexpression of miR-720. $**p < 0.01$. **c** Transwell® migration assay shows that the upregulation of miR-720 dramatically enhances cell migration ability. The *top panel* shows representative photographs of the Transwell® migration assay and the *bottom panel* shows the statistical results. $**p < 0.01$. **d** Twenty-four hours after transfection, real-time cell analysis (RTCA) experiments were performed to contrast cell migration indices between cells transfected with miR-720 mimics and the microRNA mimic negative control. The results show that after 8 h, the migration indices of cells transfected with miR-720 mimics were greater than the controls. **e** The results of qRT-PCR analysis of miR-720 expression show that the miR-720 inhibitors can effectively knockdown miR-720 in HeLa cells. $**p < 0.01$. The (3-4,5-dimethyl-2-thiazolyl)-2,5-diphenyl-2-H-tetrazolium bromide (MTT) assays show upregulation (**f**) or downregulation (**g**) of miR-720, does not show an effect on cell proliferation viability in HeLa cells

transfected for 24 h with the miR-720 mimic (M-720) or the miR-mimic negative control (M-NC). Overexpression of miR-720 in HeLa cells significantly promoted migration ability, as determined by wound healing assays, showing that the abilities of migrated cells filling a scratch was significantly enhanced in miR-720-overexpressed cells than the M-NC cells ($p < 0.01$) (Fig. 1b). The induction effect of miR-720 on cell migration was further confirmed by Transwell® assays. The representative photographs of Transwell® migration, plus the histogram of the results, both showed that the M-720 had a significant improvement on cell migration (Fig. 1c). A real-time cell analysis is a new method to accurately detect cell migration in real time. Using this method, we further demonstrated that upregulation of miR-720 could induce cell migration in HeLa cells (Fig. 1d).

In addition, inhibition by miR-720 inhibitors resulted in a dramatic decrease in miR-720 expression (Fig. 1e). We therefore used these transfected cells to conduct 3-4,5-dimethyl-2-thiazolyl)-2,5-diphenyl-2-H-tetrazolium bromide (MTT) assays to assess the effects of miR-720 on cell proliferation. The results showed that neither the miR-720 mimic nor the miR-720 inhibitor had significant effects on cell proliferation (Fig. 1f, g). Thus, we next studied the role of miR-720 in cell migration of HeLa cells.

Identification of the miR-720 targets by integrative bioinformatics analysis

In order to characterize the molecular mechanism of miR-720 on cell migration, the potential mRNA targets of miR-720 were identified. To investigate the potential target genes and their binding sites on the seed region of miR-720, we used the TargetScan program (http://www.targetscan.org/) [7, 38, 39] and the miRanda program (http://www.microrna.org/) [40]. The TargetScan and miRanda program predicted respectively 827 and 1328 candidate genes, which were possible targets of miR-720 (Fig. 2b).

Recent studies have shown that miRNAs can reduce the levels of many of their target transcripts, and not just protein expression deriving from these transcripts [41]. Based on these observations, we used a high throughout genome mRNA microarray to identify potential target genes of miR-720. We performed global microarray gene expression profiling using the Human Genome U133 Plus 2.0 Array (Affymetrix, Santa Clara, CA, USA) in HEK293T cells transfected with pre-miR-720 or negative control mimics. Twenty-four hours after transfection, the expression level of miR-720 (relative to endogenous U6 RNA) in HEK293T cells was determined by qRT-PCR. The expression level of miR-720 was increased about 550-fold as compared to the negative control. The microarray results showed that when compared with the controls, 216 probes, representing 195 genes (three of these genes are still unnamed and not included) were downregulated by ≥2-fold ($p < 0.05$) in pre-miR-720 transfected HEK293T cells (Fig. 2a; Additional file 1: Table S1). Using a Gene List Venn Diagram, we identified 10 potential target genes as *CHP, INSIG1, INTS7, KCTD15, METTL2B, NRXN3, PER2, RAB35, SGK3,* and *TET2* among the microarray results and the putative miR-720 target gene list (as predicted by TargetScan and miRanda) (Fig. 2c).

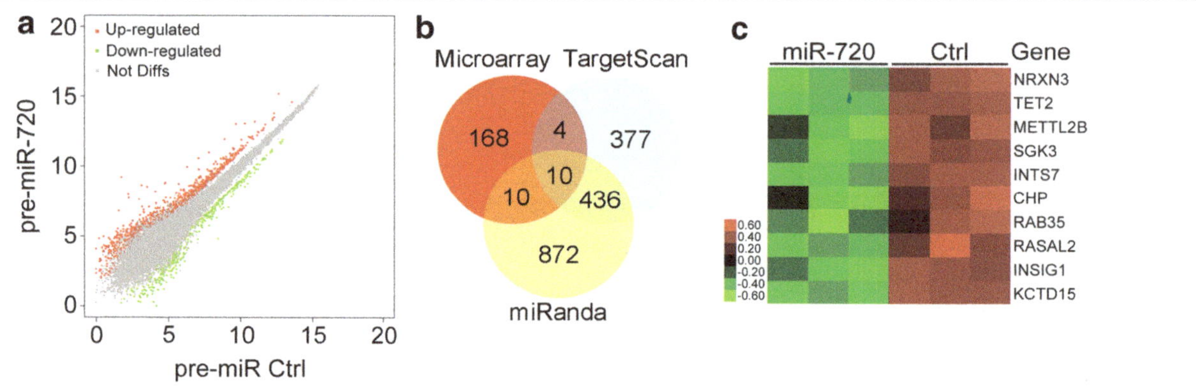

Fig. 2 Identification of miR-720 targets. **a** Microarray assays were performed on HEK293T cells transfected with pre-miR-720 and the pre-miR-control. The *red dots* represent genes upregulated with a ≥2-fold change, the *green dots* represent genes downregulated with a >0.5-fold change, and the *gray dots* indicate genes with expression levels ranging from −0.5-fold change to +2-fold change in the scatterplot. **b** The *Venn diagram* shows the relationships between the mRNA microarray and two miRNA-target prediction algorithms on the quantity of miR-720 targets. The TargetScan program and the miRanda program predicted that 827 candidate genes and 1328 candidate genes, respectively, were possible targets of miR-720. Expressions of 192 genes in HEK293T cells were changed ≥2-fold with a p value cut-off of 0.05 by ectopic expression of pre-miR-720. Among these 192 genes, 14 and 20 were predicted by TargetScan 5.1 and miRanda, respectively. Among these 20 genes, 10 were classified as the intersection targets. **c** The heat map shows the change in expression levels of 10 genes with overexpression of miR-720

Identification of miR-720 targets by the luciferase reporter assay

Using luciferase reporter assays, we next sought to verify direct regulation of these candidate targets by miR-720. Among these candidate target genes, except for *KCTD15* with two predicted miR-720 binding sites in 3′-UTR, the rest of the target genes had only a predicted target site in 3′-UTR. We subcloned the partial 3′-UTRs containing the miR-720-binding sites of these candidate target genes, such as Rab35, into the luciferase-based reporter vector pMIR-REPORT (Ambion, Austin, Texas, US), and cotransfected the reporter constructs in HEK293T cells with the pre-miR-720 precursor or negative control (Fig. 3a). Among these reporter constructs, miR-720 significantly suppressed the luciferase activity of the reporter vector containing binding sites in *INSIG1, KCTD15, METTL2B, NRXN3, Rab35, RASAL2,* or *TET2*, but not in *CHP, PER2,* or *SGK3* for miR-720 targeting (Fig. 3b). To further confirm the predicted miRNA binding sites, seven base pair mutations of the miR-720 binding sites on the *INSIG1, KCTD15, METTL2B, NRXN3, Rab35, RASAL2,* and *TET2* genes were generated by site-directed mutagenesis. Because *KCTD15* has two predicted binding sites in its 3′-UTR, we performed molecular cloning for single site mutations to obtain vectors named MUT1-KCTD15, MUT2-KCTD15, and double site mutation vectors named MUT1,2-KCTD15. As expected, once the miR-720 binding sites in the 3′-UTR of these candidate target mRNAs were mutated, the luciferase activities could not be suppressed by miR-720 (Fig. 3c). Taken together, the results of these reporter assays showed that miR-720 could directly bind to the 3′-UTR of *INSIG1, KCTD15,* and *RAB35.*

Rab35 is a target of miR-720 in HeLa cells

The studies suggested that *INSIG1* is an insulin-induced gene and encodes an endoplasmic reticulum (ER) membrane protein that plays a critical role in regulating cholesterol concentrations in cells [42–46]; and Kctd15 has a role in regulating the neural crest formation in the embryo [47, 48]. And Rab35 was involved in breast cancer cell migration processes [36] and promotes cell–cell adhesion [37]. Because miR-720 could induce cell migration in HeLa cells, we focus our initial research emphasis on Rab35. Firstly we further confirmed whether the mRNA and protein expression levels of *Rab35* could have been regulated by miR-720 in cervical cancer HeLa cells. The results showed that mRNA expression of Rab35 was not significantly affected by both the overexpression and suppressed expression of miR-720 (Fig. 4a, b). However, the protein level of Rab35 was negatively regulated by miR-720 in HeLa cells as expected (Fig. 4c). Thus, we propose that miR-720 plays a role in the regulation of Rab35 at the translational level in HeLa cells.

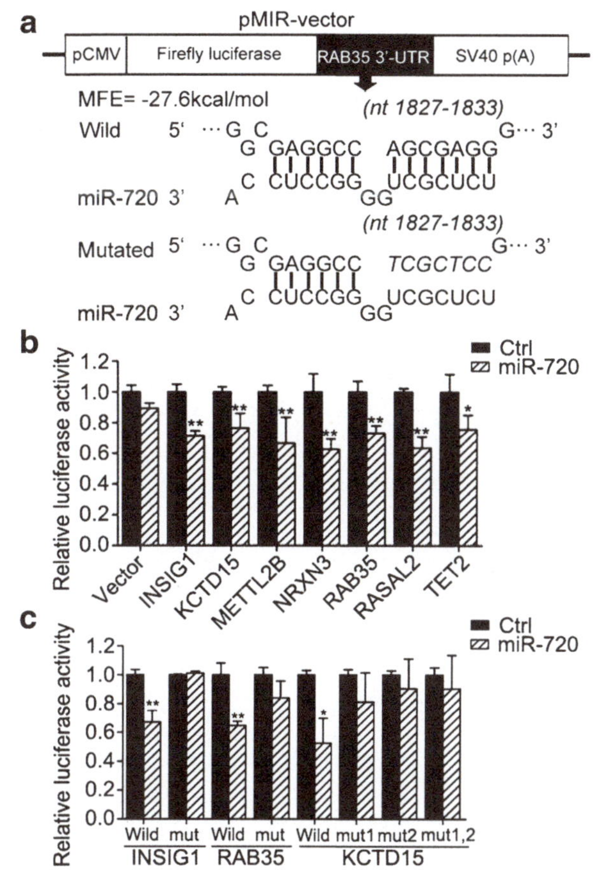

Fig. 3 Dual luciferase reporter assays verify that miR-720 regulates its targets by binding directly to their 3′-UTR. **a** The diagram shows that 3′-UTR of Rab35 was cloned downstream into the open reading frame of the pcDNA3.0-Vector, and also displays the detailed binding sites or the mutated binding sites of the 3′-UTR for miR-720 targeting; **b** The results of analysis indicate that the relative luciferase activities of the pMIR-REPORT vector containing wide-type 3′-UTR of *INSIG1, KCTD15, METTL2B, NRXN3, Rab35, RASAL2,* or *TET2* could be decreased by upregulating miR-720; Firefly luciferase activity was normalized to Renilla luciferase activity. The relative luciferase expression level is expressed as the mean ± standard deviation (SD). Three independent experiments were performed, and representative data are shown. $*p < 0.05$ shows the significant difference. **c** Normalized luciferase activity in cells transfected with reporter vector containing mutant type 3′-UTR of *KCTD15, INSIG1,* or *RAB35* could not be affected by overexpression of miR-720 compared with cells transfected with wild type 3′-UTR. The relative luciferase expression level is expressed as the mean ± standard deviation (SD). Three independent experiments were performed, and representative data are shown. $*p < 0.05$ shows the significant difference

Rab35 can suppress cell migration of HeLa cells

Then we wondered whether Rab35 had negative effects on cell migration in HeLa cells compared with miR-720. So we constructed a miR-720 insensitive Rab35 expression vector (pcDNA3.0-Rab35) that only included the coding sequence of Rab35 on the base of the

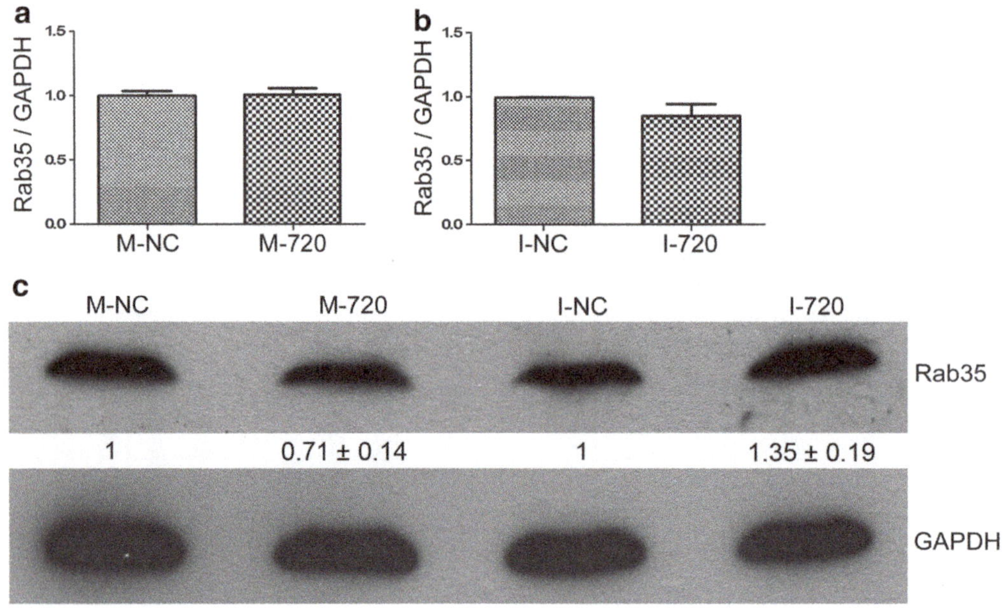

Fig. 4 Rab35 is negatively regulated by miR-720 at the translational level in HeLa cells. Transfection of miR-720 mimics (**a**) or miR-720 inhibitors (**b**) in HeLa cells did not significantly affect Rab35 mRNA expression levels, as assessed by qRT-PCR analysis. **c** Representative photographs of Rab35 protein expression detected by western blotting, and the results of gray intensity analysis using Image J software showed that Rab35 protein levels were negatively regulated by miR-720

pcDNA3.0-Vector, to escape miR-720 targeting. The overexpression level of this vector was assessed by western blotting, and the results showed that the vector successfully induced Rab35 overexpression (Fig. 5a). Then, we assayed the impact of forced expression of Rab35 on cell migration of HeLa cells. Using the wound healing assay, the overexpression of Rab35 inhibited the healing of the scratch when compared to the control group transfected with the empty pcDNA3.0-Vector (Fig. 5b). In the other two types of cell migration assays (Transwell® migration assay and real-time cell analysis), we consistently found that Rab35 had the ability to inhibit cell migration of HeLa cells (Fig. 5c, d). These results showed that Rab35 has an opposite effect on HeLa cell migration, in comparison with miR-720, indicating that it may be a functional target of miR-720 in HeLa cells.

miR-720 mediates cell migration by targeting Rab35 in HeLa cells

In the previous experiments, overexpression of miR-720 could promote cell migration of HeLa, and forced expression of Rab35 could suppress cell migration. To further demonstrate whether Rab35 is the actual functional target of miR-720 acting on cell migration of HeLa cells, we cotransfected the miR-720 mimic and the miR-720 insensitive Rab35 vector into HeLa cells, then conducted a Transwell® migration assay. Even though there is overexpression of miR-720, the miR-720 insensitive Rab35 vector can still restore Rab35 expression and antagonize the positive effect of miR-720 on cell migration of HeLa cells, finally resulting in inhibition of cell migration, compared with the negative control group transfected with the miR-720 mimic and the empty pcDNA3.0-Vector (Fig. 6a, b). Thus, we postulate that miR-720 exerts its positive function on cell migration of HeLa cells by negatively regulating Rab35, which can suppress cell migration of HeLa cells.

Molecular mechanism of the miR-720 effect on cell migration of HeLa cells

We next sought to characterize the mechanism of action involved in miR-720 induction of HeLa cell migration. Epithelial-to-mesenchymal transition (EMT) is an important process in morphogenesis and tissue repair, and this process is often abnormally activated in cancer cells, which will promote their malignant and stem cell characteristics and finally accelerate cell migration [49]. To determine if EMT was aberrantly changed, we assessed the alterations in E-cadherin protein expression, which is a well-established marker for epithelial cells, and vimentin, which is a marker of mesenchymal cells, in the transfected HeLa cells used in the previous functional study [50]. The results showed that the forced expression of miR-720 upregulated vimentin and downregulated E-cadherin (Fig. 7a). Correspondingly, miR-720 inhibition and overexpression of Rab35 had the opposite effects on E-cadherin and

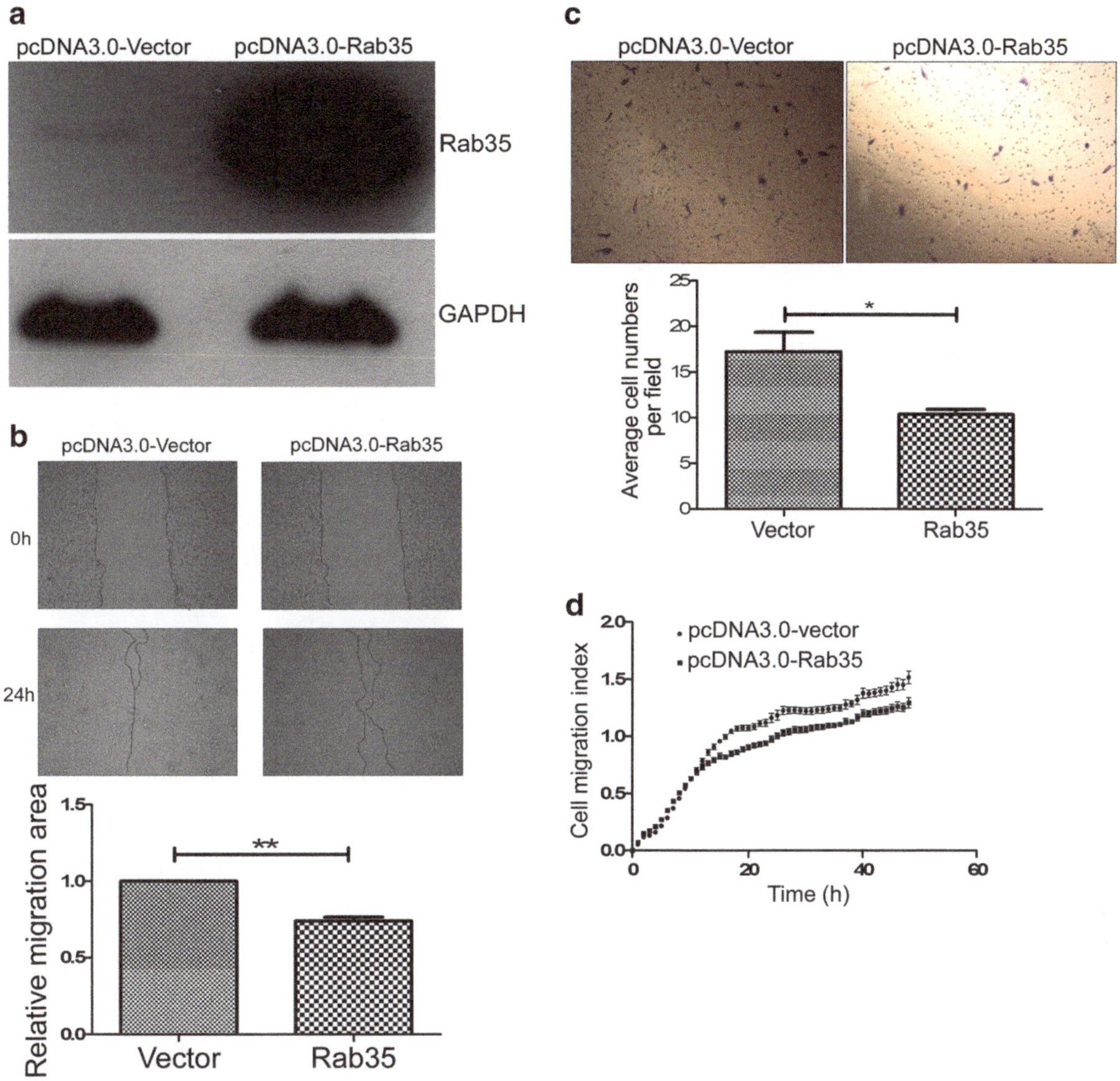

Fig. 5 Rab35 has the opposite effect on the migration of HeLa cells, relative to miR-720. **a** Representative western blot assays show that transfection with the constructed vector pcDNA3.0-Rab35 results in a high expression level of Rab35. **b** Representative photographs of wound healing assays show that the forced expression of Rab35 decreased cell wound healing ability. The statistical results of cell migration area measured by Image J software demonstrate a significant reduction in cell migration caused by overexpression of Rab35. $^{**}p < 0.01$. **c** Representative photographs of Transwell® migration assays and the statistical results show that the forced expression of Rab35 led to a dramatic decrease in cell migration. $^{*}p < 0.05$. **d** Real-time cell analysis shows that overexpression of Rab35 decreased the cell migration index when compared with the corresponding negative control

vimentin levels; E-cadherin was increased and vimentin was decreased (Fig. 7b, c). Collectively, these results suggest that the intrinsic mechanism of miR-720 promotion on cell migration by downregulation of Rab35 is essentially through the activation of the EMT in HeLa cells.

Discussion

Tumor metastasis remains a major cause of cancer-related death. Metastasis is comprised of various sequential steps, involving cancer cell dissemination, cancer cell spreading, and formation of secondary tumors in other organs and tissues [51, 52]. The first essential step of tumor metastasis and invasion is the change in the expression of cell adhesion molecules (CAM), and the breakdown and remodeling of the extracellular matrix (ECM), resulting in the ability of cancer cells to metastasize. Increasing evidence suggests that miRNAs play critical roles in the regulation of cell migration and invasion,

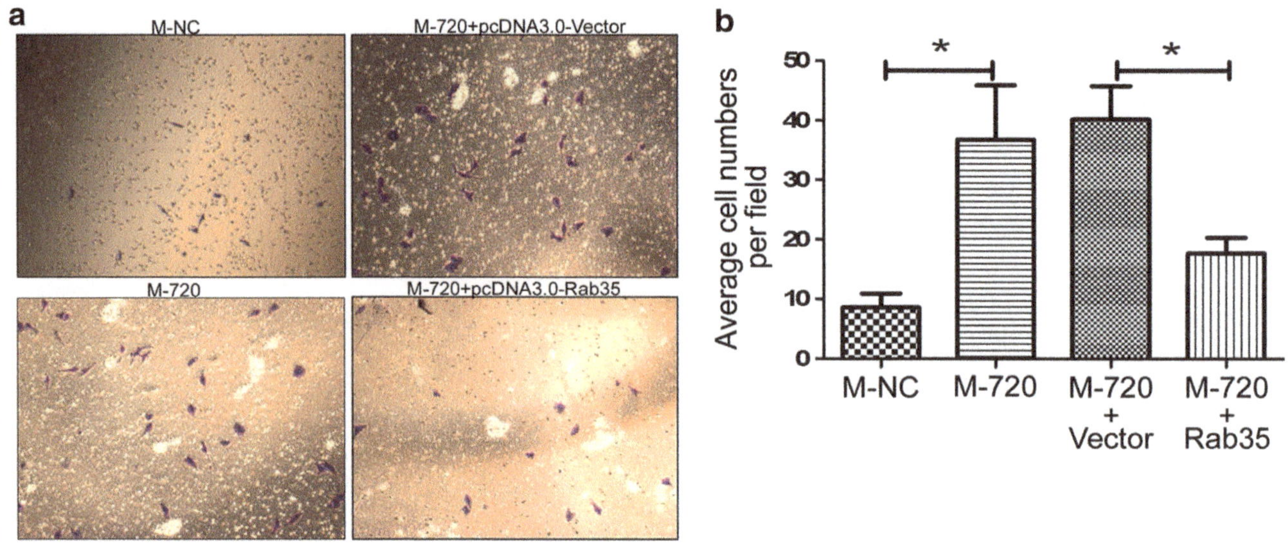

Fig. 6 Restoration of Rab35 expression reverses the promoting effect of miR-720 on cell migration. Representative photographs (**a**) and statistical results (**b**) of Transwell® assays show that while transfecting miR-720 mimics could lead to a significant increase in cell migration ability compared with cells transfected with the microRNA mimic negative control, cotransfecting pcDNA3.0-Rab35 and miR-720 mimics resulted in a dramatic decrease in cell migration ability compared with the negative group cotransfected with miR-720 mimics and the pcDNA3.0-Vector. *$p < 0.05$

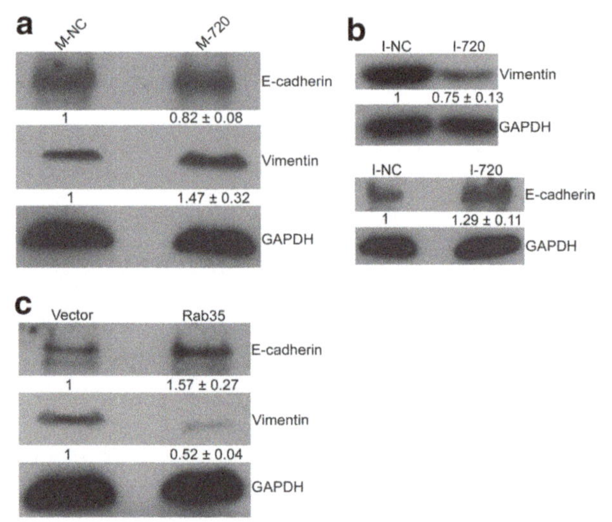

Fig. 7 Detection of E-cadherin and vimentin expression by western blotting. **a** HeLa cells transfected with miR-720 mimics show a significant increase in vimentin protein expression and a dramatic decrease in E-cadherin protein expression. Transfection of miR-720 inhibitors (**b**) or pcDNA3.0-Rab35 (**c**) had a negative effect (E-cadherin was increased and vimentin was decreased), in contrast to transfection of miR-720 mimics in HeLa cells

as coordinated regulators of ECM remodeling during cancer cell migration and invasion [53]. We previously reported that miR-720 expression is significantly upregulated in cervix uteri squamous cell carcinoma tissue when compared to normal cervix uteri tissue, indicating that miR-720 is closely related to the pathological processes of cervical cancer [17]. Some studies have reported that miR-720 impedes cell invasion and migration, and then inhibits metastasis in breast cancer by directly targeting TWIST1 [16]. In the present study, we showed that overexpression of miR-720 leads to a reduction of E-cadherin and an increase of vimentin protein levels in cervical cancer cell lines, which indicates that miR-720 can induce EMT in cervical cancer cells and promote cell migration. In combination with our previous studies and reports from other investigators, we propose that miR-720 may be an important regulator of cell migration and invasion in various cancers, in spite of its functional differences that are dependent on distinct cellular microenvironments. It was reported that individual miRNA has the potential to regulate hundreds of targets [54]. In addition, a miRNA can not only directly affect the levels of target mRNA but also indirectly affect the levels of target mRNA, in other words, a miRNA can have secondary effects or even tertiary effects on its target mRNA [55]. Besides, the effects of a miRNA on regulating its targets crucially depends on its expression levels and the regulation happened to have a cell-type dependent effect [56–58]. Therefore, we propose that miR-720 may regulate the cell migration processes in various cancer cells by distinct molecular mechanism.

Since miR-720 was discovered, it has been widely studied as a miRNA. A study showed that miR-720 could negatively regulate p63 involved in an autoregulatory feedback loop, which then contributed to epithelial development processes [59]. The miR-720 could suppress cell migration and invasion in breast cancer by directly targeting TWIST1 [16]. Furthermore, miR-720 participates in the control of the stem cell phenotype of human dental pulp cells by directly repressing NANOG levels [12]. miR-720 is closely related to the pathological processes of various tumors [17]. A more recent study showed that overexpression of miR-720 in primary human CD8+ T cells inhibits the T cell receptor (TCR) stimulation-induced proliferation in patients with chronic hepatitis B virus (HBV) infection, which suggests that therapies targeting miR-720 may help restore impaired immunity in chronic HBV-infected patients [60]. However, another study reported that miR-720 is probably a fragment from a tRNA, rather than an miRNA [11]. And other report showed that, as a tRNA-derived miRNA, miR-720 is one of the four most abundant MCF7 extracellular vesicle miRNAs, suggesting that miR-720 may be a new biomarker in breast cancer cells [61]. Although there is controversy over whether miR-720 is a miRNA or a tRNA-derived RNA fragment (tRF), functional studies of miR-720 will provide valuable information concerning the possible clinical significance of this small non-RNA molecule.

As a key regulator of endosomal membrane trafficking and the actin cytoskeleton, Rab35 in this study was found to be directly regulated by miR-720 at the posttranscriptional level. The small GTPase, Rab35, a member of the RAS oncogene family, regulates many essential cellular processes, such as recycling from endosomes, exosome release, cytokinesis, and actin cytoskeleton organization by cycling between a GTP-bound active form and a GDP-bound inactive form. Active Rab35 controls recycling pathways to increase cell adhesion and decrease cell migration [32]. It is noteworthy that many studies have demonstrated a close relationship between Rab35 and Arf6, which is also a small GTPase. Both these two small GTPases are involved in functionally related cell processes, such as cell migration and cytokinesis, endocytosis, actin remodeling, sorting, and recycling of adhesion molecules. However, the activities of Rab35 and Arf6 are inversely coordinated [24, 27, 62, 63]. To the best of our knowledge, this is the first study to provide experimental evidences that Rab35 is posttranscriptionally regulated by miR-720, which then contributes to the regulation of cell migration. Based upon these observations, it is important to further validate the functions of the miR-720/Rab35 axis in tumor metastasis and invasion in animal models and clinical tissues in future studies.

Conclusions

Our results show that miR-720 promotes cell migration in cervical cancer cells by directly targeting Rab35. Targeting the miR-720/Rab35 axis is therefore a promising therapeutic strategy for cervical cancer treatment.

Methods

Cell culture

HeLa cells and HEK293T cells were obtained from the Type Culture Collection of the Chinese Academy of Sciences (Shanghai, China). HeLa cells were cultured in Minimum Essential Medium (Gibco/Life Technologies, US) and HEK293T cells were incubated in Dulbecco's Modified Eagle's Medium (Gibco/Life Technologies, US). The base medium was supplemented with 10 % fetal bovine serum (Gibco/Life Technologies, US) to make the complete growth medium, and the cells were incubated at 37 °C with 5 % CO_2.

Oligonucleotide transfection

The pre-miR-720, miR-720 mimics, inhibitor, and corresponding controls were designed and synthesized by RiboBio (Guangzhou, China). HEK293T cells were transfected with pre-miR-720 or pre-miR-control at a final concentration of 100 nM. HeLa cells were transfected with mimics at a final concentration of 100 nM, or transfected with inhibitor at a final concentration of 200 nM using Lipofectamine® RNAiMAX reagent (Invitrogen, US), following the manufacturer's instructions. After 48 h, the cells were harvested for further analysis.

RNA extraction and quantitative real-time PCR

Total RNA was extracted using TRIzol® Reagent (Life Technologies, US) according to the manufacturer's protocol. One μg of total RNA was reverse transcribed into cDNA with a FastQuant RT Kit (Tiangen Biotech, Beijing, China). Quantitative analyses of miR-720 were performed using the Bulge-LoopTM miRNA quantitative RT-PCR primer (RiboBio, Guangzhou, China) and/or a S-Poly(T) real-time PCR assay of microRNAs assays [64], and SYBR Select Master Mix (Life Technologies) on an ABI Prism 7500 real-time PCR system (Applied Biosystems, Foster City, CA, USA). Quantitative analysis of Rab35 was performed using designed qPCR primers (forward, 5′-ACGACCACCTCTTCAAGCTG-3′; reverse, 5′-CCGGATCTTGAAATCCACTC-3′) and the same SYBR Select Master Mix with miR-720 qPCR. PCR was performed using 20 μL reaction mixture in triplicate at 95 °C, for 10 min, followed by 40 cycles of 95 °C for 10 s, 60 °C for 34 s, and 72 °C for 30 s. U6 snRNA was used as an internal control for miRNA analysis, and glyceraldehyde 3-phosphate dehydrogenase (GAPDH) mRNA was used as an internal control for quantitative analysis of mRNA. The results were calculated using the $2^{-\Delta\Delta CT}$ method.

Microarray analysis

After the experimental HEK293T group was transfected with pre-miR-720 and the control HEK293T group was transfected with the pre-miR-control for 24 h, the HEK293T cells were lysed with TRIzol® reagent (Life Technologies, US) and total RNA was extracted according to the manufacturer's protocol. The RNA samples were then sent to the Shanghai Biotechnology Corporation to perform microarray analysis (Affymetrix GeneChip® Human Genome U133 Plus 2.0 Array). Each group sample set was comprised of three replicates. The Affymetrix GeneChip® system was used for hybridization, staining, scanning, and imaging of the arrays. Raw data were analyzed with the Affymetrix GeneChip® Operating Software (GCOS1.4) using the manufacturer's default analysis settings and global scaling as the normalization method. One-way analysis of variance (ANOVA) was performed with GeneSpring 7.31 software (Agilent, Santa Clara, CA, USA) to identify genes whose expression changed significantly between the pre-miR-720 group and the control.

Luciferase reporter assay

The putative binding sites of the 3′-UTR of the human genes for miR-720 targeting were predicted by TargetScan Human (http://www.targetscan.org/) computational methods.

The partial 3′-UTR fragment (about 250 bp) of these potential targets, including predicted binding sites, as our previous report [65], were separately cloned into the pMIR-REPORT™ miRNA Expression Reporter Vector (Applied Biosystems) at the *Mlu* I/*Hin*d III site. The primers were designed as Table 1.

The mutant 3′UTR inserts, with an opposite mutation in the miRNA seed sequence binding sites, were generated by overlapping PCR methods [66] using the mutated primers, listed as Table 1.

Wild-type and mutation inserts were confirmed by DNA sequencing. HEK293T cells were seeded in triplicate at a density of 2×10^5 cells per 24-well plate. The following day, cells were transfected with 100 ng wild-type or mutated firefly reporter vector, 10 ng of the control vector containing Renilla luciferase, and pRL-TK (Promega, US), at a final concentration of 50 nM miRNA, or negative control (NC) precursors, using 1.5 μL Lipofectamine® 2000 (Invitrogen) per well. Cells were assayed 48 h after transfection with the Dual Luciferase Assay (Promega) according to the manufacturer's instructions. Each experiment was repeated at least in triplicate. The efficiency of transfection was normalized using the Renilla luciferase activity.

The pcDNA expression plasmids and plasmid transfection

The coding sequence of Rab35 was amplified from HeLa cell cDNA by PCR using primers: forward, 5′-CGCGGATCCATGGCCCGGGACTACGACCA-3′; reverse, 5′-CCGCTCGAGTTAGCAGCAGCGTTTCTTTC-3′. The PCR fragment was inserted using *Bam*H I/*Xho* I into the pcDNA3.0-Vector to generate pcDNA3.0-Rab35. The empty pcDNA3.0-Vector was used as the negative control. HeLa cells were transfected with plasmid using the Lipofectamine® 2000 Transfection Reagent (Invitrogen) according to the manufacturer's protocol. After 48 h, the cells were harvested for further analysis.

Western blot analysis

Total cell extracts (40 μg) were resolved on a 10 % SDS-PAGE and transferred to nitrocellulose membranes (Millipore, Germany). Membranes were blocked with 5 % skim milk (BioSharp, US) and further incubated with the following primary antibodies: Rab35 and the mesenchymal cell marker vimentin (1:2000; San Ying Biotechnology, China), the epithelial cell marker E-cadherin (1:200; BD Biosciences, US), and GAPDH (1:10,000; Ray Antibody Beijing, China). After washing, membranes were incubated with a 1:10,000 dilutions of HRP-conjugated secondary antibodies (Santa Cruz Biotechnology, Santa Cruz, CA, USA). After washing six times with TTBS, with each wash lasting 5 min, the membranes were incubated with Pierce ECL western blotting substrate (Thermo Fisher Scientific, US), and the protein bands were visualized by autoradiography and quantified by Image J software (NIH, Bethesda, MD, USA).

Cell proliferation assay

For the HeLa cell proliferation assay, cells were transiently transfected for 24 h, and then seeded into 96-well plates (6×10^3 cells/well), with each group comprised of six replicates. The cell growth was regarded as the initial value when the cells had been seeded for 2 h. At indicated times, cells were incubated with 10 μL of 5 mg/mL 3-4,5-dimethyl-2-thiazolyl)-2,5-diphenyl-2-H-tetrazolium bromide (MTT) for 4 h at 37 °C, and then the generated crystals were dissolved by dimethyl sulfoxide (DMSO). Absorbance was measured at 450 nm using a microplate reader (Biotech) every 24 h for four consecutive days.

Wound healing assay

After transfection for 24 h in 6-well plates, cells were replated into 12-well plates (2.5×10^5 cells per well), in triplicate, for the wound healing assay. When the cells reached ~90 % confluency, a 10 μL pipette tip was used to scrap across the confluent cell layer, followed by gentle washing three times with phosphate-buffered saline (PBS), and then addition of culture medium containing 2.5 % fetal bovine serum. The scratch was immediately

Table 1 Primers used in this study

Name	Sequences (5′–3′)
3′UTR-CHP-S	CAAAACGCGTCTGTCAACACAAACCTGC
3′UTR-CHP-A	CGTAAAGCTTGCCAGACCCCTGAACTAT
3′UTR-INSIG1-S	GCTTACGCGTGAGGGAAATGTCTTGGAG
3′UTR-INSIG1-A	CGCCAAGCTTGATGTTCAAATCTGGTAG
3′UTR-INTS7-S	ATCGACGCGTACAGTTTGGTTTTTCATA
3′UTR-INTS7-A	ACTCAAGCTTAAACAAGAAAGAACAATC
3′UTR-KCTD15-S	CAACACGCGTATCGTCACAGGAGAAGGT
3′UTR-KCTD15-A	AGACAAGCTTTCCAACCCCGCCCCAAC
3′UTR-METTL2B-S	ATATACGCGTCCCGTTGTGTTTCCGAGC
3′UTR-METTL2B-A	CGGCAAGCTTAGCCCTTCACTAACCCCT
3′UTR-NRXN3-S	ACTTACGCGTCTGAGGGGAAAAATGGCT
3′UTR-NRXN3-A	TAACAAGCTTTGGCTGGGTGAATGGAC
3′UTR-RAB35-S	TTAAACGCGTAAGGAGGGTGCTGTGGAG
3′UTR-RAB35-A	ACACAAGCTTCCCATAACCCCCATTCAT
3′UTR-SGK3-S	ATATACGCGTGAGACCATCCTGGGCAAC
3′UTR-SGK3-A	CCGCAAGCTTCCAGTTATTCTCCTTTAC
3′UTR-RASAL2-S	ACTAACGCGTCGACTTCCAAGGTCAATG
3′UTR-RASAL2-A	CAGAAAGCTTGTCCAACCAGAACCAGTC
3′UTR-TET2-S	CGAGACGCGTAGACTGGTAAAGTGTGGT
3′UTR-TET2-A	CACCGAAGCTTATTCACTATTTCTGCCA
INSIG1-MUT-F	GAAGTTATTAGATGAAAGGTCGCTCTGAATCTTTAAAACAGAC
INSIG1-MUT-R	GTCTGTTTTAAAGATTCAGAGCGACCTTTCATCTAATAACTTC
KCTD15-site1-MUT-F	TGTGGACTCCTCCCAGTTGTCGCTCTATGTGCTTTGCCGGGAG
KCTD15-site1-MUT-R	CTCCCGGCAAAGCACATAGAGCGACAACTGGGAGGAGTCCACA
KCTD15-site2-MUT-F	GAGGGTCCAAAGCTGGCCGTCGCTCCACCAGGGTCCCAGGTGT
KCTD15-site2-MUT-R	ACACCTGGGACCCTGGTGGAGCGACGGCCAGCTTTGGACCCTC
METTL2B-MUT-F	GTCCAGCCTGGGCAAAATTCGCTCTGACCCTGAATCTGAAAGT
METTL2B-MUT-R	ACTTTCAGATTCAGGGTCAGAGCGAATTTTGCCCAGGCTGGAC
NRXN3-MUT-F	AGGAAAAAAAACTCAAAACAAATCGCTCTGAGACTATTGCCATA
NRXN3-MUT-R	TATGGCAATAGTCTCAGAGCGATTTGTTTTGAGTTTTTTTTCCT
RAB35-MUT-F	CCTCTGAGCGATCAGGCCTCCGGTCGCTCCGTGTGCTTGCAAATTC
RAB35-MUT-R	GAATTTGCAAGCACACGGAGCGACCGGAGGCCTGATCGCTCAGAGGC
RASAL2-MUT-F	AGTAGGAACTGTTGTGTGTCGCTCTCATGAGCCTGTAGGTTCA
RASAL2-MUT-R	TGAACCTACAGGCTCATGAGAGCGACACACAACAGTTCCTACT
TET2-MUT-F	ATGTAGAAGACTCTTATGTCGCTCTTAATGCAGAGAAGGCCTT
TET2-MUT-R	AAGGCCTTCTCTGCATTAAGAGCGACATAAGAGTCTTCTACAT

Underlined characters indicate regions of the miR-720 seed sequences for mutation in luciferase reporter assay

subjected to photography using a light microscope. After incubation for 24 h, additional photographs were taken. Wound healing ability was determined by measuring the scraped area alteration because of cell migration using Image J software.

Transwell® assay

After transfection for 24 h, HeLa cells (2.5×10^4 cells) were suspended in 300 μL of Minimal Essential Medium (MEM) without serum and then reseeded into the upper chamber of the Transwell® inserts (8 μm pore size; Corning, USA) of a companion 24-well plate in pre-warmed containing 10 % FBS. After incubating at 37 °C for 24 h, cells on the top surface of the insert were removed by gentle wiping with a cotton swab, and the cells which migrated to the bottom surface of the insert were fixed in 4 % paraformaldehyde for 15 min, stained with 0.1 % crystal violet (Sigma-Aldrich, St. Louis, MO, USA) for 15 min, rinsed in PBS, and then photographed. Cell migration ability was determined by counting the stained cells in the bottom surface of the insert under a light microscope (100×) in eight randomly selected fields. The average number of cells in the eight fields was taken as the final result. Each group had three replicates and each experiment was repeated three times.

Real-time cell analysis

For real-time cell analysis (RTCA), HeLa cells were transiently transfected for 24 h, and 6×10^4 cells were suspended in 100 μL of MEM without serum in the upper chamber (ACEA Biosciences; Hangzhou, China) according to the basic cell migration assay protocol of the RTCA xCELLigence system (ACEA Biosciences). Each group had four replicates, and the cell migration index was calculated by real-time detection for 48 h.

Statistical analysis

Data were expressed as mean ± SEM. Student's *t* test (unpaired, two tailed) was used in the analysis of differences between the experimental groups and control groups, with $p < 0.05$ considered statistically significant. Statistical analyses were performed using GraphPad Prism, version 5.0 software.

Authors' contributions

MG and YT designed experiments and analyzed data; YT, YLin, CL, XH, YLiu, MH and JL performed experiments; MG, YT and GS wrote the manuscript; MG, WL, TW and GS supervised the project. All authors read and approved the final manuscript.

Author details

[1] College of Life Sciences and State Key Laboratory of Virology, Wuhan University, 430072 Wuhan, People's Republic of China. [2] Department of Pathology, Zhongnan Hospital, Wuhan University, 430071 Wuhan, People's Republic of China. [3] School of Basic Medical Sciences, Wuhan University, 430071 Wuhan, People's Republic of China. [4] Department of Respiratory and Critical Care Medicine, Tongji Hospital, Tongji Medical College, Huazhong University of Science and Technology, 430030 Wuhan, China.

Acknowledgements

This work was supported by National Natural Science Foundation of China Grants 30871245 and 31271511 (to M. Guo), 81170049 and 81470252 (to T. Wang), 31370187 (to G. Sun) and Fundamental Research Funds for the Central Universities Grant 2042014KF0243 (to M. Guo).

Compliance with ethical guidelines

Competing interests

The authors declare that they have no competing interests.

References

1. Bushati N, Cohen SM. microRNA functions. Annu Rev Cell Dev Biol. 2007;23:175–205.
2. Bartel DP. MicroRNAs: genomics, biogenesis, mechanism, and function. Cell. 2004;116(2):281–97.
3. Ambros V. The functions of animal microRNAs. Nature. 2004;431(7006):350–5.
4. Wightman B, Ha I, Ruvkun G. Posttranscriptional regulation of the heterochronic gene lin-14 by lin-4 mediates temporal pattern formation in *C. elegans*. Cell. 1993;75(5):855–62.
5. Lee RC, Feinbaum RL, Ambros V. The *C. elegans* heterochronic gene lin-4 encodes small RNAs with antisense complementarity to lin-14. Cell. 1993;75(5):843–54.
6. Bartel DP. MicroRNAs: target recognition and regulatory functions. Cell. 2009;136(2):215–33.
7. Lewis BP, Burge CB, Bartel DP. Conserved seed pairing, often flanked by adenosines, indicates that thousands of human genes are microRNA targets. Cell. 2005;120(1):15–20.
8. Croce CM. Causes and consequences of microRNA dysregulation in cancer. Nat Rev Genet. 2009;10(10):704–14.
9. Garzon R, Calin GA, Croce CM. MicroRNAs in cancer. Annu Rev Med. 2009;60:167–79.
10. Alvarez-Garcia I, Miska EA. MicroRNA functions in animal development and human disease. Development. 2005;132(21):4653–62.
11. Schopman NC, Heynen S, Haasnoot J, Berkhout B. A miRNA-tRNA mix-up: tRNA origin of proposed miRNA. RNA Biol. 2010;7(5):573–6.
12. Hara ES, Ono M, Eguchi T, Kubota S, Pham HT, Sonoyama W, Tajima S, Takigawa M, Calderwood SK, Kuboki T. miRNA-720 controls stem cell phenotype, proliferation and differentiation of human dental pulp cells. PLoS One. 2013;8(12):e83545.
13. Nonaka R, Miyake Y, Hata T, Kagawa Y, Kato T, Osawa H, Nishimura J, Ikenaga M, Murata K, Uemura M et al. Circulating miR-103 and miR-720 as novel serum biomarkers for patients with colorectal cancer. Int J Oncol. 2015;47(3):1097–102.
14. Jones CI, Zabolotskaya MV, King AJ, Stewart HJ, Horne GA, Chevassut TJ, Newbury SF. Identification of circulating microRNAs as diagnostic biomarkers for use in multiple myeloma. Br J Cancer. 2012;107(12):1987–96.
15. Wang X, Kuang Y, Shen X, Zhou H, Chen Y, Han Y, Yuan B, Zhou J, Zhao H, Zhi Q, et al. Evaluation of miR-720 prognostic significance in patients with colorectal cancer. Tumour Biol J Int Soc Oncodev Biol Med. 2015;36(2):719–27.
16. Li LZ, Zhang CZ, Liu LL, Yi C, Lu SX, Zhou X, Zhang ZJ, Peng YH, Yang YZ, Yun JP. miR-720 inhibits tumor invasion and migration in breast cancer by targeting TWIST1. Carcinogenesis. 2014;35(2):469–78.
17. Lin Y, Zeng Y, Zhang F, Xue L, Huang Z, Li W, Guo M. Characterization of microRNA expression profiles and the discovery of novel microRNAs involved in cancer during human embryonic development. PLoS One. 2013;8(8):e69230.
18. Jemal A, Bray F, Center MM, Ferlay J, Ward E, Forman D. Global cancer statistics. CA Cancer J Clin. 2011;61(2):69–90.
19. Etoh K, Fukuda M. Structure-function analyses of the small GTPase Rab35 and its effector protein centaurin-beta2/ACAP2 during neurite outgrowth of PC12 cells. J Biol Chem. 2015;290(14):9064–74.
20. Kobayashi H, Fukuda M. Rab35 establishes the EHD1-association site by coordinating two distinct effectors during neurite outgrowth. J Cell Sci. 2013;126(Pt 11):2424–35.
21. Kanno E, Ishibashi K, Kobayashi H, Matsui T, Ohbayashi N, Fukuda M. Comprehensive screening for novel Rab-binding proteins by GST pull-down assay using 60 different mammalian Rabs. Traffic (Copenhagen, Denmark). 2010;11(4):491–507.
22. Kobayashi H, Etoh K, Ohbayashi N, Fukuda M. Rab35 promotes the recruitment of Rab8, Rab13 and Rab36 to recycling endosomes through MICAL-L1 during neurite outgrowth. Biol Open. 2014;3(9):803–14.
23. Kobayashi H, Etoh K, Fukuda M. Rab35 is translocated from Arf6-positive perinuclear recycling endosomes to neurite tips during neurite outgrowth. Small GTPases. 2014;5:e29290.
24. Kobayashi H, Fukuda M. Rab35 regulates Arf6 activity through centaurin-beta2 (ACAP2) during neurite outgrowth. J Cell Sci. 2012;125(Pt 9):2235–43.

25. Chevallier J, Koop C, Srivastava A, Petrie RJ, Lamarche-Vane N, Presley JF. Rab35 regulates neurite outgrowth and cell shape. FEBS Lett. 2009;583(7):1096–101.
26. Hsu C, Morohashi Y, Yoshimura S, Manrique-Hoyos N, Jung S, Lauterbach MA, Bakhti M, Gronborg M, Mobius W, Rhee J, et al. Regulation of exosome secretion by Rab35 and its GTPase-activating proteins TBC1D10A-C. J Cell Biol. 2010;189(2):223–32.
27. Chesneau L, Dambournet D, Machicoane M, Kouranti I, Fukuda M, Goud B, Echard A. An ARF6/Rab35 GTPase cascade for endocytic recycling and successful cytokinesis. Curr Biol CB. 2012;22(2):147–53.
28. Zhang J, Fonovic M, Suyama K, Bogyo M, Scott MP. Rab35 controls actin bundling by recruiting fascin as an effector protein. Science. 2009;325(5945):1250–4.
29. Dambournet D, Machicoane M, Chesneau L, Sachse M, Rocancourt M, El Marjou A, Formstecher E, Salomon R, Goud B, Echard A. Rab35 GTPase and OCRL phosphatase remodel lipids and F-actin for successful cytokinesis. Nat Cell Biol. 2011;13(8):981–8.
30. Chua CE, Lim YS, Tang BL. Rab35–a vesicular traffic-regulating small GTPase with actin modulating roles. FEBS Lett. 2010;584(1):1–6.
31. Marat AL, Ioannou MS, McPherson PS. Connecdenn 3/DENND1C binds actin linking Rab35 activation to the actin cytoskeleton. Mol Biol Cell. 2012;23(1):163–75.
32. Chaineau M, Ioannou MS, McPherson PS. Rab35: GEFs, GAPs and effectors. Traffic (Copenhagen, Denmark). 2013;14(11):1109–17.
33. Egami Y, Fukuda M, Araki N. Rab35 regulates phagosome formation through recruitment of ACAP2 in macrophages during FcgammaR-mediated phagocytosis. J Cell Sci. 2011;124(Pt 21):3557–67.
34. Shim J, Lee SM, Lee MS, Yoon J, Kweon HS, Kim YJ. Rab35 mediates transport of Cdc42 and Rac1 to the plasma membrane during phagocytosis. Mol Cell Biol. 2010;30(6):1421–33.
35. Charrasse S, Comunale F, De Rossi S, Echard A, Gauthier-Rouviere C. Rab35 regulates cadherin-mediated adherens junction formation and myoblast fusion. Mol Biol Cell. 2013;24(3):234–45.
36. Zhu Y, Shen T, Liu J, Zheng J, Zhang Y, Xu R, Sun C, Du J, Chen Y, Gu L. Rab35 is required for Wnt5a/Dvl2-induced Rac1 activation and cell migration in MCF-7 breast cancer cells. Cell Signal. 2013;25(5):1075–85.
37. Allaire PD, Seyed Sadr M, Chaineau M, Seyed Sadr E, Konefal S, Fotouhi M, Maret D, Ritter B, Del Maestro RF, McPherson PS. Interplay between Rab35 and Arf6 controls cargo recycling to coordinate cell adhesion and migration. J Cell Sci. 2013;126(Pt 3):722–31.
38. Friedman RC, Farh KK, Burge CB, Bartel DP. Most mammalian mRNAs are conserved targets of microRNAs. Genome Res. 2009;19(1):92–105.
39. Grimson A, Farh KK, Johnston WK, Garrett-Engele P, Lim LP, Bartel DP. MicroRNA targeting specificity in mammals: determinants beyond seed pairing. Mol Cell. 2007;27(1):91–105.
40. John B, Enright AJ, Aravin A, Tuschl T, Sander C, Marks DS. Human MicroRNA targets. PLoS Biol. 2004;2(11):e363.
41. Lim LP, Lau NC, Garrett-Engele P, Grimson A, Schelter JM, Castle J, Bartel DP, Linsley PS, Johnson JM. Microarray analysis shows that some microRNAs downregulate large numbers of target mRNAs. Nature. 2005;433(7027):769–73.
42. Ren R, Zhou X, He Y, Ke M, Wu J, Liu X, Yan C, Wu Y, Gong X, Lei X, et al. Crystal structure of a mycobacterial Insig homolog provides insight into how these sensors monitor sterol levels. Science. 2015;349(6244):187–91.
43. Burg JS, Powell DW, Chai R, Hughes AL, Link AJ, Espenshade PJ. Insig regulates HMG-CoA reductase by controlling enzyme phosphorylation in fission yeast. Cell Metab. 2008;8(6):522–31.
44. Sun LP, Seemann J, Goldstein JL, Brown MS. Sterol-regulated transport of SREBPs from endoplasmic reticulum to Golgi: Insig renders sorting signal in Scap inaccessible to COPII proteins. Proc Natl Acad Sci USA. 2007;104(16):6519–26.
45. Radhakrishnan A, Ikeda Y, Kwon HJ, Brown MS, Goldstein JL. Sterol-regulated transport of SREBPs from endoplasmic reticulum to Golgi: oxysterols block transport by binding to Insig. Proc Natl Acad Sci USA. 2007;104(16):6511–8.
46. Goldstein JL, DeBose-Boyd RA, Brown MS. Protein sensors for membrane sterols. Cell. 2006;124(1):35–46.
47. Zarelli VE, Dawid IB. The BTB-containing protein Kctd15 is SUMOylated in vivo. PLoS One. 2013;8(9):e75016.
48. Zarelli VE, Dawid IB. Inhibition of neural crest formation by Kctd15 involves regulation of transcription factor AP-2. Proc Natl Acad Sci USA. 2013;110(8):2870–5.
49. Polyak K, Weinberg RA. Transitions between epithelial and mesenchymal states: acquisition of malignant and stem cell traits. Nat Rev Cancer. 2009;9(4):265–73.
50. Miettinen PJ, Ebner R, Lopez AR, Derynck R. TGF-beta induced transdifferentiation of mammary epithelial cells to mesenchymal cells: involvement of type I receptors. J Cell Biol. 1994;127(6 Pt 2):2021–36.
51. Quail DF, Joyce JA. Microenvironmental regulation of tumor progression and metastasis. Nat Med. 2013;19(11):1423–37.
52. Chaffer CL, Weinberg RA. A perspective on cancer cell metastasis. Science. 2011;331(6024):1559–64.
53. Zhou L, Liu F, Wang X, Ouyang G. The roles of microRNAs in the regulation of tumor metastasis. Cell Biosci. 2015;5:32.
54. Vidigal JA, Ventura A. The biological functions of miRNAs: lessons from in vivo studies. Trends Cell Biol. 2015;25(3):137–47.
55. Cloonan N, Brown MK, Steptoe AL, Wani S, Chan WL, Forrest AR, Kolle G, Gabrielli B, Grimmond SM. The miR-17-5p microRNA is a key regulator of the G1/S phase cell cycle transition. Genome Biol. 2008;9(8):R127.
56. Lu LF, Gasteiger G, Yu IS, Chaudhry A, Hsin JP, Lu Y, Bos PD, Lin LL, Zawislak CL, Cho S, et al. A Single miRNA-mRNA Interaction Affects the Immune Response in a Context- and Cell-Type-Specific Manner. Immunity. 2015;43(1):52–64.
57. Tay Y, Tan SM, Karreth FA, Lieberman J, Pandolfi PP. Characterization of dual PTEN and p53-targeting microRNAs identifies microRNA-638/Dnm2 as a two-hit oncogenic locus. Cell Rep. 2014;8(3):714–22.
58. Denzler R, Agarwal V, Stefano J, Bartel DP, Stoffel M. Assessing the ceRNA hypothesis with quantitative measurements of miRNA and target abundance. Mol Cell. 2014;54(5):766–76.
59. Chikh A, Matin RN, Senatore V, Hufbauer M, Lavery D, Raimondi C, Ostano P, Mello-Grand M, Ghimenti C, Bahta A, et al. iASPP/p63 autoregulatory feedback loop is required for the homeostasis of stratified epithelia. EMBO J. 2011;30(20):4261–73.
60. Wang Y, Zhang Z, Ji D, Chen GF, Feng X, Gong LL, Guo J, Li ZW, Chen CF, Zhao BB, et al. Regulation of T cell function by microRNA-720. Sci Rep. 2015;5:12159.
61. Guzman N, Agarwal K, Asthagiri D, Yu L, Saji M, Ringel MD, Paulaitis ME. Breast Cancer-Specific miR Signature Unique to Extracellular Vesicles Includes "microRNA-like" tRNA Fragments. Mol Cancer Res MCR. 2015;13(5):891–901.
62. Uytterhoeven V, Kuenen S, Kasprowicz J, Miskiewicz K, Verstreken P. Loss of skywalker reveals synaptic endosomes as sorting stations for synaptic vesicle proteins. Cell. 2011;145(1):117–32.
63. Hanono A, Garbett D, Reczek D, Chambers DN, Bretscher A. EPI64 regulates microvillar subdomains and structure. J Cell Biol. 2006;175(5):803–13.
64. Kang K, Zhang X, Liu H, Wang Z, Zhong J, Huang Z, Peng X, Zeng Y, Wang Y, Yang Y, et al. A novel real-time PCR assay of microRNAs using S-Poly(T), a specific oligo(dT) reverse transcription primer with excellent sensitivity and specificity. PLoS One. 2012;7(11):e48536.
65. Lin Y, Li D, Liang Q, Liu S, Zuo X, Li L, Sun X, Li W, Guo M, Huang Z. miR-638 regulates differentiation and proliferation in leukemic cells by targeting cyclin-dependent kinase 2. J Biol Chem. 2015;290(3):1818–28.
66. Ho SN, Hunt HD, Horton RM, Pullen JK, Pease LR. Site-directed mutagenesis by overlap extension using the polymerase chain reaction. Gene. 1989;77(1):51–9.

Co-administration with DNA encoding papillomavirus capsid proteins enhances the antitumor effects generated by therapeutic HPV DNA vaccination

Benjamin Yang[1], Andrew Yang[1], Shiwen Peng[1], Xiaowu Pang[5], Richard B.S. Roden[1,2,4], T.-C. Wu[1,2,3,4] and Chien-Fu Hung[1,4*]

Abstract

Background: DNA vaccines have emerged as attractive candidates for the control of human papillomavirus (HPV)-associated malignancies. However, DNA vaccines suffer from limited immunogenicity and thus strategies to enhance DNA vaccine potency are needed. We have previously demonstrated that for DNA vaccines encoding HPV-16 E7 antigen (CRT/E7) linkage with calreticulin (CRT) linked enhances both the E7-specific $CD8^+$ T cell immune responses and antitumor effects against E7-expressing tumors. In the current study, we aim to introduce an approach to elicit potent $CD4^+$ T cell help for the enhancement of antigen-specific $CD8^+$ T cell immune responses generated by CRT/E7 DNA vaccination by using co-administration of a DNA vector expressing papillomavirus major and minor capsid antigens, L1 and L2.

Result: We showed that co-administration of vectors containing codon-optimized bovine papillomavirus type 1 (BPV-1) L1 and L2 in combination with DNA vaccines could elicit enhanced antigen-specific $CD8^+$ in both CRT/E7 and ovalbumin (OVA) antigenic systems. We also demonstrated that co-administration of vectors expressing BPV-1 L1 and/or L2 DNA with CRT/E7 DNA led to the generation of L1/L2-specific $CD4^+$ T cell immune responses and L1-specific neutralizing antibodies. Furthermore, we showed that co-administration with DNA encoding BPV1 L1 significantly enhances the therapeutic antitumor effects generated by CRT/E7 DNA vaccination. In addition, the observed enhancement of $CD8^+$ T cell immune responses by DNA encoding L1 and L2 was also found to extend to HPV-16 L1/L2 system.

Conclusion: Our strategy elicits both potent neutralizing antibody and therapeutic responses and may potentially be extended to other antigenic systems beyond papillomavirus for the control of infection and/or cancer.

Keywords: Capsid, DNA vaccine, Human papillomavirus (HPV)

Background

The knowledge that high risk human papillomavirus (HPV) is a necessary etiological factor for the development of cervical cancer provides the opportunity for control of cervical cancer and/or other HPV-associated malignancies through vaccination against HPV. Currently, the two commercially available prophylactic vaccines, Gardasil and Cervarix, based upon virus-like particles (VLP) derived from the major capsid protein L1 effectively protect against infection by the two most common HPV types found in cervical cancer (for review see [1]). The minor capsid antigen L2 also shows promise for preventive vaccination in animal models, although it is less immunogenic than L1 VLP. However, neither L1 VLP nor L2-based vaccines generate therapeutic effects against established HPV infection [2]. Therefore, given the significant burden of HPV-associated lesions worldwide, there is an urgent need to develop therapeutic HPV vaccines for the control of existing HPV infection and associated malignancies.

* Correspondence: chung2@jhmi.edu
[1]Departments of Pathology, School of Medicine, Johns Hopkins University, CRBII Room 307, 1550 Orleans Street, Baltimore, MD 21231, USA
[4]Oncology, Johns Hopkins Medical Institutions, Baltimore, MD, USA
Full list of author information is available at the end of the article

Quite different from preventive vaccines which target the viral capsid proteins L1 and/or L2, therapeutic HPV vaccines focus on targeting the HPV E6 and E7, since only these oncoproteins are consistently expressed in HPV-associated cancers and are responsible for the malignant transformation.

Among the various therapeutic HPV vaccines currently being tested, DNA vaccines have emerged as attractive candidates for the treatment of cervical cancer and associated malignancies. Naked DNA is relatively safe, stable, and easy to produce and transport (for review see [3]). Furthermore, DNA vaccines are capable of sustained cellular gene expression, promote MHC class I antigen presentation, and have the capacity for repeated administration since they do not lead to the generation of neutralizing antibodies. However, an important limitation of DNA vaccines is limited potency since they lack the intrinsic ability to amplify and spread *in vivo*. Therefore, it is important to consider strategies to improve DNA vaccine potency strategies (for review, see [4, 5]).

One strategy to enhance DNA vaccine potency is to improve antigen expression, processing, and presentation in antigen-presenting cells using intracellular targeting strategies (for review, see [4, 5]). Several of our previous studies have employed DNA vaccines encoding calreticulin (CRT) linked to HPV-16 E7 antigen (CRT/E7) [6–11] because this fusion greatly enhances the E7-specific $CD8^+$ T cell immune responses in vaccinated mice. This phenomenon likely reflects the efficient recognition of calreticulin by dendritic cells and improved targeting to the MHCI pathway by targeting to the endoplasmic reticulum [6].

Activation and proliferation of $CD4^+$ T cells is crucial to the success of both humoral and cell-mediated responses to viral infection. Although the fusion of E7 with CRT enables such DNA vaccines to elicit significant E7-specific CD8 T cell immunity in the absence of CD4 T cell help [12], approaches to boost $CD4^+$ T cell help are likely to enhance DNA vaccine potency. Indeed, CD4 $^+$ T cells play a significant role in priming effector $CD8^+$ T cells, thus augmenting the $CD8^+$ T cell responses, as well as generation of memory T cell populations (for review see [13]). $CD4^+$ T cells help to differentiate naïve $CD8^+$ T cells into effector cells by providing activation signals to dendritic cells (DCs), most notably IL-2, thus promoting $CD8^+$ T cell proliferation. Thus, strategies to induce $CD4^+$ T helper cells at sites of $CD8^+$ T cell priming can potentially enhance CTL immune responses.

In the current study, we aim to combine intracellular targeting strategies using CRT with a strategy to enhance $CD4^+$ T help for the development of a therapeutic HPV DNA vaccine. Since papillomavirus L1 or L2 antigens likely contain $CD4^+$ T cell epitopes [14–18], we reasoned that co-administration of vectors containing codon-optimized bovine papillomavirus (BPV) L1 and L2 may provide $CD4^+$ T cell help and enhance the antigen-specific $CD8^+$ T cell immune responses generated by DNA vaccines. An additional potential benefit would be the induction of neutralizing antibody and protective immunity [19, 20]. We showed that co-administration of vectors containing BPV L1 or L2 DNA in combination with DNA vaccines could elicit enhanced antigen-specific $CD8^+$ in both CRT/E7 and ovalbumin (OVA) antigenic systems. We also demonstrated that co-administration of vectors containing BPV1 L1 ± L2 DNA with CRT/E7 DNA led to the generation of L1/L2-specific $CD4^+$ T cell immune responses as well as L1-specific neutralizing antibodies. Furthermore, we showed that co-administration with BPV1 L1 significantly enhances the therapeutic antitumor effects generated by CRT/E7 DNA vaccination. In addition, the observed enhancement of $CD8^+$ T cell immune responses by DNA encoding L1 and L2 was also found to extend to HPV-16 L1/L2 system. Overall, our data suggest that co-administration of DNA encoding papillomavirus L1 or L2 can be used to enhance antigen-specific $CD8^+$ T cell immune responses generated by therapeutic HPV DNA vaccination for the control of HPV infection and HPV-associated tumors. Furthermore, our approach can also generate neutralizing antibodies against papillomavirus for potential prevention against infection. This strategy also provides the opportunity to combine preventive and therapeutic approaches. Our strategy may potentially be extended to other antigenic systems for the control of infection and/or cancer.

Results

Co-administration with vectors encoding papillomavirus L1 or L2 significantly enhances the antigen-specific $CD8^+$ T cell immune responses generated by CRT/E7 or OVA DNA vaccination

In order to characterize the antigen-specific $CD8^+$ T cell immune responses generated by vaccination with CRT/E7 or OVA DNA in combination with vectors containing codon-optimized BPV1 L1 or L2 DNA, C57BL/6 mice (five per group) were vaccinated intradermally via gene gun with CRT/E7 or OVA DNA with or without BPV1 L1 or L2 DNA twice at 1-week intervals. Splenocytes from vaccinated mice were collected 1 week after last immunization and the E7 or OVA-specific T cell immune responses were characterized using intracellular cytokine staining followed by flow cytometry analysis. As shown in Fig. 1, mice vaccinated with CRT/E7 or OVA DNA vaccine in combination with BPV1-L1 or L2 DNA generated significantly higher E7-specific and OVA-specific $CD8^+$ T cell immune responses compared to mice vaccinated with CRT/E7 or OVA DNA alone. To evaluate whether the enhancement of antigen-specific CD8+ T cell immune responses by co-administration of

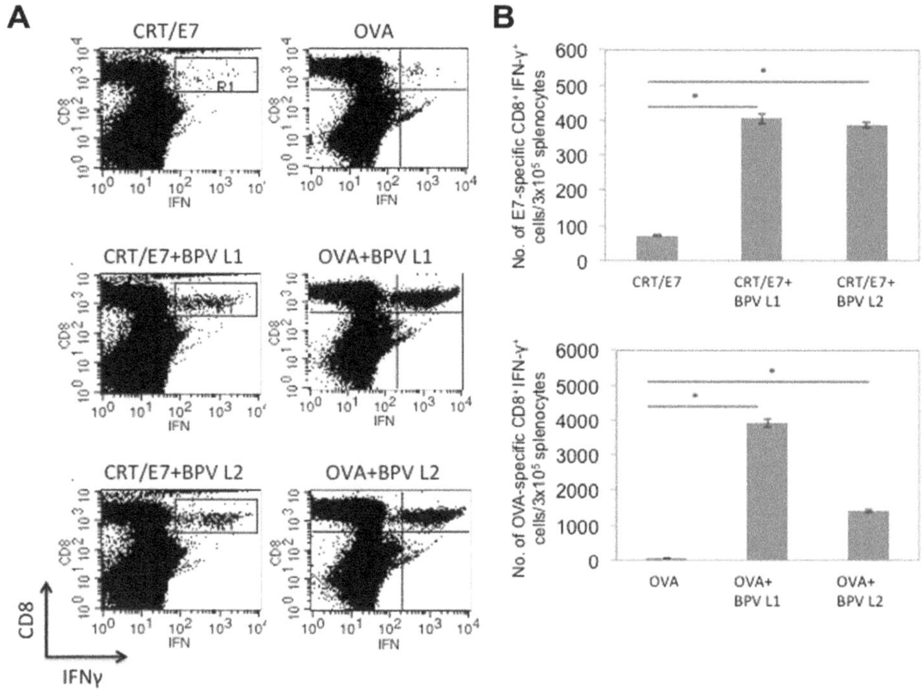

Fig. 1 Characterization of antigen-specific CD8$^+$ T cell immune responses generated by antigen-specific DNA vaccine mixed with vectors containing BPV1 L1 or L2 DNA. C57BL/6 mice (five per group) were vaccinated intradermally via gene gun with 2 μg/mouse of CRT/E7 or OVA DNA with or without BPV1 L1 or L2 DNA twice at 1-week intervals. Splenocytes from vaccinated mice were collected 1 week after last immunization and the E7 or OVA-specific T cell immune responses were characterized using intracellular cytokine staining followed by flow cytometry analysis. **a** Representative flow cytometry data depicting the number of E7 (upper panel) or OVA(lower panel)-specific CD8$^+$ T cells. **b** Bar graph representing the number of E7 (upper panel) or OVA (lower panel) -specific CD8$^+$ T cells/3x10^5 splenocytes (mean ± SD). Data shown are representative of two experiments performed. * indicates $p < 0.05$

BPV1 L1 or L2 DNA is also observed in other papillomavirus systems, we co-administered HPV16 L1 or L2 DNA with CRT/E7 or OVA DNA vaccination. Of note, co-administration of HPV16 L1 or L2 DNA with CRT/E7 or OVA DNA vaccination also generated significantly higher E7-specific CD8+ T cell responses compared to CRT/E7 or OVA DNA vaccination alone in mice (Fig. 2). Thus, our data indicate that co-administration with papillomavirus L1 or L2 DNA significantly enhances the antigen-specific CD8$^+$ T cell immune responses generated by DNA vaccination.

Co-administration of papillomavirus L1 or L2 DNA with CRT/E7 or OVA DNA led to the generation of L1/L2-specific CD4$^+$ T cell immune responses

In order to determine whether the co-administration with BPV1 L1 or L2 DNA with CRT/E7 DNA will lead to the generation of L1 or L2-specific CD4$^+$ T cell immune responses, C57BL/6 mice (five per group) were vaccinated intradermally via gene gun with CRT/E7 DNA with BPV1 L1 or L2 DNA. Mice vaccinated with CRT/E7 DNA alone were used as negative controls. Splenocytes from vaccinated mice were collected 1 week after last immunization and incubated with BPV1 L1/L2 virus-like particles (VLPs). The L1 or L2-specific CD4$^+$ T cell immune responses were characterized using intracellular cytokine staining followed by flow cytometry analysis. As shown in Fig. 3a and b, mice vaccinated with BPV1 L1 in combination with CRT/E7 DNA led to the generation of L1-specific CD4$^+$ T cell immune responses. Similarly, vaccination with BPV1 L2 with CRT/E7 DNA led to significant level of L2-specific CD4$^+$ T cell immune responses compared to vaccination with CRT/E7 alone. Again, to observe whether the CD4+ T cell responses elicited by this vaccination strategy extend to other papillomavirus systems, we co-administered HPV16 L1 or L2 DNA with CRT/E7 or OVA DNA vaccination. As shown in Fig. 3c and d, compared to vaccination with CRT/E7 or OVA DNA alone, mice vaccinated with HPV-16 L1 or L2 DNA in combination with CRT/E7 or OVA DNA led to the generation of L1 or L2-specific CD4$^+$ T cell immune responses. These results suggest that co-administration with DNA encoding papillomavirus L1 or L2 with

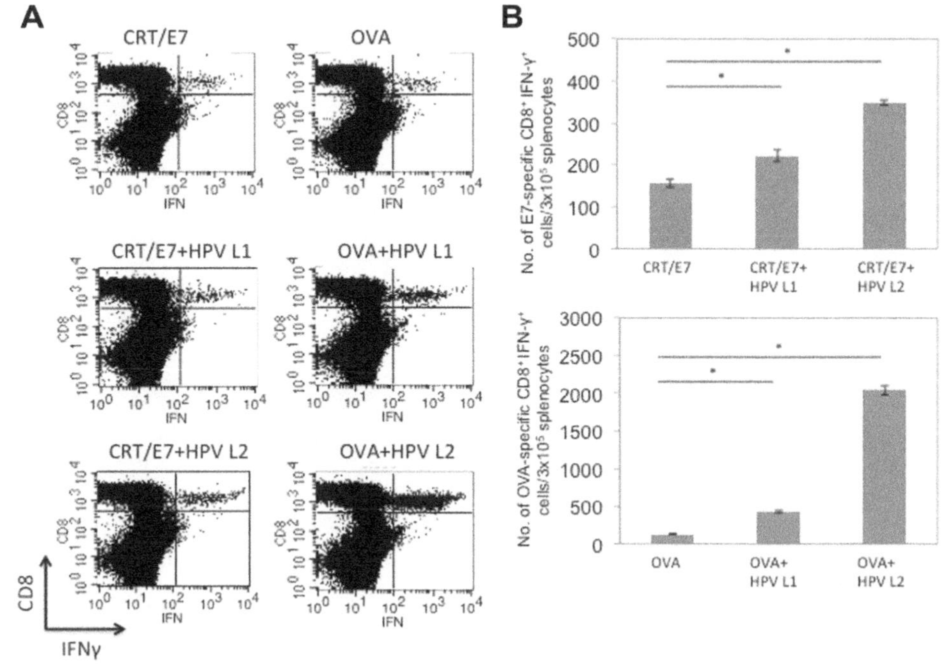

Fig. 2 Characterization of antigen-specific $CD8^+$ T cell immune responses generated by antigen-specific DNA vaccine mixed with HPV-16 L1 or L2 DNA. C57BL/6 mice (five per group) were vaccinated intradermally via gene gun with 2 μg/mouse of CRT/E7 or OVA DNA with or without HPV-16 L1 or L2 DNA twice at 1-week intervals. Splenocytes from vaccinated mice were collected 1 week after last immunization and the E7 or OVA-specific T cell immune responses were characterized using intracellular cytokine staining followed by flow cytometry analysis. **a** Representative flow cytometry data depicting the number of E7 (upper panel) or OVA (lower panel)-specific $CD8^+$ T cells. **b** Bar graph representing the number of E7 (upper panel) or OVA (lower panel)-specific $CD8^+$ T cells/$3x10^5$ splenocytes (mean± SD). Data shown are representative of two experiments performed. * indicates $p < 0.05$

CRT/E7 DNA was able to generate appreciable L1 or L2-specific $CD4^+$ T cell immune responses respectively in vaccinated mice.

Co-administration with BPV1 L1 DNA significantly enhances the therapeutic antitumor effects generated by CRT/E7 DNA vaccination

In order to determine if the observed enhancement of antigen-specific $CD8^+$ T cell immune responses by co-administration of BPV1 L1 DNA can translate into potent therapeutic antitumor effects, we performed in vivo tumor treatment experiments using an HPV-16 E7-expressing murine tumor cell line, TC-1. TC-1 also expresses HPV16 E6, but does not contain either L1 or L2. C57BL/6 mice (five per group) were first challenged with TC-1 tumor cells subcutaneously. One week after tumor challenge, mice were treated intradermally via gene gun with CRT/E7 DNA alone, BPV1 L1 DNA alone or CRT/E7 DNA in combination with BPV1 L1 DNA. Vaccinated mice were boosted twice at 1-week intervals with the same dose and regimen. Tumor growth were monitored twice weekly by caliper measurements and palpations. As shown in Fig. 4, tumor-bearing mice treated with CRT/E7 DNA vaccine in combination with BPV1 L1 DNA generated significantly reduced tumor volume and prolonged survival compared to mice treated with CRT/E7 DNA alone or BPV1 L1 DNA alone. Thus, our data indicate that co-administration with BPV1 L1 DNA is capable of significantly enhancing the therapeutic antitumor effects generated by CRT/E7 DNA vaccination.

The enhancement in E7-specific CD8+ T cell immune responses are contributed by CD4+ T helper cells

In order to determine the mechanism underlying the observed enhancement of antigen-specific CD8+ T cell immune responses generated by coadministration with L1 or L2 DNA vectors, we have generated pcDNA3 encoding the reverse sequences of L1 (BPV L1 (–)) or L2 DNA (BPV L2 (–)). C57BL/6 mice (five per group) were vaccinated intradermally via gene gun with CRT/E7 DNA with or without the reverse sequence of BPV1 L1 or L2 DNA twice at 1-week intervals. Splenocytes from vaccinated mice were collected 1 week after last immunization and the E7-specific T cell immune responses were characterized using intracellular cytokine staining followed by flow cytometry analysis. We found that mice vaccinated with CRT/E7 DNA vaccine in combination with the reverse sequence BPV1-L1 or L2 DNA did not lead to the increased frequency of E7-specific $CD8^+$ T cell immune responses observed in mice

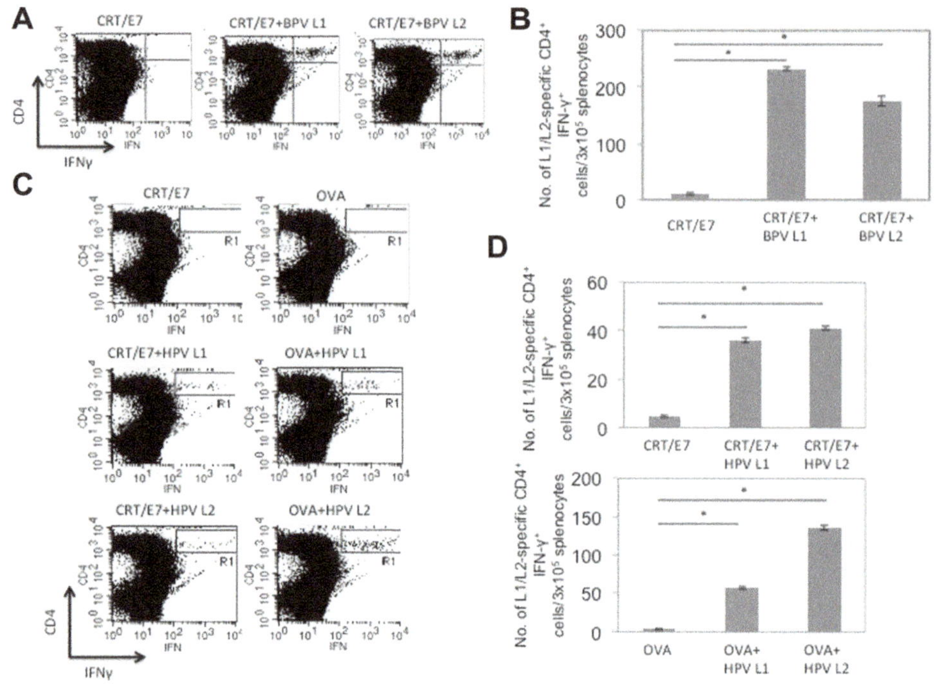

Fig. 3 Characterization of BPV1 and HPV-16 L1 or L2-specific $CD4^+$ T cell immune responses generated by CRT/E7 or OVA DNA mixed with DNA encoding BPV1 or HPV-16 L1 or L2. C57BL/6 mice (five per group) were vaccinated intradermally via gene gun with 2 μg/mouse of CRT/E7 with or without BPV1 or HPV-16 L1 or L2 DNA twice at 1-week intervals. Splenocytes from vaccinated mice were collected 1 week after last immunization and pulsed with 5 μg/mL of BPV1 or HPV-16 L1/L2 VLPs. The BPV1 L1/ L2-specific $CD4^+$ T cell immune responses were characterized using intracellular cytokine staining followed by flow cytometry analysis. **a** Representative flow cytometry data depicting the number of BPV1 L1/L2-specific $CD4^+$ T cells. **b** Bar graph representing the number of BPV1 L1/L2-specific $CD4^+$ T cells/$3x10^5$ splenocytes (mean± SD). **c** Representative flow cytometry data depicting the number of HPV-16 L1/L2-specific $CD4^+$ T cells. **d** Bar graph representing the number of HPV-16 L1/L2-specific $CD4^+$ T cells/$3x10^5$ splenocytes (mean± SD). Data shown are representative of two experiments performed. * indicates $p < 0.05$

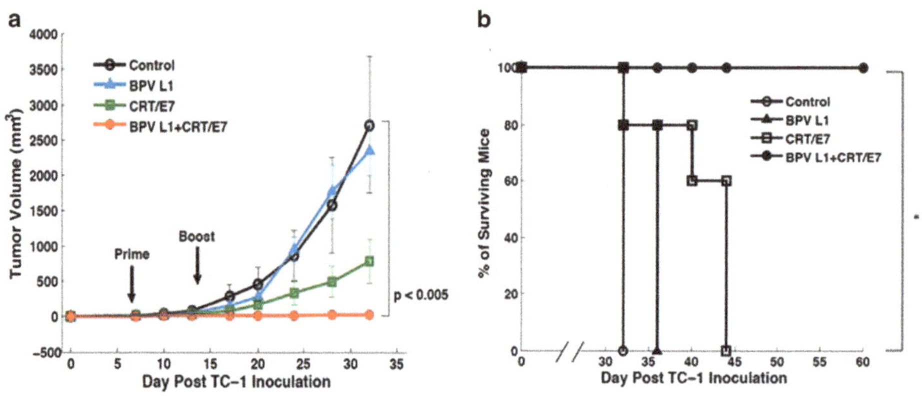

Fig. 4 *In vivo* tumor treatment experiments in mice vaccinated with CRT/E7 DNA mixed with BPV1 L1 DNA. C57BL/6 mice (five per group) were first challenged with $1x10^5$/mouse of TC-1 tumor cells subcutaneously. One week after tumor challenge, mice were treated intradermally via gene gun with 2 μg/mouse of CRT/E7 DNA alone, BPV1 L1 DNA alone or CRT/E7 DNA in combination with BPV1 L1 DNA. Vaccinated mice were boosted twice at 1-week intervals with the same dose and regimen. Mice were sacrificed on day 30 after the last vaccination. Tumor growth were monitored twice weekly by caliper measurements and palpations. **a** Line graph depicting the tumor volume over time of tumor-bearing mice treated with CRT/E7 DNA and/or BPV1 L1 DNA. **b** Kaplan-Meier survival analysis of tumor-bearing mice treated with CRT/E7 DNA and/or BPV1 L1 DNA. The data presented are from one representative experiment of the two performed. * indicates $p < 0.05$

vaccinated with CRT/E7 DNA with BPV1-L1 or L2 DNA (data not shown). The insert sequences does not express into L1 and L2 that activate CD4+ T cell help, thereby cannot enhance the E7-specific CD8+ T cell responses of the CRT/E7 vaccine. The result suggests that CD4+ T cell help generated by co-expression of L1 or L2 protein promotes E7-specific CD8+ T cell immune responses to CRT/E7 DNA vaccination.

Co-administration of BPV1 L1 DNA with CRT/E7 DNA led to the generation of L1-specific neutralizing antibodies

In order to determine if co-administration of BPV1 L1 DNA with CRT/E7 DNA will lead to the generation of BPV1 L1-specific neutralizing antibodies, C57BL/6 mice (three per group) were immunized on days 1, 15, and 30 intradermally via gene gun with CRT/E7 and/or BPV1 L1 DNA. In vitro neutralization assays were performed using BPV1 L1 pseudovirus on twofold dilutions of antisera collected from the mice 2 weeks after the final immunization. Mice vaccinated with CRT/E7 in combination with BPV1 L1 DNA were found to generate similar neutralizing antibody responses compared to mice vaccinated with BPV1 L1 DNA alone (Fig. 5).

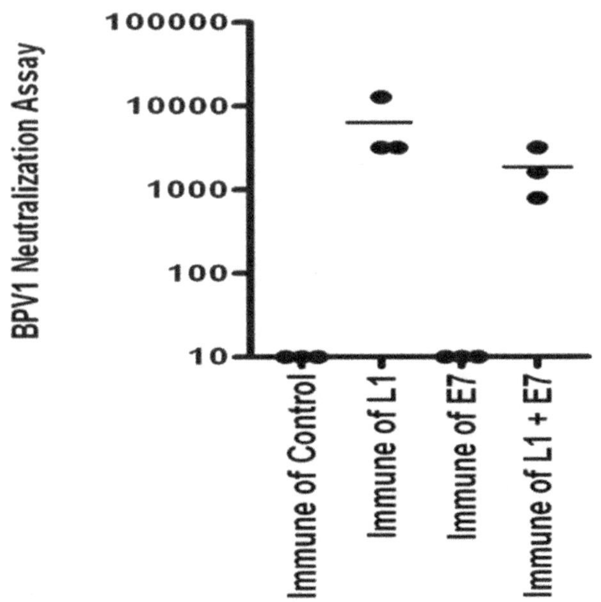

Fig. 5 Characterization of BPV1-specific neutralizing antibody responses generated by mice vaccinated with CRT/E7 and/or BPV1 L1 DNA. C57BL/6 mice (three per group) were immunized on days 1, 15, and 30 intradermally using a gene gun with 2 μg of DNA per mouse of CRT/E7 and/or BPV1 L1 DNA. In vitro neutralization assays were performed using BPV1 L1 pseudovirus on twofold dilutions of antisera collected from the mice 2 weeks after the final immunization. Endpoint titers achieving 50 % neutralization are plotted and the means shown as horizontal lines. PI = Pre Immune; L1 = BPV1 L1 DNA vaccine; E7 = CRT/E7 DNA vaccine

Co-administration of BPV1 L1 or L2 DNA with OVA DNA vaccination generated OVA-specific CD8+ T cell response through intramuscular administration

Finally, we evaluate whether co-administration with papillomavirus L1 or L2 DNA can elicit potent antigen-specific CD8+ T cell responses when applied through different route of administration. C57BL/6 mice (three per group) were vaccinated intramuscularly with OVA DNA with or without BPV1 L1 or L2 DNA twice at one-week intervals. One week after the last immunization, PBMCs were collected and the OVA-specific CD8+ T cell immune responses were characterized through flow cytometry analysis. As shown in Fig. 6, mice vaccinated intramuscularly with OVA DNA in combination with BPV1 L1 or L2 DNA generated significantly higher percentage of OVA-specific CD8+ T cells compared to mice vaccinated intramuscularly with OVA DNA alone. This data indicates that co-administration with papillomavirus L1 or L2 DNA can lead to enhanced antigen-specific CD8+ T cell immune responses through the intramuscular route of administration.

Discussion

In the current study, we showed that co-administration of vectors containing codon-optimized BPV1 or HPV-16 L1 or L2 in combination with DNA vaccines could elicit enhanced antigen-specific $CD8^+$ in both CRT/E7 and ovalbumin (OVA) antigenic systems. We also demonstrated that co-administration of BPV1 or HPV-16 L1 or L2 DNA with CRT/E7 DNA led to the generation of L1/L2-specific $CD4^+$ T cell immune responses. In addition, the observed enhancement of E7-specific $CD8^+$ T cell immune responses by L1 DNA also confers improved therapeutic antitumor effects against an E7-expressing tumor. Moreover, co-administration of BPV1 L1 DNA induced generation of L1-specific neutralizing antibodies, which may serve to prevent further papillomavirus infections. Of note, the enhanced antigen-specific CD8+ T cell responses are observed in intradermal as well as intramuscular routes of administration. Indeed, we have already shown that vaccination with vector expressing L1 is protective against vaginal challenge with papillomavirus pseudovirions [20]. Taken together, our study suggests the promise of this approach for future clinical translation, and it can potentially be applied to other antigenic systems.

Here we show that CD4+ T cell help plays an important role in the enhancement of antigen-specific CD8+ T cell immune responses observed in our vaccination regimen as co-administration with the reverse sequence of BPV1 L1 or L2 did not enhance the antigen-specific CD8+ T cell responses. Studies have shown that L1 and L2 are generally much more effective in eliciting CD4+ T cell responses [14–18]. While it is possible that BPV L1 or L2 could elicit some CD8+ T cell responses, we

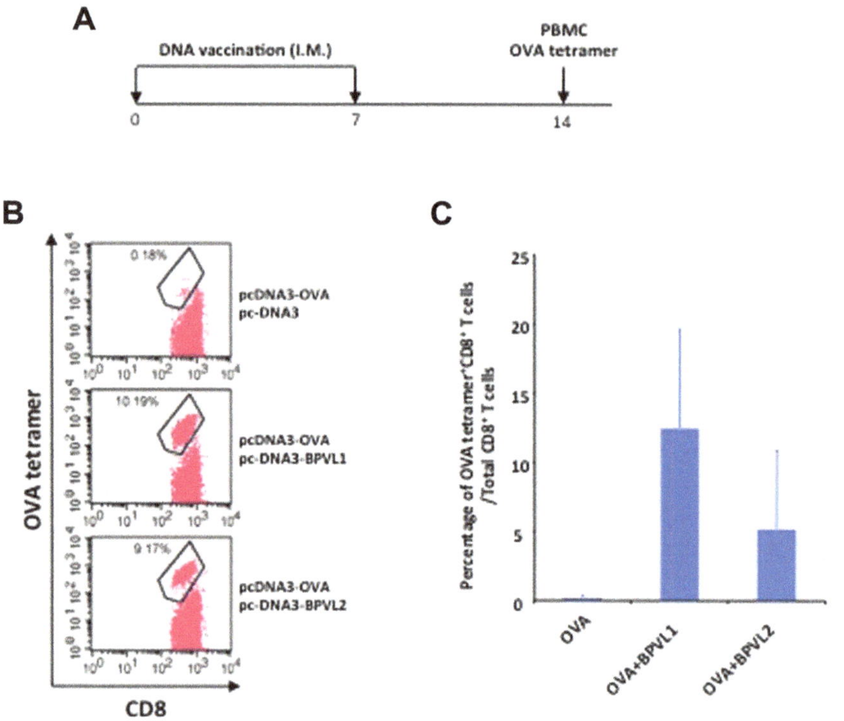

Fig. 6 Comparison of OVA-specific $CD8^+$ T cell responses induced by pcDNA3-OVA vaccination with or without co-administration of BPV L1 or L2. **a**. Schematic illustration of the experiment. Briefly, 5 ~ 8 weeks old female C57BL/6 mice (3 mice/group) were vaccinated with 10 μg/mouse of pcDNA3-OVA, with either 10 μg/mouse of pcDNA3, or pcDNA3-BPVL1, or pcDNA3-BPVL2 via intramuscular injection. The mice were boosted with the same regimen once after one week. 7 days after the last vaccination, PBMCs were collected from peripheral blood, stained with FITC-conjugated anti-mouse CD8a antibody, PE-conjugated OVA peptide (SIINFEKL) loaded $H\text{-}2K^b$ tetramer. The data were acquired with FACSCalibur and analyzed with CellQuest. **b**. Representative flow cytometry image of PBMC staining. **c**. Summary of the flow cytometry data

believe the CD4+ T cell help generated by L1 or L2 DNA is the main contributor to the enhanced antigen-specific CD8+ T cell response observed. Furthermore, it has been shown that CD4+ T cells can help generate memory T cells [21, 22]. Though the current study focuses on characterizing the antigen-specific CD8+ T cell therapeutic antitumor effect by our vaccination strategy, it will be of interest for future studies to further characterize the complete effect of CD4+ T cell and its ability to generate memory T cell responses for prolonged protection.

Our vaccination strategy was able to generate a potent therapeutic antitumor effect in tumor-bearing mice. Interestingly, co-administration of BPV1 L1 DNA with CRT/E7 DNA generated L1-specific neutralizing antibodies, which confers prophylactic value. It has also been shown that vaccination with L1 DNA induced L1-specific neutralizing antibodies in Balb/c mice [20]. Therefore, our vaccination strategy of co-administration of L1 DNA can generate potent antibody responses in more than one genetic background. Of note, studies have shown that papillomavirus L2 is generally not as effective in generating L2-specific neutralizing antibodies [20, 23], thus co-administration with L1 DNA should be prioritized in future translation.

In the current study we show that co-administration of BPV1 L1 DNA with CRT/E7 led to potent therapeutic antitumor effects and prolonged survival due to the enhanced antigen-specific CD8+ T cell responses by CD4+ T cell help. Since co-administration with HPV16 L1 DNA with CRT/E7 also significantly enhances antigen-specific CD8+ T cell responses by CD4+ T cell help, we believe that potent therapeutic antitumor effects should also be observed. To further promote clinical translation, subsequent investigations focusing on directly characterizing the antitumor effects of co-administrating HPV16 L1 with CRT/E7, and whether reversing the sequence of HPV16 L1 abolishes the antigen-specific CD8+ T cell response enhancement should be conducted. In addition, since our vaccination regimen achieved complete tumor suppression, the frequency of vaccination may be modified and further studied to determine the optimal vaccination regimen. Importantly, our data show that the current vaccination strategy can generate enhanced antigen-specific CD8+ T cell responses by both intradermal and intramuscular vaccination. Since DNA vaccines are commonly applied intramuscularly in the clinic, future translation of the current vaccination technology may focus on the intramuscular route of administration.

Several strategies have been employed to induce $CD4^+$ T helper cells to enhance antigen-specific $CD8^+$ T cell-mediated immune responses generated by therapeutic HPV DNA vaccines. We have previously demonstrated that a DNA vaccine encoding invariant chain (Ii) with the class II-associated invariant peptide (CLIP) region replaced with the pan HLA-DR binding epitope (PADRE) could elicit potent PADRE-specific $CD4^+$ T cell responses in vaccinated mice [24]. In addition, a co-administration of this DNA construct (Ii-PADRE) with DNA encoding HPV-16 E7 generated significantly greater $CD8^+$ T cell immune responses relative to a co-administration of DNA encoding HPV-16 E7 with DNA encoding unmodified Ii [24]. Thus, the current study represents another promising approach to enhance $CD4^+$ T help for the improvement of DNA vaccine potency, but with the added benefit of inducing prophylactic immunity too. It will be of interest in the future to perform a head-to-head comparison between vectors containing BPV L1/L2 DNA with Ii-PADRE DNA for their ability to enhance antigen-specific $CD8^+$ T cell responses by therapeutic HPV DNA vaccines. Such information will facilitate the selection of the most effective or desirable DNA construct for improving DNA vaccine potency.

Another potential mechanism for enhancing the therapeutic HPV DNA vaccine potency through the co-administration with L1/L2 DNA is the potential formation of VLPs in transfected cells. It has been shown that the expression of L1 can lead to the formation of VLPs in eukaryotic cells [25]. Furthermore, previous studies have demonstrated that papillomavirus VLPs can directly activate dendritic cells and thereby increase expression of costimulatory markers and MHC class I and II molecules [26–28]. Thus, the co-administration of L1 DNA may lead to the local activation of DCs, resulting in further enhancement of antigen-specific $CD8^+$ T cell immune responses generated by DNA vaccination. However, since the L2 only expression construct had a similar effect to L1 DNA, this suggests that the presence of VLP does not explain the enhanced CD8 T cell response upon co-administration with CRT-E7 or OVA constructs.

Strategies to enhance $CD4^+$ T cell help may potentially be combined with other strategies to further enhance DNA vaccine potency. We have previously demonstrated a significant enhancement of DNA vaccine potency by combining a strategy to prolong dendritic cell life and intracellular targeting strategies with a strategy to boost $CD4^+$ T cell help [29]. Since all these strategies function via different mechanisms, the combination may potentially result in significantly enhanced antigen-specific immune responses and improved antitumor effects. For clinical translation, it will be desirable to identify the best combination of the different strategies in order to achieve the best DNA vaccine potency.

Conclusions

In summary, our study demonstrates that the employment of DNA encoding papillomavirus L1 or L2 can lead to generation of antigen-specific $CD4^+$ T cells and neutralizing antibodies, resulting in the improvement of therapeutic and preventive HPV DNA vaccine potency. Our strategy may potentially be extended to other antigenic systems for the control of infection and/or cancer.

Materials & Methods

Mice

C57BL/6 mice (6–8 weeks old) were purchased from the National Cancer Institute (Frederick, MD). All animals were maintained under specific pathogen-free conditions at the Johns Hopkins Hospital (Baltimore, MD). All procedures were performed according to the Johns Hopkins Institutional Care and Use Committee approved protocols and in accordance with recommendations for the proper care of laboratory animals.

Cells and DNA constructs

TC-1 cells were obtained by co-transformation of primary C57BL/6 mouse lung epithelial cells with HPV-16 E6 and E7 and an activated ras oncogene as described previously [30]. They were maintained in RPMI medium supplemented with 2 mM glutamine, 1 mM sodium pyruvate, 20 mM 4-(2-hydroxyethyl)-1-piperazineethanesulfonic acid (HEPES), $5x10^5$ M β-mercaptoethanol, 100 IU ml^{-1} penicillin, 100 μg ml^{-1} streptomycin, 10 % fetal bovine serum, and cultured at 37 °C in a humidified incubator with 5 % CO_2. The pcDNA3-OVA and pcDNA3-CRT/E7 DNA constructs were generated as described previously [6, 31].

DNA vaccination

DNA-coated gold particles were prepared as described previously [32]. DNA-coated gold particles were delivered to the shaved abdominal region of mice using a helium-driven gene gun (Bio-Rad Laboratories Inc., Hercules, CA, USA) with a discharge pressure of 400 p.s.i. C57BL/6 mice were immunized with 2 μg of plasmid DNA to each mouse encoding pcDNA3-CRT/E7 mixed with pcDNA3-BPV1-L1 or L2 or HPV-L1 or L2 delivered to the shaved abdomen. The mice received a homologous boost 1 week later.

C57BL/6 mice were vaccinated with 10 μg of pcDNA3-OVA DNA with 10 μg of pcDNA3, pcDNA3-BPVL1, or pcDNA3-BPVL2 intramuscularly in the thigh muscle. The mice received a homologous boost 1 week later

Intracellular cytokine staining and flow cytometry analysis

Splenocytes were harvested from mice 1 week after the last vaccination. Prior to intracellular cytokine staining, $5x10^6$ splenocytes from each vaccination group were incubated for 16 h with 1 μg ml^{-1} HPV-16 E7 H-2Db epitope (RAHYNIVTF) or OVA peptide (ISQAVHAA-HAEINEAGR) [31], or 5 μg/mL BPV1 or HPV-16 L1/L2 VLPs in the presence of GolgiPlug (BD Pharmingen) (1 μl ml^{-1}). The stimulated splenocytes were then washed once with FACScan buffer and stained with phycoerythrin- conjugated monoclonal rat anti-mouse CD8α or CD4. Cells were subjected to intracellular cytokine staining using the Cytofix/Cytoperm kit according to the manufacturer's instructions (BD Pharmingen). Intracellular IFN-γ was stained with fluorescein isothiocyanate-conjugated rat anti-mouse IFN-γ to identify the immune response and cytokine levels. PBMCs were collected from peripheral blood 1 week after last intramuscular vaccination and stained with anti-mouse CD8α and OVA peptide (SIINFEKL) loaded H-$2K^b$ tetramer. Flow cytometry analysis was performed using FACSCalibur with CELLQuest software (BD Biosciences, Mountain View, CA, USA).

In vivo tumor treatment experiments

C57BL/6 mice (five per group) were inoculated subcutaneously with $1x10^5$ TC-1 tumor cells per mouse on the left flank. After 1 week, when tumor progression is usually observed, mice were vaccinated with DNA constructs pcDNA3-BPV1 L1 or L2 or pcDNA3-HPV L1 or L2 in conjunction with pCDNA3-CRT/E7 or pcDNA3-OVA or the control empty vector. A homologous boost was administered 1 week after the first immunization. Mice were monitored for tumor growth by measuring diameters with calipers twice a week.

Neutralization assays

The BPV1 L1, L2 and HPV L1, L2 pseudovirions with encapsulated secreted alkaline phosphatase (SEAP) were generated by co-transfection of 293TT cells with plasmids encoding BPV1 L1, L2 or HPV L1 and L2 and a SEAP reporter plasmid as described previously [33]. Cells collected after transfection were treated overnight with Brij 58 (0.5 %), Benzonase (0.5 %) and purified by centrifugation on an Optiprep step gradient (27, 33, and 39 %) at 40,000 rpm for 4.5 h. Pseudovirus neutralization assays were carried out as outlined previously [34]. Briefly, the pseudovirus and the pooled mouse immune sera were incubated for 1 h and the mixture was used to infect 293TT cells. 68–72 h post-infection, the supernatants were collected and SEAP activity in the supernatants was measured by colorimetric assay. Serum neutralization titers were defined as the highest dilution that caused at least a 50 % reduction in SEAP activity, compared to control pre-immune serum samples.

Statistical analysis

All data expressed as means ± s.d. are representative of at least two different experiments. Data for intracellular cytokine staining with flow cytometry analysis and tumor treatment experiments were evaluated by analysis of variance. Comparisons between individual data points were made using Student's *t*-test. All p values < 0.05 were considered significant.

Abbreviations

HPV: Human papillomavirus; CRT: Calreticulin; BPV: Bovine papillomavirus; OVA: Ovalbumin; DCs: Dendritic cells; VLPs: Virus-like particles; CLIP: Class II-associated invariant peptide; PADRE: Pan HLA-DR binding epitope; SEAP: Encapsulated secreted alkaline phosphatase.

Competing interests

Richard Roden is an inventor of L2-related patents licensed to Shantha Biotechnics Ltd., GlaxoSmithKline, PaxVax, Inc. and Acambis, Inc. Richard Roden has received research funding from Sanofi Pasteur, Shantha Biotechnic, Medigene and GlaxoSmithKline. T.-C. Wu and Richard Roden have an equity ownership interest in Papivax LLC. Richard Roden and T.-C. Wu own Papivax Biotech Inc. stock options and are members of Papivax Biotech Inc.'s Scientific Advisory Board. Under a licensing agreement between Papivax Biotech, Inc. and the Johns Hopkins University, Richard Roden, T.-C. Wu and Chien-fu Hung are entitled to royalties on technologies described in this article. This arrangement has been reviewed and approved by the Johns Hopkins University in accordance with its conflict of interest policies.

Authors' contributions

BY, RBSR, TCW, and CFH conceived and designed experiments and interpreted data. BY, AY, and SP performed and experiments. BY, SP, XP, RBSR, TCW, and CFH wrote the manuscript. All authors read and approved the final manuscript.

Acknowledgements

This work was supported by NIH/NCI grants P20CA192988, RO1CA114425, 1R21AI109259, CA118790and the Cervical Cancer SPORE Program P50 CA098252.

Author details

[1]Departments of Pathology, School of Medicine, Johns Hopkins University, CRBII Room 307, 1550 Orleans Street, Baltimore, MD 21231, USA. [2]Obstetrics and Gynecology, Johns Hopkins Medical Institutions, Baltimore, MD, USA. [3]Molecular Microbiology and Immunology, Johns Hopkins Medical Institutions, Baltimore, MD, USA. [4]Oncology, Johns Hopkins Medical Institutions, Baltimore, MD, USA. [5]Department of Oral Pathology, College of Dentistry, Howard University, Washington, DC, USA.

References

1. Roden R, Wu TC. How will HPV vaccines affect cervical cancer? Nat Rev Cancer. 2006;6:753–63.
2. Schiller JT, Castellsague X, Villa LL, Hildesheim A. An update of prophylactic human papillomavirus L1 virus-like particle vaccine clinical trial results. Vaccine. 2008;26 Suppl 10:K53–61.
3. Gurunathan S, Klinman DM, Seder RA. DNA vaccines: immunology, application, and optimization*. Annu Rev Immunol. 2000;18:927–74.
4. Hung CF, Yang M, Wu TC. Modifying professional antigen-presenting cells to enhance DNA vaccine potency. Methods Mol Med. 2006;127:199–220.
5. Tsen SW, Paik AH, Hung CF, Wu TC. Enhancing DNA vaccine potency by modifying the properties of antigen-presenting cells. Expert Rev Vaccines. 2007;6:227–39.
6. Cheng WF, Hung CF, Chai CY, Hsu KF, He L, Ling M, et al. Tumor-specific immunity and antiangiogenesis generated by a DNA vaccine encoding calreticulin linked to a tumor antigen. J Clin Invest. 2001;108:669–78.

7. Kim JW, Hung CF, Juang J, He L, Kim TW, Armstrong DK, et al. Comparison of HPV DNA vaccines employing intracellular targeting strategies. Gene Ther 2004;11(12):1011–8.
8. Peng S, Ji H, Trimble C, He L, Tsai YC, Yeatermeyer J, et al. Development of a DNA vaccine targeting human papillomavirus type 16 oncoprotein E6. J Virol. 2004;78:8468–76.
9. Peng S, Tomson TT, Trimble C, He L, Hung CF, Wu TC. A combination of DNA vaccines targeting human papillomavirus type 16 E6 and E7 generates potent antitumor effects. Gene Ther. 2006;13:257–65.
10. Peng S, Kim TW, Lee JH, Yang M, He L, Hung CF, et al. Vaccination with dendritic cells transfected with BAK and BAX siRNA enhances antigen-specific immune responses by prolonging dendritic cell life. Hum Gene Ther. 2005;16:584–93.
11. Kim TW, Lee JH, Hung CF, Peng S, Roden R, Wang MC, et al. Generation and characterization of DNA vaccines targeting the nucleocapsid protein of severe acute respiratory syndrome coronavirus. J Virol. 2004;78:4638–45.
12. Peng S, Song L, Knoff J, Wang JW, Chang YN, Hannaman D, et al. Control of HPV-associated tumors by innovative therapeutic HPV DNA vaccine in the absence of CD4+ T cells. Cell Biosci. 2014;4:11.
13. Castellino F, Germain RN. Cooperation between CD4+ and CD8+ T cells: when, where, and how. Annu Rev Immunol. 2006;24:519–40.
14. Steele JC, Mann CH, Rookes S, Rollason T, Murphy D, Freeth MG, et al. T-cell responses to human papillomavirus type 16 among women with different grades of cervical neoplasia. Br J Cancer. 2005;93:248–59.
15. Mustafa W, Maciag PC, Pan ZK, Weaver JR, Xiao Y, Isaacs SN, et al. Listeria monocytogenes delivery of HPV-16 major capsid protein L1 induces systemic and mucosal cell-mediated CD4+ and CD8+ T-cell responses after oral immunization. Viral Immunol. 2009;22:195–204.
16. Pinto LA, Edwards J, Castle PE, Harro CD, Lowy DR, Schiller JT, et al. Cellular immune responses to human papillomavirus (HPV)-16 L1 in healthy volunteers immunized with recombinant HPV-16 L1 virus-like particles. J Infect Dis. 2003;188:327–38.
17. Tobery TW, Smith JF, Kuklin N, Skulsky D, Ackerson C, Huang L, et al. Effect of vaccine delivery system on the induction of HPV16L1-specific humoral and cell-mediated immune responses in immunized rhesus macaques. Vaccine. 2003;21:1539–47.
18. Williams OM, Hart KW, Wang EC, Gelder CM. Analysis of CD4(+) T-cell responses to human papillomavirus (HPV) type 11 L1 in healthy adults reveals a high degree of responsiveness and cross-reactivity with other HPV types. J Virol. 2002;76:7418–29.
19. Leder C, Kleinschmidt JA, Wiethe C, Muller M. Enhancement of capsid gene expression: preparing the human papillomavirus type 16 major structural gene L1 for DNA vaccination purposes. J Virol. 2001;75:9201–9.
20. Kwak K, Jiang R, Jagu S, Wang JW, Wang C, Christensen ND, et al. Multivalent human papillomavirus l1 DNA vaccination utilizing electroporation. PLoS One. 2013;8:e60507.
21. Shedlock DJ, Shen H. Requirement for CD4 T cell help in generating functional CD8 T cell memory. Science. 2003;300:337–9.
22. Overstreet MG, Chen YC, Cockburn IA, Tse SW, Zavala F. CD4+ T cells modulate expansion and survival but not functional properties of effector and memory CD8+ T cells induced by malaria sporozoites. PLoS One. 2011;6:e15948.
23. Cason J, Kambo PK, Jewers RJ, Chrystie IL, Best JM. Mapping of linear B cell epitopes on capsid proteins of bovine papillomavirus: identification of three external type-restricted epitopes. J Gen Virol. 1993;74(Pt 12):2669–77.
24. Hung CF, Tsai YC, He L, Wu TC. DNA Vaccines Encoding Ii-PADRE Generates Potent PADRE-specific CD4(+) T-Cell Immune Responses and Enhances Vaccine Potency. Mol Ther. 2007;15:1211–9.
25. Zhou J, Sun XY, Davies H, Crawford L, Park D, Frazer IH. Definition of linear antigenic regions of the HPV16 L1 capsid protein using synthetic virion-like particles. Virology. 1992;189:592–9.
26. Yan M, Peng J, Jabbar IA, Liu X, Filgueira L, Frazer IH, et al. Activation of dendritic cells by human papillomavirus-like particles through TLR4 and NF-kappaB-mediated signalling, moderated by TGF-beta. Immunol Cell Biol. 2005;83:83–91.
27. Yang R, Murillo FM, Cui H, Blosser R, Uematsu S, Takeda K, et al. Papillomavirus-like particles stimulate murine bone marrow-derived dendritic cells to produce alpha interferon and Th1 immune responses via MyD88. J Virol. 2004;78:11152–60.
28. Warrino DE, Olson WC, Scarrow MI, D'Ambrosio-Brennan LJ, Guido RS, Da Silva DM, et al. Human papillomavirus L1L2-E7 virus-like particles partially mature human dendritic cells and elicit E7-specific T-helper responses from patients with cervical intraepithelial neoplasia or cervical cancer in vitro. Hum Immunol. 2005;66:762–72.
29. Kim D, Hoory T, Wu TC, Hung CF. Enhancing DNA vaccine potency by combining a strategy to prolong dendritic cell life and intracellular targeting strategies with a strategy to boost CD4+ T cell. Hum Gene Ther. 2007;18:1129–39.
30. Lin KY, Guarnieri FG, Staveley-O'Carroll KF, Levitsky HI, August JT, Pardoll DM, et al. Treatment of established tumors with a novel vaccine that enhances major histocompatibility class II presentation of tumor antigen. Cancer Res. 1996;56:21–6.
31. Kim TW, Hung CF, Ling M, Juang J, He L, Hardwick JM, et al. Enhancing DNA vaccine potency by coadministration of DNA encoding antiapoptotic proteins. J Clin Invest. 2003;112:109–17.
32. Chen CH, Wang TL, Hung CF, Yang Y, Young RA, Pardoll DM, et al. Enhancement of DNA vaccine potency by linkage of antigen gene to an HSP70 gene. Cancer Res. 2000;60:1035–42.
33. Pastrana DV, Buck CB, Pang YY, Thompson CD, Castle PE, FitzGerald PC, et al. Reactivity of human sera in a sensitive, high-throughput pseudovirus-based papillomavirus neutralization assay for HPV16 and HPV18. Virology. 2004;321:205–16.
34. Pastrana DV, Gambhira R, Buck CB, Pang YY, Thompson CD, Culp TD, et al. Cross-neutralization of cutaneous and mucosal Papillomavirus types with anti-sera to the amino terminus of L2. Virology. 2005;337:365–72.

17

Influence of partial and complete glutamine-and glucose deprivation of breast-and cervical tumorigenic cell lines

Michelle Helen Visagie[1*], Thandi Vuyelwa Mqoco[1], Leon Liebenberg[2], Edward Henry Mathews[2], George Edward Mathews[2] and Anna Margaretha Joubert[1]

Abstract

Background: Due to their high proliferative requirements, tumorigenic cells possess altered metabolic systems whereby cells utilize higher quantities of glutamine and glucose. These altered metabolic requirements make it of interest to investigate the effects of physiological non-tumorigenic concentrations of glucose and glutamine on tumorigenic cells since deprivation of either results in a canonical amino acid response in mammalian cell.

Methods: The influence of short-term exposure of tumorigenic cells to correlating decreasing glutamine- and glucose quantities were demonstrated in a highly glycolytic metastatic breast cell line and a cervical carcinoma cell line. Thereafter, cells were propagated in medium containing typical physiological concentrations of 1 mM glutamine and 6 mM glucose for 7 days. The effects on morphology were investigated by means of polarization-optical transmitted light differential interference contrast. Flow cytometry was used to demonstrate the effects of glutamine-and glucose starvation on cell cycle progression and apoptosis induction. Fluorometrics were also conducted to investigate the effects on intrinsic apoptosis induction (mitocapture), reactive oxygen species production (2,7-dichlorofluorescein diacetate) and acidic vesicle formation (acridine orange).

Results: Morphological data suggests that glutamine-and glucose deprivation resulted in reduced cell density and rounded cells. Glutamine-and glucose starvation also resulted in an increase in the G_2M phase and a sub-G_1 peak. Complete starvation of glutamine and glucose resulted in the reduction of the mitochondrial membrane potential in both cell lines with MDA-MB-231 cells more prominently affected when compared to HeLa cells. Further, starved cells could not be rescued sufficiently by propagating since cells possessed an increase in reactive oxygen species, acidic compartments and vacuole formation.

Conclusion: Starvation from glutamine and glucose for short periods resulted in decreased cell density, rounded cells and apoptosis induction by means of reactive oxygen species generation and mitochondrial dysfunction. In addition, the metastatic cell line reacted more prominently to glutamine-and glucose starvation due to their highly glycolytic nature. Satisfactory cellular rescue was not possible as cells demonstrated oxidative stress and depolarized mitochondrial membrane potential. This study contributes to the knowledge regarding the *in vitro* effects and signal transduction of glucose and/or L-glutamine deprivation in tumorigenic cell lines.

Keywords: Metabolism, Apoptosis, Morphology, Reactive oxygen species, Glycolysis, Glutamine, Glucose

* Correspondence: michelle.visagie@up.ac.za
[1]Department of Physiology, University of Pretoria, Private Bag X323, Arcadia 0007, South Africa
Full list of author information is available at the end of the article

Introduction

Tumorigenic tissue possesses altered metabolic activities when compared to differentiated, non-proliferating tissue. These modified metabolic activities exerted by the tumors are necessary for the highly proliferative nature of transformed-and tumorigenic tissue [1]. In tumorigenic cells, a shift occurs from adenosine triphosphate (ATP) production through phosphorylation to generation by means of glycolysis even in the presence of oxygen [2]. Cancer-associated aerobic glycolysis which results in the production of lactic acid and pyruvate was described nearly 100 years ago and is known as the Warburg effect [2, 3]. Initially it was reported that the effect was due to mitochondrial dysfunction, however, further research indicates that cancer cells prefer glucose catabolism via glycolysis over oxidative phosphorylation even if the mitochondria is competent [3]. Since glucose is thus mainly utilized for glycolysis, glutamine is used as the mitochondrial tricarboxylic acid cycle (TCA) substrate and for nicotinamide adenine dinucleotide phosphate (NADPH) and fatty acids synthesis [4].

Besides glycolysis, tumorigenic cells are also addicted to glutaminolysis for proliferation purposes. Glutaminolysis is defined as the conversion of glutamine to glutamate. This process provides carbon and nitrogen used for the production of energetic, biosynthetic and reductive precursor for tumorigenic cells [5]. Thus, tumorigenic cells clearly utilize higher quantities of glutamine and glucose when compared to non-tumorigenic and senescent cells.

Glucose and glutamine are the most crucial building blocks required for metabolism and subsequent proliferation and tumorigenic processes [1]. However, due to the largely different metabolic requirements of tumorigenic cells it is of interest and importance to investigate the physiological effects of non-tumorigenic concentrations of glucose and glutamine on tumorigenic cells. This is especially significant since deprivation of either results in a canonical amino acid response (ASS) in mammalian cells [6]. In addition, gene expression studies conducted on primary and metastatic tumors demonstrated that metastatic cells are more prominently dependent on glycolysis when compared to oxidative phosphorylation [7].

This study thus investigated the influence of correlating decreasing quantities of glutamine and glucose on morphology, mitochondrial membrane potential, reactive oxygen species (ROS) and acidic vesicle formation after short-term exposures (2 h, 4 h, 6 h) in a highly glycolytic estrogen receptor metastatic negative breast cell line and a cervical carcinoma cell line. In addition, after exposure, medium was replaced with medium containing a typical physiological concentration of glutamine-and glucose (1 mM and 6 mM respectively) whereby cells were allowed to proliferate for 7 days after which the influence of this exposure was also investigated.

Materials and methods

Cell lines

Human cervical adenocarcinoma cell line (HeLa) and a highly metastatic breast adenocarcinoma cell line (MDA-MB-231) were chosen to demonstrate the effects of medium consisting of varying metabolic states. The HeLa cell line was purchased through Sterilab Services (Pty) Ltd, Johannesburg, South Africa, from the American Tissue Culture Collection (ATCC), Maryland, United States of America. The HeLa cell line is the oldest and most distributed immortalized cell line that presents with aggressive growth and doubles on average every 24 h [8]. The primary source of energy in HeLa cells is glutamine rather than glucose, thus demonstrating that oxidative phosphorylation is preferential to generate ATP [9]. Furthermore, HeLa cells are capable of adapting their mitochondrial network, structure and function depending on substrate basis to generate energy exclusively from oxidative phosphorylation by remodelling its mitochondria [10].

The MDA-MB-231 cell line was provided by Microsep (Pty) Ltd Johannesburg, South Africa. MDA-MB-231 is a triple negative tumorigenic breast cell line. This indicates that MDA-MB-231 cells do not express receptors for steroid hormones (estrogen and progesterone), type II receptor tyrosine kinase (RTK) Her-2, but do possess upregulation of basal cytokeratins and epidermal growth factor response [11–13]. Further, the MDA-MB-231 cell line is highly metastatic and presents with elevated glycolytic activity under normoxic conditions [14]. MDA-MB-231 cells mainly use glycolysis rather than mitochondrial respiration to produce energy required for cell functioning and proliferation [15]. Furthermore, MDA-MB-231 cells contain mitochondria presenting with deoxyribonucleic acid (DNA) mutations resulting in decreased oxidative metabolism [16].

General reagents

Actinomycin D, glucose, L-glutamine and sodium pyruvate free-Dulbecco's minimum essential medium eagle (DMEM), as well as high glucose (25.52 mM, 4500 mg/L), L-glutamine (4 mM) and sodium pyruvate (1 mM, 110 mg/L) containing DMEM, bicarbonate, L-glutamine, glucose, trypsin, crystal violet, NaCl, KCl, KH_2PO_4 and Na_2HPO_4, acridine orange and 2,7-dichlorofluorescein diacetate (DCF-DA) were supplied by Sigma Chemical Co. (St. Louis, United States of America). Heat-inactivated fetal calf serum (FCS), sterile cell culture flasks and plates were obtained through Sterilab Services (Kempton Park, Johannesburg, South Africa). Penicillin, streptomycin and fungizone were purchased from Highveld Biological Ltd (Pty). (Sandringham, Gauteng, South Africa).

General cell culture procedures

Cells were grown and maintained in 25 cm^2 tissue culture flasks in a humidified atmosphere at 37 °C, 5 % CO_2 in a Forma Scientific water-jacketed incubator (Ohio, United States of America). Cells were cultured in DMEM with 25.52 mM glucose, 4 mM L-glutamine, and 1 mM sodium pyruvate supplemented with 10 % heat-inactivated fetal calf serum (56 °C, 30 min), 100 U/ml penicillin G, 100 µg/ml streptomycin and fungizone (250 µg/l). The media according to metabolic state were prepared 24 h before exposure and autoclaved to ensure sterility.

Cells were exposed to varying metabolic conditions as described below:

Control: DMEM with 25.52 mM glucose, 4 mM L-glutamine, and 1 mM sodium pyruvate supplemented with 10 % heat-inactivated FCS (56 °C, 30 min), 100 U/ml penicillin G, 100 µg/ml streptomycin and fungizone (250 µg/l).

Experimental Condition 1: DMEM with 6 mM glucose, 1 mM L-glutamine, and 0 mM sodium pyruvate supplemented with 10 % heat-inactivated FCS (56 °C, 30 min), 100 U/ml penicillin G, 100 µg/ml streptomycin and fungizone (250 µg/l).

Experimental condition 2: DMEM with 3 mM glucose, 0.5 mM L-glutamine, and 0 mM sodium pyruvate supplemented with 10 % heat-inactivated FCS (56 °C, 30 min), 100 U/ml penicillin G, 100 µg/ml streptomycin and fungizone (250 µg/l).

Experimental Condition 3: DMEM with 0 mM glucose, 0 mM L-glutamine, and 0 mM sodium pyruvate supplemented with 10 % heat-inactivated FCS (56 °C, 30 min), 100 U/ml penicillin G, 100 µg/ml streptomycin and fungizone (250 µg/l).

Positive control: Growth medium containing 0.1 µg/ml actinomycin D was used as a positive control to induce cell death via apoptosis.

General experimental procedures for short term exposures and recovery experiments:

Short term exposure: Cells were seeded at 500 000 cells per 25 cm^2 flask or 5 000 cells/well into Nunc F96 microwell plates (AEC-Amersham Soc (Ltd), Kyalami, South Africa). After 24 h, cells were exposed to varying metabolic conditions for 2 h, 4 h and 6 h. Thereafter, all experimental methods were conducted as described below.

Recovery experiment: Cells were seeded at 60 000 cells per 25 cm^2 flask or 850 cells/well into Nunc F96 microwell plates (AEC-Amersham Soc (Ltd), Kyalami, South Africa). After 24 h, cells were exposed to the varying metabolic conditions for 2 h, 4 h and 6 h. Subsequently, cells were washed with PBS and medium was replaced with DMEM containing 6 mM glucose and 1 mM L-glutamine. Medium was subsequently replaced every 2 days. Subsequently, all experimental methods were conducted as described below.

Polarization-optical transmitted light differential interference contrast

Polarization-optical transmitted light differential interference contrast (PlasDIC) is a contrast method used to view morphology. PlasDIC displays the required phase profile which is relative to the product of the section thickness and the refractive index difference between the environment and the average refractive index of quartz. PlasDIC has high-quality DIC imaging of individual cells, cell clusters and thick individual cells in plastic cell-culture vessels [16, 17]. PlasDIC was conducted according to Visagie, et al. [17].

Cell cycle progression and apoptosis induction

Flow cytometry was employed to measure the DNA content of cells after exposure to the various metabolic conditions and to monitor the effect on cell cycle progression [18]. The latter was accomplished by means of ethanol fixation and propidium iodide staining which was conducted according to Mqoco, et al. [16]. Cell cycle Propidium iodide fluorescence was measured with fluorescence activated cell sorting (FACS) FC500 System flow cytometer (Beckman Coulter South Africa (Pty) Ltd). Data from at least 10 000–30 000 events were analyzed with CXP software (Beckman Coulter South Africa (Pty) Ltd. (Pretoria, Gauteng, South Africa). Cell cycle distributions was calculated with Cyflogic 1.2.1 released 2008/11/19 (Perttu Terho & Cyflo Ltd) by assigning relative DNA content per cell to sub-G_1, G_1, S and G_2M fractions.

Mitochondrial membrane potential

A reduction in mitochondrial membrane potential is an early indicator of apoptosis induction [19]. Changes in the mitochondrial membrane potential were investigated using the mitocapture antibody BIOCOM biotech Pty (Ltd) (Clubview, South Africa. Mitocapture is a cationic dye that accumulates in the mitochondria of healthy cells. However, the Mitocapture is unable to accumulate in the mitochondria of apoptotic cells due to the altered mitochondrial membrane potential and therefor the Mitocapture remains in the cytoplasm in its monomer form (green) [20]. After above-mentioned general experimental procedures were followed, diluted Mitocapture solution (mixed according to suppliers' instructions) was pipetted to all samples. Samples were then incubated for 60 min in a humidified atmosphere (37 °C, 5 % CO_2). Samples were then incubated the fluorescence was measured at excitation wavelength of 485 nm and emission wavelength of 520 nm using fluorometrics (Department of Pharmacology, University of Pretoria).

Hydrogen peroxide generation

Hydrogen peroxide generation was measured using 2, 7-dichlorofluorescein diacetate (DCFDA). DCFDA, a non-fluorescent probe, which upon oxidation by ROS and peroxides is converted to the highly fluorescent derivative DCF [21]. After above-mentioned general experimental procedures were followed, DCF-DA (200 µl; 10 µM) was pipetted to all the samples and were subsequently incubated for 60 min in a humidified atmosphere (37 °C, 5 % CO_2. Fluorescence was measured at excitation wavelength of 485 nm and emission wavelength of 520 nm using fluorometrics (Department of Pharmacology, University of Pretoria).

Acridine orange staining

Acridine orange is a lysosomotropic fluorescent compound that moves freely across cell membranes when uncharged [22]. However, acridine orange accumulates in its protonated form in acidic compartments and thus serves as a tracer for acidic vesicular organelles including autophagic vacuoles and lysosomes [22]. After above-mentioned general experimental procedures were followed, PBS containing acridine orange (200 µl; 5 mg/ml) was added to all the samples and samples were incubated for 60 min in a humidified atmosphere (37 °C, 5 % CO_2). Fluorescence was measured at excitation wavelength of 485 nm and emission wavelength of 520 nm using fluorometrics (Department of Pharmacology, University of Pretoria).

Statistics

At least three independent experiments were conducted for all techniques. Each independent fluorometrical experiment had a sample size of 3. Averages of each experiment were represented in bar charts, with T-bars referring to standard deviations. P-values < 0.05 were regarded as statistically significant and were indicated by an asterisk (*). Cell cycle progression data from at least 10 000–30 000 events were analyzed using CXP software (Beckman Coulter South Africa (Pty) Ltd. (Pretoria, Gauteng, South Africa)). Cell cycle distributions was calculated with Cyflogic 1.2.1 released 2008/11/19 (Perttu Terho & Cyflo Ltd).

Results

Glucose and L-glutamine deprivation results in decreased cell density and round shrunken cells

Polarization-optical transmitted light differential interference contrast (PlasDIC) was used to demonstrate the effects of glucose-and glutamine deprivation on morphology in the cervical HeLa epithelial cell line and metastatic estrogen receptor negative breast cell line. Glucose-and glutamine deprivation, regardless of individual medium concentrations, for 2 h resulted in a slight decrease in cell density in both cell lines when compared to cells propagated in growth medium (Fig. 1). Cells were still attached with most cells present in metaphase. Rounded-and shrunken cells were also observed in cells propagated in medium with 0–3 mM glucose-and 0–0.05 mM glutamine. In addition, the lower the quantities of glucose-and glutamine, the lower the cell density when compared to cells propagated in growth medium, implying that glucose and glutamine both have essential roles in proliferation and morphology.

PlasDIC was also utilized to demonstrate the 4 h deprivation of glucose-and glutamine on cell morphology in HeLa-and MDA-MB-231 cells (Fig. 1). After 4 h exposure to DMEM containing 6 mM glucose and 1 mM L-glutamine, cell density is decreased with the presence of some rounded cells in both cell lines. Further reductions to 3 mM glucose and 0.5 mM L-glutamine accompanied with exposure for 4 h demonstrated decreased cell density and increased number of rounded and shrunken cells. Complete deprivation of glutamine and glucose for 4 h resulted in a further reduction in cell density accompanied with the presence of rounded and shrunken cells. However, all cells remained attached after exposure and the majority of cells occupied interphase. Furthermore, cell density was reduced more prominently after 4 h exposure to the metabolic media when compared to 2 h of exposure.

The effects of glutamine-and glucose deprivation on morphology were also investigated after 6 h (Fig. 1). Cells propagated in DMEM containing 3–6 mM glucose and 0.5-1 mM L-glutamine for 4 h period demonstrated decreased cell density and the presence of some rounded shrunken cells. The cells propagated in medium containing no glutamine and glucose also demonstrated the presence of some rounded shrunken cells and decreased cell density. The latter was more pronounced when compared to cells propagated in DMEM containing 3–6 mM glucose and 0.5-1 mM L-glutamine. As with the exposures for 2 h-and 4 h, cells were mostly present in interphase with cells still attached.

Cell morphology was also investigated with regard to possible recuse and long term effects of typical physiological concentrations of glucose and L-glutamine. HeLa and MDA-MB-231 cells were exposed according to varying metabolic conditions for 2 h and 4 h and 6 h after which cells were washed and subsequently medium was replaced with DMEM containing 6 mM glucose and 1 mM L-glutamine for a 7 day period (Fig. 2). Morphology and cell density after 7 days presented with shrunken cells and elongated shape often accompanied with cell protrusions. MDA-MB-231-and HeLa cells propagated in medium containing 6 mM glucose and 1 mM L-glutamine for 2 h and 4 h, and allowed 7 days prior recovery demonstrated decreased cell size and the

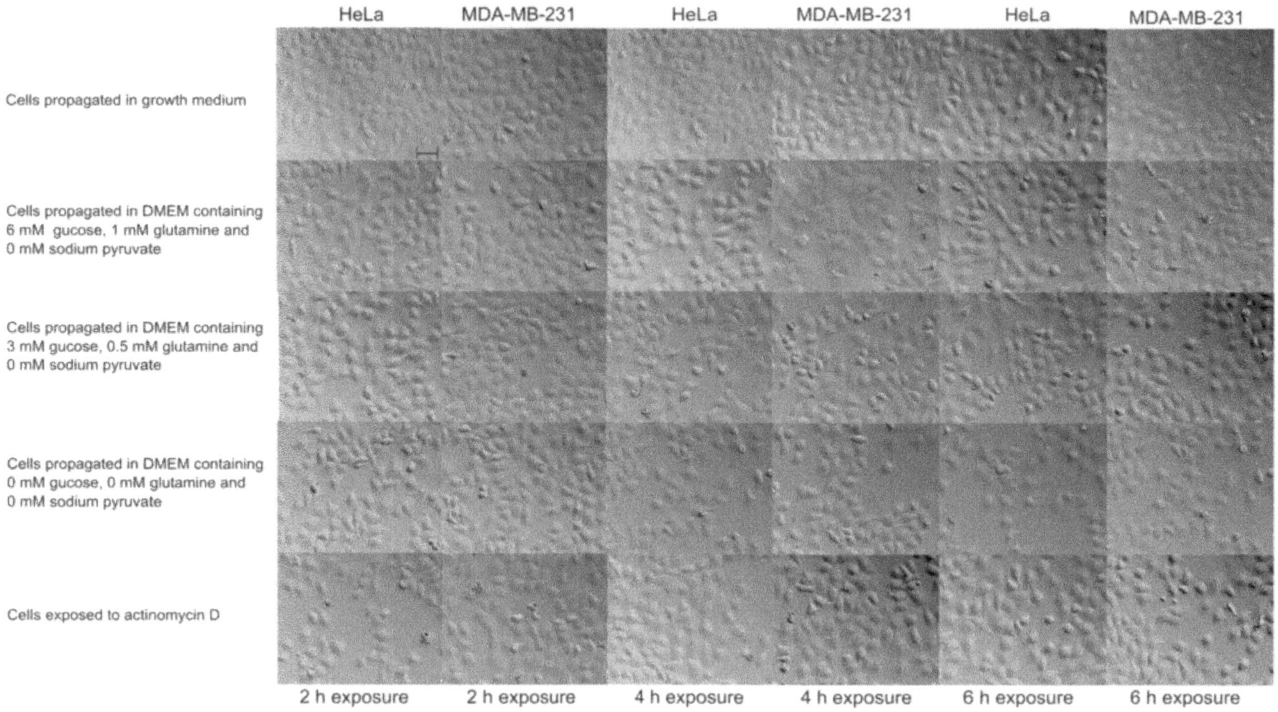

Fig. 1 PlasDIC images after short-term exposures (2 h, 4 h, 6 h) glutamine- and glucose starvation. PlasDIC images of HeLa and MDA-MB-231 cells propagated in media according to metabolic state and cells exposed to actinomycin D for 2 h, 4 h and 6 h. Exposure to DMEM containing 6 mM glucose and 1 mM L-glutamine for 2 h resulted in decreased cell density. Exposure to DMEM containing 0 mM-3 mM glucose and 0 mM-0.5 mM L-glutamine for 2 h resulted in decreased cell density and rounded shrunken cells. After 4 h cells propagated in medium containing 6 mM glucose and 1 mM L-glutamine exhibited decreased cell density and rounded shrunken cells. Cells propagated in medium containing low quantities of glucose and glutamine or no glucose and glutamine for 4 h demonstrated decreasing cell density and increased number of cells appearing rounded and shrunken when compared to cells exposed to DMEM containing 6 mM glucose and 1 mM L-glutamine and cells propagated in growth medium. Cells propagated in DMEM containing 6 mM glucose and 1 mM L-glutamine for 6 h demonstrated decreased cell density and the presence of some rounded shrunken cells. The latter was also observed with cells propagated in DMEM containing 3 mM glucose and 0.5 mM L-glutamine for 6 h. The cells propagated in DMEM containing 0 mM glucose and 0 mM L-glutamine for 6 h also demonstrated the presence of some rounded shrunken cells and decreased cell density. The latter was more pronounced when compared to cells propagated in DMEM containing 3–6 mM glucose and 0.5-1 mM L-glutamine growth medium for 6 h. After 6 h exposure, cells were mostly present in interphase with cells still attached. The scale bar in all images represents 50 μm

MDA-MB-231 cells were elongated. Cells propagated in DMEM containing 6 mM glucose and 1 mM L-glutamine for 6 h and allowed 7 days prior recovery demonstrated more prominent decreased cell size and elongated cell morphology in both cell lines. Cells exposed to medium containing 0–0.5 mM L-glutamine and 3 mM glucose also demonstrated decreased cell density and reduced cell size in both cell lines. The MDA-MB-231 cells exposed to these conditions also demonstrated elongated cells. This trend became more and more prominent with increased exposure to both metabolic conditions with both cell lines possessing elongated morphology at 4 h and 6 h of exposure after 7 days recovery when previously accompanied with unattached cells.

All the morphological characteristics of shrunken cell size and elongation increased with decreasing quantities of L-glutamine and glucose and longer exposure periods. However, all of the above-mentioned effects appeared earlier in the MDA-MB-213 cell line when compared to the HeLa cell line indicating that the metabolic states influences the highly metastatic cell line more prominently. Furthermore, this morphological data suggest that there are lasting effects after cells are deprived of nutrients, even after the medium was replaced with medium containing physiological concentrations of the nutrients.

Dose-dependent glucose and L-glutamine deprivation results in apoptosis induction and cell cycle changes

The influence of these different mediums on cell cycle progression was investigated using ethanol fixation, propidium iodide staining and flow cytometry. Exposure in Hela-and MDA-MB-231 cells to medium containing 6 mM glucose and 1 mM L-glutamine resulted in an increased number of cells in the sub-G_1 phase, a decreased number of cells occupying the G_1 phase and an increase in cells in the G_2M phase with statistically insignificant changes between exposure for 2 h, 4 h and 6 h (Table 1

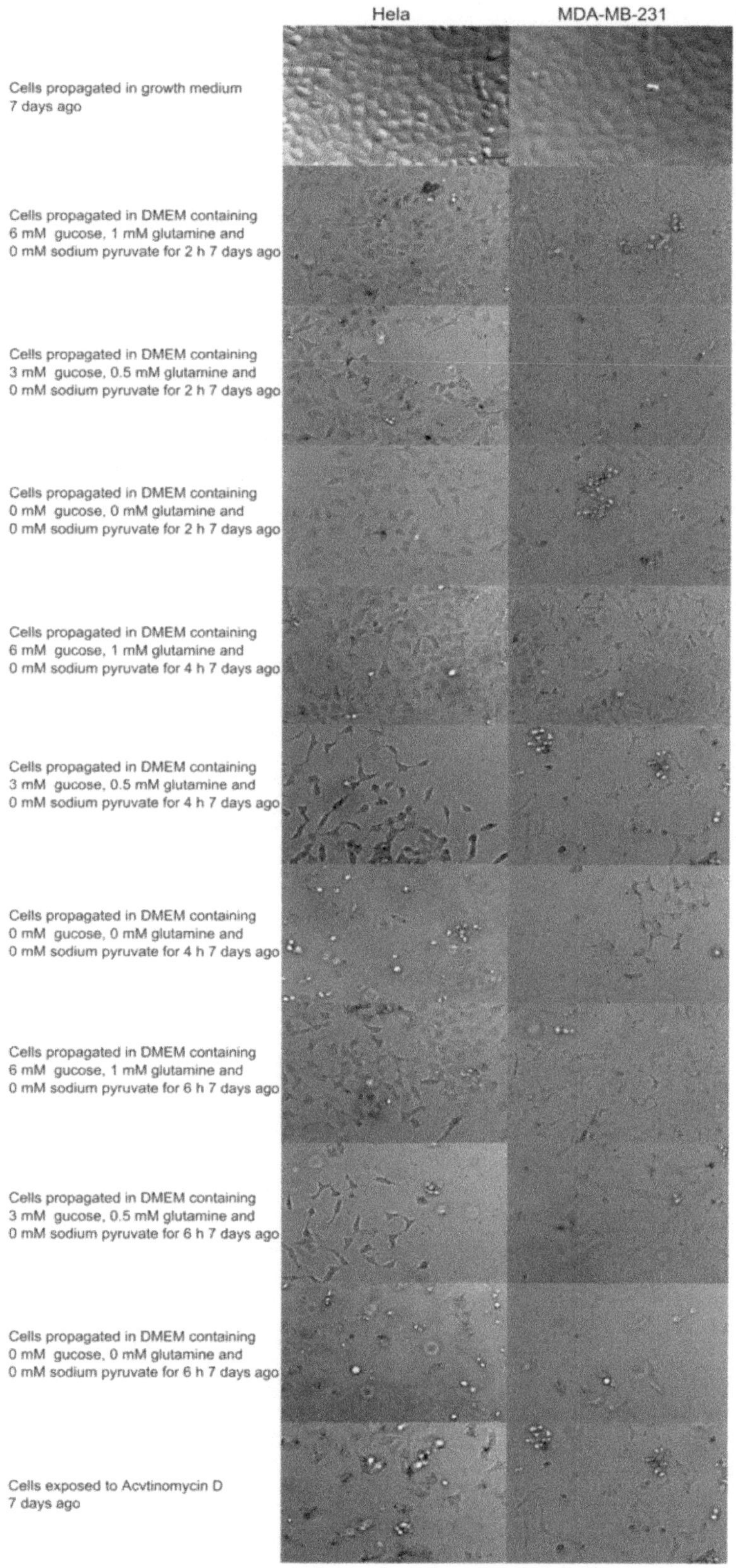

Fig. 2 (See legend on next page.)

(See figure on previous page.)

Fig. 2 Unsuccessful rescue of HeLa and MDA-MB-231 after 7 days. HeLa and MDA-MB-231 cells propagated in media according to metabolic state for 2 h, 4 h and 6 h, 7 days ago, which after cells were washed and medium was replaced with DMEM containing 6 mM glucose and 1 mM L-glutamine. The effects of the decreasing L-glutamine and glucose concentrations were more pronounced 7 days after the exposure when compared to those on the day of exposure self. Effects on decreased cell density were also more severe. Morphological characteristics observed included decreased cell density, reduced cell size and elongation. All of the above-mentioned morphological characteristics were more prominent in the DMEM containing 0 mM glucose and 0 mM L-glutamine when compared to cells propagated in DMEM containing 3 mM-6 mM glucose and 0.5 mM-1 mM L-glutamine. The same applies for the 6 h exposures compared to the 2 h and 4 h exposures. However, all of the above-mentioned effects appeared earlier in the MDA-MB-213 cell line when compared to the HeLa cell line (20x magnification). The scale bar in all images represents 50 μm

and Fig. 3). The changes in cell cycle progression were progressively more pronounced when cells were exposed to medium containing lower glucose-and L-glutamine quantities. In addition, the influence of the media according to metabolic state on cell cycle progression was progressively greater between different exposure periods when the media contains decreasing quantities of glucose and L-glutamine.

Exposure to medium containing 3 mM glucose and 0.5 mM L-glutamine in Hela cells for 2 h resulted in 11 % of cells being present in sub-G_1 phase, 63 % in the G_1 phase, 7 % in the S phase, and 19 % in the G_2M phase. However, after 4 h, 14 % of cells were in the sub-G_1 phase, 48 % in the G_1 phase, 8 % in the S phase, and 31 % in the G_2M phase. After 6 h of exposure 15 % of cells were in the sub-G_1 phase, 34 % in the G_1 phase, 8 % in the S phase, and 43 % in the G_2M phase. Exposure medium containing 3 mM glucose and 0.5 mM L-glutamine in MDA-MB-231 for 2 h resulted in 9 % of cells being present in the sub-G_1 phase, 46 % in the G_1 phase, 15 % in the S phase, and 30 % in the G_2M phase. After exposure to medium containing 3 mM glucose and 0.5 mM L-glutamine for 4 h, 10 % of cells were in the Sub-G_1 phase, 59 % in the G_1 phase, 10 % in the S phase, and 21 % in the G_2M phase. After 6 h of exposure 21 % of cells were in the sub-G_1 phase, 54 % in the G_1 phase, 10 % in the S phase, and 16 % in the G_2M phase. These trends continued with the exposure of cells to medium containing 0 mM glucose and 0 mM L-glutamine.

In addition, the rescue and long-term effects of physiological concentrations of glucose and L-glutamine was also investigated. This was accomplished by exposing the cell lines to medium according to varying metabolic conditions for the appropriate period before cells were washed with PBS and medium was replaced with 6 mM glucose and 1 mM L-glutamine (medium was replaced every 2 days). The effects on the cell cycle and apoptosis induction on day 7 are demonstrated in Table 2 and Fig. 3. Cells pertaining to this exposure group demonstrated cell cycle progression data indicating significant apoptosis induction. The sub-G_1 fractions increased with the decreasing glucose and L-glutamine quantities and increasing exposure periods (2 h, 4 h and 6 h).

Hela and MDA-MB-231 cells propagated in DMEM containing 6 mM glucose and 1 mM L-glutamine for 7 days demonstrated both an increase in apoptotic cells (sub-G_1 phase) and an increase in the S phase. MDA-MB-231 cells also presented with an increased G_2M phase when exposed to DMEM containing 6 mM glucose and 1 mM L-glutamine throughout. Hela cells propagated in DMEM containing 3 mM glucose and 0.05 mM L-glutamine and allowed 7 days recovery propagated in DMEM containing 6 mM glucose and 1 mM L-glutamine also presented with an apoptotic sub-G1 peak and an increased G_2M phase. The MDA-MB-231 cells exposed to DMEM containing 3 mM glucose and 0.5 mM L-glutamine showed a very prominent increase in the S phase. All of the above-mentioned increases in number of cells occupying the respective cell cycle phases were associated with a corresponding decrease of cells occupying the G_1 phase. HeLa cells exposed to DMEM containing no glucose or L-glutamine for short exposure periods and allowed 7 days recovery in DMEM containing 6 mM glucose and 1 mM L-glutamine showed an increase in the number of cells occupying the S phase. MDA-MB-231 cells exposed to DMEM containing no glucose or L-glutamine for short exposure periods and allowed 7 days recovery in DMEM containing 6 mM glucose and 1 mM L-glutamine resulted in an increase in the number of cells in the S phase; most prominently in the 2 h, followed by 4 h and lastly by 6 h accompanied by a steady increase in the number of apoptotic (sub-G_1) cells and the number of cells in the G_1 phase.

Glucose and L-glutamine deprivation results in depolarisation of the mitochondrial membrane potential

This study further investigated the induction of apoptosis by demonstrating the effect of the varying metabolic conditions on the mitochondrial membrane potential. The intrinsic apoptotic pathway involves the loss of mitochondrial membrane potential resulting in cytochrome *c* release and subsequent caspase activation [9]. The results indicated that the mitochondrial membrane potential of cells exposed to DMEM containing no glucose or L-glutamine was affected the most in both cells lines (Fig. 4a and b). In addition, MDA-MB-231 cells were

Table 1 Cell cycle progression histograms of HeLa and MDA-MB-231 cells propagated in media according to metabolic state for the appropriate exposure period (2 h, 4 h and 6 h) (*P*-value < 0.05)

Sample	Histogram profile
HeLa cells propagated in growth medium for 2 h	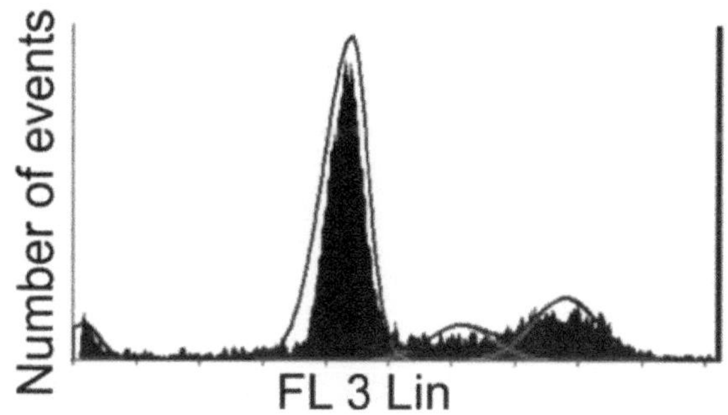
HeLa cells propagated in growth medium for 4 h	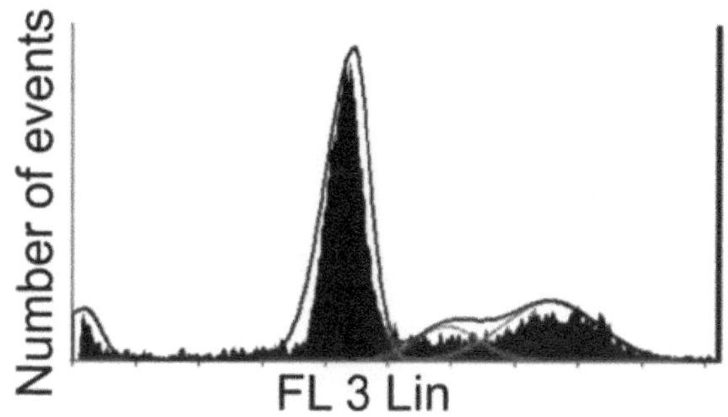
HeLa cells propagated in growth medium for 6 h	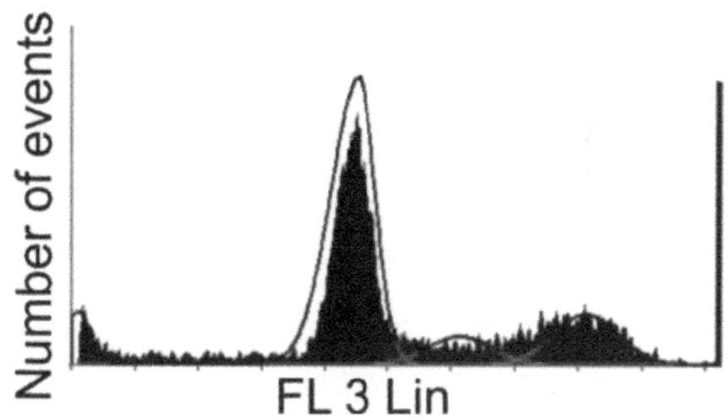
HeLa cells propagated in medium containing 6 mM glucose and 1 mM L-glutamine for 2 h	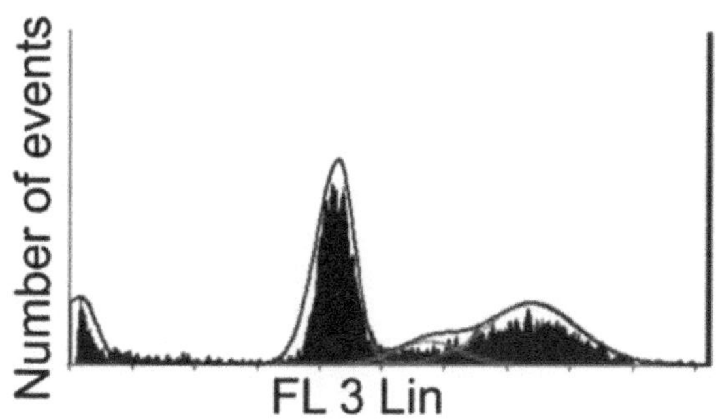

Table 1 Cell cycle progression histograms of HeLa and MDA-MB-231 cells propagated in media according to metabolic state for the appropriate exposure period (2 h, 4 h and 6 h) (P-value < 0.05) *(Continued)*

HeLa cells propagated in medium containing 6 mM glucose and 1 mM L-glutamine for 4 h	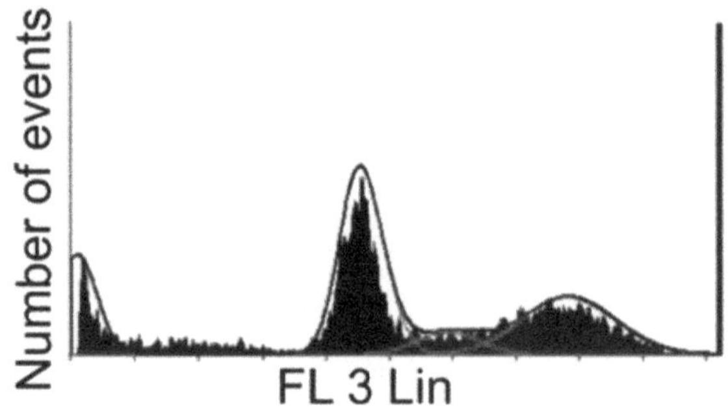
HeLa cells propagated in medium containing 6 mM glucose and 1 mM L-glutamine for 6 h	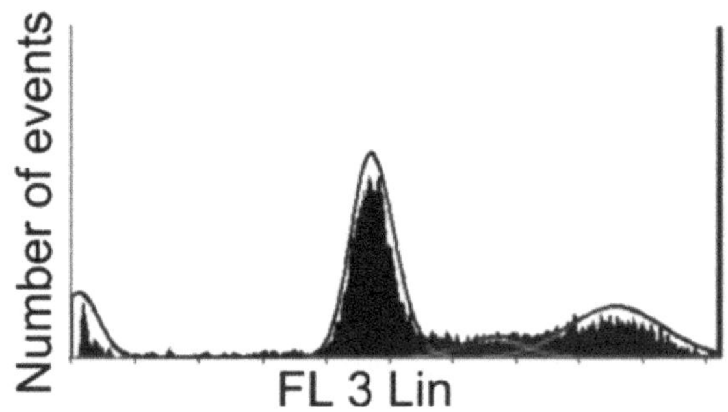
HeLa cells propagated in medium containing 3 mM glucose and 0.5 mM L-glutamine for 2 h	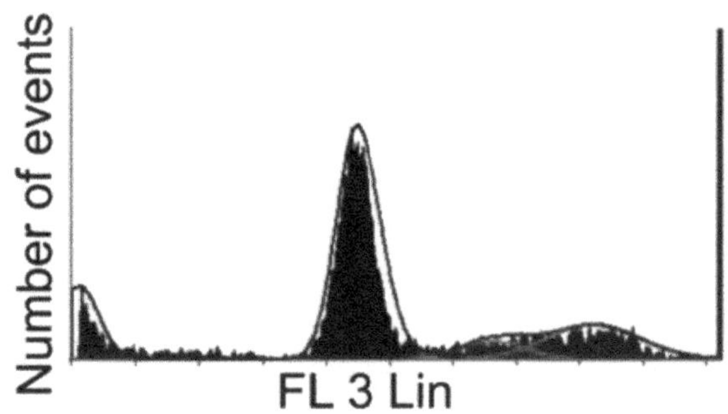
HeLa cells propagated in medium containing 3 mM glucose and 0.5 mM L-glutamine for 4 h	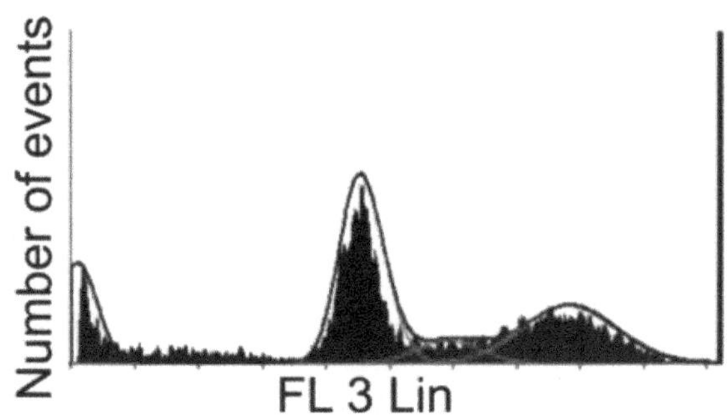

Table 1 Cell cycle progression histograms of HeLa and MDA-MB-231 cells propagated in media according to metabolic state for the appropriate exposure period (2 h, 4 h and 6 h) (*P*-value < 0.05) *(Continued)*

HeLa cells propagated in medium containing 3 mM glucose and 0.5 mM L-glutamine for 6 h	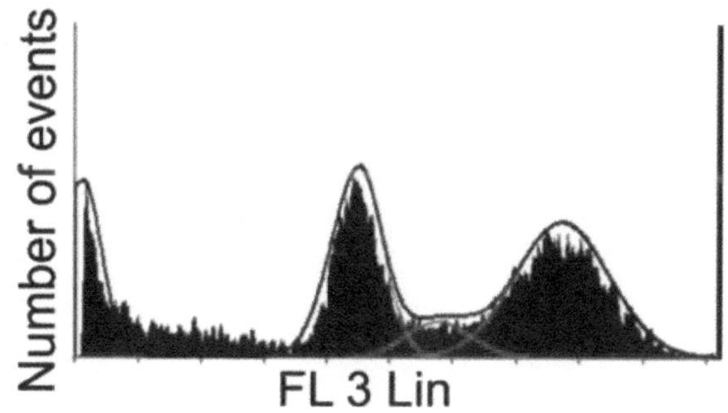
HeLa cells propagated in medium containing 0 mM glucose and 0 mM L-glutamine for 2 h	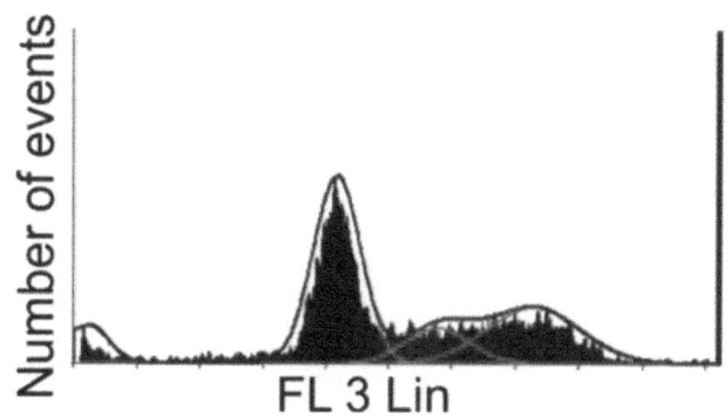
HeLa cells propagated in medium containing 0 mM glucose and 0 mM L-glutamine for 4 h	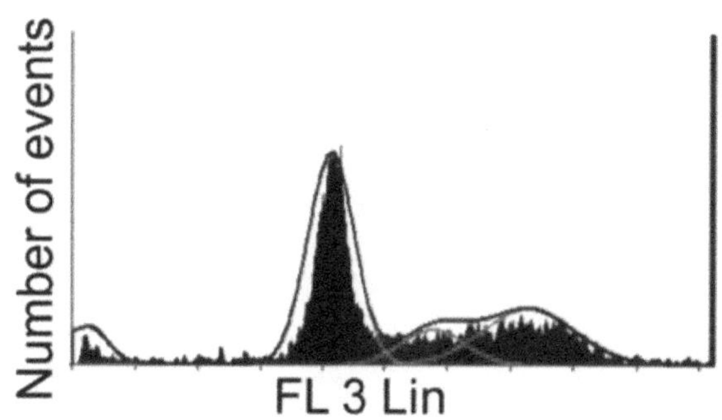
HeLa cells propagated in medium containing 0 mM glucose and 0 mM L-glutamine for 6 h	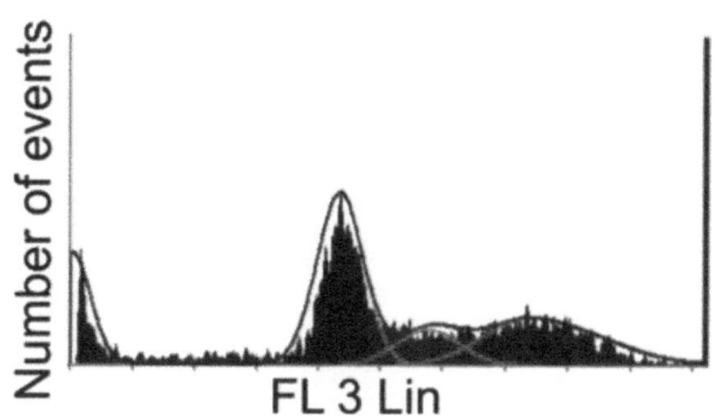

Table 1 Cell cycle progression histograms of HeLa and MDA-MB-231 cells propagated in media according to metabolic state for the appropriate exposure period (2 h, 4 h and 6 h) (*P*-value < 0.05) *(Continued)*

MDA-MB-231 cells propagated in growth medium for 2 h	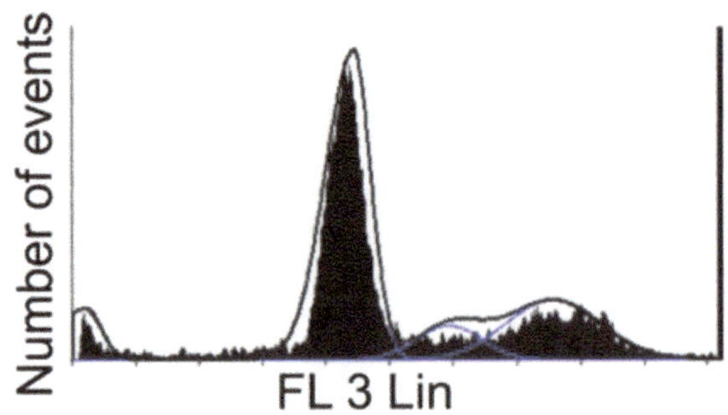
MDA-MB-231 cells propagated in growth medium for 4 h	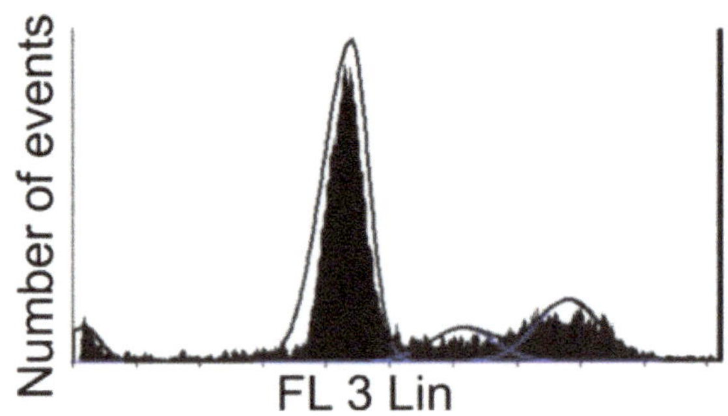
MDA-MB-231 cells propagated in growth medium for 6 h	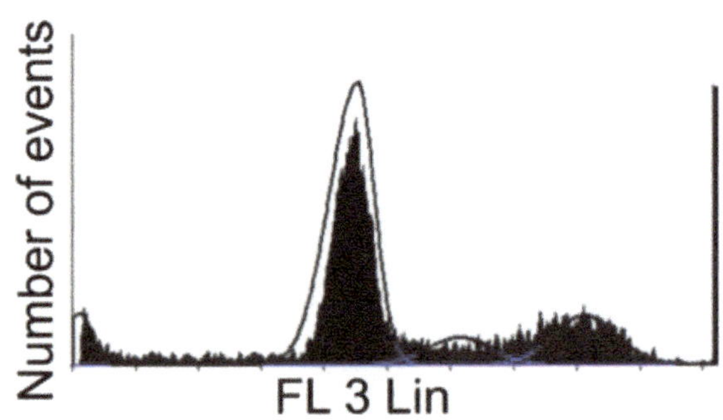
MDA-MB-231 cells propagated in medium containing 6 mM glucose and 1 mM L-glutamine for 2 h	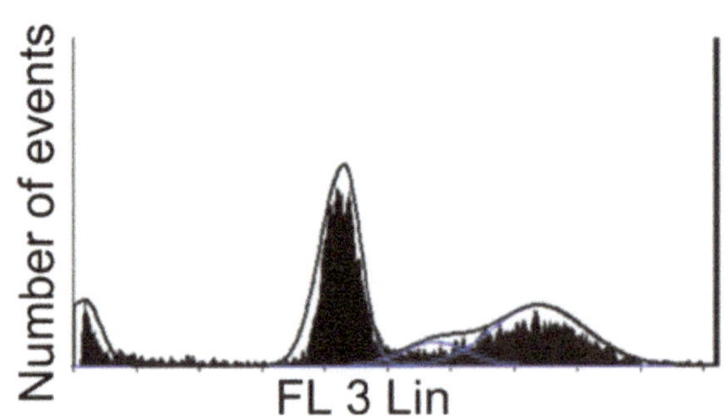

Table 1 Cell cycle progression histograms of HeLa and MDA-MB-231 cells propagated in media according to metabolic state for the appropriate exposure period (2 h, 4 h and 6 h) (*P*-value < 0.05) *(Continued)*

MDA-MB-231 cells propagated in medium containing 6 mM glucose and 1 mM L-glutamine for 4 h	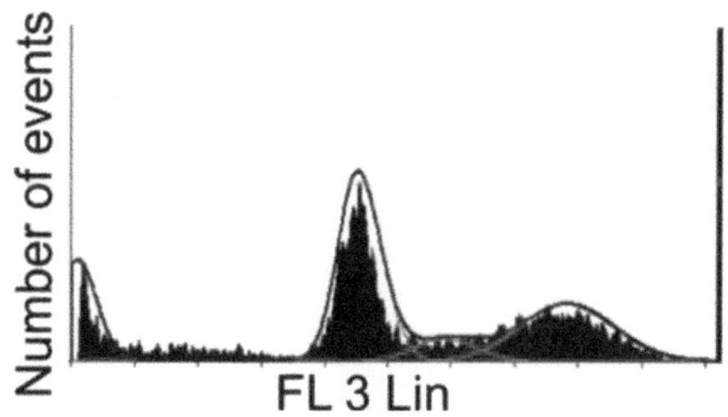
MDA-MB-231 cells propagated in medium containing 6 mM glucose and 1 mM L-glutamine for 6 h	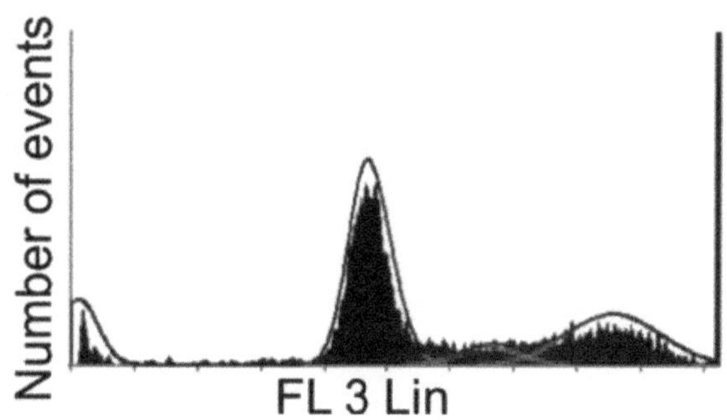
MDA-MB-231 cells propagated in medium containing 3 mM glucose and 0.5 mM L-glutamine for 2 h	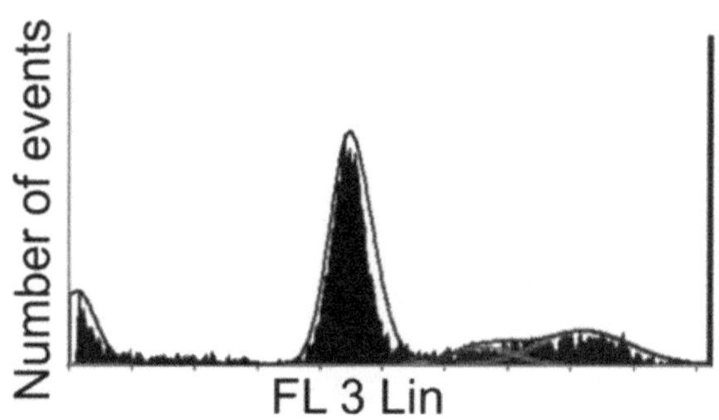
MDA-MB-231 cells propagated in medium containing 3 mM glucose and 0.5 mM L-glutamine for 4 h	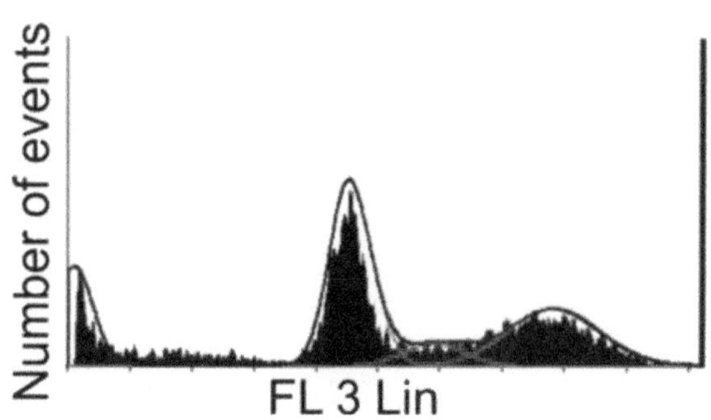

Table 1 Cell cycle progression histograms of HeLa and MDA-MB-231 cells propagated in media according to metabolic state for the appropriate exposure period (2 h, 4 h and 6 h) (*P*-value < 0.05) *(Continued)*

MDA-MB-231 cells propagated in medium containing 3 mM glucose and 0.5 mM L-glutamine for 6 h	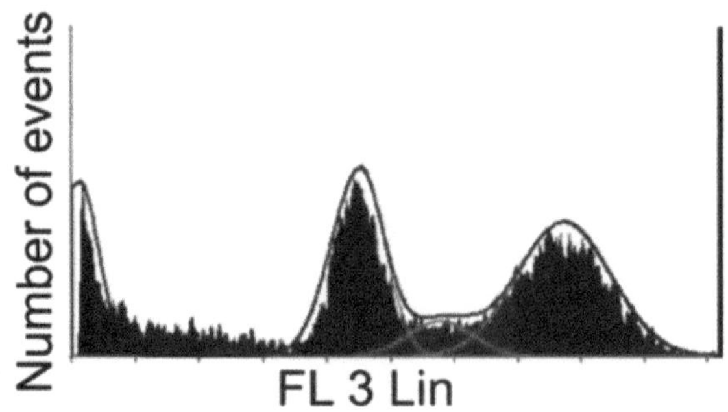
MDA-MB-231 cells propagated in medium containing 0 mM glucose and 0 mM L-glutamine for 2 h	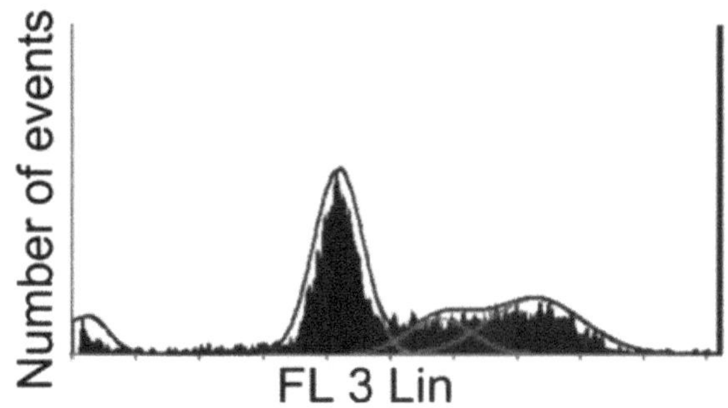
MDA-MB-231 cells propagated in medium containing 0 mM glucose and 0 mM L-glutamine for 4 h	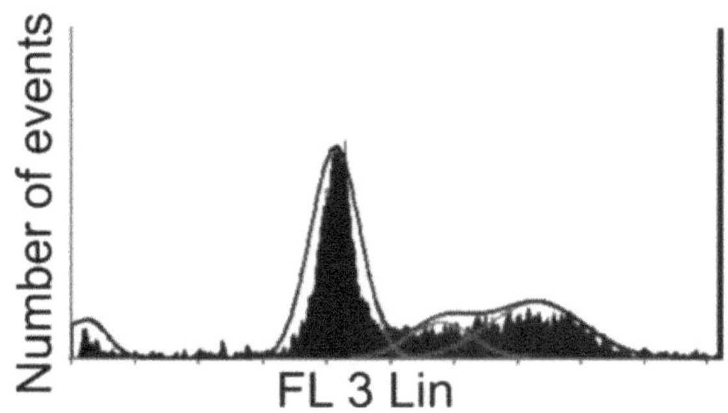
MDA-MB-231 cells propagated in medium containing 0 mM glucose and 0 mM L-glutamine for 6 h	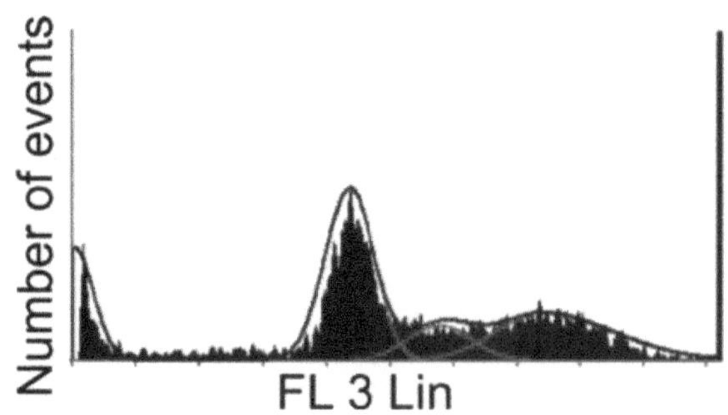

also more prominently affected overall when compared to HeLa cells. Recovery and colony formation after 7 days propagation in DMEM containing 6 mM glucose and 1 mM L-glutamine indicated that MDA-MB-231 cells are still more prominently affected (Fig. 4c and d). HeLa cells were also presenting with a significant number of cells possessing a reduced mitochondrial membrane potential after exposure to medium containing no glucose or

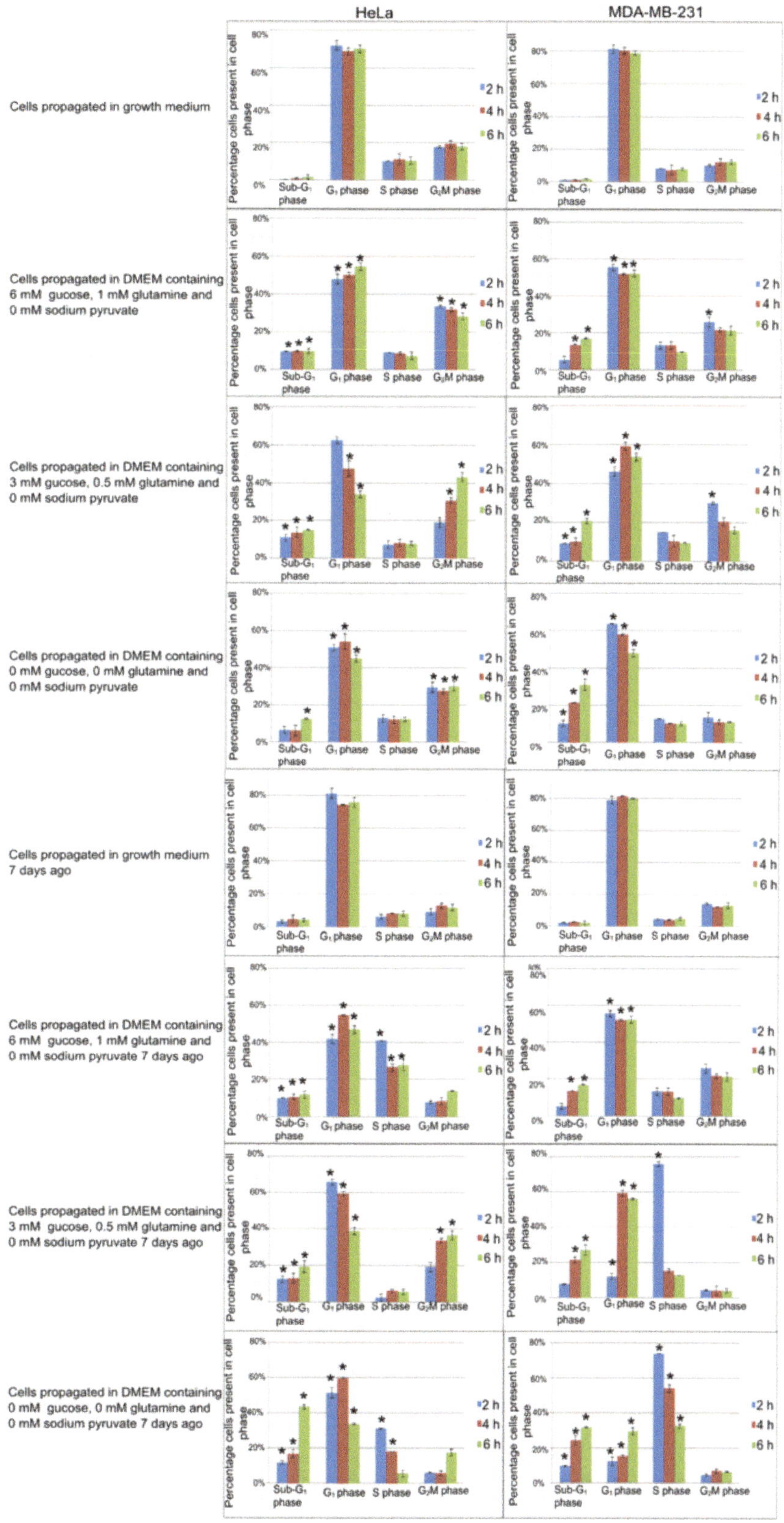

Fig. 3 (See legend on next page.)

(See figure on previous page.)
Fig. 3 Cell cycle progression after partial- and complete glutamine- and glucose starvation for short term exposures and after 7 days. Percentage of cells occupying each cell cycle phase after cells was propagated in media according to metabolic state for the appropriate exposure period (2 h, 4 h and 6 h). Hela cells propagated in medium containing 6 mM glucose and 1 mM L-glutamine demonstrated an increased sub-G_1- and G_2M faction. MDA-MB-231 cells propagated in medium containing 6 mM glucose and 1 mM L-glutamine also showed an increased sub-G_1 fraction. MDA-MB-231 and HeLa cells propagated in medium containing 6 mM glucose and 1 mM L-glutamine demonstrated an increased sub-G_1 and G_2M fraction. HeLa- and MDA-MB-231 cells propagated in media containing no glucose or L-glutamine demonstrated an increase in the number of apoptotic cells and the HeLa cells also showed an increase in the G_2M fraction. The effects on the cell cycle and apoptosis induction on day 7 by means of flow cytometry using propidium iodide staining showed significant induction of apoptosis in all treated samples. Hela- and MDA-MB-231 cells propagated in medium containing 6 mM glucose and 1 mM L-glutamine 7 days before also demonstrated an increase in the number of cells occupying the S phase. The MDA-MB-231 cells also showed a G_2M increase. The HeLa cells propagated in medium containing 3 mM glucose and 0.5 mM L-glutamine also presented with increased G_2M fraction. MDA-MB-231 cells propagated in DMEM containing 0 mM-3 mM glucose and 0 mM-0.5 mM L-glutamine demonstrated an increased number of cells in the S phase. The Hela cells propagated in medium containing 0 mM glucose and 0 mM L-glutamine for 2 h and 4 h also showed an increased S phase. An asterisk (*) indicates P-value < 0.05

L-glutamine, even 7 days after withdrawing the media and replacing with DMEM containing 6 mM glucose and 1 mM L-glutamine. MDA-MB-231 was affected with any variance in the metabolic state of the media with DMEM containing 0–3 mM glucose and 0–0.5 mM L-glutamine resulting in the most prominently presented reduced mitochondrial membrane potential.

Unsuccessful cell recovery demonstrating increased hydrogen peroxide generation

Hydrogen peroxide production was determined by means of a DCFDA which, upon oxidation by ROS and peroxides, is converted to the highly fluorescent derivative DCF [21, 22]. Exposure to the various mediums did not change the hydrogen peroxide production in the first six hours after exposure (Fig. 5a and b). However, the results from the cell lines allowed 7 days recovery after 7 days propagation in DMEM containing 6 mM glucose and 1 mM L-glutamine demonstrated that the effects of the different metabolic media still affected the cell functioning and ROS production after being replaced with DMEM containing 6 mM glucose and 1 mM L-glutamine as indicated by the increased ROS production in all cell lines exposed to the varied metabolic mediums (Fig. 5c and d). In the HeLa cell line, ROS production was increased more prominently when exposed to DMEM containing 6 mM glucose and 1 mM L-glutamine followed by decreasing glucose- and glutamine amounts. Results also indicated that MDA-MB-231 cells propagated in growth medium produced larger quantities of ROS possibly owing to their highly glycolytic- and metastatic nature. However, the metabolic media also increased their ROS production, most prominently by DMEM containing 3 mM glucose and 0.05 mM L-glutamine.

Unsuccessful cell recovery demonstrating increased lysosomal staining

Acridine orange is a lysosomotropic fluorescent compound that moves freely across cell membranes when uncharged. However, acridine orange accumulates in its protonated forming acidic compartments and thus serves as a tracer for acidic vesicular organelles including autophagic vacuoles and lysosomes [23]. The initial 6 h exposure to the medium consisting of various metabolic states did not result in a significant increased lysosomal staining in either cell line (Fig. 6a and b). Cells lines that were exposed to various metabolic states followed by 7 days recovery in DMEM containing 6 mM glucose and 1 mM L-glutamine demonstrated increased lysosomal staining indicating an increase in acidic compartments and vacuole formation (Fig. 6c and d).

Discussion

Cancer cells exert several intrinsic gene mutations (affecting p53, MYC, AMPK, PI3K and HIF1) and extrinsic responses to the tumour environment (hypoxia and acidity). This results in an altered cellular metabolism generating high amounts of ATP resulting in enhanced proliferation, increased macromolecule synthesis and the balance of a delicate redox homeostasis [2].

Many tumorigenic cells metabolize much higher amounts of glucose than lactate in aerobic glycolysis. This is known as the Warburg effect and this occurs even in the presence of mitochondrial respiration [24]. A major source of energy in cell metabolism is glucose that is metabolised to pyruvate in glycolysis and further oxidized to form carbon dioxide generating ATP in the tricarboxylic acid cycle. Glutamine metabolism contributes to biomass precursors as it is a major carbon and nitrogen source [25].

This study investigated the necessity of glucose and L-glutamine in cell proliferation and functioning. This was accomplished by demonstrating the effects of media with different metabolic states, containing decreasing glucose or L-glutamine concentrations, in a human cervical adenocarcinoma cell line (HeLa) and a highly metastatic breast adenocarcinoma cell line (MDA-MB-231) on morphology, cell cycle progression, hydrogen peroxide

Table 2 Cell cycle progression histograms of HeLa and MDA-MB-231 cells propagated in media according to metabolic state for the appropriate exposure period (2 h, 4 h and 6 h) 7 days ago, which after cells were washed and medium was replaced with condition 1 media (P-value < 0.05)

Sample	Histogram profile
HeLa cells propagated in growth medium for 2 h	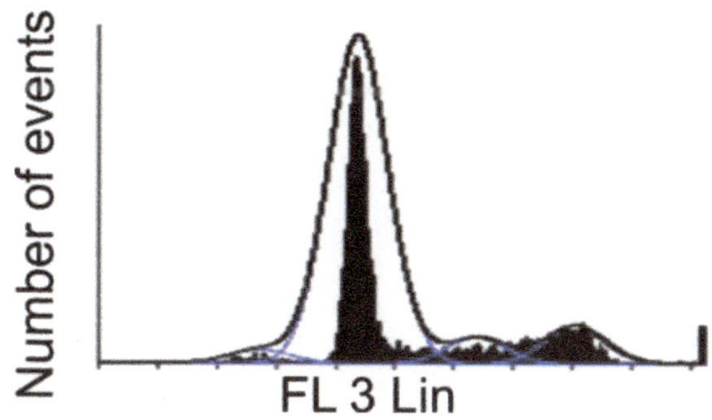
HeLa cells propagated in growth medium for 4 h	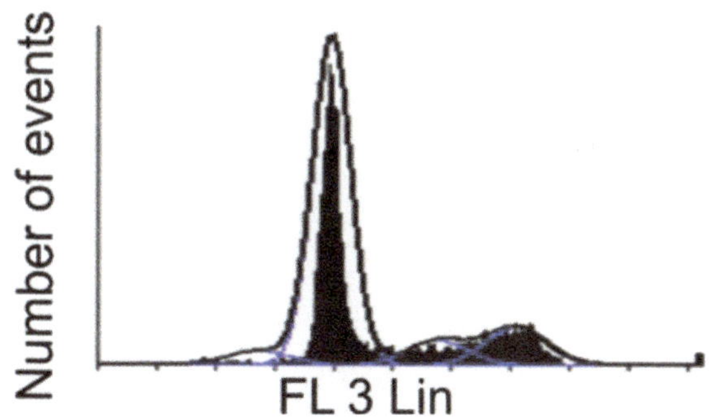
HeLa cells propagated in growth medium for 6 h	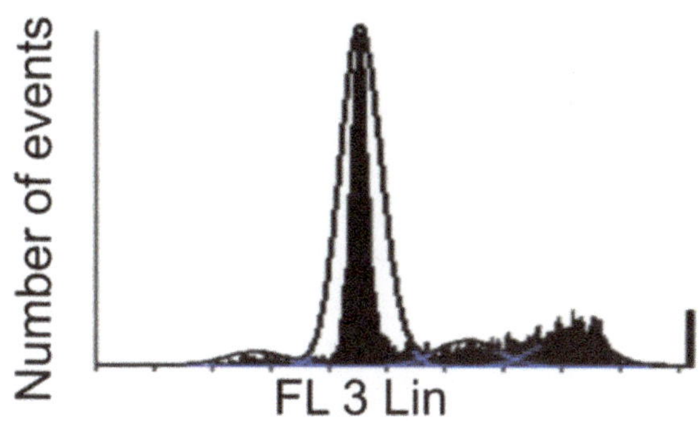
HeLa cells propagated in medium containing 6 mM glucose and 1 mM L-glutamine for 2 h	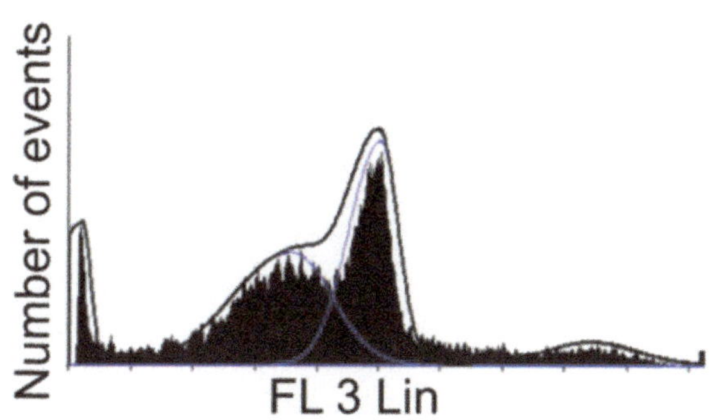

Table 2 Cell cycle progression histograms of HeLa and MDA-MB-231 cells propagated in media according to metabolic state for the appropriate exposure period (2 h, 4 h and 6 h) 7 days ago, which after cells were washed and medium was replaced with condition 1 media (*P*-value < 0.05) *(Continued)*

HeLa cells propagated in medium containing 6 mM glucose and 1 mM L-glutamine for 4 h	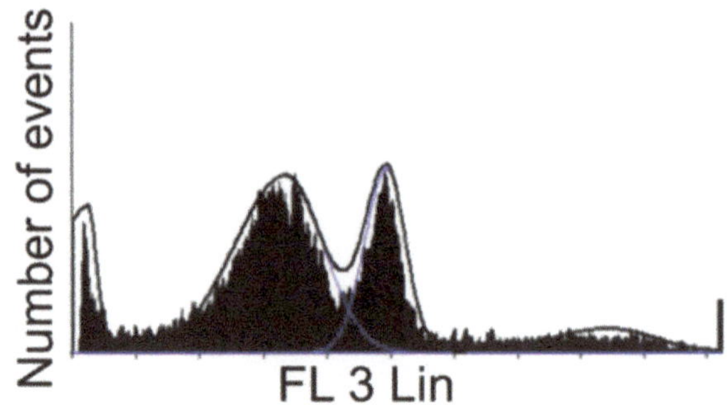
HeLa cells propagated in medium containing 6 mM glucose and 1 mM L-glutamine for 6 h	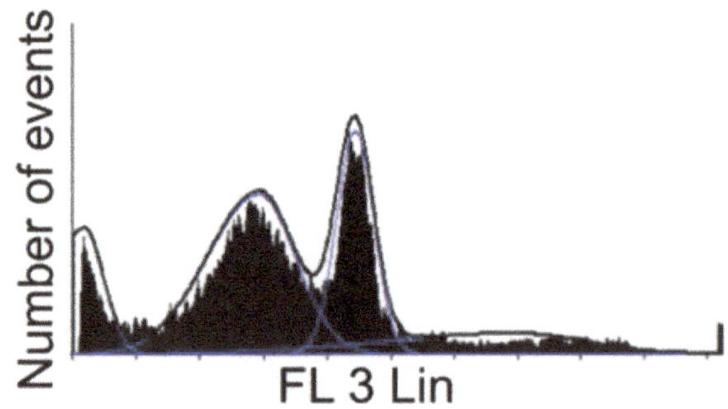
HeLa cells propagated in medium containing 3 mM glucose and 0.5 mM L-glutamine for 2 h	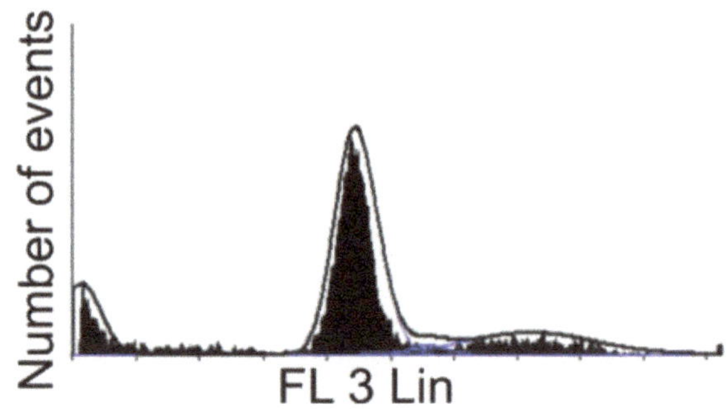
HeLa cells propagated in medium containing 3 mM glucose and 0.5 mM L-glutamine for 4 h	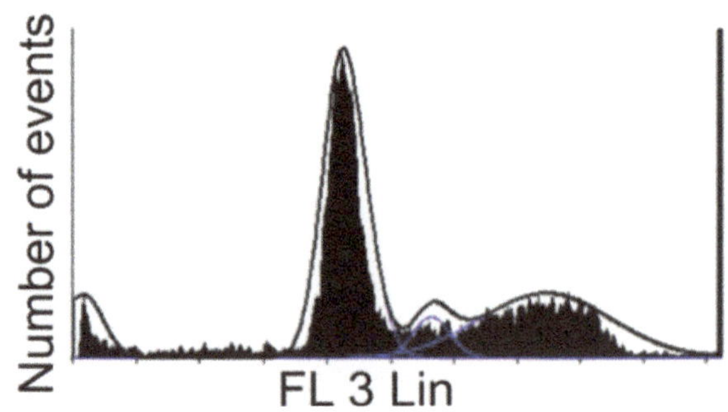

Table 2 Cell cycle progression histograms of HeLa and MDA-MB-231 cells propagated in media according to metabolic state for the appropriate exposure period (2 h, 4 h and 6 h) 7 days ago, which after cells were washed and medium was replaced with condition 1 media (P-value < 0.05) *(Continued)*

HeLa cells propagated in medium containing 3 mM glucose and 0.5 mM L-glutamine for 6 h	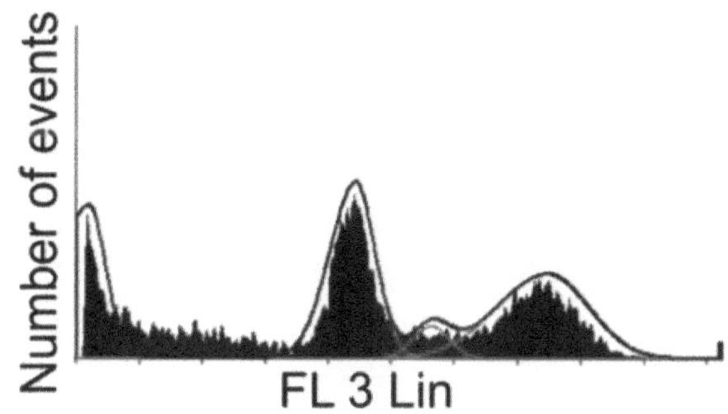
HeLa cells propagated in medium containing 0 mM glucose and 0 mM L-glutamine for 2 h	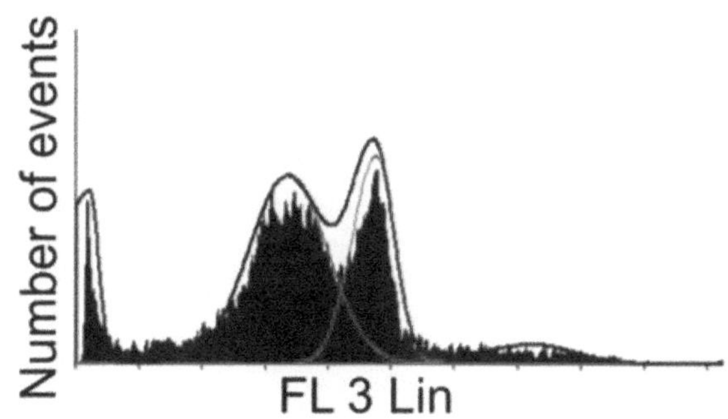
HeLa cells propagated in medium containing 0 mM glucose and 0 mM L-glutamine for 4 h	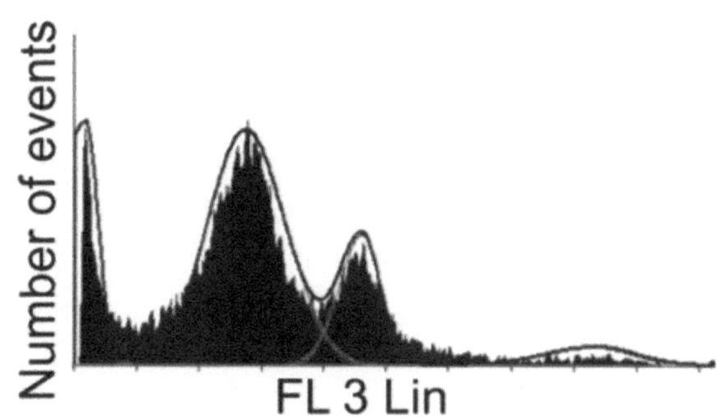
HeLa cells propagated in medium containing 0 mM glucose and 0 mM L-glutamine for 6 h	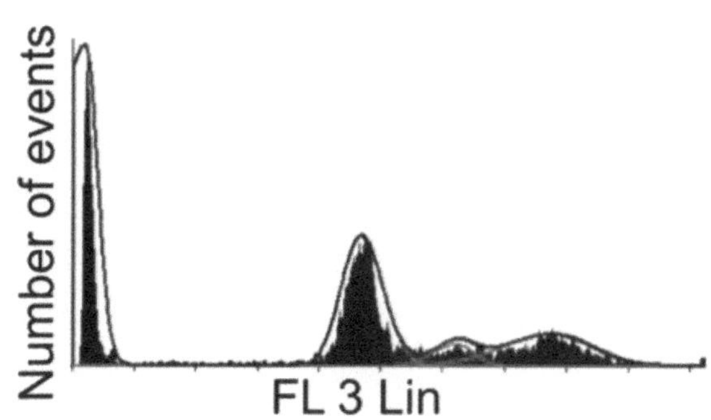

Table 2 Cell cycle progression histograms of HeLa and MDA-MB-231 cells propagated in media according to metabolic state for the appropriate exposure period (2 h, 4 h and 6 h) 7 days ago, which after cells were washed and medium was replaced with condition 1 media (*P*-value < 0.05) *(Continued)*

MDA-MB-231 cells propagated in growth medium for 2 h	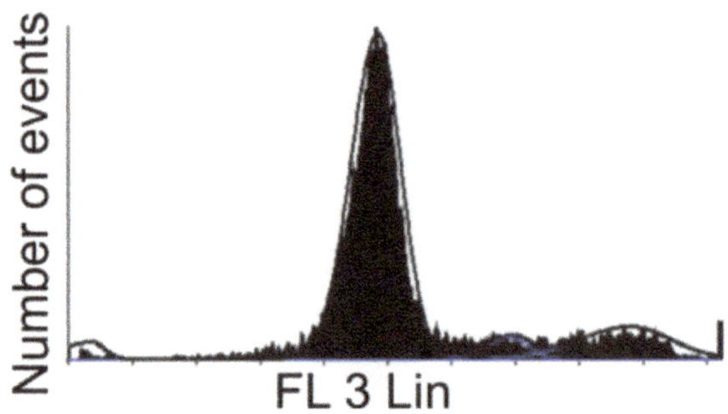
MDA-MB-231 cells propagated in growth medium for 4 h	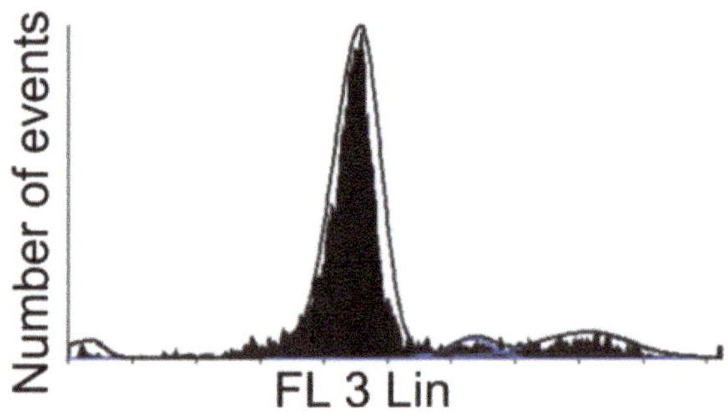
MDA-MB-231 cells propagated in growth medium for 6 h	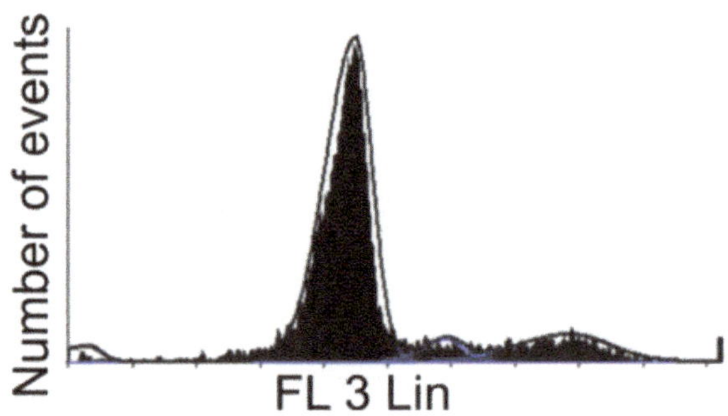
MDA-MB-231 cells propagated in medium containing 6 mM glucose and 1 mM L-glutamine for 2 h	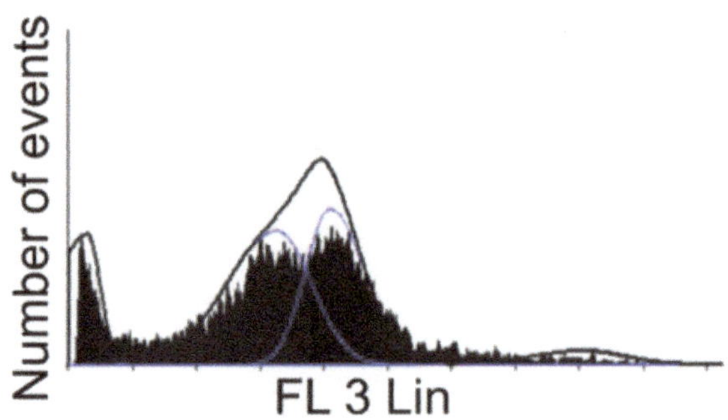

Table 2 Cell cycle progression histograms of HeLa and MDA-MB-231 cells propagated in media according to metabolic state for the appropriate exposure period (2 h, 4 h and 6 h) 7 days ago, which after cells were washed and medium was replaced with condition 1 media (*P*-value < 0.05) *(Continued)*

MDA-MB-231 cells propagated in medium containing 6 mM glucose and 1 mM L-glutamine for 4 h	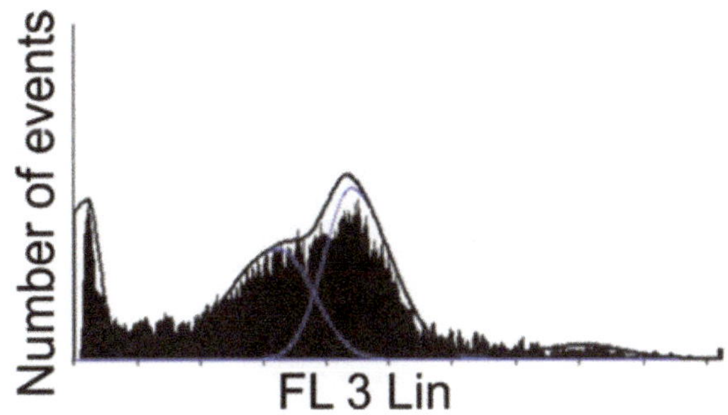
MDA-MB-231 cells propagated in medium containing 6 mM glucose and 1 mM L-glutamine for 6 h	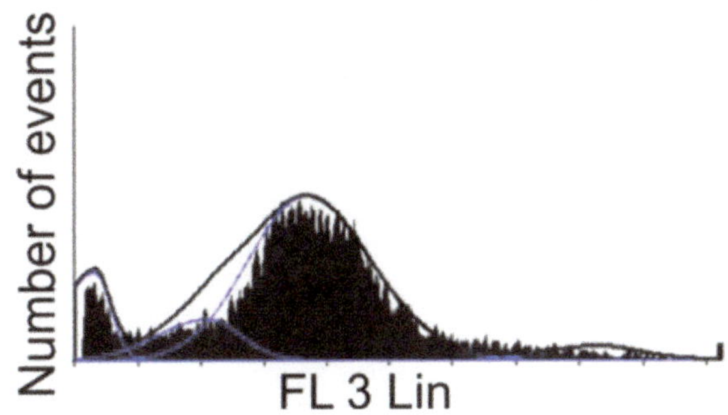
MDA-MB-231 cells propagated in medium containing 3 mM glucose and 0.5 mM L-glutamine for 2 h	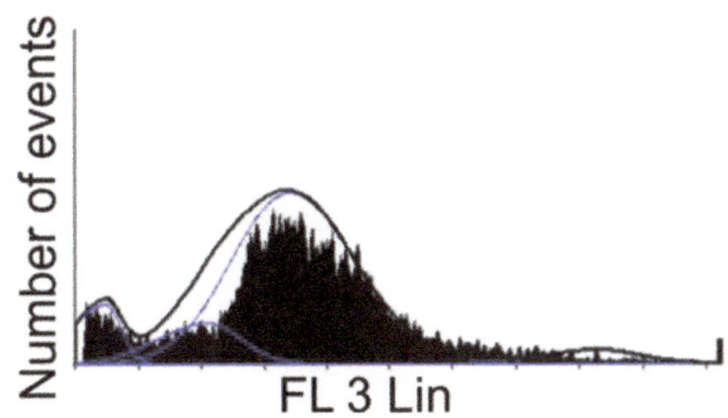
MDA-MB-231 cells propagated in medium containing 3 mM glucose and 0.5 mM L-glutamine for 4 h	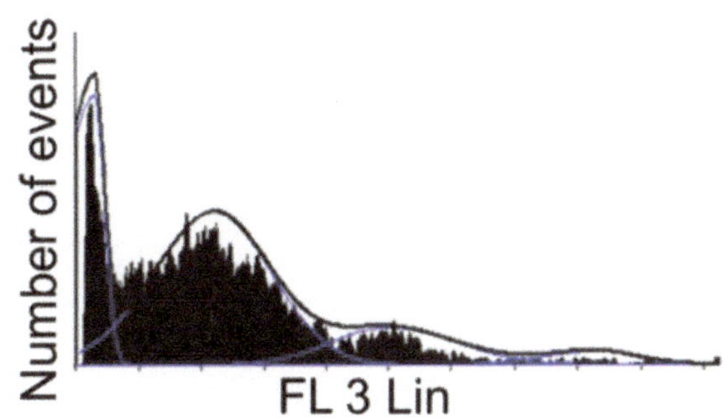

Table 2 Cell cycle progression histograms of HeLa and MDA-MB-231 cells propagated in media according to metabolic state for the appropriate exposure period (2 h, 4 h and 6 h) 7 days ago, which after cells were washed and medium was replaced with condition 1 media (*P*-value < 0.05) *(Continued)*

MDA-MB-231 cells propagated in medium containing 3 mM glucose and 0.5 mM L-glutamine for 6 h	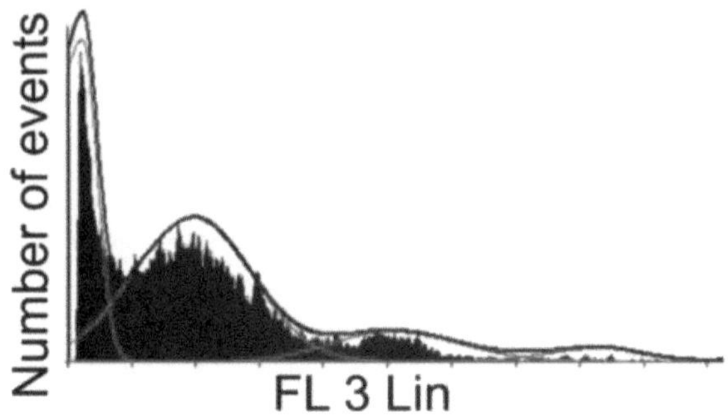
MDA-MB-231 cells propagated in medium containing 0 mM glucose and 0 mM L-glutamine for 2 h	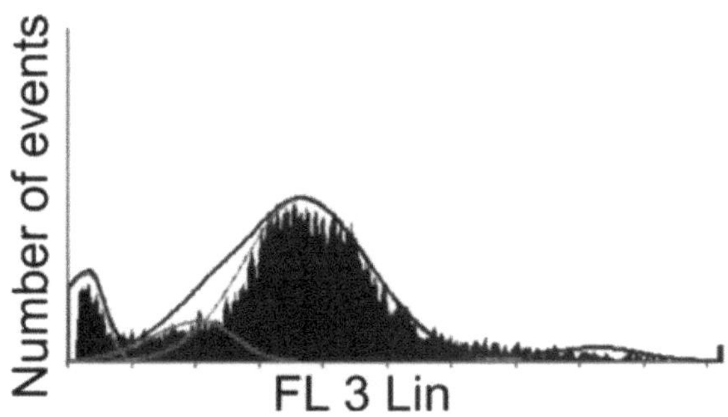
MDA-MB-231 cells propagated in medium containing 0 mM glucose and 0 mM L-glutamine for 4 h	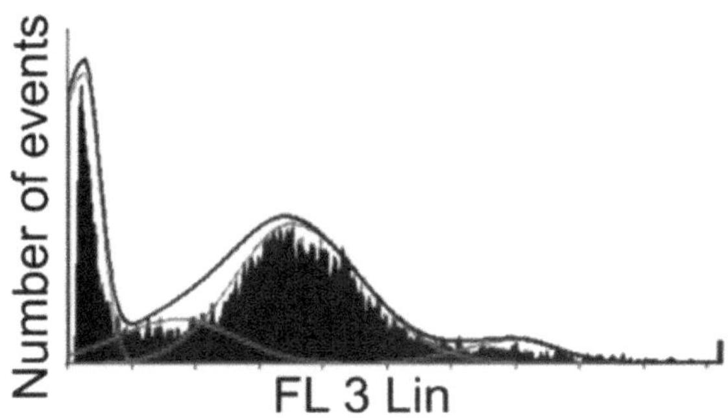
MDA-MB-231 cells propagated in medium containing 0 mM glucose and 0 mM L-glutamine for 6 h	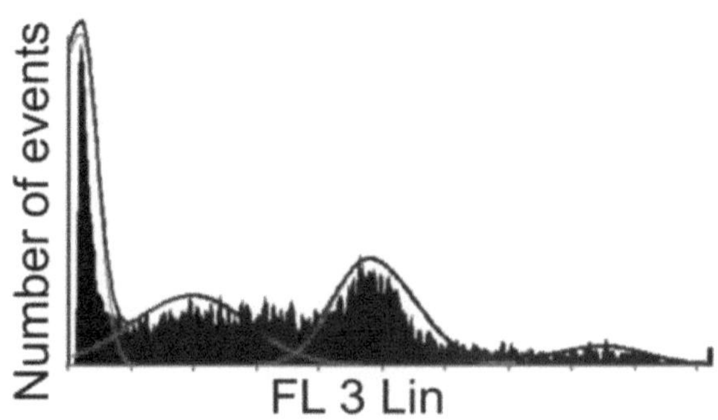

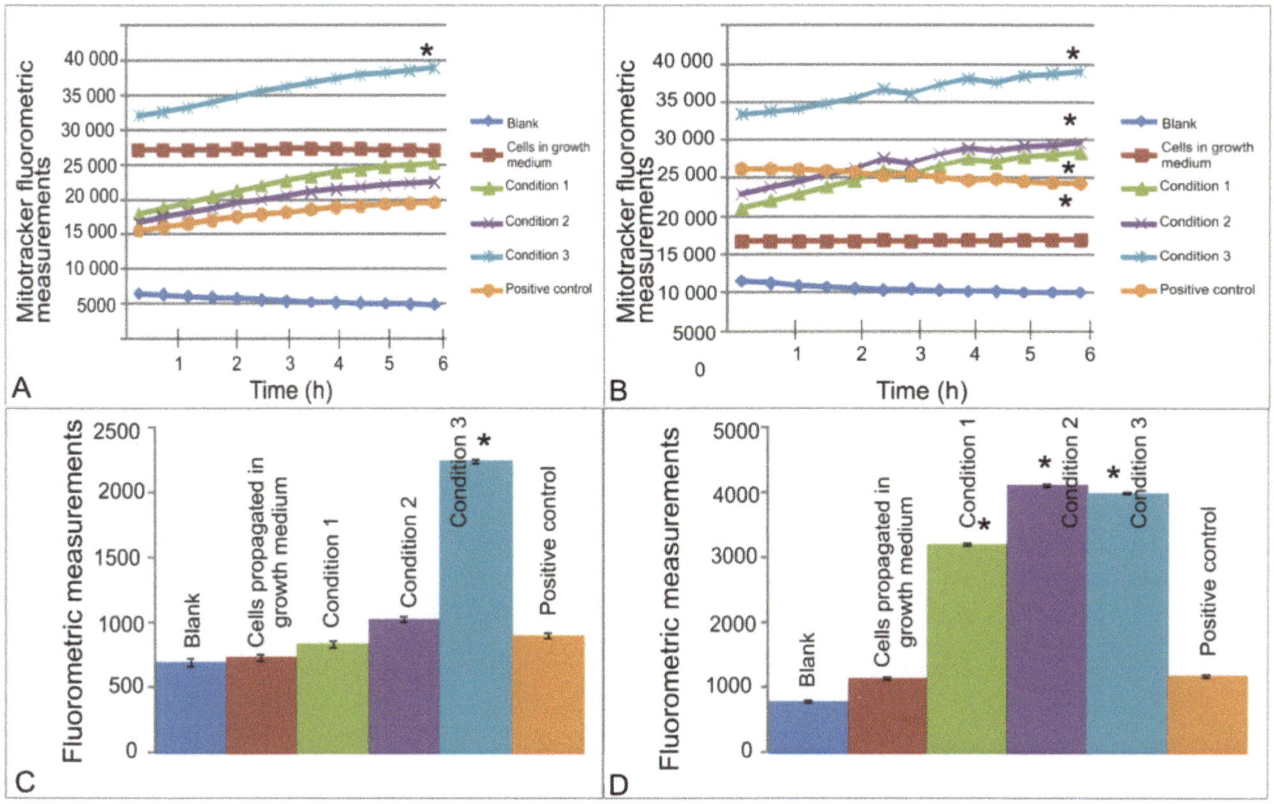

Fig. 4 Mitochondrial membrane potential after partial- and complete glutamine- and glucose starvation for short term exposures and after 7 days. Mitochondrial membrane potential of HeLa cells (**a**) and MDA-MB-231 cells (**b**) exposed to medium consisting of varying metabolic conditions. Cells exposed to medium containing no glucose or L-glutamine were the only samples with reduced mitochondrial membrane potential indicating apoptosis induction. Fluorometrics and mitocapture demonstrated unsuccessful recovery and colony formation demonstrated that the HeLa (**c**) cell line was less prominently affected than the MDA-MB-231 (**d**) cell line. Little changes were observed in HeLa cells exposed to DMEM containing 3 mM-6 mM glucose and 0.5 mM-1 mM L-glutamine. However, cells exposed to medium containing 0 mM glucose and 0 mM L-glutamine demonstrated a statistically significant change in the mitochondrial membrane potential. With regard to the MDA-MB-231 cell lines, all three metabolic conditions affected the mitochondrial membrane potential cells exposed to DMEM containing 0 mM- 3 mM glucose and 0 mM-0.5 mM L-glutamine the most prominent. An asterisk (*) indicates *P*-value < 0.05

generation and cell death via apoptosis- and autophagy induction.

Morphological findings demonstrate that decreasing amounts of glucose and L-glutamine in the growth medium resulted in decreased cell density in both cell lines. These effects were more pronounced 7 days after the exposure medium was replaced with medium containing 6 mM glucose and 1 mM L-glutamine. Since glucose is an essential source of carbon and energy required for cell survival and proliferation, glucose deprivation results in a failure of glycolytic enzyme induction with subsequent cessation of cell division [26]. Glucose deprivation was also found to induce cytotoxicity in the multidrug-resistant carcinoma cell line (MCF-7/ADR). Within 10 min, several signaling pathways including extracellular regulated protein kinases (ERK1/2), Lyn Kinase (a *src* family kinase) and c-Jun N-terminal kinase (JNK) were activated. ERK1/2 activation results in subsequent increased ROS generation. ERK1/2 are members of the mitogen activated protein kinase (MAPK) family [27]. MAPK is responsible for the phosphorylation of nuclear substrates including redox regulated transcription factors (*c*-Myc and *c*-fos) involved in cellular responses to oxidative stress [28].

Cell progression data suggested that glucose- and glutamine deprivation resulted in a G_2M block after 2–6 h in the HeLa cell line and 2–4 h in the MDA-MB-231 cell line accompanied with an increased induction of apoptosis in both cell lines. Glucose deprivation in a non-leukemic murine cell line (32Dcl23), transformed 32Dcl23 cell line and fibrosarcoma cell line (KHT-C2-LP1) also resulted in G_2M arrest [29, 30]. Further, it has been widely reported that glutamine deprivation results in G_1 cell cycle arrest in non-transformed cells. Glutamine deprivation in a human hepatocarcinoma (Hep3B) cell line resulted in significant altered gene expression

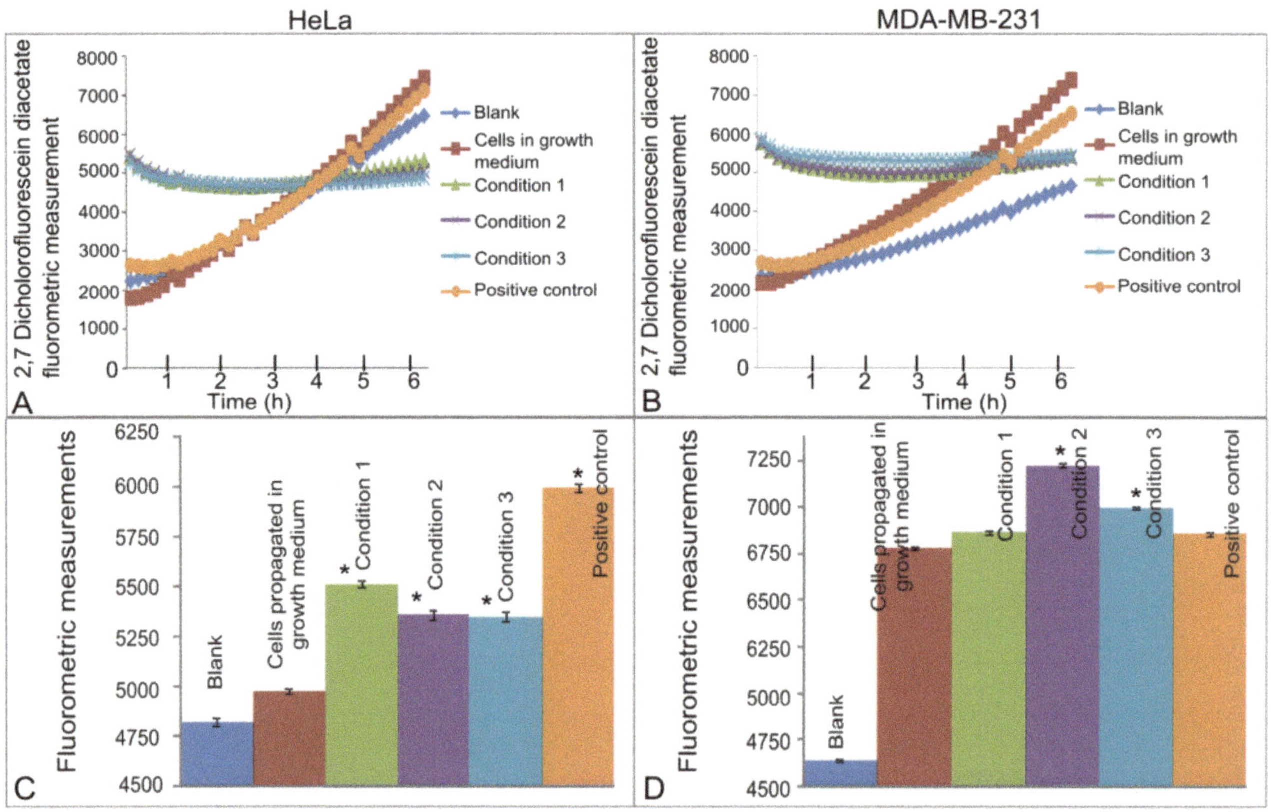

Fig. 5 Hydrogen peroxide production after partial- and complete glutamine- and glucose starvation for short term exposures and after 7 days. Hydrogen peroxide generation in HeLa cells (**a**) and MDA-MB-231 (**b**) after exposure to media presenting with different metabolic conditions did not change in any statistically significant manner (*P*-value > 0.05). In addition, cell recovery by propagating exposed HeLa cells (**c**) and MDA-MB-231 (**d**) in DMEM containing 6 mM glucose and 1 mM L-glutamine for 7 days was unsuccessful and demonstrating increased hydrogen peroxide production. An asterisk (*) indicates *P*-value < 0.05

related to the G_2M phase and DNA damage checkpoint including growth arrest and DNA-damage-inducible 45, gamma (GADD45G) [31]. Abcouver, et al. [32] also reported that glutamine deprivation in primary ductal carcinoma breast cells (TSE) and breast epithelial cells (HBL) resulted in rapid increase in GADD45 and DNA damage-inducible transcript 3 (GADD153). Cell cycle progression data also demonstrated an increased number of cells occupying the G_2M phase after glutamine deprivation. K-Ras-driven tumorigenic cells arrest in either the S phase or G_2M phase upon glutamine deprivation [32, 33]. Glutamine or glucose deprivation also results in synthetic lethality of various antitumor cell phase specific compounds. For example, glutamine deprivation in combination with capecitabine or paclitaxel resulted in enhanced cell death [5]. The increase of cells occupying G_1 phase after exposure to growth media containing decreased glutamine and glucose quantities suggests apoptosis induction. Various reports verify the induction of apoptosis by glucose or glutamine deprivation observed here including human embryonic kidney cells (HA1E) and mouse embryonic fibroblast cell line (NIH3T3) [34].

During the intrinsic apoptotic pathway, cellular stress signaling leads to permeabilization of the mitochondrial outer membrane resulting cytochrome *c* release into the cytosol caspase activation [31]. This is supported by previous reports where glucose deprivation in hemapoietic FL5.12 cells, human- and rat neutrophils resulted in mitochondrial membrane potential depolarisation [35, 36]. Thus, apoptosis induction was verified by additional flow cytometry findings demonstrating that exposure to the medium containing decreased glucose and L-glutamine quantities resulted in a reduction of the mitochondrial membrane potential. Mitochondrial ultrastructure studies revealed that complete glucose starvation for 6 h-9 h resulted in increased mitochondrial fragmentation, while reduced glucose or complete glutamine starvation resulted in mitochondrial elongation. Simultaneously, starvation of glucose and glutamine also lead to fused mitochondria [35]. Glutamine deprivation in human lung carcinoma cells (A549) demonstrated dense mitochondria

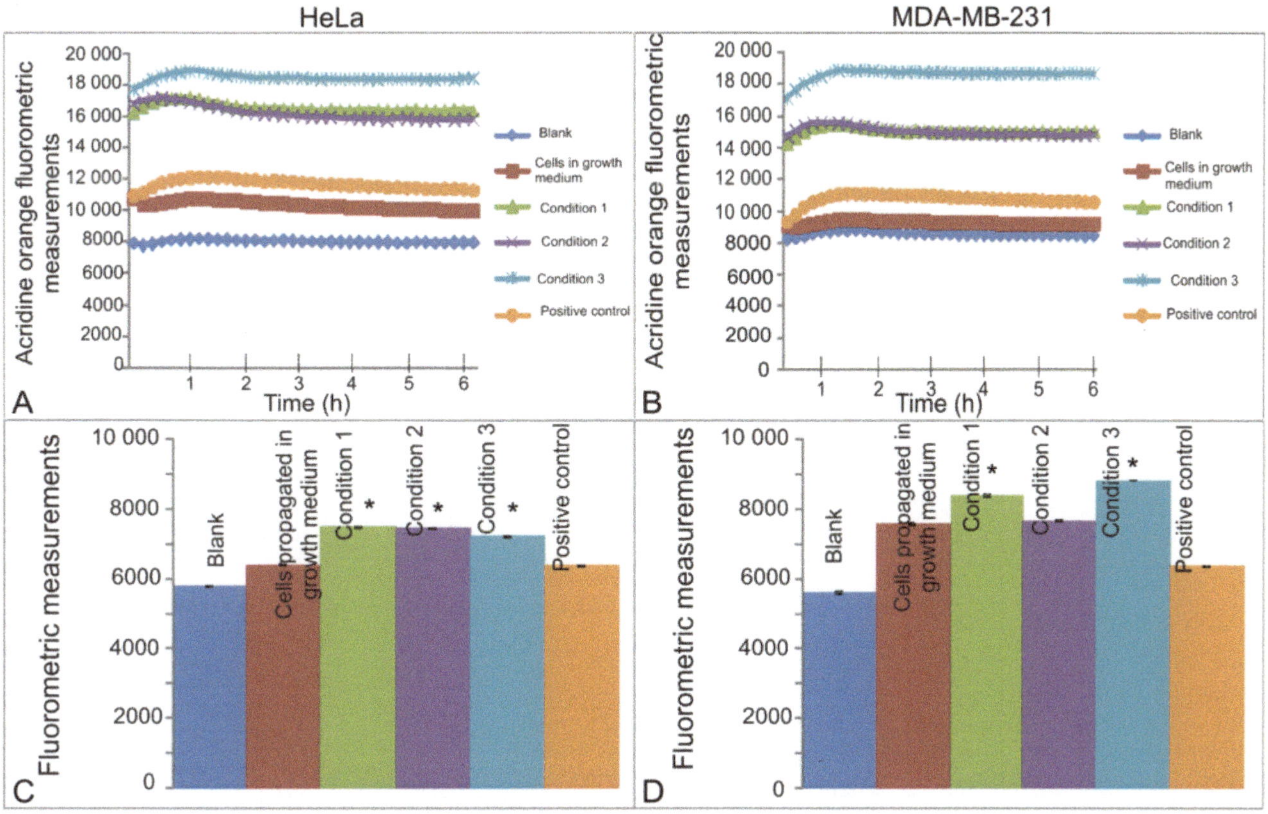

Fig. 6 Acridine orange staining after partial- and complete glutamine- and glucose starvation for short term exposures and after 7 days. Acridine orange staining of HeLa cells (**a**) and MDA-MB-231 (**b**) after exposure to media presenting with different metabolic conditions. Acridine orange production did not change in any statistically significant manner when exposed to these metabolic conditions (P-value > 0.05). Acridine orange staining and colony formation after 7 days in HeLa (**c**) and MDA-MB-231 cells (**d**). Results demonstrated that glucose-and glutamine deprivation effects cell functioning days after exposure was terminated with all the exposure to conditioned media demonstrating increased acridine orange staining suggesting an increase in acidity. An asterisk (*) indicates P-value < 0.05

with no further abnormal mitochondrial structural changes. Glutamine supplementation (1 mM) resulted in an increase of mitochondria number accompanied with large mitochondria size. The potential sensitive chloromethyltetramethylrosamine (CMTMRos) stain in the same study demonstrated that complete glutamine deprivation resulted in less round mitochondria and not as densely located around the nucleus when compared to cells cultured in medium containing 1 mM glutamine. Mitochondria in both conditions possessed thin filamentous structures [36].

Cytochrome *c* release is another hallmark of the intrinsic apoptotic pathway and was observed after glutamine deprivation in FL5.12 cells, KB26.5 murine hybridomas [37, 38]. Another study reported that glutamine deprivation in murine hybridoma cell line (Sp20) lead to the release of cytochrome *c* and SMAC/DIABLO accompanied with Bax translocation to the mitochondria and caspase 9 activation which is all characteristics of the intrinsic pathway [39]. Further, glutamine deprivation in myc-transformed fibroblasts has demonstrated that bcl-2 and caspase 9 inhibition prevented cell death verifying the induction of the intrinsic pathway [37]. Glutamine deprivation in the lymphoblastic leukemia CD4^{+} (CEM clone 13) cells, human lymphoblastic leukeumia (CEM-CCRF) cells and human promyeloblast (HL-60) cells also led to cell shrinkage and activation of CD95 receptors suggesting extrinsic pathway involvement [40].

This study demonstrated that glucose- and L-glutamine deprivation resulted in increased hydrogen peroxide production after a 7 day recovery period in both cell lines. An environment low in glucose results in increased oxidative phosphorylation for adequate ATP supply; this would lead to an additional oxygen electron reduction (electron transport chain) with subsequent increased ROS. The increased ROS (hydrogen peroxide and superoxide) is due to less reduced nicotinamide adenine dinucleotide- and pyruvate production in the pentose phosphate system and glycolysis, respectively [41].

Several reports have also indicated that glucose deprivation also caused increased hydrogen peroxide production in several cell lines including Chinese hamster ovary cell line (CHO), human liver carcinoma cell line (Hep2G), human pancreatic carcinoma (PANC1) and human fibroblasts [42–45]. Glucose deprivation resulting in oxidative stress also increased association between death associated protein 6 (DAXX), apoptosis signal-regulating kinase 1 (ASK1) and DAXX relocation from the nucleus to the cytoplasm. This is of importance since DAXX mediates the recruitment of ASK1 to FAS necessary for Fas-mediated apoptosis. [44]. Owada, et al. [43] also demonstrated that increased hydrogen peroxide resulting from glucose deprivation in Hep2G and PANC1 cells demonstrated subsequent AKT phosphorylation and activation [43, 45].

Conclusion

This study demonstrated that exposure to decreasing quantities glucose or L-glutamine resulted in decreased cell density, G_2M block and apoptosis induction within a few hours. After 7 days of being cultured in DMEM containing 6 mM glucose and 1 mM L-glutamine the above-mentioned effects are more prominent accompanied with a reduction in the mitochondrial membrane potential and increased acridine orange staining in both cell lines. In addition, the highly glycolytic- and metastatic cell line was more prominently affected when compared to the cervical carcinoma cell line. This study thus contributes the knowledge regarding the *in vitro* effects and signal transduction of glucose or L-glutamine deprivation in tumorigenic cell lines. Further research is imperative since it can potentially identify new targets for chemotherapy in the ongoing battle against cancer.

Competing interests

The authors declare that no competing interests exist.

Authors' contributions

TVM and MHV were involved in the project design, interpretation of data and conducted the experiments. MHV did the statistical analysis in this project and drafted the manuscript. AMJ was involved in the planning of this project, project supervision and editing of the manuscript. LL, EHM, GEM and AMJ contributed towards the planning and funding required for this project. GEM also assisted in editing the manuscript. All authors read and approved the final manuscript.

Acknowledgements

This study was supported by grants from the Cancer Association of South Africa, the Struwig Germeshuysen Trust, RESCOM (Research Council of the University of Pretoria), the South African National Research Foundation and Medical Research Council. L Liebenberg, EH Matthews and GE Mathews assisted in acquiring additional funding.

Author details

[1]Department of Physiology, University of Pretoria, Private Bag X323, Arcadia 0007, South Africa. [2]Centre for Research and Continued Engineering Development, North-West University, Lynnwood Ridge, South Africa.

References

1. Hensley CT, Wasti AT, BeBeradinis RJ. Glutamine and cancer: cell biology, physiology and clinical opportunities. J Clin Invest. 2015;123:3678–94.
2. Cairns RA, Harris IS, Mak TW. Regulation of cancer cell metabolism. Nat Rev Cancer. 2011;11:85–95.
3. Shanware NP, Bray K, Abraham RT. The PI3K, metabolic, and autophagy networks: interactive partners in cellular health and disease. Annu Rev Pharmacol Toxicol. 2013;53:89–106.
4. Lozy F, Karantza VG. Autophagy and cancer cell metabolism. Semin Cell Dev Biol. 2012;23:395–401.
5. Qie S, Liang D, Yin C, Gu W, Meng M, Wang C, et al. Glutamine deprivation and glucose depletion trigger growth inhibition via distinctive gene expression reprogramming. Cell Cycle. 2012;11:3679–90.
6. Kung H-N, Marks JR, Chi J-T. Glutamine synthetase is a genetic determinant of cell type-specific glutamine independence in breast epithelia. PLoS Genet. 2011;7:e1002229.
7. Sottnik JL, Lori JC, Rose BJ, Thamm DH. Glysolysis inhibition by 2-deoxy-D-glucose reverts the metastatic phenotype in vitro and in vivo. Clin Exp Metastasis. 2011;28:865–75.
8. Rahbari R, Sheahan T, Modes V, Collier P, Macfarlane C, Badge RM. A novel L1 retrotransposon marker for HeLa cell line identification. Biotechniques. 2009;46:277–84.
9. Jose C, Bellance N, Rossignoi R. Choosing between glycolysis and oxidative phosphorylation: a tumor's dilemma? Biochim Biophys Acta. 1807;2011:552–61.
10. Rossignol R, Gilkerson R, Aggeler R, Yamagata K, Remington SJ, Capaldi RA. Energy substrate modulates mitochondrial structure and oxidative capacity in cancer cells. Cancer Res. 2014;64:986–93.
11. Corkery B, Crown J, Clynes M, Donovan N. Epidermal growth factor receptor as a potential therapeutic target in triple-negative breast cancer. Ann Oncol. 2009;20:862–7.
12. Hall DD, Wu Y, Domann FE, Spitz DR, Anderson ME. Mitochondrial calcium uniporter activity is dispensable for MDA-MB-231 breast carcinoma cell survival. PLoS One. 2014;9:e96866.
13. Liu B, Fan Z, Edgerton SM, Deng XS, Alimova IN, Lind SE, et al. Metformin induces unique biological and molecular responses in triple negative breast cancer cells. Cell Cycle. 2009;8:2031–40.
14. Robey IF, Lien AD, Welsh SJ, Baggett BK, Gillies RJ. Hypoxia-inducible factor-1α and glycolytic phenotype in tumors. Neoplasia. 2005;7:324–30.
15. Palorini R, Simonetto T, Cirulli C, Chiaradonna F. Mitochondrial complex 1 inhibitors and forced oxidative phosphorylation synergize in inducing cancer cell death. Int J Cell Biol. 2013; doi:10.1155/2013/243876.
16. Mqoco TV, Visagie MH, Albrecht C, Joubert AM. Differential cellular interaction of *Sutherlandia frutescens* extracts on tumorigenic and non-tumorigenic breast cells. S Afr J Bot. 2014;90:59–67.
17. Visagie MH, Birkholtz LM, Joubert AM. 17-Beta-estradiol analog inhibits cell proliferation by induction apoptosis in breast cell lines. Microsc Res Tech. 2014;77:236–42.
18. Ekim B, Magnuson B, Acosta-Jaquez HA, Keller JA, Feener EP, Fingar DC. mTOR Kinase domain phosphorylation promotes mTORC1 signaling, cell growth, and cell cycle progression. Mol Cell Biol. 2011;31:2878–01.
19. Yoon JC, Ling AJY, Isik M, Lee DD, Steinbaugh MJ, Sack LM, et al. GLTSCR2/PICT1 links mitochondrial stress and Myc signaling. Proc Natl Acad Sci U S A. 2014;11:3781–6.
20. Takai N, Ueda T, Nishida M, Nasu K, Nahara H. Bufalin induces growth inhibition, cell cycle arrest and apoptosis in human endometrial and ovarian cancer cells. Int J Mol Med. 2008;21:637–43.
21. Costa A, Scholer-Dahirel A, Mechta-Grigoriou F. The role of reactive oxygen species and metabolism on cancer cells and their microenvironment. Semin Cancer Biol. 2014;26:23–32.
22. Yao ZF, Cao J, Xu LM, Sun XC, Kang J, Yang G, et al. Perfluorooctane sulfonate blocked autophagy flux and induced lysosome membrane permeabilization in HepG2 cells. Food Chem Toxicol. 2014;67:96–104.
23. Kusuzaki K, Murata H, Takeshita H, Hashiguchi S, Nozaki T, Emoto K, et al. Intracellular binding sites of acridine orange in living osteosarcoma cells. Anticancer Res. 2000;20:971–5.
24. Koppenol WH, Bounds PL, Dang CV. Otto Warburg's contributions to current concepts of cancer metabolism. Nat Rev Cancer. 2011;11:325–37.
25. Lunt SY, Vander Heiden MG. Aerobic glycolysis: meeting the metabolic requirements of cell proliferation. Annu Rev Cell Dev Biol. 2011;27:441–64.

26. Brand K. Aerobic glycolysis by proliferating cells: protection against oxidative stress at the expense of energy yield. J Bioenerg Biomembr. 1997;29:355–64.
27. Spitz DRS, Sim J, Didnour LA, Galforo SS, Lee YJ. Glucose deprivation-induced oxidative stress in human tumor cells: a fundamental defect in metabolism. Ann NY Acad Sci. 2006;899:349–62.
28. Lee YJ, Galoforo SS, Berns CM, Chen JC, Davis BH, Sim JE, et al. Glucose deprivation-induced cytotoxicity and alterations in mitogen-activated protein kinase activation are mediated by oxidative stress in multidrug-resistant human breast carcinoma cells. J Biol Chem. 1998;273:5294–9.
29. Kansara M, Berridge MV. Oncogenes modulate cell sensitivity to apoptosis induced by glucose deprivation. Anticancer Res. 2004;24:2503–10.
30. Schlappack OK, Zimmermann A, Hill RP. Glucose starvation and acidosis: effect on experimental metastatic potential, DNA content and MTX resistance of murine tumor cells. Br J Cancer. 1991;64:663–70.
31. Landes T, Martinou JC. Mitochondrial outer membrane permeabilization during apoptosis: the role of mitochondrial fission. Biochim Biophys Acta. 2011;1813:540–5.
32. Abcouwer SF, Schwarz C, Mequid RA. Glutamine deprivation induces the expression of GADD45 and GADD153 primarily by mRNA stabilization. J Biol Chem. 1999;274:28645–51.
33. Saqcena, S Mukhopadhyay S, Hosny C, Alhamed A, Chatterjee A, Foster DA. Blocking anelerotic entry of glutamine into the TCA cycle sensitizes K-Ras mutant cancer cells to cytotoxic drugs. Oncogene. 2014; doi:10.1038/onc.2014.207.
34. Yuneva M. Finding an "Achilles heel" of cancer. Cell Cycle. 2008;7:2083–9.
35. Rambold AS, Kostelecky B, Elia N, Lippincott-Swartz J. Tubular network formation protects mitochondria from autophagosomal degradation during nutrient starvation. Proc Natl Acad Sci U S A. 2011;108(5):101902–10195.
36. Ahmad S, White CW, Chang L-Y, Schneider BK, Allen CB. Glutamine protects mitochondria structure and function in oxygen toxicity. Am J Physiol. 2001;280(4):L779–91.
37. Maldonado AC, Muñoz-Pinedo C. Dying for something to eat: how cells respond to starvation. Open Cell Sign J. 2011;3:13–23.
38. Fuchs BC, Bode BP. Stressing out over survival: glutamine as an apoptotic modulator. J Surg Res. 2006;131:26–40.
39. Paquette JC, Guérin PJ, Gauthier ER. Rapid induction of the intrinsic apoptotic pathway by L-glutamine starvation. J Cell Physiol. 2004;202:912–21.
40. Fumarola C, Zerbini A, Guidotti GG. Glutamine deprivation-mediated cell shrinkage induces ligand-independent CD95 receptor signaling and apoptosis. Cell Death Differ. 2001;8:1004–13.
41. Blackburn RV, Spitz D, Liu X, Galoforo SS, Sim JE, Ridnour LA, et al. Metabolic oxidative stress activates signal transduction and gene expression during glucose deprivation in human tumor cells. Free Radic Biol Med. 1999;26:419–30.
42. Lord-Fontaine S, Averill-Bates DA. Heat shock inactivates cellular antioxidant defences against hydrogen peroxide: protection by glucose. Free Radic Biol Med. 2002;32:762–6.
43. Owada S, Shimoda Y, Tsuchihara K, Esumi H. Critical role of H2O2 generated by NOX4 during cellular response under glucose deprivation. PLoS One. 2013;8:e56628.
44. Song JJ, Lee YL. Catalase but not MNSOD, inhibits glucose-activated ASK1-MEK-MAPK signal transduction pathway and prevents relocalization of DAXX: hydrogen peroxide as a major second messenger of metabolic oxidative stress. J Cell Biochem. 2003;90:304–14.
45. Aki T, Yamaguchi K, Fujimiya T, Mizukami Y. Phosphoinositide 3-kinase accelerates autophagic cell death during glucose deprivation in rat cardiomyocyte-derived cell line H9c2. Oncogene. 2003;22:8529–35.

Unveiling the hidden function of long non-coding RNA by identifying its major partner-protein

Yongfang Yang, Liwei Wen and Hongliang Zhu*

Abstract

Tens of thousands of long non-coding RNAs (lncRNAs) have been discovered in eukarya, but their functions are largely unknown. Fortunately, lncRNA–protein interactions may offer details of how lncRNAs play important roles in various biological processes, thus identifying proteins associated with lncRNA is critical. Here we review progress of molecular archetypes that lncRNAs execute as guides, scaffolds, or decoys for protein, focusing on advantages, shortcomings and applications of various conventional and emerging technologies to probe lncRNAs and protein interactions, including protein-centric biochemistry approaches such as nRIP and CLIP, and RNA-centric biochemistry approaches such as ChIRP, CHART and RAP. Overall, this review provides strategies for probing interactions between lncRNAs and protein.

Keywords: Long non-coding RNA, Function, Interaction, Protein, Biochemistry approaches

Background

Recently, an explosion of microarray tiling and high-throughput deep sequencing analysis has led to the discovery of thousands of previously presumed non-coding transcripts [1, 2]. Global transcriptional analyses of the human genome have revealed that non-coding RNA far exceed the protein-coding mRNAs which account for only about two percent of the human genome [3]. Non-coding RNA include many small regulatory RNAs and tens of thousands of polyadenylated and nonpolyadenylated lncRNAs which have been shown to be essential for many rapidly growing research areas [4]. Although only a few lncRNA have been documented to have important biological functions, increasing evidences suggest that the regulation of lncRNAs on target genes is complicated [5].

lncRNAs, through interactions with protein, DNA and RNA, regulate gene expression at multiple levels, including chromatin remodeling and nuclear transcription, pre-mRNA splicing and cytoplasmic mRNA translation [6]. Moreover, virtually all functional RNA molecules interact with protein complexes and protein is confirmed to be the first and principal partner of lncRNA [7]. Thus, understanding lncRNA functions can be accomplished by identification of lncRNA-bound proteomes. Substantial effort is being devoted to depicting RNA–protein interactions for gaining insight into molecular mechanisms, but lncRNA–protein interplay is poorly understood [8–10]. In this review, we highlight molecular modes and functions of lncRNA–protein interactions and summarize conventional and emerging techniques to probe these interactions, with hopes of illuminating hidden lncRNA regulatory mechanisms.

Characteristics and function of lncRNA

LncRNA are a group of non-coding RNAs defined as being larger than 200 nucleotides in length, which distinguish them from small RNAs such as microRNAs, small nucleolar RNAs (snoRNAs) and small interfering RNAs (siRNAs) [11]. According to the relative position of the coding gene, lncRNA exist in four groups: intergenic, introngenic, overlap and antisense [12]. Compared with protein coding RNA, lncRNAs are typically shorter

*Correspondence: hlzhu@cau.edu.cn
Department of Food Biotechnology, College of Food Science and Nutritional Engineering, China Agricultural University, 100083 Beijing, China

with fewer exons, less abundance, less coding potential and more restrictions to particular tissues or cells [13]. Moreover, lncRNAs sequences are less conserved than mRNA among related species. Recently, secondary structures of lncRNAs have been shown to be conserved, having 'repeat A' region in lncRNA Xist (X inactive-specific transcript) and a 'roX-boxes' sequence motif comprised of two lncRNAs roX1 and roX2 [14, 15]. Research that lncRNAs have various important regulatory effect on target gene expression contributing to epigenetic modification, transcription and post-transcriptional processing via specific interactions with proteins and other cellular factors [16–18].

LncRNAs mediate epigenetic changes by recruiting chromatin remodeling complexes to specific genomic loci [16]. For example, the lncRNA HOX antisense intergenic RNA (HOTAIR)which is initiated from the HOXC cluster interacts with ploycomb repressive complex 2 (PRC2) to silence transcription across 40 kb of the HOXC locus in trans by inducing a repressive chromatin state [19]. lncRNAs, Xist, RepA and Kcnqot1 all recruit the polycomb complex to the target genome and they trimethylate lysine 27 residues (me3K27) of histone H3 to induce heterochromatin formation and repress gene expression [20, 21]. In addition, lncRNA also regulate target gene at transcriptional [18]. Proximal promoters can be transcribed into long ncRNAs that recruit and integrate RNA binding proteins function into the transcriptional process [22]. For example, an lncRNA induced by DNA damage and transcribed from the *cyclin D1* gene promoter, recruits and integrates RNA binding protein TLS to silence *cyclin D1* gene expression [22]. LncRNAs could act as co-factors to modulate transcription factor activity. LncRNA Evf-2 is transcribed from an enhancer and recruits transcription factor DlX2 to this same enhancer to induce expression of adjacent protein-coding genes [23]. Moreover, post-transcriptional regulation of lncRNAs is being revealed. Normally, lncRNAs are involved in splicing regulation and translational control [17]. The lncRNA MALAT1 (metastasis-associated long adenocarcinoma transcript 1) interacts with serine–arginine splicing factor to regulate its distribution in nuclear speckle domains and to modulate pre-mRNA alternative splicing [24]. A neuron-specific antisense lncRNA, AS Uchl1, could specifically induce the translation of ubiquitin carboxyl-terminal esterase L1(*Uchl1*) under certain stress conditions through its complementarity with target mRNA [25]. LncRNA brain cytoplasmic RNA 1 (BC1) blocks protein complex assembly to repress translation initiation in neurons and germ cells [26].

Molecular archetypes of the lncRNA–protein interaction

Recently, how lncRNAs control gene expression and molecular function archetypes of lncRNAs have been concerned. Wang's group discussed four emerging archetypes of molecular functions that lncRNAs execute as signals, decoys, guides, and scaffolds via proteins, DNA and RNA interaction [27]. Here, we distill the myriad functions of lncRNA into three archetypes of molecular mechanisms to illustrate how lncRNAs directly interacting with proteins and serve as 'guide' to recruit protein complexes to target genes, serve as 'scaffold' to assemble proteins into RNPs, and serve as 'decoy' to sequester regulatory proteins away from target gene [28]. We then offer examples of each archetype's lncRNA–protein interactions.

LncRNAs act as protein guides

First, lncRNA acts as guide to recruit proteins to chromatin sites through RNA-DNA base pairing, to regulate downstream gene expression (Fig. 1a). For example, lncRNA fetal-lethal non-coding developmental regulatory RNA (Fendrr), which is specifically transcribed in nascent lateral plate mesoderm of the developing mouse embryo, guides PRC2 to target genes to increase PRC2 occupancy and trimethylate of H3K27me3, subsequently leading to attenuation of target gene expression [29]. Cold assisted intronic non-coding RNA (COLDAIR), a cold-induced lncRNA with a capped 5′ end lacking a 3′ poly A tail, is transcribed from the intron of the *FLC* locus gene in *Arabidopsis thaliana* and recruits PRC2 to establish and maintain stable repressive chromatin of *FLC* through H3K27 trimethylation during vernalization [30]. Other than recruiting PCR2 to repress target gene expression, some lncRNAs, such as lincRNA-p21 can guide hnRNP-K protein to the promoter of the *p21* gene and act as a co-activator for p53-dependent *p21* transcription [31]. Most known human proteins have nucleic acid binding domains [32], so potential lncRNA–protein interactions may act as adaptors to link lncRNA to target loci (Fig. 1a). The telomere complex is a classical model for proteins serving as adaptors between RNA and DNA [33, 34]. The telomere repeat factor TRF2 forms a stable complex with telomere-repeat-encoding RNA (TERRA) and telomere DNA repeats [35]. These interactions could be applied to lncRNA to illustrate archetypes for lncRNA and protein interactions. A well-studied protein that acts as an adaptor between regulatory lncRNA and chromatin is through YY1 tethering lncRNA of Xist to the inactive X nuclear center through repeat C. YY1 protein can bind both RNA and DNA through different sequence motifs and may serve as an adaptor for Xist [36].

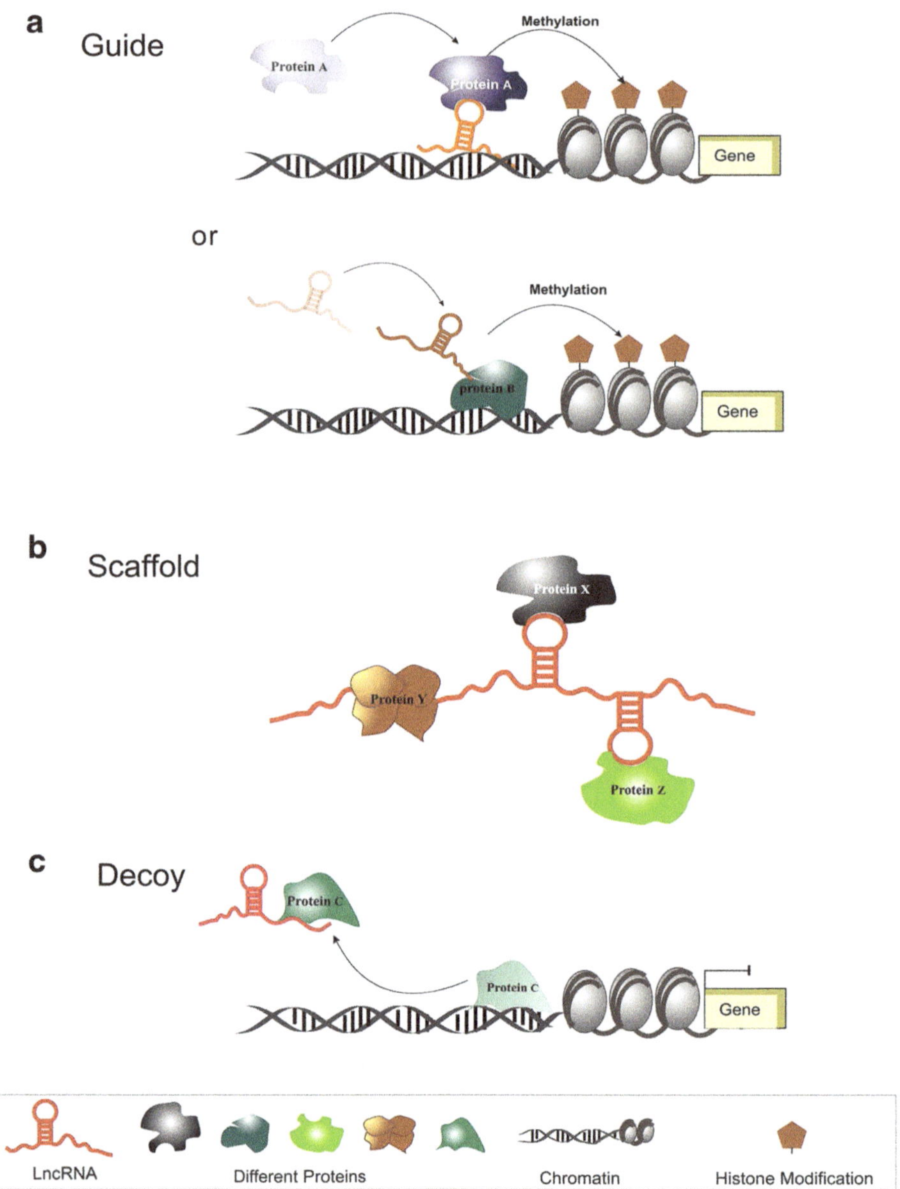

Fig. 1 Schematic illustration of possible molecular archetypes of lncRNA–protein. **a** lncRNA guides protein to target genomic loci or the protein acts as an adaptor for lncRNA to link lncRNA to the target gene. **b** lncRNA brings two or three proteins together to form discrete complexes of lncRNA–RNPs. **c** lncRNA act as decoys to draw proteins away from t target genes

LncRNAs scaffolds bring proteins together

lncRNA can be scaffolds to create discrete protein complexes: lncRNA–RNPs (Fig. 1b). HOTAIR could both bind to PRC2 and LSD1 to repress gene transcription and the catalytic methyl-transferase subunit EZH2 of PRC2 is confirmed to be recruited via a structural domain at the 5′-end of HOTAIR to impart repressive histone modifications. Meanwhile the 3′-end of HOTAIR associates with LSD1, inducing H3K4 demethylated modification [37]. Another nascent antisense lncRNA, ANRIL, which is transcribed by RNA polymerase II at the TSS of the $p16^{INK4a}$ gene, recruits PRC2 and PRC1 to mediate protein-coding gene repression *in cis* [38]. LncRNA roX is transcribed from the *Drosophila X* genome, which is thought to be critical scaffold for assembly of a functional MSL dosage compensation complex to activate transcription through acetylation of H4K16 [15, 39]. Moreover, lncRNAs act as protein scaffolds to control gene expression by modulation of nuclear architecture. The subnuclear structure-specific lncRNAs taurine upregulated gene 1 (TUG1) and nuclear-enriched autosomal transcript 2 (NEAT2)bind to methylated and unmethylated polycomb 2 protein (Pc2) respectively to mediate assembly of multiple corepressor or coactivator protein complexes [40], which switch non-histone protein methylated mark recognition to relocation of transcription units in the nuclear three-dimensional space, achieving coordinated gene expression regulation.

LncRNAs act as decoys to titrate away proteins

lncRNAs act as decoys to remove proteins away from target loci (Fig. 1c). The lncRNA p21 associated ncRNA DNA damage activated (PANDA) is a well-studied lncRNA that acts as a decoy for transcription factors. PANDA is located 5 kb upstream of the *CDKN1A* with a 5′-cap and a 3′-polyadenylated but non-spliced tail. PANDA binds to and sequestrates NF-YA transcription factor from target gene promoters to repress gene expression [41]. Also, lncRNA could also be decoy of other proteins. LncRNA growth arrest-specific 5 (Gas5) has been identified to interact with glucocorticoid receptor (GR) to prevent binding to DNA response elements, thereby blocking glucocorticoid signal pathway [42]. The lncRNA metastasis-associated lung adenocarcinoma transcript 1 (MALAT1) binds to and sequesters several serine/arginine splicing factors to modulate their nuclear distribution and phosphorylation states to ensure splicing factor regulation of alternative splicing of cellular pre-mRNAs at a precise time, place, and concentration [24].

Technologies to probe the lncRNA–protein interactions

AS the significance of lncRNA–protein interactions is better understood, their biochemistry attributes are being discovered and novel bioinformatics approaches are being developed to identify and predict proteins that interact with target lncRNA. Previously, most methods to study RNA–protein interactions are protein-centric, including native RNA immunoprecipitation (nRIP), cross-linking and immunoprecipitation (CLIP) [43, 44]. Recently, the discovery of numerous non-coding RNA has led to concern about RNA-centric approaches, such as the RNA pull-down assay, chromatin isolation by RNA purification (ChIRP), capture hybridization analysis of RNA targets (CHART), and RNA antisense purification (RAP) [45–48]. So other methods are being sought [49, 50], and here we depict detailed strategies for identifying lncRNA–protein interactions.

Protein-centric approach to probing lncRNA–protein interactions

nRIP and nRIP-seq

nRIP is used to detect the association of individual proteins with specific RNA species in vivo. An antibody-based technology, this can be used to immunoprecipitate an RNA binding protein complex from a heterogeneous cellular homogenate in vivo. RNAs stably associated with the protein complex will immunoprecipitated together and associated RNAs including lncRNA and small RNA or even coding RNA can be measured with real-time PCR or be identified by RNA sequencing [51]. One important consideration prior to commencing RIP-based approaches designed to identify protein–RNA interactions is whether cross-linking is necessary. Native RIP is the method without crosslinking before cell lysis, which is a more appropriate for proteins that bind RNA directly. To reduce RNA recovery rates and identify the proteins that bind RNA indirectly, RIP assay is performed to crosslink cells with formaldehyde before cell lysis step [52]. nRIP is economical, requiring no specialized equipment and can be carried out under native conditions and thus allows identification of kinetically stable interactions [43]. However, the nRIP approach has limitations. First, differentiating direct from indirect interactions is difficult and. the read length of associated RNA is too large for identifying the actual binding site. Finally, nRIP assays are commonly known to have variability (reproducibility of 60 % or more) [53]. Thus, multiple biological replicates for nRIP are required. Thus, RIP-based approaches have been used to identify many lncRNA–protein interactions (see Table 1). Zhao's group discovered that Xist, Tsix, and RepA interacted with PRC2 by native RIP [14]. Recently, Fendrr was identified to bind to PCR2 complex and WDR5 protein by nRIP [29]. Previously, RNA isolated by native RIP was analyzed with microarray technologies (RIP-ChIP) [54], but this is naturally limited by array design and coverage, so nRIP has recently been coupled with high-throughput sequencing (nRIP-seq) to capture the genome-wide RNA pools bound to target proteins [55]. Recent studies suggest that a genome-wide pool of thousands of PRC2-interacting RNAs including some characterized lncRNA, and many unannotated RNAs were identified in embryonic stem cells by nRNA-seq [56].

CLIP and CLIP-seq

CLIP is a powerful protein-centric tool used to isolate cross-linked RNA and protein complexes in tissues or cultured cells and subsequently purify the RNA targets. CLIP overcomes the drawbacks of nRIP by cross-linking RNA–protein complexes with ultraviolet light. Based on strong cross-links, followed by RNase treatment of the cell lysate to shorten RNA fragments, immunoprecipitation is performed to purify the covalently cross-linked lncRNA–protein. Importantly, covalent cross-linking permits stringent washing of immunoprecipitates, and this reduces background noise [44]. CLIP has been

Table 1 Summary of lncRNA analyzed by several biochemistry approaches

LncRNAs	RBP	Biological function	Methods	Ref
ANRIL	PCR2, PCR1	Influences $p16^{INK4a}$ gene expression and cell senescence	CLIP	[38]
Air	G9a	Targets G9a in cis for imprinting	CLIP	[57]
Fendrr	PRC2, WDR5	Regulates gene in cis and in trans	RIP	[29]
FIRRE	hnPNPU	Modulation of nuclear architecture across chromosomes	RAP	[58]
HOTAIR	PCR2, LSD1	Silences transcription in trans via its modular architecture	RNA pull-down	[37]
Hottip	MLL-WDR5	Activates gene expression via chromosomal looping	RIP	[59]
lincRNA-p21	hnRNP-K	Mediates p53-dependent gene repression	RNA pull down-MS	[31]
MALAT1	PSPC1, PSF, PURA	Sequesters splicing factor to regulate alternative splicing	CHART-MS	[60]
NEAT1	PSPC1, SRSF1, ESRP2	Plays roles in RNA processing and transcriptional regulation	CHART-MS	[60]
Rox1	MLE, MSL	Mediates X chromosome upregulated to rescue male lethality	dChIRP	[61]
TERC	TCAB1	Functions as the template and scaffold for the telomerase complex	ChIRP	[47]
Xist	81 proteins (Hnrnpk, Spen)	Mediates chromatin modifications and Polycomb targeting	ChIRP-MS	[62]
Xist	10 proteins (SHARP, HDAC3)	Interacts directly with SHARP to silence transcription through HDAC3	RAP-MS	[63]

used to reveal that many intronic lncRNA directly bind to the PRC2 complex (see Table 1) [64]. For instance, Takashi's group reported that lncRNA Air interacted with the H3K9 histone methyl-transferase G9a by CLIP [57], but their data suggest that the post-assay RNA quantity is small and the assay is tedious steps. Consequently, CLIP combined with high-throughput sequencing (HITS-CLIP or CLIP-seq) is used to identify many RBPs, such as Nova, Ago2, and TDP-43 [65–67]. The CLIP assay occasionally produces false–positive interactions and it determining the exact binding sites is not always straightforward [68]. Therefore, modified protocols have been developed to define cross-linking events, such as photoactivatable-ribonucleoside-enhanced CLIP (PAR-CLIP) and individual-nucleotide resolution CLIP (iCLIP) [69, 70]. With PAR-CLIP, cells are cultured in the presence of 4-SU (4-thiouridine) or 6-SG (6-thioguanosine), which are incorporated into RNA and induce strong cross-linking between RNAs and RBPs. Thus, this method can eliminate nonspecific targets and identify exact binding sites at a single nucleotide resolution [71]. Disadvantage of PAR-CLIP is difficulties in the use of 4-SU and 6-SG in living animals due to the toxicity. Thus, the PAR-CLIP method has been successfully applied to RBPs, such as HuR, FMRP, and Ataxin-2 [72–74]. To identify RNA binding motifs and novel functions, iCLIP introduces an adapter at the 5′ end through the primer used for reverse transcription by cDNA circularization and subsequent linearization. Thus, both truncated and read-through cDNAs are captured. Importantly, iCLIP also provides information about the cross-link site that permits precise mapping of RNA–protein contacts at a nucleotide resolution [70]. Rossbach's group performed iCLIP combined with deep-sequencing (iCLIP-Seq) to reveal global regulatory roles of hnRPN L protein [75].

RNA-centric approach to dissecting lncRNA–protein interactions

RNA pull-down assay

RNA pull-down assay is a preliminary RNA-centric in vitro method that enabling identification and characterization of various proteins which interact with a given lncRNA of interest. First, lncRNA probes were synthesized and labeled with high affinity tags, such as biotin, then cell lysate was prepared from a in vitro sample. Next, the lncRNA probe was incubated with lysate or recombinant protein to form a specific lncRNA–protein complex. Subsequently, the protein complex was pulled down with streptavidin agarose or magnetic beads. Finally, the retrieved protein was identified with Western blot or mass spectrometry (MS) [45]. Rinn's group used RNA pull-down to discover that HOTAIR was directly associated with the PCR2 complex, which repressed transcription of the *HOXD* loci in trans [19].

ChIRP and ChIRP-MS

Advances in RNA-centric biochemical purification offer new opportunities for systematically mapping lncRNA interactions with proteins and chromatin. The ChIRP method is based on using the biotinylated oligonucleotides complementary to the lncRNA of interest as a "handle" to pull down lncRNA-associated proteins and chromatin DNA. In brief, cultured cells are cross-linked, chromatin is extracted and sonicated, and then biotinylated tilling oligos that tile whole lncRNA were added and hybridized. Finally, the hybrids including target lncRNA, proteins and chromatin DNA were eluted with magnetic streptavidin beads and subjected to q-PCR or deep sequencing for DNA analysis, or to Western blotting or MS for protein analysis (Fig. 2) [46]. In addition, the recently developed ChIRP-seq method allows global and high-throughput discovery of genomic DNA associated with lncRNA. Chu's group used ChIRP-seq to reveal the precision genomic occupancy of roX2, TERC, and HOTAIR: three rather different lncRNAs in two species successfully (see Table 1) [47]. To dissect the lncRNA functional domains in situ, domain-specific chromatin isolation by RNA purification (dChIRP) has been developed based on the ChIRP method and with dChIRP, biotinylated oligos are used as specific pools to recover specific domains of target RNA that improve the RNA genomic localization signal-to-noise ratio by >20-fold over traditional ChIRP [61]. dChIRP allowed lncRNA to be characterized at the domain level and revealed the lncRNA architecture and function with high precision and sensitivity [76]. Recently, Quinn's group reported a 'three-fingered hand' topology of roX1 and that the three D domains of roX1 bind directly to the MSL protein complex to individually rescue male lethality by dChIRP [77].

MS based proteomics is a common tool for studying cellular interactions. Baltz and colleagues and Castello's group used MS to identify hundreds of novel RBPs in human cells [78, 79]. Recently, to enable quantitation and accurate discovery of novel RNA–protein interactions from complexes assembled in vivo, Klass and colleagues used quantitative MS combined with RNase treatment of affinity-purified RNA–protein complexes to identify proteins that bind to RNA concurrently with an RBP of interest [80]. Kramer's group developed an experimental and computational workflow method combining photo-induced cross-linking, high-resolution MS and automated analysis of the resulting spectra for identification of RNA interactions with proteins [81]. This MS-based workflow based on MS can be applied to map any RNA–protein complex of interest. Recently, ChIRP-MS, an optimized ChIRP method for systematically discovering lncRNA-bound proteome in vivo proteomes by MS was developed to identify 81 endogenous proteins that associated with Xist in two waves to coordinate X chromatin spreading and silencing. Interestingly, HrnpK protein participates in Xist-mediated gene silencing and chromatin modifications, but not Xist biogenesis or localization. Thus, the results suggested ChIRP-MS assay achieved high output and specificity regarding lncRNA–protein interactions in vivo [62].

CHART and CHART-MS

Another hybridization-based purification strategy is CHART which is used to confirmed the genome-wide localization of lncRNA in chromatin and isolate the protein associated with the lncRNA of interest. CHART is more similar than different with ChIRP (Fig. 2), but one significant difference is the design criteria of the oligonucleotide probe. With ChIRP, short antisense DNA oligonucleotides tile across the entire target lncRNA without a priori knowledge of target RNA function domain cover all potential hybridization spots [47]. In contrast, probes of CHART are empirically determined after RNase H assay which determines the candidate hybridization region [82]. CHART is a useful method for biochemically defining DNA and proteins associated with lncRNAs. CHART-seq, which combines CHART and RNA-seq, was applied to discover hundreds of trans-genomic binding sites for NEAT1 and MALAT1 [60]. Moreover, West's group initially adapted the CHART assay to identify the full complement of proteins associated with RNAs in vivo with MS. CHART-MS was performed for two human lncRNAs, NEAT1 and MALAT1, to identify many nuclear speckle and para-speckle components and several new proteins not previously associated with them (see Table 1) [60].

RAP and RAP-MS

Similar to ChIRP and CHART, the RAP method is also used to capture a target lncRNA of interest through hybridization with antisense biotinylated oligos (Fig. 2) [47]. With RAP, various cross-linking conditions can be performed to identify different molecules that interact with the target RNA via different mechanisms. For direct RNA–RNA interactions, psoralens are used for cross-linking, but for protein–RNA interactions, formaldehyde or ultraviolet (UV) light is applied to crosslink. Compared to ChIRP and CHART, the most distinctive feature of RAP is its use of long capture probes (>60 nucleotides), which form very stable RNA-DNA hybrids [7]. Such a probe design strategy robustly captures any RNA and enables the use of stringent hybridization and washing conditions that dramatically reduce nonspecific interactions of off-target nucleic acids or proteins. Long DNA probes are considerably more costly but the background signals may be reduced due to the fewer probes used compared with short probes [48]. Hacisuleyman's group applied RAP to discover the genomics sites and proteins that associated with lincRNA FIREE. And confirmed that it interacts with hnPNPU protein in an RRD-dependent manner and localizes across several trans-chromosomal binding sites (see Table 1) [58]. To developed a high-throughput method to identify proteins associated with a specific lncRNA in vivo, McHugh and colleagues combined RAP with MS to obtain high yields of RNA complex and identified ten proteins associated with lncRNA Xist, including SHARP, RBM15, MYEF2, CELF1, HNRNPC,

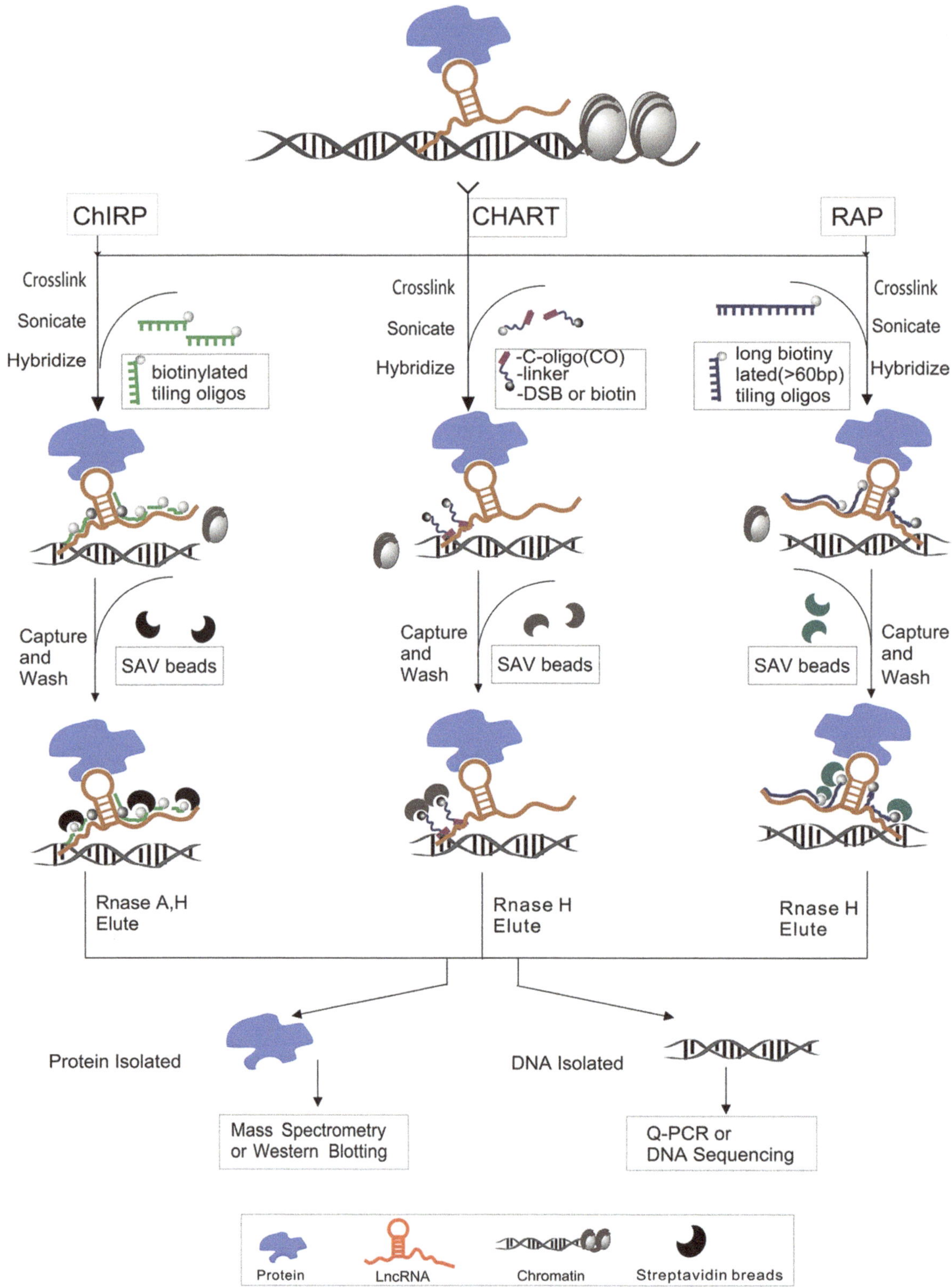

Fig. 2 Schematic representation of ChIRP, CHART and RAP to identify associated proteins and chromatin DNA. RNA–protein–DNA complexes were cross-linked in vivo and solubilized by sonication. Corresponding biotinylated oligonucleotides of three methods were designed and synthesized to be hybridized to target lncRNAs under stringent conditions. Associated proteins and chromatin DNA were efficiently pulled down with streptavidin magnetic beads. Co-purified RNA, protein and DNA were isolated with RNase elution and subjected analyzed downstream analysis. Isolated proteins were analyzed by mass spectrometry or Western blotting and chromatin DNA was used for q-PCR, deep sequencing

LBR, SAF-A, RALY, HNRNPM, and PTBP1 (see Table 1). Also, they reported that the Xist interacts directly with SHARP to silence transcription through HDAC3 and that the recruitment of PCR2 by Xist depended on SHARP and HDAC3. These data is contrasted with previous work indicating that Xist directly interacted with PCR2 across the X chromosome [63]. Thus, the RAP-MS can be useful for investigating lncRNA regulation mechanism.

Bioinformatics approach to predicting lncRNA–protein interactions

Biochemical approaches to identify the lncRNA–protein complexes are constantly expanding along with computational technologies. Compared with biochemical assays, the bioinformatics is more convenient and rapid for large-scale predictions of protein–lncRNA associations. Tartaglia's group developed the algorithm, 'fast predictions of RNA and protein interactions and domains at the Center for Genomic Regulation, Barcelona, Catalonia' (catRAPID), which evaluates interaction propensities of polypeptide and nucleotide chains using their physicochemical properties [49]. catRAPID was used to predict RNA–protein interactions in neurodegenerative disorders, in which RNA-binding proteins apparently have a major role [83]. Recently, this method was used to predict protein interactions in the Xist regulatory network [84], and data show that catRAPID is powerful for predicting RNA–protein interactions from sequences. However, prediction of lncRNAs function is generally hampered by poor sequence homology and lack of interaction data. Consequently, Lu and colleagues developed a new computational method, lncPro, to predict lncRNA–protein interactions. Compared to CatRAPID, lncPro is computational-friendly and does not lead to nonsensical cross terms. Applying lncPro to all human proteins, this laboratory reported that long non-coding RNAs tend to interact with nuclear and RNA-binding proteins [50]. However, this technique is limited for finding the direct lncRNA–protein interaction s due to the volume of proteins. Recently, to gain insights into global relationships between lncRNAs and their binding proteins, Shang and colleagues constructed an lncRNA–protein network (LPN) including 177 lncRNAs, 92 proteins and confirmed 683 relationships between them, based on experimentally determined functional interactions [85]. Therefore, bioinformatics approaches to predicting lncRNA–protein interactions may guide future experimental approaches and facilitate a deeper understanding of the role of lncRNAs.

Conclusions and perspectives

Given the multitude of non-coding transcripts discovered by second-generation deep sequencing, lncRNAs arouse interest to biological and bio-medical researchers. Recently, evidence has accumulated to support the idea that lncRNAs are critical to numerous biological processes, whereas the mechanisms by which lncRNA are poorly understood. Protein, an important partner for RNA in vivo, has been associated with molecular archetypes of lncRNA and we observed scaffolds, guides and decoys in these associations. However, some lncRNA interact with protein through more than one kind molecular mechanism. For example, HOTAIR is a scaffold for PCR2 and LSD1 as well as a guide to recruit PCR2 to target loci. Therefore molecular mechanisms behind lncRNA–protein interactions are complicated and rarely described. Study of lncRNAs interaction partners and the use of technologies to isolate and identify molecules associated with lncRNA are assisting researchers with the study of proteins and genomic DNA that directly and indirectly interplay with target lncRNAs. However, these interactions have not been studied across diverse species. As technologies improve, we may 1 day better understand evolution and functional mechanisms of lncRNAs.

Abbreviations

lncRNA: long non-coding RNA; RBP: RNA binding protein; RIP: RNA immunoprecipitation; PRC2: ploycomb repressive complex 2; HOTTIP: HOXA transcript at the distal tip; HOTAIR: HOX antisense intergenic RNA; BC1: brain cytoplasmic RNA 1; Fendrr: fetal-lethal non-coding developmental regulatory RNA; COLDAIR: cold assisted intronic non-coding RNA; TUG1: taurine upregulated gene 1; NEAT2: nuclear-enriched autosomal transcript 2; Pc2: polycomb 2 protein; PANDA: p21 associated ncRNA DNA damage activated; Gas5: growth arrest-specific 5; MALAT1: metastasis-associated lung adenocarcinoma transcript 1; CLIP: cross-linking and immunoprecipitation; ChIRP: chromatin isolation by RNA purification; CHART: capture hybridization analysis of RNA targets; RAP: RNA antisense purification; PAR-CLIP: photoactivatable-ribonucleoside-enhanced CLIP; iCLIP: individual-nucleotide resolution CLIP; HITS-CLIP: high-throughput sequencing of CLIP; MS: mass spectrometry; LPN: lncRNA–protein network.

Authors' contributions

HZ and YY planned the manuscript outline and wrote the draft. YY generated figures and tables. LW and HZ revised and edited the manuscript. All authors read and approved the final manuscript.

Acknowledgements

We thank Chen-Guang Zhou and Jing Shi for stimulating discussions and critical review of the manuscript.

Competing interests

The authors declared that they have no competing interests.

References

1. Johnson JM, Edwards S, Shoemaker D, Schadt EE. Dark matter in the genome: evidence of widespread transcription detected by microarray tiling experiments. Trends Genet. 2005;21:93–102.
2. Trapnell C, Williams BA, Pertea G, Mortazavi A, Kwan G, Van Baren MJ, Salzberg SL, Wold BJ, Pachter L. Transcript assembly and quantification by

RNA-Seq reveals unannotated transcripts and isoform switching during cell differentiation. Nat Biotechnol. 2010;28:511–5.

3. Djebali S, Davis CA, Merkel A, Dobin A, Lassmann T, Mortazavi A, Tanzer A, Lagarde J, Lin W, Schlesinger F. Landscape of transcription in human cells. Nature. 2012;489:101–8.
4. Novikova IV, Hennelly SP, Sanbonmats KY. Sizing up long non-coding RNAs: do lncRNAs have secondary and tertiary structure? Bioarchitecture. 2012;2:189–99.
5. Wilusz JE, Sunwoo H, Spector DL. Long noncoding RNAs: functional surprises from the RNA world. Gene Dev. 2009;23:1494–504.
6. Yoon J, Abdelmohsen K, Gorospe M. Functional interactions among microRNAs and long noncoding RNAs. Seminars in cell and developmental biology. Elsevier; 2014. p. 9–14.
7. Chu C, Spitale RC, Chang HY. Technologies to probe functions and mechanisms of long noncoding RNAs. Nat Struct Mol Biol. 2015;22:29–35.
8. Rinn JL, Ule J. Oming in on RNA–protein interactions. Genome Biol. 2014;15:401.
9. Buenrostro JD, Araya CL, Chircus LM, Layton CJ, Chang HY, Snyder MP, Greenleaf WJ. Quantitative analysis of RNA–protein interactions on a massively parallel array reveals biophysical and evolutionary landscapes. Nat Biotechnol. 2014;32:562–8.
10. Tome JM, Ozer A, Pagano JM, Gheba D, Schroth GP, Lis JT. Comprehensive analysis of RNA–protein interactions by high-throughput sequencing-RNA affinity profiling. Nat Methods. 2014;11:683–8.
11. Wang S, Tran E. Unexpected functions of lncRNAs in gene regulation. Commun Integr Biol. 2013; 6.
12. Zhu B, Yang Y, Li R, Fu D, Wen L, Luo Y, Zhu H. RNA sequencing and functional analysis implicate the regulatory role of long non-coding RNAs in tomato fruit ripening. J Exp Bot. 2015;66:4483–95.
13. Derrien T, Johnson R, Bussotti G, Tanzer A, Djebali S, Tilgner H, Guernec G, Martin D, Merkel A, Knowles DG. The GENCODE v7 catalog of human long noncoding RNAs: analysis of their gene structure, evolution, and expression. Genome Res. 2012;22:1775–89.
14. Zhao J, Sun BK, Erwin JA, Song J, Lee JT. Polycomb proteins targeted by a short repeat RNA to the mouse X chromosome. Science. 2008;322:750–6.
15. Ilik IA, Quinn JJ, Georgiev P, Tavares-Cadete F, Maticzka D, Toscano S, Wan Y, Spitale RC, Luscombe N, Backofen R. Tandem stem-loops in roX RNAs act together to mediate X chromosome dosage compensation in *Drosophila*. Mol Cell. 2013;51:156–73.
16. Lee JT. Epigenetic regulation by long noncoding RNAs. Science. 2012;338:1435–9.
17. Yoon J, Abdelmohsen K, Gorospe M. Posttranscriptional gene regulation by long noncoding RNA. J Mol Biol. 2013;425:3723–30.
18. Ponting CP, Oliver PL, Reik W. Evolution and functions of long noncoding RNAs. Cell. 2009;136:629–41.
19. Rinn JL, Kertesz M, Wang JK, Squazzo SL, Xu X, Brugmann SA, Goodnough LH, Helms JA, Farnham PJ, Segal E. Functional demarcation of active and silent chromatin domains in human HOX loci by noncoding RNAs. Cell. 2007;129:1311–23.
20. Terranova R, Yokobayashi S, Stadler MB, Otte AP, van Lohuizen M, Orkin SH, Peters AH. Polycomb group proteins Ezh2 and Rnf2 direct genomic contraction and imprinted repression in early mouse embryos. Dev Cell. 2008;15:668–79.
21. Pandey RR, Mondal T, Mohammad F, Enroth S, Redrup L, Komorowski J, Nagano T, Mancini-DiNardo D, Kanduri C. Kcnq1ot1 antisense noncoding RNA mediates lineage-specific transcriptional silencing through chromatin-level regulation. Mol Cell. 2008;32:232–46.
22. Wang X, Arai S, Song X, Reichart D, Du K, Pascual G, Tempst P, Rosenfeld MG, Glass CK, Kurokawa R. Induced ncRNAs allosterically modify RNA-binding proteins in cis to inhibit transcription. Nature. 2008;454:126–30.
23. Feng J, Bi C, Clark BS, Mady R, Shah P, Kohtz JD. The Evf-2 noncoding RNA is transcribed from the Dlx-5/6 ultraconserved region and functions as a Dlx-2 transcriptional coactivator. Gene Dev. 2006;20:1470–84.
24. Tripathi V, Ellis JD, Shen Z, Song DY, Pan Q, Watt AT, Freier SM, Bennett CF, Sharma A, Bubulya PA. The nuclear-retained noncoding RNA MALAT1 regulates alternative splicing by modulating SR splicing factor phosphorylation. Mol Cell. 2010;39:925–38.
25. Carrieri C, Cimatti L, Biagioli M, Beugnet A, Zucchelli S, Fedele S, Pesce E, Ferrer I, Collavin L, Santoro C. Long non-coding antisense RNA controls Uchl1 translation through an embedded SINEB2 repeat. Nature. 2012;491:454–7.
26. Lin D, Pestova TV, Hellen CU, Tiedge H. Translational control by a small RNA: dendritic BC1 RNA targets the eukaryotic initiation factor 4A helicase mechanism. Mol Cell Biol. 2008;28:3008–19.
27. Wang KC, Chang HY. Molecular mechanisms of long noncoding RNAs. Mol Cell. 2011;43:904–14.
28. Rinn JL, Chang HY. Genome regulation by long noncoding RNAs. Annu Rev Biochem. 2012;81:145–66.
29. Grote P, Wittler L, Hendrix D, Koch F, Währisch S, Beisaw A, Macura K, Bläss G, Kellis M, Werber M. The tissue-specific lncRNA Fendrr is an essential regulator of heart and body wall development in the mouse. Dev Cell. 2013;24:206–14.
30. Heo JB, Sung S. Vernalization-mediated epigenetic silencing by a long intronic noncoding RNA. Science. 2011;331:76–9.
31. Huarte M, Guttman M, Feldser D, Garber M, Koziol MJ, Kenzelmann-Broz D, Khalil AM, Zuk O, Amit I, Rabani M. A large intergenic noncoding RNA induced by p53 mediates global gene repression in the p53 response. Cell. 2010;142:409–19.
32. Venter JC, Adams MD, Myers EW, Li PW, Mural RJ, Sutton GG, Smith HO, Yandell M, Evans CA, Holt RA. The sequence of the human genome. Science. 2001;291:1304–51.
33. Zappulla DC, Cech TR. RNA as a flexible scaffold for proteins: yeast telomerase and beyond. Cold Spring Harbor symposia on quantitative biology. Cold Spring Harbor Laboratory Press; 2006. p. 217–24.
34. Cech TR. Life at the end of the chromosome: telomeres and telomerase. Angew Chem Int Ed. 2000;39:34–43.
35. Bilaud T, Brun C, Ancelin K, Koering CE, Laroche T, Gilson E. Telomeric localization of TRF2, a novel human telobox protein. Nat Genet. 1997;17:236–9.
36. Jeon Y, Lee JT. YY1 tethers Xist RNA to the inactive X nucleation center. Cell. 2011;146:119–33.
37. Tsai M, Manor O, Wan Y, Mosammaparast N, Wang JK, Lan F, Shi Y, Segal E, Chang HY. Long noncoding RNA as modular scaffold of histone modification complexes. Science. 2010;329:689–93.
38. Wang H, Wang L, Erdjument-Bromage H, Vidal M, Tempst P, Jones RS, Zhang Y. Role of histone H2A ubiquitination in Polycomb silencing. Nature. 2004;431:873–8.
39. Maenner S, Müller M, Fröhlich J, Langer D, Becker PB. ATP-dependent roX RNA remodeling by the helicase maleless enables specific association of MSL proteins. Mol Cell. 2013;51:174–84.
40. Yang L, Lin C, Liu W, Zhang J, Ohgi KA, Grinstein JD, Dorrestein PC, Rosenfeld MG. ncRNA-and Pc2 methylation-dependent gene relocation between nuclear structures mediates gene activation programs. Cell. 2011;147:773–88.
41. Hung T, Wang Y, Lin MF, Koegel AK, Kotake Y, Grant GD, Horlings HM, Shah N, Umbricht C, Wang P. Extensive and coordinated transcription of noncoding RNAs within cell-cycle promoters. Nat Genet. 2011;43:621–9.
42. Kino T, Hurt DE, Ichijo T, Nader N, Chrousos GP. Noncoding RNA Gas5 is a growth arrest and starvation-associated repressor of the glucocorticoid receptor. Sci Signal. 2010;3:a8.
43. Gong C, Popp MW, Maquat LE. Biochemical analysis of long non-coding RNA-containing ribonucleoprotein complexes. Methods. 2012;58:88–93.
44. Darnell R. CLIP (cross-linking and immunoprecipitation) identification of RNAs bound by a specific protein. Cold Spring Harb Protoc. 2012;2012:t72132.
45. Feng Y, Hu X, Zhang Y, Zhang D, Li C, Zhang L. Methods for the Study of Long Noncoding RNA in Cancer Cell Signaling. Cancer Cell Signaling. Springer; 2014. p. 115–43.
46. Chu C, Quinn J.Chang HY. Chromatin isolation by RNA purification (ChIRP). J Vis Exp. 2012;61. doi:10.3791/3912.
47. Chu C, Qu K, Zhong FL, Artandi SE, Chang HY. Genomic maps of long noncoding RNA occupancy reveal principles of RNA–chromatin interactions. Mol Cell. 2011;44:667–78.
48. Engreitz J, Lander ES, Guttman M. RNA antisense purification (RAP) for mapping rna interactions with chromatin. Nuclear bodies and noncoding RNAs. Springer; 2015. p. 183–97.
49. Bellucci M, Agostini F, Masin M, Tartaglia GG. Predicting protein associations with long noncoding RNAs. Nat Methods. 2011;8:444–5.
50. Lu Q, Ren S, Lu M, Zhang Y, Zhu D, Zhang X, Li T. Computational prediction of associations between long non-coding RNAs and proteins. BMC Genom. 2013;14:651.

51. Selth LA, Close P, Svejstrup JQ. Studying RNA–protein interactions in vivo by RNA immunoprecipitation. Epigenetics protocols. Springer; 2011. p. 253–64.
52. Niranjanakumari S, Lasda E, Brazas R, Garcia-Blanco MA. Reversible cross-linking combined with immunoprecipitation to study RNA–protein interactions in vivo. Methods. 2002;26:182–90.
53. Khalil AM, Guttman M, Huarte M, Garber M, Raj A, Morales DR, Thomas K, Presser A, Bernstein BE, van Oudenaarden A. Many human large intergenic noncoding RNAs associate with chromatin-modifying complexes and affect gene expression. Proc Natl Acad Sci. 2009;106:11667–72.
54. Keene JD, Komisarow JM, Friedersdorf MB. RIP-Chip: the isolation and identification of mRNAs, microRNAs and protein components of ribonucleoprotein complexes from cell extracts. Nat Protoc Electron Ed. 2006;1:302.
55. Cloonan N, Forrest AR, Kolle G, Gardiner BB, Faulkner GJ, Brown MK, Taylor DF, Steptoe AL, Wani S, Bethel G. Stem cell transcriptome profiling via massive-scale mRNA sequencing. Nat Methods. 2008;5:613–9.
56. Zhao J, Ohsumi TK, Kung JT, Ogawa Y, Grau DJ, Sarma K, Song JJ, Kingston RE, Borowsky M, Lee JT. Genome-wide identification of polycomb-associated RNAs by RIP-seq. Mol Cell. 2010;40:939–53.
57. Nagano T, Mitchell JA, Sanz LA, Pauler FM, Ferguson-Smith AC, Feil R, Fraser P. The Air noncoding RNA epigenetically silences transcription by targeting G9a to chromatin. Science. 2008;322:1717–20.
58. Hacisuleyman E, Goff LA, Trapnell C, Williams A, Henao-Mejia J, Sun L, McClanahan P, Hendrickson DG, Sauvageau M, Kelley DR. Topological organization of multichromosomal regions by the long intergenic noncoding RNA Firre. Nat Struct Mol Biol. 2014;21:198–206.
59. Wang KC, Yang YW, Liu B, Sanyal A, Corces-Zimmerman R, Chen Y, Lajoie BR, Protacio A, Flynn RA, Gupta RA. A long noncoding RNA maintains active chromatin to coordinate homeotic gene expression. Nature. 2011;472:120–4.
60. West JA, Davis CP, Sunwoo H, Simon MD, Sadreyev RI, Wang PI, Tolstorukov MY, Kingston RE. The long noncoding RNAs Neat1 and Malat1 bind active chromatin sites. Mol Cell. 2014;55:791–802.
61. Quinn JJ, Chang HY. In situ dissection of RNA functional subunits by domain-specific chromatin isolation by RNA purification (dChIRP). Nuclear bodies and noncoding RNAs. Springer; 2015. p. 199–213.
62. Chu C, Zhang QC, Da Rocha ST, Flynn RA, Bharadwaj M, Calabrese JM, Magnuson T, Heard E, Chang HY. Systematic discovery of Xist RNA binding proteins. Cell. 2015;161:404–16.
63. McHugh CA, Chen C, Chow A, Surka CF, Tran C. The Xist lncRNA interacts directly with SHARP to silence transcription through HDAC3. Nature. 2015;521:232–6.
64. Ule J, Jensen K, Mele A, Darnell RB. CLIP: a method for identifying protein–RNA interaction sites in living cells. Methods. 2005;37:376–86.
65. Licatalosi DD, Mele A, Fak JJ, Ule J, Kayikci M, Chi SW, Clark TA, Schweitzer AC, Blume JE, Wang X. HITS-CLIP yields genome-wide insights into brain alternative RNA processing. Nature. 2008;456:464–9.
66. Chi SW, Zang JB, Mele A, Darnell RB. Argonaute HITS-CLIP decodes microRNA–mRNA interaction maps. Nature. 2009;460:479–86.
67. Lagier-Tourenne C, Polymenidou M, Hutt KR, Vu AQ, Baughn M, Huelga SC, Clutario KM, Ling S, Liang TY, Mazur C. Divergent roles of ALS-linked proteins FUS/TLS and TDP-43 intersect in processing long pre-mRNAs. Nat Neurosci. 2012;15:1488–97.
68. Li Q, Uemura Y, Kawahara Y. Cross-linking and immunoprecipitation of nuclear RNA-binding proteins. nuclear bodies and noncoding RNAs. Springer; 2015. p. 247–63.
69. Hafner M, Landthaler M, Burger L, Khorshid M, Hausser J, Berninger P, Rothballer A, Ascano M, Jungkamp A, Munschauer M. Transcriptome-wide identification of RNA-binding protein and microRNA target sites by PAR-CLIP. Cell. 2010;141:129–41.
70. König J, Zarnack K, Rot G, Curk T, Kayikci M, Zupan B, Turner DJ, Luscombe NM, Ule J. iCLIP reveals the function of hnRNP particles in splicing at individual nucleotide resolution. Nat Struct Mol Biol. 2010;17:909–15.
71. Hafner M, Landthaler M, Burger L, Khorshid M, Hausser J, Berninger P, Rothballer A, Ascano M, Jungkamp A, Munschauer M. PAR-CliP-a method to identify transcriptome-wide the binding sites of RNA binding proteins. J Vis Exp. 2010;41. doi:10.3791/2034.
72. Ascano M, Mukherjee N, Bandaru P, Miller JB, Nusbaum JD, Corcoran DL, Langlois C, Munschauer M, Dewell S, Hafner M. FMRP targets distinct mRNA sequence elements to regulate protein expression. Nature. 2012;492:382–6.
73. Lebedeva S, Jens M, Theil K, Schwanhäusser B, Selbach M, Landthaler M, Rajewsky N. Transcriptome-wide analysis of regulatory interactions of the RNA-binding protein HuR. Mol Cell. 2011;43:340–52.
74. Yokoshi M, Li Q, Yamamoto M, Okada H, Suzuki Y, Kawahara Y. Direct binding of Ataxin-2 to distinct elements in 3′ UTRs promotes mRNA stability and protein expression. Mol Cell. 2014;55:186–98.
75. Rossbach O, Hung L, Khrameeva E, Schreiner S, König J, Curk T, Zupan B, Ule J, Gelfand MS, Bindereif A. Crosslinking-immunoprecipitation (iCLIP) analysis reveals global regulatory roles of hnRNP L. RNA Biol. 2014;11:146–55.
76. Lau E. Non-coding RNA: zooming in on lncRNA functions. Nat Rev Genet. 2014;15:574–5.
77. Quinn JJ, Ilik IA, Qu K, Georgiev P, Chu C, Akhtar A, Chang HY. Revealing long noncoding RNA architecture and functions using domain-specific chromatin isolation by RNA purification. Nat Biotechnol. 2014;32:933–40.
78. Baltz AG, Munschauer M, Schwanhäusser B, Vasile A, Murakawa Y, Schueler M, Youngs N, Penfold-Brown D, Drew K, Milek M. The mRNA-bound proteome and its global occupancy profile on protein-coding transcripts. Mol Cell. 2012;46:674–90.
79. Castello A, Fischer B, Eichelbaum K, Horos R, Beckmann BM, Strein C, Davey NE, Humphreys DT, Preiss T, Steinmetz LM. Insights into RNA biology from an atlas of mammalian mRNA-binding proteins. Cell. 2012;149:1393–406.
80. Klass DM, Scheibe M, Butter F, Hogan GJ, Mann M, Brown PO. Quantitative proteomic analysis reveals concurrent RNA–protein interactions and identifies new RNA-binding proteins in *Saccharomyces cerevisiae*. Genome Res. 2013;23:1028–38.
81. Kramer K, Sachsenberg T, Beckmann BM, Qamar S, Boon K, Hentze MW, Kohlbacher O, Urlaub H. Photo-cross-linking and high-resolution mass spectrometry for assignment of RNA-binding sites in RNA-binding proteins. Nat Methods. 2014;11:1064–70.
82. Simon MD, Wang CI, Kharchenko PV, West JA, Chapman BA, Alekseyenko AA, Borowsky ML, Kuroda MI, Kingston RE. The genomic binding sites of a noncoding RNA. Proc Natl Acad Sci. 2011;108:20497–502.
83. Cirillo D, Agostini F, Klus P, Marchese D, Rodriguez S, Bolognesi B, Tartaglia GG. Neurodegenerative diseases: quantitative predictions of protein–RNA interactions. RNA. 2013;19:129–40.
84. Agostini F, Cirillo D, Bolognesi B, Tartaglia GG. X-inactivation: quantitative predictions of protein interactions in the Xist network. Nucleic Acids Res. 2013;41:e31.
85. Shang D, Yang H, Xu Y, Yao Q, Zhou W, Shi X, Han J, Su F, Su B, Zhang C. A global view of network of lncRNAs and their binding proteins. Mol Biosyst. 2015;11:656–63.

19

Exogenous hydrogen sulfide restores cardioprotection of ischemic post-conditioning via inhibition of mPTP opening in the aging cardiomyocytes

Hongzhu Li[1,3*], Chao Zhang[2], Weiming Sun[1], Lina Li[1], Bo Wu[1], Shuzhi Bai[1], Hongxia Li[1], Xin Zhong[1,3], Rui Wang[4], Lingyun Wu[5] and Changqing Xu[1,3*]

Abstract

The physiological and pathological roles of hydrogen sulfide (H_2S) in the regulation of cardiovascular functions have been recognized. H_2S protects against the hypoxia/reoxygenation (H/R)-induced injury and apoptosis of cardiomyocytes, and ischemic post-conditioning (PC) plays an important role in cardioprotection from H/R injury in neonatal cardiomyocytes but not in aging cardiomyocytes. Whether H_2S is involved in the recovery of PC-induced cardioprotection in aging cardiomyocytes is unclear. In the present study, we found that both H/R and PC decreased cystathionine-γ-lyase (CSE) expression and the production rate of H_2S. Supplementation of NaHS protected against H/R-induced apoptosis, the expression of cleaved caspase-3 and cleaved caspase-9, the release of cytochrome *c* (Cyt *c*), and mPTP opening. The addition of NaHS also counteracted the reduction of cell viability caused by H/R and increased the phosphorylation of ERK1/2, PI3K, Akt, GSK-3β and mitochondrial membrane potential. Additionally, NaHS increased Bcl-2 expression, promoted PKC-ε translocation to the cell membrane, and activated mitochondrial ATP-sensitive K channels ($mitoK_{ATP}$). PC alone did not provide cardioprotection in H/R-treated aging cardiomyocytes, which was significantly restored by the supplementation of NaHS. In conclusion, our results suggest that exogenous H_2S restores PC-induced cardioprotection via the inhibition of mPTP opening by the activation of the ERK1/2-GSK-3β, PI3K-Akt-GSK-3β and PKC-ε-$mitoK_{ATP}$ pathways in aging cardiomyocytes. These findings provide a novel target for the treatment of aging ischemic cardiomyopathy.

Keywords: Hydrogen sulfide, Post-conditioning, Mitochondrial permeability transition pore, Aging cardiomyocytes

Background

Myocardial ischemia (hypoxia)/reperfusion (reoxygenation) causes cardiomyocyte injury, including cardiomyocyte apoptosis and necrosis. Free radical generation, calcium overload and the adhesion of leukocytes are the main mechanisms of ischemia/reperfusion (I/R) injury. In 1986, Murry et al. first reported that ischemic preconditioning (IPC) plays an important cardioprotective role against ischemia-induced injuries [1, 2]. However, IPC must be applied before the ischemic event, which is unpredictable, and is impractical in the clinical setting of acute myocardial infarction [3]. According to a similar regimen of brief periods of ischemia applied just after, instead of just before, sustained ischemia was shown to be as protective as preconditioning. In 2003, Zhao et al. [4] first proposed the concept of ischemic post-conditioning (PC). PC is defined as repetitive cycles of briefly interrupted reperfusion applied at the onset of establishing reflow and has been shown to significantly improve outcome following an episode of ischemia [4]. The main theories of PC-induced protection are the preservation of mitochondrial integrity via regulation of

*Correspondence: hongzhuli61@163.com; xucq45@126.com
[1] Department of Pathophysiology, Harbin Medical University, Baojian Road, Harbin 150081, China
Full list of author information is available at the end of the article

the mitochondrial permeability transition pore (mPTP) [2]. Inhibition of mPTP opening is considered to be the final step in a complex series of cellular signalling events preventing cell death [2]. It is thought that PC activates a signal transduction pathway involving the pro-survival kinases phosphatidylinositol-3-OH kinase (P13K) and protein kinase B (Akt) and the p42/p44 extracellular signal-regulated kinases (ERK1/2), and it has been termed the reperfusion injury salvage kinase (RISK) pathway [5–9]. Meanwhile, PC also activates protein kinase C (PKC)-mitochondrial ATP-sensitive potassium ($mitoK_{ATP}$) channels (PKC-$mitoK_{ATP}$ pathway) [5, 9–11]. The RISK and PKC-$mitoK_{ATP}$ pathways terminate with the inhibition of mPTP opening at reperfusion, thus affording cardioprotection in PC [2, 12].

The degeneration, decrease of autophagic capacity and mitochondrial function (mtDNA mutation), increase of oxidative stress and reduced production of endogenous protective substances in ageing cardiomyocytes, leads to a weakening or disappearance of sensitivity of aging cardiomyocytes to PC [13, 14]. Aging hearts are also resistant to the powerful endogenous protections provided by PC. In other words, PC loses its myocardial protective effect in aging hearts [15].

Hydrogen sulfide (H_2S) is a highly diffusible gasotransmitter that influences cellular and organ functions through a number of different mechanisms [16]. Endogenous production of H_2S is mainly catalysed by cystathionine β-synthase (CBS), cystathionine-γ-lyase (CSE) and 3-mercaptosulphurtransferase (3-MPST) [17]. CBS and CSE have been consistently shown to produce H_2S in mammalian tissues, with L-cysteine and/or homocysteine as the main substrate [18, 19]. Recently, 3-MPST, which uses both L-cysteine and alpha ketoglutarate as substrates along with cysteine aminotransferase to produce H_2S, was identified [20]. Among them, CSE is the major H_2S-producing enzyme in vascular tissues. The abnormal metabolism and functions of the CSE/H_2S pathway have been linked to various cardiovascular diseases, including I/R injury, atherosclerosis, hypertension, and oxidative stress [21–26].

It was previously reported that H_2S is involved in PC-induced cardioprotection [21–26]. Our previous study indicated that exogenous H_2S recovered cardioprotection from PC in isolated aging rat hearts [27]. However, whether H_2S plays a key role in the recovery of PC-induced cardioprotection in aging cardiomyocytes is unknown. This study investigated the effect of exogenous H_2S on the recovery of PC-induced cardioprotection and its possible mechanisms, including the ERK1/2-GSK-3β, PI3K-Akt-GSK-3β and PKC-ε-$mitoK_{ATP}$ pathways and mPTP opening, in aging cardiomyocytes.

Methods

Drugs and reagents

Sodium hydrogen sulfide (NaHS), the anti-CSE antibody, PD98059 (an inhibitor of ERK), LY294002 (a PI3K inhibitor), 5-hydroxydecanoate (5-HD, a mK_{ATP} inhibitor), Chelerythrine chloride (Che, a PKC inhibitor) were purchased from Sigma Chemical Co. (St. Louis, MO, USA). The primary antibodies for anti-PKC-ε, anti-cleaved caspase-3 and -9, Bcl-2, cytochrome *c* (Cyt *c*), Na^+/K^+-ATPase, cyclin D1, $p21^{Cip/WAF-1}$ and GAPDH were from Santa Cruz (Bergheimer, Germany). Hoechst 33342, JC-1 kit and Calcein-AM were also from Santa Cruz. The anti-ERK1/2 and PI3K-Akt-GSK-3β antibodies were obtained from Cell Signaling Technology (Danvers, USA). Senescence *β*-galactosidase (*β*-gal) staining kit was purchased from Beyotime Institute of Biotechnology (Shanghai, China). Rat advanced glycation end products (AGEs) ELISA kit was purchased from Proteintech Group (Wuhan, China). All other chemicals were from Sigma or Santa Cruz.

Primary culture of cardiomyocytes

Primary cultures of neonatal cardiomyocytes were prepared as previously described [8, 27]. Newborn Wistar rats, aged 1–3 days and weighing 5–8 g, were used for this study. All animal experiments were conducted in compliance with the Guide for the Care and Use of Laboratory Animals published by the China National Institutes of Health and approved by the Animal Care Committees of Harbin Medical University, China. Briefly, cells were dissociated from minced hearts of 1- to 3-day neonatal Wistar rats with a 0.25% solution of crude trypsin. Cells were cultured as monolayers at a density of 5×10^4 cells/cm^2 in Dulbecco's modified Eagle medium (DMEM) equilibrated with humidified air containing 5% CO_2 at 37°C. The medium contained 10% calf serum and 2 μM fluorodeoxyuridine, the latter to prevent proliferation of non-myocytes.

Aging of myocardial cells induced by D-galactose

The treatment for D-galactose induction was as previously described [28, 29]. Once the attached cardiomyocytes were beating spontaneously, the DMEM supplemented with 20% fetal calf serum was removed, and DMEM supplemented with different concentrations (0, 0.1, 1, 10, 100 g/L) D-galactose was added to the cardiomyocytes in the culture cluster for a further different incubation period (0, 12, 24, 48, 72 h). The degree of cell aging was observed through SA *β*-Gal Staining and AGEs ELISA Assay. In the present study, we selected 10 g/L D-galactose concentrations for 48 h incubation period.

Established aging cardiomyocytes model of hypoxia/reoxygenation

A hypoxic condition was produced by D-Hank solution (in mM: 5.37 KCl, 0.44 KH_2PO_4, 136.89 NaCl, 4.166 $NaHCO_3$, 0.338 Na_2HPO_4, 5 D-glucose, pH 7.3–7.4 at 37°C) saturated with 95% N_2 and 5% CO_2. The pH was regulated to 6.8 with lactate to mimic ischemic solution. The aging cardiomyocytes were put into a hypoxic incubator that was equilibrated with 1% O_2/5% CO_2/94% N_2. After hypoxia, the culture medium was rapidly replaced with fresh DMEM with 10% fetal bovine serum (normoxic culture solution) for initiating reoxygenation [9].

Experimental protocols

The aging cardiomyocytes were randomly divided into the following seven groups. Each group included eight samples (n = 8) (Fig. 1): (1) control group (Control): the aging cardiomyocytes were cultured for 9 h with 10% fetal bovine serum-DMEM; (2) hypoxia/reoxygenation group (H/R): the aging cardiomyocytes were exposed to hypoxic culture medium for 3 h and reoxygenated for 6 h by replacing the hypoxic culture medium with fresh DMEM with 10% fetal bovine serum; (3) H/R + H_2S group: the procedure was similar to that for group 2, except that 100 μM NaHS were added in 6 h reoxygenation; (4) PC group: at the end of 3 h of hypoxia, the aging cardiomyocytes were exposed to normoxic culture solution for 5 min, after which cells were placed in hypoxic solution for 5 min. The PC cycle was repeated three times and followed by 6 h of reoxygenation; (5) PC + H_2S group: at the end of 3 h of hypoxia, initiated immediately at the onset of reoxygenation, 100 μM NaHS were given at the onset of reoxygenation for 5 min following with 5 min hypoxia. This protocol was repeated for another two times. The cells were then treated as those of group 3; (6) PC + PD98059 (or LY294002, or 5-HD, or Che) group: 10 μM PD98059 (or 10 μM LY294002 or 100 μM 5-HD or 100 μM Che) were added to the medium 40 min before the end of hypoxia. The cells were then treated as those of group 4; (7) PC + PD98059 (or LY294002, or 5-HD, or Che) + H_2S group: 10 μM PD98059 (or 10 μM LY294002 or 100 μM 5-HD or 100 μM Che) were added to the medium 40 min before the end of hypoxia. The cells were then treated as those of group 5.

The normal cultured cardiomyocytes (without D-galactose-treated cardiomyocytes) were randomly divided into three groups. Each group included eight samples (n = 8): Control group; H/R group; PC group. The cells were treated as those of group 1, 2 and 4, respectively.

AGEs ELISA Assay

The rat advanced glycation end products (AGEs) assay was performed with AGEs ELISA kit according to the instructions from the manufacturer and was as previously described [29, 30]. The reagents of the test kit were placed at room temperature for 30 min and diluted 1:20 with distilled water. Aliquots of 100 μL of the standards and samples were added to blank micropores and 50 μL enzyme marker solution was added. Microtiter plates were incubated at 37°C for 60 min and then washed five times and put aside for 10–20 s each time. The A and B substrate solutions (50 μL) were added into the microtiter plates for 15 min dark reactions at 37°C. The reaction was terminated by the addition of 50 μL stop solution, and the optical density (OD) at 450 nm was determined by an ultra microplate reader (Bio-Rad Laboratories, Hercules, CA, USA). An AGEs standard curve was generated and the AGEs values of the samples were calculated from the standard curve.

SA β-Gal staining

Senescence-associated β-gal (SA β-gal) activity was measured with the β-gal staining kit at pH 6.0 according to the instructions from the manufacturer [29, 30]. Briefly, the cells were washed in phosphate buffered saline (PBS), fixed for 10–15 min at room temperature with 1 mL of fixative solution and incubated overnight at 37°C with the staining solution mix. Cells were observed for development of the blue coloration with a microscope at a magnification of 400×. Aging cardiomyocytes were assessed by counting the number of cells that displayed blue coloration.

Observation of cell division index

Briefly, the cells were washed in phosphate buffered saline (PBS) for three times, fixed for 30 min at room temperature with methanol:ice acetic acid (3:1) and incubated for 10 min with Giemsa. Cells were observed with a microscope at a magnification of 400×. Five fields (at least 100 cells of each field) were randomly selected and the percentage of cell division was calculated.

Detection of cell viability

Cell viability was determined by the 3-(4,5-dimethylthiazol-2-yl)-2,5-diphenyltetrazolium bromide (MTT) assay, as described previously [9, 25, 31]. Cells were cultured in 96-well plates. MTT (final concentration, 0.5 mg/mL) was added to each well under sterile conditions, and the plates were incubated for 4 h at 37°C. The supernatant was removed, and dimethyl sulfoxide (150 μl/well) was added. The plates were then agitated on a plate shaker. The absorbance of each well was measured at 490 nm with a Bio-Rad automated EIA analyser (Bio-Rad Laboratories, Hercules, CA, USA). The viability of control cells was considered 100%, and the others were expressed as percentages of control.

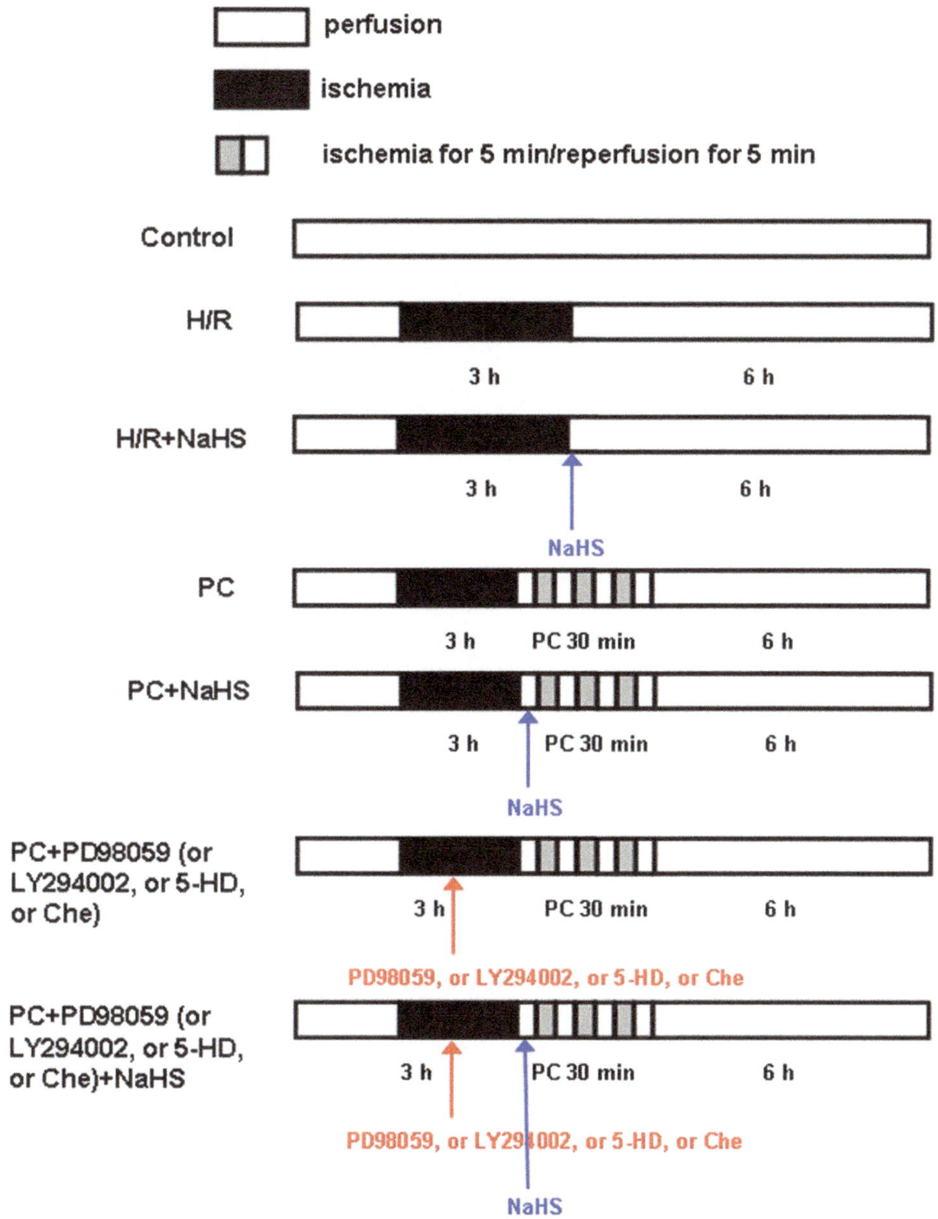

Fig. 1 Summary of experimental treatments protocol. The aging cardiomyocytes were exposed to hypoxic culture medium for 3 h and reoxygenated for 6 h by replacing the hypoxic culture medium with fresh DMEM with 10% fetal bovine serum. For details of ischemic postconditioning, NaHS, PD98059, LY294002, 5-HD and Che treatments *see text*.

Determination of H_2S production

H_2S production rate was measured as described previously [25]. In brief, after different treatments, the H9C2 cells (cardiomyocytes line) were collected and homogenized in 50 mM ice-cold potassium phosphate buffer (pH 6.8). The flasks containing the reaction mixture (100 mM potassium phosphate buffer, 10 mM L-cysteine, 2 mM pyridoxal 5-phosphate, and 10% cell homogenates) and center wells containing 0.5 mL 1% zinc acetate and a piece of filter paper (2 × 2.5 cm) were flushed with N_2 gas and incubated at 37°C for 90 min. The reaction was stopped by adding 0.5 mL of 50% trichloroacetic acid, and the flasks were incubated at 37°C for another 60 min. The contents of the center wells were transferred to test tubes, each containing 3.5 mL of water. Then 0.5 mL of 20 mM N, *N*-dimethyl-*p*-phenylenediamine sulfate in 7.2 M HCl and 0.5 mL 30 mM $FeCl_3$ in 1.2 M HCl was added. The absorbance of the resulting solution at 670 nm was measured 20 min later with a FLUOstar OPTIMA microplate spectrophotometer.

Apoptotic rate of cells by flow cytometry assay

The apoptotic rate was measured by flow cytometry as described previously [9, 28, 31]. Cells were washed three times with ice-cold PBS, and then stained with annexin V-fluorescein isothiocyanate for 15 min at room temperature in 200 μl binding buffer. Next, 300 μl binding buffer was added, and the cells were stained with propidium iodide for 30 min at 4°C. The fluorescence of the cells was analyzed by flow cytometry. The percentage of apoptotic cells was determined using Mod Fit LT software (Verity Software House Inc., Topsham, ME, USA).

Hoechst 33342 staining

Cells were analyzed for apoptosis after visualization of nuclei morphology with fluorescent DNA-binding dye Hoechst 33342, as described previously [9]. After treatment, cells were rinsed with PBS and incubated with 5 μg/mL Hoechst 33342 for 10 min. Nuclei were visualized at 400× magnification using fluorescent microscopy (Nikon Corporation, Tokyo, Japan) at an excitation wavelength of 330–380 nm. Apoptotic nuclei of cells were assessed by counting the number of cells that displayed nuclear morphology changes, such as chromatin condensation and fragmentation.

Real-time PCR analysis

Total RNA was isolated using an RNeasy Mini Kit (Qiagen, Germantown, MD, USA) and converted to cDNA with an iScriptTM cDNA Synthesis Kit (Bio-Rad, Hercules, CA, USA). Real-time PCR was performed in an iCycler iQ5 apparatus (Bio-Rad) associated with the iCycler optical system software (version 3.1) using SYBR Green PCR Master Mix. The primers of Bcl-2 were 5′-GGCATCTTCTCCT TCCAG-3′ (forward) and 5′-CATCCCAGCCTCCGT TAT-3′ (reverse). Caspase-3 primers were 5′-CAGACA-GTGGAACTGACGATGA-3′ (forward) and 5′-AACAGAA ACATGCCCCTACCCC-3′ (reverse). Caspase-9 primers were 5′-CCCGTGAAGCAAGGATTT-3′ (forward) and 5′-ACTGTGGGTCTGGGAAGC-3′ (reverse). P-ERK1/2 primers were 5′-ATCCCCCATGGAACGACCTG-3′ (forward) and 5′-ACCCGCCAGGGACAAAAATG-3′ (reverse). The primers of p-PI3K were 5′-CCCTTCTG AACTGGCTTAAAGA-3′ (forward) and 5′-GGACAGTG TAAATTCCTCAATGG-3′ (reverse). The primers for p-Akt were 5′-TGTGACCATGAACGAGTTTGA-3′ (forward) and 5′-GTCGTGGGTCTGGAATGA-3′ (reverse). P-GSK-3β primers were 5′-CGGGACCCAAATGTCA AACA-3′ (forward) and 5′-CGTGACCAGTGTTGCTG AGT-3′ (reverse). The primers of PKC-ε were 5′-CATGGA AGGATAAGCGTTGGT-3′ (forward) and 5′-CCCA AGTCCCGTGTTAAGA-3′ (reverse). The primers for GAPDH were 5′-CTCAACTACATGGTCTACATG-3′ (forward) and 5′-TGGCATGGACTGTGGTCATGAG-3′ (reverse). The cycling conditions were: one cycle of 94°C for 2 min; 30 cycles of 94°C for 30 s, 60°C for 40 s and 72°C for 1 min; and 72°C for 4 min. Relative mRNA quantification was calculated by using the arithmetic formula "2−ΔΔCT", where ΔCT is the difference between the threshold cycle of a given target cDNA and an endogenous reference GAPDH cDNA.

Detection of Cyt *c* release from mitochondrial

Western blot analysis of Cyt *c* in the cytosolic fraction was performed as described previously [9, 25, 28, 31]. Briefly, cells were harvested, washed twice with ice-cold PBS, and incubated in ice-cold Tris-sucrose buffer (0.35 mM sucrose, 10 mM Tris–HCl at pH 7.5, 1 mM EDTA, 0.5 mM dithiothreitol, 0.1 mM phenylmethylsulphonyl fluoride). After a 40 min incubation, cells were centrifuged at 1,000×*g* for 5 min at 4°C and the supernatant was further centrifuged at 40,000×*g* for 30 min at 4°C. The supernatant was retained as the cytosolic fraction and analyzed by Western blot with a primary rat anti-Cyt *c* monoclonal antibody and a secondary goat anti-rat immunoglobulin G (Promage). GAPDH expression was used as the control.

Translocation of PKC-ε

Cardiomyocytes were lysed immediately after different treatment by resuspending in lysis buffer [50 mM Tris–HCl, pH 8.0, 150 mM NaCl, 5 mM EDTA, 1% Triton X-100, 0.26% sodium deoxycholate, 50 mM sodium fluoride, 10 mM β-glycerophosphate, 0.1 mM sodium orthovanadate, 10 μg/mL leupeptin, and 1 mM phenylmethylsulfonyl fluoride (PMSF)] and incubating on ice for 20 min. Cell debris and insoluble material were cleared by centrifugation at 10,000×*g* for 10 min. The supernatant is called the detergent-solubilized cell lysate. For the preparation of membrane-enriched fractions and subcellular fractions, cells were resuspended in 25 mM Tris–HCl, pH 7.5, 250 mM sucrose, 5 mM $MgCl_2$, 100 mM KCl, 10 μg/mL each of aprotinin and leupeptin, and 1 mM PMSF. Cells were disrupted by Dounce homogenization and fractionated by differential velocity centrifugation as previously described [7, 9]. Cell membrane fractions were analyzed by Western blotting with primary rabbit polyclonal isoform specific anti-PKC-ε and secondary goat anti-rat IgG. Na^+/K^+-ATPase was used a membrane fractions loading control. The volume of protein bands was quantified using a Bio-Rad Chemi DocTM EQ densitometer and Bio-Rad Quantity One software (Bio-Rad Laboratories, Hercules, USA).

Measurement of mitochondrial membrane potential ($\Delta\psi m$)

Changes in mitochondrial transmembrane potential ($\Delta\psi m$) were measured with the dye 5,5′,6,6′-tetrachloro-1,1′,3,3′-tetraethylbenzimidazolcarbocyanine iodide (JC-1). Mitochondrial membrane potential was determined as previously described [9]. Briefly, neonatal rat cardiomyocytes (2.5×10^5 cells/60 mm^2 dishes) were seeded, incubated, and treated for 48 h at 37°C. After experimentation, cells were stained with JC-1 (2 μg/mL, Invitrogen) at 37°C in the dark for 15 min and rinsed three times with cold PBS. Observations were made using a Zeiss LSM 510 inverted confocal scanning microscope. JC-1 monomer (green) fluorescence was observed by excitation with 514 nm and examination of emission at 529 nm. JC-1 aggregate (red) fluorescence was observed by examination of emission at 585/590 nm. At least 100 areas were selected from each image, and the average intensity for each region was quantified. The ratio of JC-1 aggregate to monomer (red/green) intensity for each region was calculated. A decrease in this ratio was interpreted as decrease of $\Delta\psi m$, whereas an increase in this ratio was interpreted as gain in $\Delta\psi m$.

Assay of mitochondrial permeability transition pore (mPTP) opening

Changes of mitochondrial permeability transition pore (mPTP) opening were measured with coincubation of calcein-AM and cobalt chloride as previously described [9, 32]. Cardiomyocytes were plated in 24-well plates (0.5×10^6 cells/well). After different the treatments, the cells were loaded with calcein-AM 2 μM in presence of 5 mM of cobalt chloride in the dark for for 15 min at 37°C. Fluorescence was measured in a Zeiss LSM 510 inverted confocal scanning microscope at 488 nm excitation and 505 nm emission. Fluorescence intensity of individual cells was measured using SigmaScan Pro 5 software. The fluorescence intensity in control group was considered 100% viable.

Western blotting analysis

Cells were homogenized in ice-cold lysis buffer containing 50 mM Tris–HCl (pH, 8.0), 150 Mm NaCl, 5 mM EDTA, 1% Triton X-100, 0.26% sodium deoxycholate, 50 mM sodium fluoride, 10 mM β-glycerophosphate, 0.1 mM sodium orthovanadate, 10 μg/mL leupeptin, and 50 μg/mL phenylmethylsulfonyl fluoride (PMSF), and incubated on ice for 40 min. The homogenate was centrifuged at 15,000×g for 15 min at 4°C to remove cellular debris and isolate total protein. Protein concentrations were determined using a Bradford assay kit (Bio-Rad Laboratories; Hercules, USA). Equal amounts of proteins were boiled and separated with SDS-PAGE and electrophoretically transferred to a nitrocellulose membrane, as described previously [9, 25]. In each lane of a 10% sodium dodecyl sulfate–polyacrylamide gel electrophoresis, equal amounts of proteins were applied, electrophoresed and transferred to a polyvinylidene fluoride membrane. Membranes were blocked with Tris-buffered saline containing 5% non-fat milk at room temperature for 1 h, then incubated overnight at 4°C with primary antibody. The primary antibody dilutions were 1:1,000 for CSE, phosphorylated or total ERK1/2, PI3K, Akt or GSK-3β, and 1:500 for Bcl-2, cleaved caspase-3 and -9, GAPDH, Na^+-K^+-ATPase, cyclin D1 and $p21^{Cip/WAF-1}$. The membrane was then washed three times with 1× Tris-buffer saline-Tween 20 (TBST) buffer and incubated in TBST solution with horseradish peroxidase-conjugated secondary antibody (diluted 1:500) for 1 h at room temperature on a shaker. Finally, the membrane was washed with TBST solution for three times. Antibody–antigen complexes were detected using Western Blue Stabilized Substrate for alkaline phosphatase. GAPDH expression was used as the control. The intensities of the protein bands were quantified by a Bio-Rad ChemiDoc™ EQ densitometer and Bio-Rad Quantity One software (Bio-Rad Laboratories).

Statistical analysis

All data were expressed as the mean ± SE and represented at least three independent experiments. Statistical comparisons were made using student's t test or one-way ANOVA followed by a post hoc analysis (Tukey test) where applicable. Significance level was set at $p < 0.05$.

Results

PC plays cardioprotection in primary cultured neonatal cardiomyocytes

To observe the protective role of PC on the H/R-induced injury in primary cultured neonatal cardiomyocytes, we detected cell viability, cell apoptosis, mRNA level of caspase-3, caspase-9 and Bcl-2. Our data showed that H/R decreased cell viability ($p = 0.0003$), increased the percentage of apoptotic cells ($p = 0.0008$) and mRNA level of caspase-3 ($p = 0.0006$), caspase-9 ($p = 0.0001$) and Bcl-2 ($p = 0.0002$) compared with control group ($p < 0.05$). Compared with H/R group, PC increased cell viability ($p = 0.0005$) and Bcl-2 mRNA level ($p = 0.0007$), decreased the percentage of apoptotic cells ($p = 0.0007$) and mRNA level of caspase-3 ($p = 0.0003$) and caspase-9 ($p = 0.0009$) ($p < 0.05$), suggesting that PC decreased apoptosis by H/R (Additional file 1: Figures S1, S2).

D-Galactose induces aging in cardiomyocytes

To investigate whether D-galactose successfully induces the aging phenotype in cardiomyocytes, we examined the AGE content, which is considered to be an important marker of cardiac aging. Our results showed that incubation of cardiomyocytes with 10 g/L D-galactose for 48 h significantly increased the AGE content compared with other all groups. Cell viability was not changed by treating the cells with 10 g/L D-galactose for 48 h (Table 1).

To further confirm this phenomenon, we performed SA β-Gal staining and evaluated the H9C2 cell division index (primary cultured neonatal cardiomyocytes do not divide) and the expression of cyclin D1 and $p21^{Cip/WAF-1}$. We found that the number of SA β-gal-positive cardiomyocytes and the expression of $p21^{Cip/WAF-1}$ were significantly increased while the H9C2 cell division index and cyclin D1 expression were markedly decreased after incubation with 10 g/L D-galactose for 48 h ($p < 0.05$ vs 0 g/L D-galactose for 48 h group) (Fig. 2).

H_2S production rate and CSE expression changes using the D-galactose age-induced cardiomyocytes

CSE is a H_2S-producing key enzyme in the cardiovascular system. In order to detect whether the loss of PC cardioprotection in the aging cardiomyocytes may be related with the decrease of endogenous H_2S, we examined H_2S production rate and CSE expression changes using D-galactose age-induced cardiomyocytes and H9C2 cells. Compared with the control group, the H_2S production rate ($p = 0.0004$) and CSE expression (CSE-C: $p = 0.006$; CSE-H: $p = 0.004$) (CSE-C, primary cultures of neonatal cardiomyocytes; CSE-H, H9C2 cells) were significantly decreased in both the H/R and PC groups ($p < 0.05$). The difference in the H_2S production rate and CSE expression between the H/R and PC groups was not significant (Fig. 3).

Table 1 The AGEs content and cell viability of different concentrations of D-galactose for different times

	AGEs content (pg/mL)	Cell viability (%)
D-Galactose concentration (g/L)[a]		
0	88 ± 13	100 ± 23
0.1	191 ± 22*	92 ± 12
1	389 ± 90*	93 ± 34
10	924 ± 93*	95 ± 18
100	230 ± 45*	93 ± 26
Time (h)[b]		
0	95 ± 12	100 ± 13
12	448 ± 82*	94 ± 21
24	577 ± 75*	91 ± 19
48	939 ± 79*	96 ± 25
72	668 ± 102*	93 ± 18

[a] The AGEs content and cell viability of different concentrations of D-galactose for 48 h. * $p < 0.05$ vs. 0 g/L D-galactose group.

[b] The AGEs content and cell viability of 10 g/L D-galactose for different times. All data were from eight independent experiments. * $p < 0.05$ vs. 0 h group.

Exogenous H_2S increases cell viability and decreases apoptosis in the D-galactose age-induced primary cultured neonatal cardiomyocytes

To assay whether exogenous H_2S restores PC-induced cardioprotection, we observed cell viability through MTT mothed in the D-galactose age-induced cardiomyocytes. Cell viability was markedly reduced in the H/R group and could be reversed by NaHS co-treatment. The cell viability of the PC group was similar to the H/R group. Compared with the H/R + NaHS and PC groups, cell viability was obviously increased in the PC + NaHS group ($p = 0.003$, $p < 0.05$), indicating that exogenous H_2S restored the PC-induced increase in cell viability (Fig. 4a).

To investigate whether exogenous H_2S protects against PC-induced cardiac apoptosis, we examined cardiomyocyte apoptosis by flow cytometry. H/R significantly increased the percentage of apoptotic cells ($p = 0.0003$, $p < 0.05$ vs. control group). Compared with the H/R group, H/R + NaHS reduced the apoptotic rate ($p = 0.0006$, $p < 0.05$). The apoptotic rate of the PC group was similar to the H/R group. The percentage of apoptotic cells in the PC + NaHS group was significantly decreased compared with the H/R + NaHS and PC groups ($p = 0.005$, $p < 0.05$) (Fig. 4b). We further looked for the morphological changes in the nuclei of cardiomyocytes with Hoechst 33342. The number of apoptotic nuclei showing the typical features of fragmentation and condensation in the H/R group was significantly increased compared to the control group ($p = 0.0003$, $p < 0.05$). The number of apoptotic nuclei was significantly decreased in the H/R + NaHS group compared with that in the H/R group ($p = 0.0002$, $p < 0.05$). The number of apoptotic nuclei in the PC group was similar to the H/R group. Compared with the H/R + NaHS and PC groups, the number of apoptotic nuclei was significantly decreased in the PC + NaHS group ($p = 0.009$, $p < 0.05$), suggesting that exogenous H_2S prevented PC-inhibited apoptosis by H/R (Fig. 4c).

Exogenous H_2S inhibits pro-apoptotic factors and promotes anti-apoptotic factors in the D-galactose age-induced primary cultured neonatal cardiomyocytes

H/R damages mitochondria, then the release of pro-apoptotic factors (cleaved caspase-3, cleaved caspase-9 and Cyt *c*) from injured mitochondria is increased, which finally lead to apoptosis. To further indicate exogenous H_2S restores PC-induced cardioprotection via inhibition of apoptosis, we examined the expression of cleaved caspase-3, cleaved caspase-9 and Bcl-2 in the whole cell

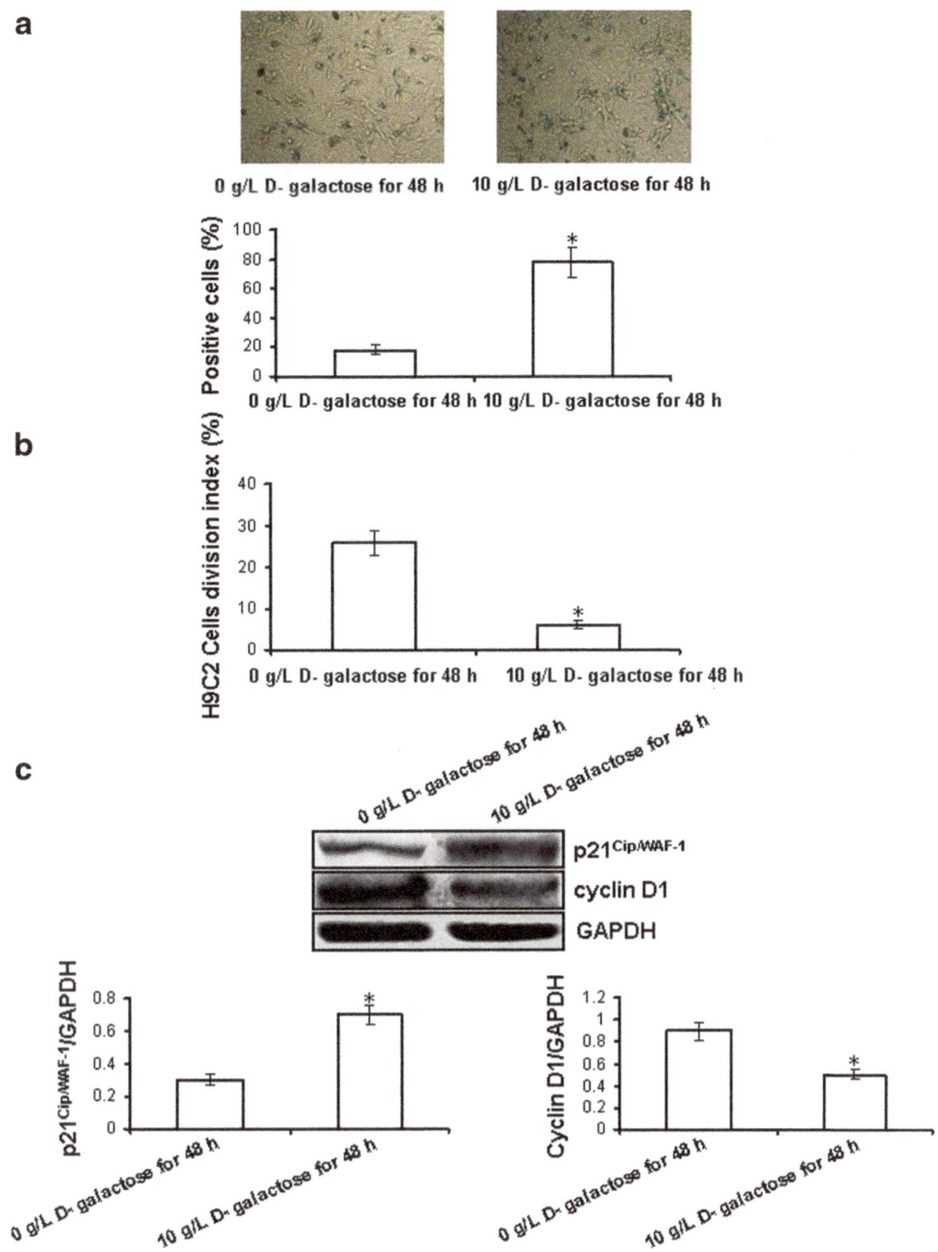

Fig. 2 Response of neonatal rat cardiomyocytes to 10 g/L D-galactose for 48 h. **a** The number of SA β-gal-positive cardiomyocytes. Phase-contrast images showing morphologic changes and stained cells. (SA-β-gal positive cells; *Blue*, magnification ×400). The aging cardiomyocytes in at least five random fields were counted. **b** H9C2 cells division index. Five fields (at least 100 cells of each field) were randomly selected and the percentage of cell division was calculated. **c** The expression of $p21^{Cip/WAF-1}$ and cyclin D1. The intensity of each band was quantified by densitometry, and data were normalized to the GAPDH signal. All data were from four independent experiments. *$p < 0.05$ vs. 0 g/L D-galactose for 48 h group.

lysates as well as Cyt *c* in the cytosolic fraction by western blot in the D-galactose age-induced cardiomyocytes.

Figure 5 shows that the expression of cleaved caspase-3 ($p = 0.0009$), cleaved caspase-9 ($p = 0.0007$) and Cyt *c* ($p = 0.0005$) and Bcl-2 ($p = 0.0004$) was increased in the H/R group compared with the control group ($p < 0.05$). Compared with H/R, H/R + NaHS showed decreased expression of cleaved caspase-3 ($p = 0.004$), cleaved caspase-9 ($p = 0.009$) and Cyt *c* ($p = 0.008$) but increased expression of Bcl-2 ($p = 0.0007$) ($p < 0.05$). The results of the PC group were similar to those of the H/R group. PC + NaHS treatment markedly decreased the expression of cleaved caspase-3 ($p = 0.004$), cleaved caspase-9 ($p = 0.009$) and Cyt *c* ($p = 0.0008$) and increased the expression of Bcl-2 ($p = 0.0007$) in comparison with the H/R + NaHS and PC groups ($p < 0.05$). These results

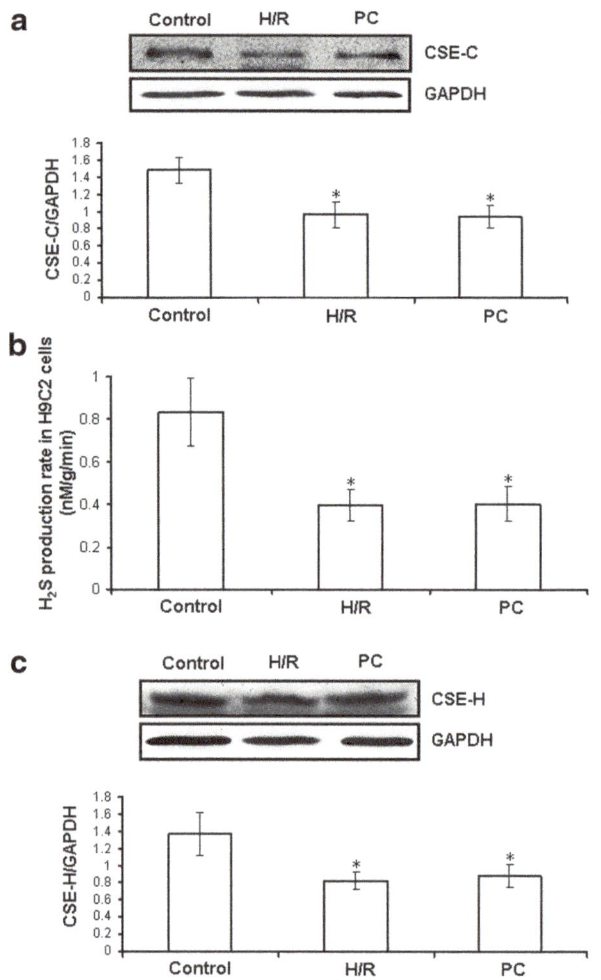

Fig. 3 H_2S production rate and CSE expressions changes using the D-galactose age-induced cardiomyocytes. **a** The expression of CSE protein (CSE-C) in primary cultures of neonatal cardiomyocytes. H_2S production rate (**b**) and CSE (CSE-H) expressions (**c**) in H9C2 cells. The intensity of each band was quantified by densitometry, and data were normalized to the GAPDH signal. All data were from four independent experiments. *$p < 0.05$ vs. control group.

suggest that exogenous H_2S restores the anti-apoptotic effect of PC against H/R by preventing the mitochondrial apoptotic pathway (Cyt *c*–caspase-9–caspase-3).

Exogenous H_2S up-regulates ERK1/2-GSK-3β and PI3K-Akt-GSK-3β pathways in the D-galactose age-induced primary cultured neonatal cardiomyocytes

ERK1/2-GSK-3β and PI3K-Akt-GSK-3β pathways play an important role in the cellular metabolism and gene expression related to growth and apoptosis. To detect whether exogenous H_2S restores PC protective role by activating ERK1/2-GSK-3β and PI3K-Akt-GSK-3β pathways, we observed the mRNA level and activity of phosphorylated ERK1/2, GSK-3β, PI3K and Akt in the D-galactose age-induced cardiomyocytes.

The activity and the mRNA level of phosphorylated ERK1/2 ($p = 0.0005$) and GSK-3β ($p = 0.0003$) in the H/R group was significantly lower than that in the control group ($p < 0.05$). The activity and the mRNA level of phosphorylated ERK1/2 ($p = 0.0009$) and GSK-3β ($p = 0.0004$) was significantly higher in the H/R + NaHS group than in the H/R group ($p < 0.05$). The changes in phosphorylated ERK1/2 and GSK-3β activities and mRNA levels in the PC group were similar to those in the H/R group. In the PC + NaHS group, the activity and the mRNA level of phosphorylated ERK1/2 ($p = 0.004$) and GSK-3β ($p = 0.006$) was increased to a larger extent than that in the H/R + NaHS and PC groups ($p < 0.05$), but an ERK1/2 inhibitor (PD98059) abolished these effects of NaHS. The total amount of ERK1/2 and GSK-3β protein remained unchanged with the different stimulations. These data demonstrate that exogenous H_2S restores the cardioprotection of PC through the activation of the ERK1/2-GSK-3β pathway (Fig. 6; Additional file 1: Figure S3).

Figure 7 and Additional file 1: Figure S4 showed that the activity and the mRNA level of phosphorylated PI3K ($p = 0.0003$), Akt ($p = 0.0005$) and GSK-3β ($p = 0.0009$) were decreased in the H/R group compared with those in the control group ($p < 0.05$). The activity and the mRNA level of PI3K ($p = 0.0008$), Akt ($p = 0.0004$) and GSK-3β ($p = 0.0006$) was increased in the H/R + NaHS group compared with that in the H/R group ($p < 0.05$). Their changes in the PC group were similar to the H/R group. PC + NaHS significantly increased the activity and the mRNA level of PI3K ($p = 0.008$), Akt ($p = 0.003$) and GSK-3β ($p = 0.007$) in comparison with the H/R + NaHS and PC groups ($p < 0.05$), and an inhibitor of PI3K (LY294002) significantly suppressed the NaHS-induced phosphorylation of PI3K, Akt and GSK-3β. The total amount of PI3K, Akt and GSK-3β protein remained unchanged with different stimulations. These results suggest that exogenous H_2S restored the protective effects of PC by the up-regulation of the PI3K-Akt-GSK-3β pathway.

Exogenous H_2S promotes translocation of PKC-ε to the cell membrane in the D-galactose age-induced primary cultured neonatal cardiomyocytes

The PKC-ε activates the mK_{ATP} and then inhibits mPTP opening, which finally plays protection during PC. In this study, we examined the translocation of PKC-ε in the cell membrane. Our results demonstrated that the novel PKC-ε isoform is activated by NaHS. Figure 8 and Additional file 1: Figure S5 showed that PKC-ε translocated to the cell membrane in the H/R + NaHS and PC + NaHS

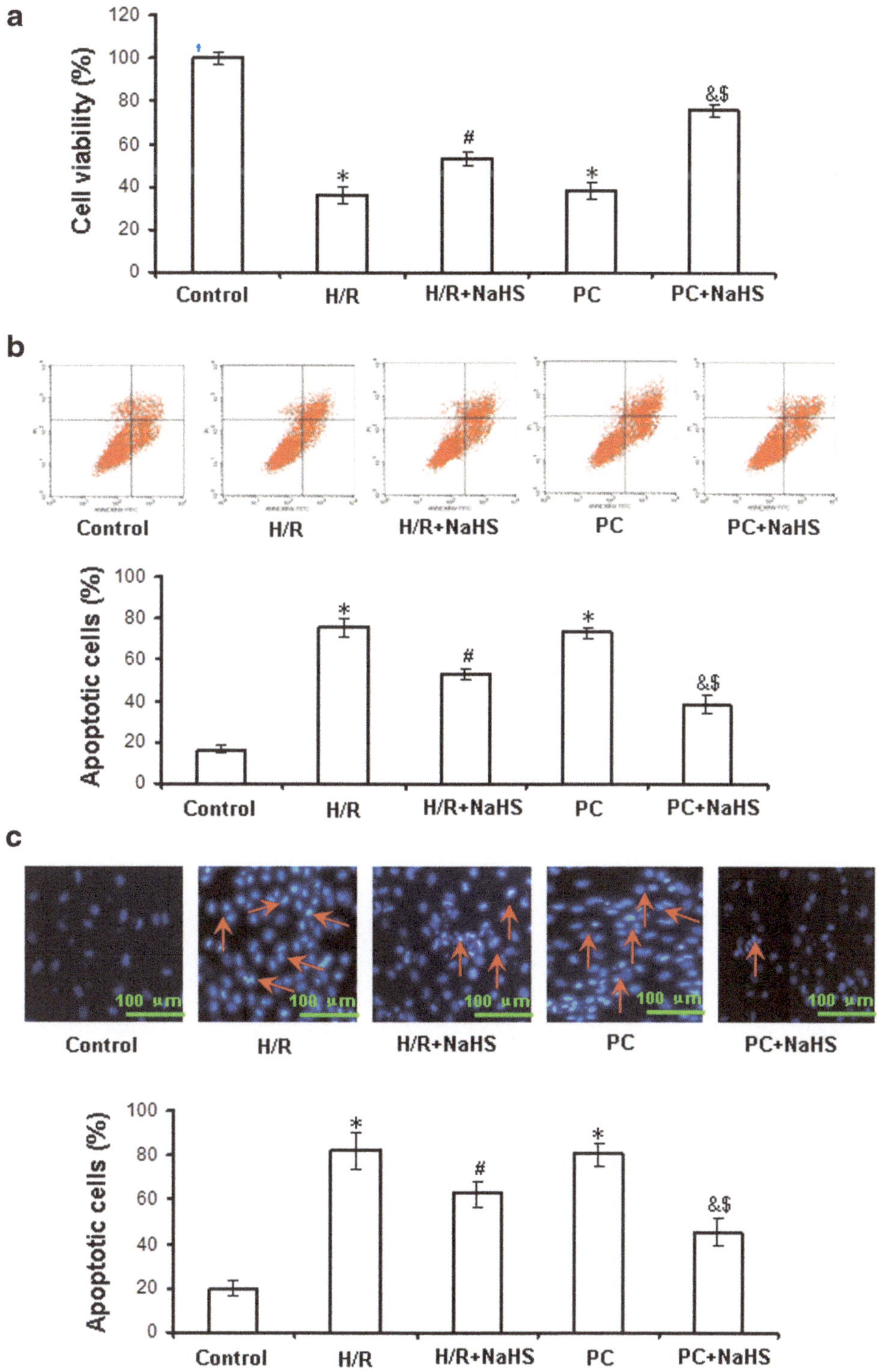

Fig. 4 The effect of exogenous H_2S on the cell viability and apoptosis in the D-galactose age-induced primary cultured neonatal cardiomyocytes. **a** Cell viability was measured by MTT assay. The cells incubated with control medium were considered 100% viable. **b** Apoptosis analyzed by flow cytometry. **c** Detection of nuclear morphology in apoptotic cells by Hoechst 33342 staining. Apoptotic cells were identified as cells with condensed, disrupted nuclei (*arrow*, Hoechst staining, ×400). *Scale bar* 100 μm. Apoptotic cells in at least five random fields were counted. All data were from four independent experiments. *$p < 0.05$ vs. control group; $^{\#}p < 0.05$ vs. H/R group; $^{\&}p < 0.05$ vs. PC group; $^{\$}p < 0.05$ vs. H/R + NaHS group.

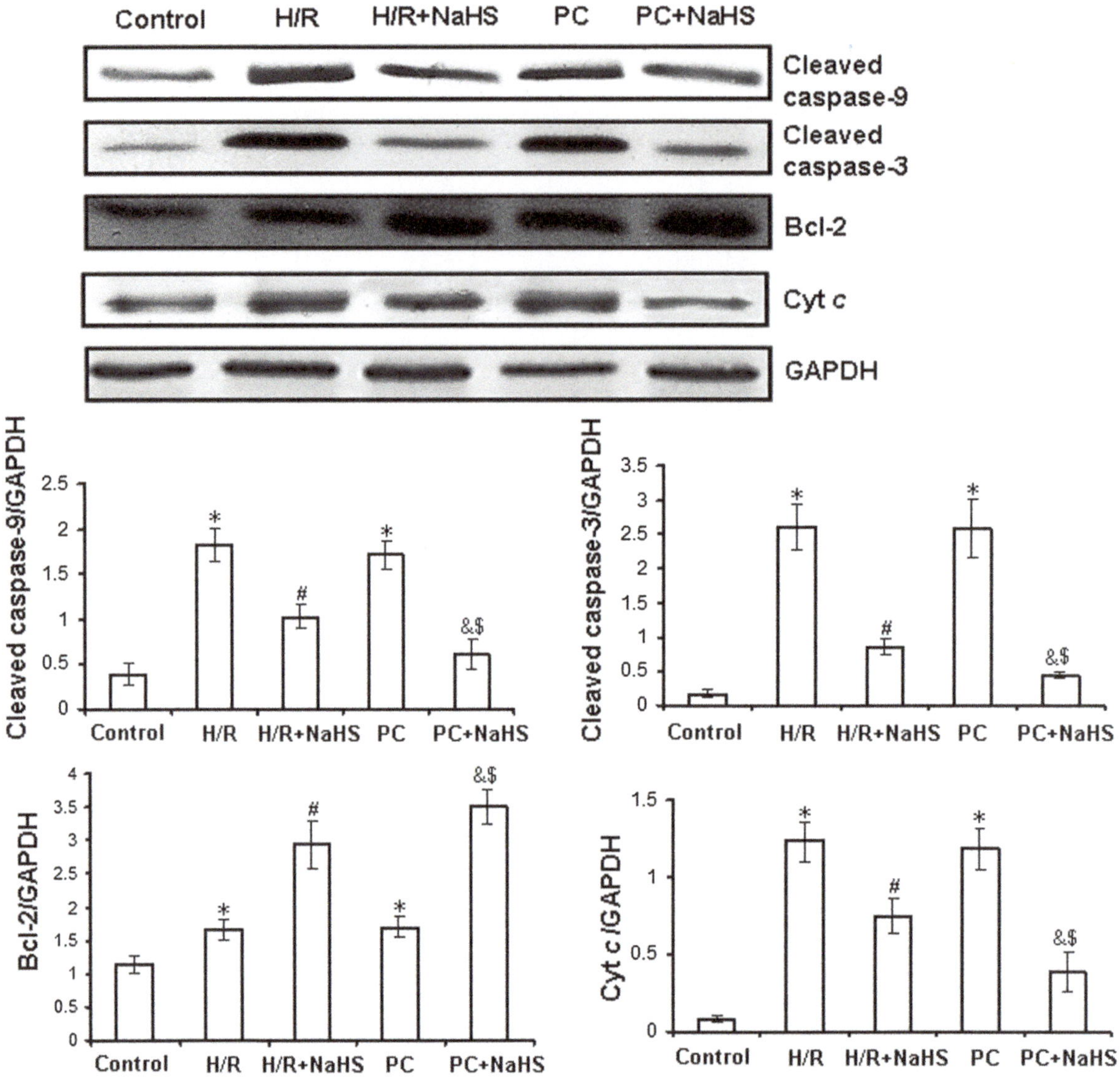

Fig. 5 Expression of Bcl-2, cleaved caspase-3 and cleaved caspase-9, cytosolic Cyt *c* in the D-galactose age-induced primary cultured neonatal cardiomyocytes by western blot analysis. The intensity of each band was quantified by densitometry, and data were normalized to the GAPDH signal. All data were from four independent experiments. *$p < 0.05$ vs. control group; #$p < 0.05$ vs. H/R group; &$p < 0.05$ vs. PC group; $$p < 0.05$ vs. H/R + NaHS group.

groups but not in the Control, H/R, H/R + Che (a specific inhibitor of PKC), H/R + Che + NaHS, PC, PC + Che and PC + Che + NaHS groups.

Exogenous H_2S increases mitochondrial membrane potential (Δψm) and inhibits mPTP opening in the D-galactose age-induced primary cultured neonatal cardiomyocytes

The decreased Δψm induces mPTP opening and then damages celles. To explore the effect of exogenous H_2S on the recovery of PC-induced cardioprotection, we observed the changes of Δψm and mPTP. As shown in Fig. 9a, the Δψm in the H/R group was significantly decreased (vs. the control group, $p = 0.0003$, $p < 0.05$). The Δψm in the H/R + NaHS group was significantly increased (vs. the H/R group, $p = 0.0008$, $p < 0.05$). The Δψm of the PC group was similar to that in the H/R group. The Δψm in the PC + NaHS group was higher than that of the H/R + NaHS and PC groups ($p = 0.0009$, $p < 0.05$). PD98059, LY294002, 5-HD (an inhibitor of mK_{ATP}) and Che reversed the increase of the Δψm by NaHS.

At the same time, we assessed mPTP opening with calcein-AM in the different groups. As shown in Fig. 9b, the fluorescence intensity was reduced in the H/R group ($p = 0.0007$, $p < 0.05$ vs. control group). H/R + NaHS resulted in increased fluorescence intensity as compared

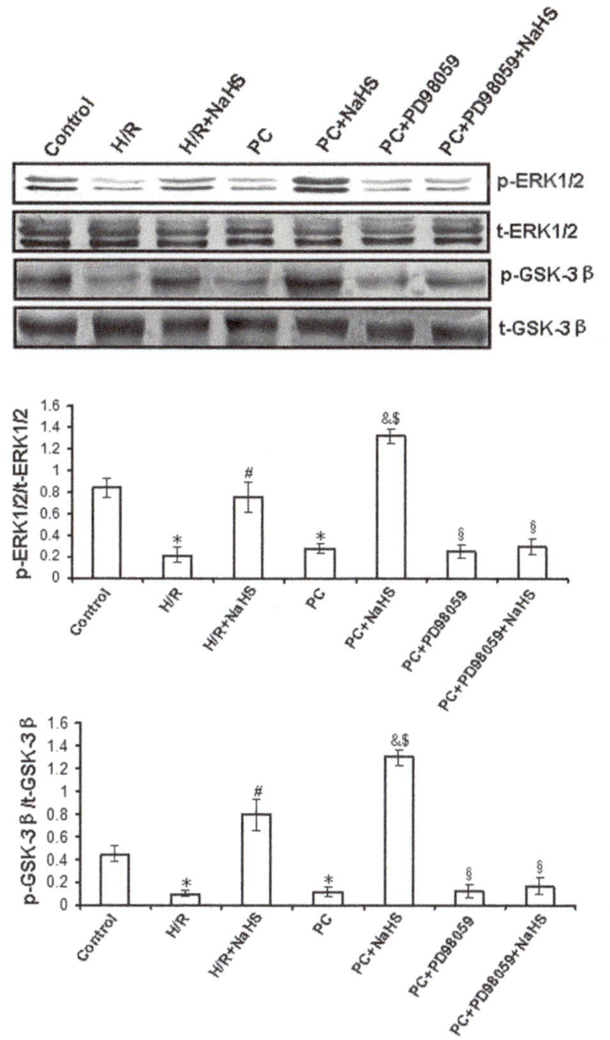

Fig. 6 The change of ERK1/2 and GSK-3β activities in the D-galactose age-induced primary cultured neonatal cardiomyocytes. The different cells were collected and subjected to western blot. The *graphs* represent the optical density of the band of phosphorylated ERK1/2 and GSK-3β normalized with that of total ERK1/2 and GSK-3β, respectively. All data were from four independent experiments. *$p < 0.05$ vs. control group; #$p < 0.05$ vs. H/R group; &$p < 0.05$ vs. PC group; $p < 0.05 vs. H/R + NaHS group; §$p < 0.05$ vs. PC + NaHS group.

to the H/R group ($p = 0.0006$, $p < 0.05$). The fluorescence intensity of the PC group was similar to the H/R group. PC + NaHS further increased the fluorescence as compared to the H/R + NaHS and PC groups ($p = 0.0008$, $p < 0.05$), while PD98059, LY294002, 5-HD and Che blocked the increase in fluorescence intensity caused by PC + NaHS.

Discussion

The senescent phenotype is associated with a typical gene expression profile and higher SA *β*-gal activity [28, 33]. At same time, AGE content is also considered to be one of the most important markers in aging [34]. Cell cycle progression is determined by the formation of protein complexes between cyclins and cyclin-dependent kinases (cdk), and cyclin D associates with cdk2, cdk4, and cdk6 for the determination of early G1 progression [35]. Also involved in the control of cyclin–cdk activity in all phases of the cell cycle is $p21^{Cip/WAF-1}$ [35]. The increase of cyclin D1 and the decrease of $p21^{Cip/WAF-1}$ reflect cell growth and division. It is well known that the cell division index reflects cell growth, and senescent cells cannot undergo cell division. Our data showed that the number of SA *β*-gal-positive cells, the AGE content and the expression of $p21^{Cip/WAF-1}$ were increased and cyclin D1 expression was decreased in cardiomyocytes, while the H9C2 cell division index was markedly decreased, in treated with 10 g/L D-galactose for 48 h (Table 1; Fig. 1). This indicates the successful establishment of the D-galactose-induced cardiomyocyte aging model used in the present study. As primary cultured neonatal cardiomyocytes cannot divide, the cell division index was assessed using H9C2 cells (cardiomyocytes line).

I/R can induce tissue and organ injury, as well as apoptosis. The mechanisms of apoptosis include the activation of mitochondrial death receptors and/or endoplasmic reticulum stress pathways [9]. The mitochondrial pathway is the major apoptosis-inducing pathway. The intrinsic or mitochondrial pathway transduces a wide spectrum of death signals that originate from both outside and inside the cells. The stimulation of these pathways triggers the translocation of death-promoting proteins (e.g., Cyt *c*) from the mitochondria to the cytoplasm [36, 37] and the activation of a class of cysteine proteases called caspases, which initiate apoptosis [37]. PC protects cardiac against I/R injury and apoptosis by improving cardiac function, decreasing infarct size and inhibiting apoptosis, among other mechanisms [5, 7, 38]. However, it was recently reported that PC loses its myocardial protective effect in ageing hearts [13–15]. The main reason is that, during ageing, cardiomyocytes undergo complex changes, which finally result in loss of contractile function and loss of endogenous protection against irreversible injury [13–15]. Aging affects cardiomyocytes at several subcellular and molecular levels, including alterations at the level of the DNA, increased oxidative stress, changes in gene/protein expression and posttranslational modifications, and the handling of cellular 'waste' material by autophagy [13–15]. All these alterations decrease the tolerance of cardiomyocytes to stress [13–15]. Our data showed that in the normal primary cultured neonatal cardiomyocytes, compared with H/R group, PC increased cell viability and Bcl-2 mRNA level, decreased the percentage of apoptotic cells and mRNA level of caspase-3 and caspase-9 (Additional file 1: Figures S1, S2).

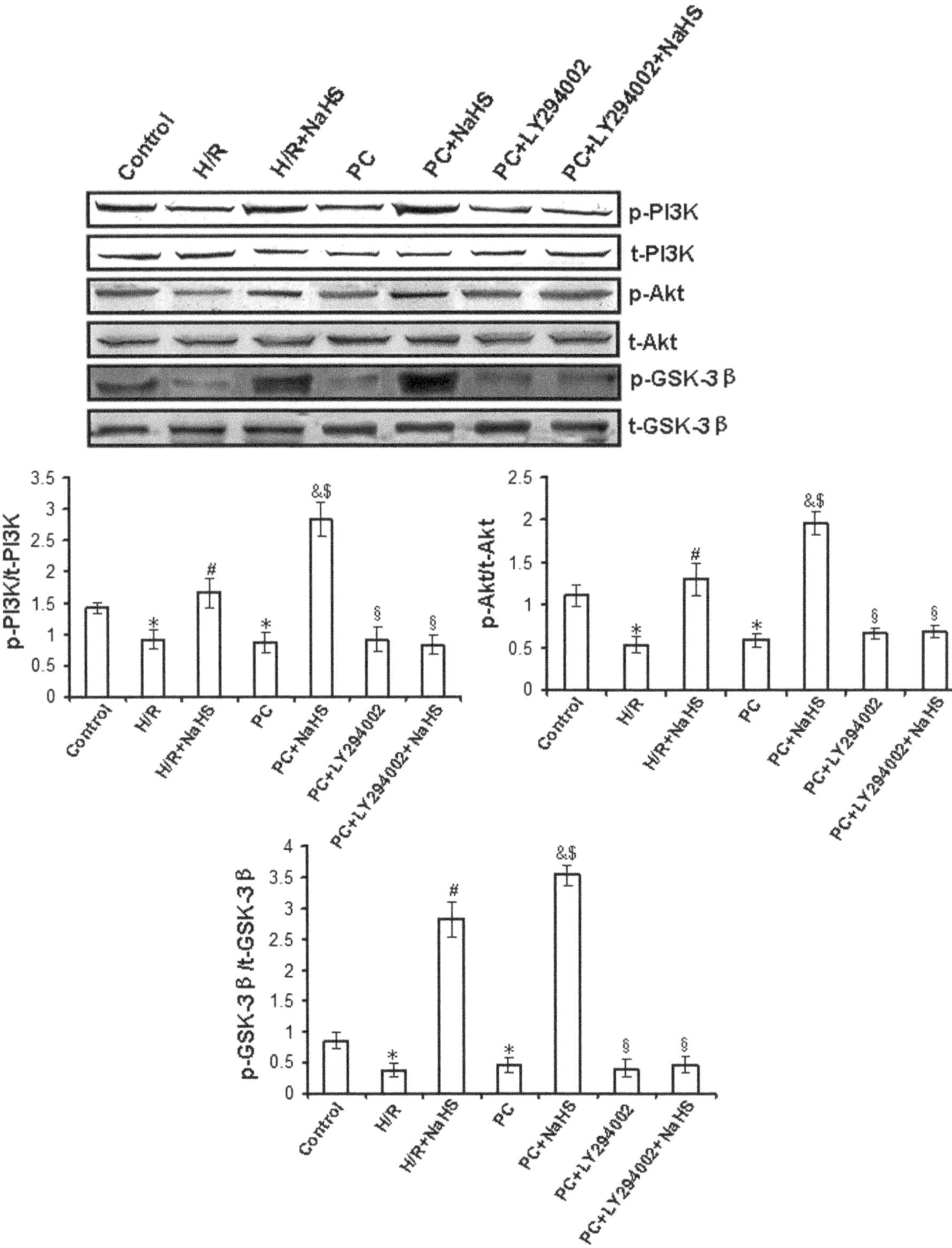

Fig. 7 The change of PI3K, Akt and GSK-3β activities in the D-galactose age-induced primary cultured neonatal cardiomyocytes. The different cells were collected and subjected to western blot. The *graphs* represent the optical density of the band of phosphorylated PI3K, Akt and GSK-3β normalized with that of total PI3K, Akt and GSK-3β, respectively. All data were from four independent experiments. *$p < 0.05$ vs. control group; #$p < 0.05$ vs. H/R group; &$p < 0.05$ vs. PC group; $$p < 0.05$ vs. H/R + NaHS group; §$p < 0.05$ vs. PC + NaHS group.

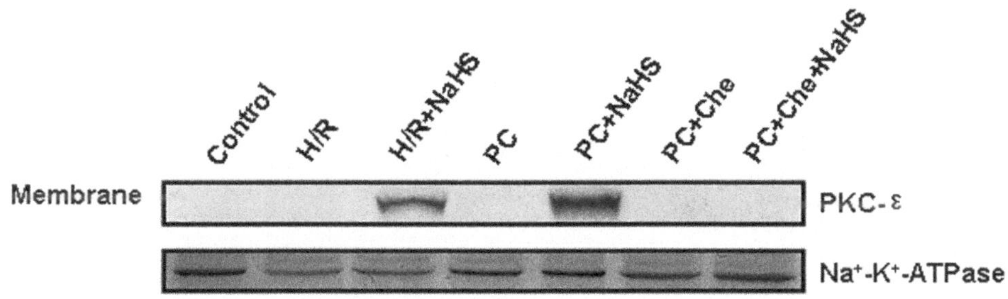

Fig. 8 Translocation of PKC-ε to cell membrane by Western blot in the D-galactose age-induced primary cultured neonatal cardiomyocytes. Control, H/R, PC, PC + Che and PC + Che + NaHS groups showed no translocation of PKC-ε to cell membrane. H/R + NaHS and PC + NaHS groups showed translocation of PKC-ε to cell membrane. Na^+/K^+-ATPase was used a membrane fraction loading control.

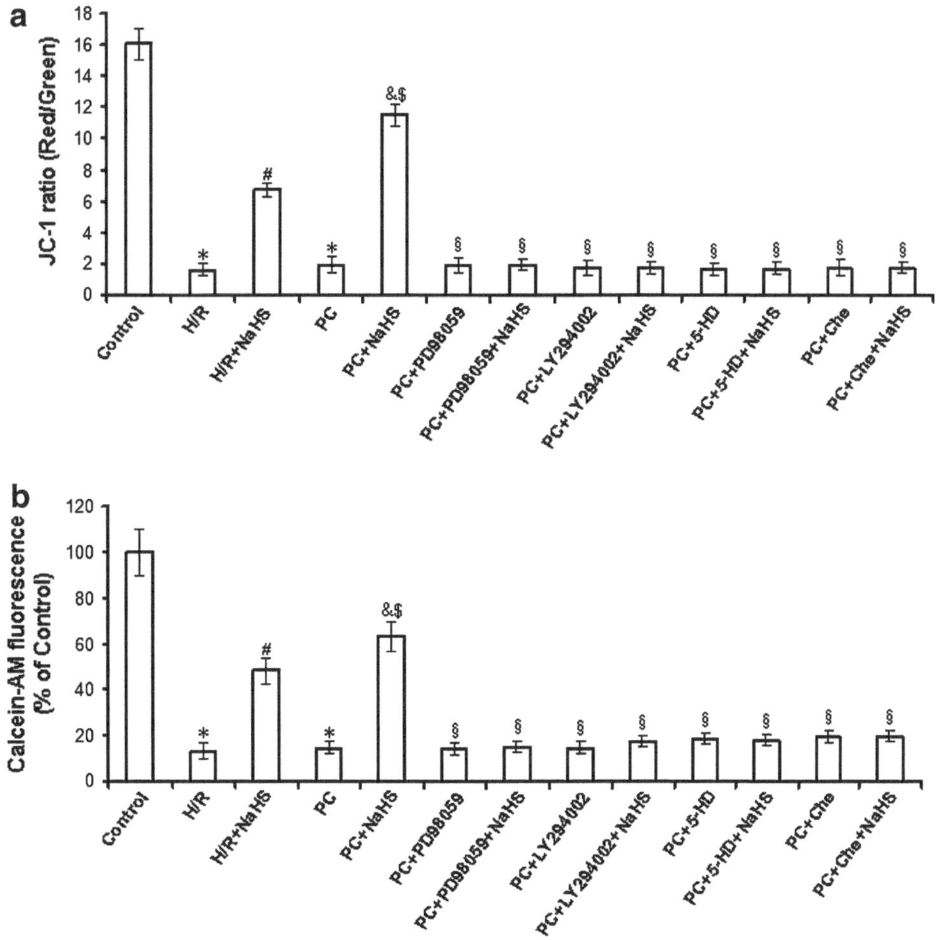

Fig. 9 Analysis of the mitochondrial membrane potential ($\Delta\psi m$) and mPTP opening in the D-galactose age-induced primary cultured neonatal cardiomyocytes. **a** JC-1 measured the mitochondrial membrane potential ($\Delta\psi m$). The cells of different groups were stained with JC-1 probe and imaged by fluorescent microscope. JC-1 spontaneously forms J-aggregate and exhibits red fluorescence under a high potential. The JC-1 monomeric form shows green fluorescence under a low potential. The individual red and green average fluorescence intensities are expressed as the ratio of red to green fluorescence. **b** Changes of mPTP opening were measured with calcein-AM. The fluorescence intensity in control group were considered 100% viable. The changes of fluorescence intensity are inversely proportional with degree of the mPTP opening. All data were from four independent experiments. *$p < 0.05$ vs. control group; $^{\#}p < 0.05$ vs. H/R group; $^{\&}p < 0.05$ vs. PC group; $^{\$}p < 0.05$ vs. H/R + NaHS group; $^{\S}p < 0.05$ vs. PC + NaHS group.

In the D-galactose age-induced cardiomyocytes, the difference in cell viability, the apoptotic rate, and cleaved caspase-9, cleaved caspase-3, Bcl-2 and Cyt *c* expression between the H/R and PC groups in aging cardiomyocytes was not significant (Figs. 3, 4). These results indicate that PC plays protective role in the normal primary cultured neonatal cardiomyocytes but no in the aging cardiomyocytes.

H_2S has long been considered as a pungent cytotoxic gas but now is regarded as the third endogenous signalling gasotransmitter. H_2S is generated in mammalian tissues from homocysteine and cysteine in a reaction catalysed by CBS and CSE, the key enzymes of the transulphuration pathway of methionine metabolism [17–19, 37]. CBS is mainly expressed in the brain and peripheral nervous system, whereas CSE is mostly found in vascular and nonvascular smooth muscle cells [17–19, 37]. Yang and colleagues [24] generated mice lacking CSE (CSE knockout) that had much lower H_2S concentrations in the aorta and heart, and their findings suggested that CSE is the major enzyme that maintains H_2S concentrations in the cardiovascular system. Recent studies have shown that increased endogenous CSE/H_2S pathway expression or exogenous H_2S is involved in PC-induced cardioprotection [39]. Therefore, we proposed that the loss of cardioprotection from PC in ageing cardiomyocytes is associated with changes in the CSE/H_2S pathway. In the present study, we found that compared with the control group, the H_2S production rate of H9C2 cells and CSE expression in ageing cardiomyocytes and H9C2 cells were significantly decreased in both the H/R and PC groups. The difference in the H_2S production rate and CSE expression between the H/R and PC groups was not significant (Fig. 2). We then used NaHS solution as a source of H_2S and observed that compared with the H/R group, cell viability and Bcl-2 expression were significantly increased, while the apoptotic rate and expression of cleaved caspase-9, cleaved caspase-3 and Cyt *c* were obviously decreased in the H/R + NaHS group, demonstrating that exogenous H_2S reduced H/R-induced cardiomyocyte injury. This is consistent with previous reports [23, 24]. Meanwhile, we also found that PC + NaHS further enhanced the cardioprotective roles of H/R + NaHS. These data suggest that exogenous H_2S restored PC-induced cardioprotective effects in ageing cardiomyocytes.

To further explore the mechanisms by which exogenous H_2S restored PC-induced cardioprotective effects, we assessed changes in mitochondrial membrane potential, mPTP opening and relevant signalling pathways. ERK1/2 is a member of the mammalian mitogen-activated protein kinase family (MAPK), which has a unique role in the regulation of cellular metabolism and gene expression (such as GSK-3β) related to growth and apoptosis [9, 39, 40]. The PI3K-Akt pathway is proximal to endothelial nitric oxide synthase [9, 41, 42], and its activation also results in the phosphorylation of downstream GSK-3β and, consequently, regulating cell biological and pathological functions. The current study suggests that the up-regulation of the ERK1/2-GSK-3β and PI3-Akt-GSK-3β pathways may contribute to the protective effect of PC through the inhibition of mPTP opening [43, 44]. In addition, PKC-ε activates $mitoK_{ATP}$ and inhibits mPTP opening, which is involved in cardioprotection during PC [45]. We showed here that H/R + NaHS promoted the phosphorylation of the ERK1/2-GSK-3β and PI3K-Akt-GSK-3β pathways and the translocation of PKC-ε to the cell membrane, increased the mitochondrial membrane potential and inhibited mPTP opening (Figs. 5, 6, 7, 8; Additional file 1: Figures S3, S4, S5). PC + NaHS further enhanced the effects of H/R + NaHS. PD98059 (an inhibitor of ERK1/2 signalling), LY 294002 (a PI3K inhibitor), Che (a PKC inhibitor) and 5-HD (a $mitoK_{ATP}$ inhibitor) abolished the effects of PC + NaHS, respectively (Figs. 5, 6, 7, 8; Additional file 1: Figures S3, S4, S5). Taken together,

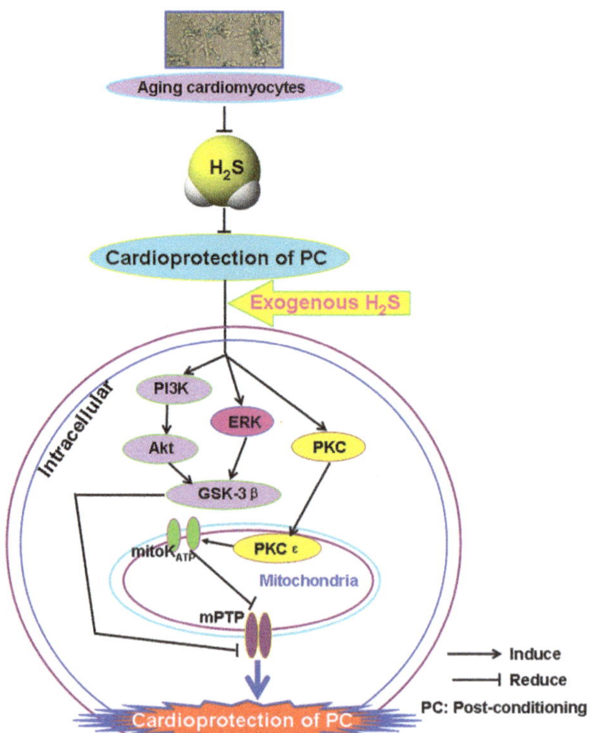

Fig. 10 Involvement of exogenous H_2S in recovery of PC-induced cardioprotection in aging cardiomyocytes. Exogenous H_2S mediates recovery of PC-induced cardioprotection via inhibition of mPTP opening by up-regulation of ERK1/2-GSK-3β, PI3K-Akt-GSK-3β and PKC-mK_{ATP} pathways.

these findings suggest that exogenous H_2S plays an important role in the recovery of PC-induced cardioprotection by inhibiting mPTP opening through the phosphorylation of the ERK1/2-GSK-3β and PI3K-Akt-GSK-3β pathways, as well as the activation of the PKC-ε-mitoK_{ATP} pathway.

In summary (Fig. 10), the present research demonstrated that (1) H/R causes injury to aging cardiomyocytes and that exogenous H_2S reduces H/R injury. (2) In aging cardiomyocytes, PC loses its cardioprotective effects on H/R injury and exogenous H_2S recovers PC-induced cardioprotection by inhibiting mPTP opening via the activation of the ERK1/2-GSK-3β, PI3K-Akt-GSK-3β and PKC-ε-mK_{ATP} pathways. Dissection of the mechanisms underlying H_2S protection should facilitate novel preventive and therapeutic approaches for ischemic cardiomyopathy in the aging process.

Additional file

Additional file 1: Figure S1. The change of the cell viability and apoptosis in the normal primary cultured neonatal cardiomyocytes. **Figure S2.** The change of caspase-3, caspase-9 and Bcl-2 mRNA levels in the normal primary cultured neonatal cardiomyocytes. **Figure S3.** The effect of exogenous H_2S on p-ERK1/2 and p-GSK-3β mRNA levels in the D-galactose age-induced cardiomyocytes. **Figure S4.** The effect of exogenous H_2S on p-PI3K, p-Akt and p-GSK-3β mRNA levels in the D-galactose age-induced cardiomyocytes. **Figure S5.** The effect of exogenous H_2S on PKC-ε mRNA levels in the cell membrane in the D-galactose age-induced cardiomyocytes.

Authors' contributions
HL and CX conceived and designed the research, and drafted the manuscript, CZ, WS, LL and SB performed the experiments. HL, BW, XZ, RW and LW revised the paper and gave some suggestions. All authors read and approved the final manuscript.

Author details
[1] Department of Pathophysiology, Harbin Medical University, Baojian Road, Harbin 150081, China. [2] Department of Emergency, Heilongjiang Provincial Hospital, Harbin 150036, China. [3] The Key Laboratory of Cardiovascular Medicine Research (Harbin Medical University), Ministry of Education, Harbin 150086, China. [4] Department of Biology, Lakehead University, Thunder Bay, ON P7B 5E1, Canada. [5] Department of Health Science, Lakehead University, Thunder Bay, ON P7B 5E1, Canada.

Acknowledgements
This research is supported by the National Natural Science Foundation of China (No. 81270273, No. 81000059, No. 81270311, No. 81400210), the Natural Science Foundation of Heilongjiang (No. LC201430).

Compliance with ethical guidelines

Competing interests
The authors declare that they have no competing interests.

References
1. Murry CE, Jennings RB, Reimer KA. Preconditioning with ischemia: a delay of lethal cell injury in ischemic myocardium. Circulation. 1986;74:1124–36.
2. Mockford KA, Girn HR, Homer-Vanniasinkam S. Postconditioning: current controversies and clinical implications. Eur J Vasc Endovasc Surg. 2009;37:437–42.
3. Chen YH, Wu XD, Yao ST, Sun S, Liu XH. Calcineurin is involved in cardioprotection induced by ischemic postconditioning through attenuating endoplasmic reticulum stress. Chin Med J (Engl). 2011;124:3334–40.
4. Zhao ZQ, Corvera JS, Halkos ME, Kerendi F, Wang NP, Guyton RA, et al. Inhibition of myocardial injury by ischemic postconditioning during reperfusion: comparison with ischemic preconditioning. Am J Physiol Heart Circ Physiol. 2003;285:H579–88.
5. Yong QC, Lee SW, Foo CS, Neo KL, Chen X, Bian JS. Endogenous hydrogen sulphide mediates the cardioprotection induced by ischemic postconditioning. Am J Physiol Heart Circ Physiol. 2008;295:H1330–40.
6. Tsang A, Hausenloy DJ, Mocanu MM, Yellon DM. Postconditioning: a form of "modified reperfusion" protects the myocardium by activating the phosphatidylinositol 3-kinase-Akt pathway. Circ Res. 2004;95:230–2.
7. Zhu M, Feng J, Lucchinetti E, Fischer G, Xu L, Pedrazzini T, et al. Ischemic postconditioning protects remodeled myocardium via the PI3K-PKB/Akt reperfusion injury salvage kinase pathway. Cardiovasc Res. 2006;72:152–62.
8. Darling CE, Jiang R, Maynard M, Whittaker P, Vinten-Johansen J, Przyklenk K. Postconditioning via stuttering reperfusion limits myocardial infarct size in rabbit hearts: role of ERK1/2. Am J Physiol Heart Circ Physiol. 2005;289:H1618–26.
9. Li H, Wei C, Gao J, Bai S, Li H, Zhao Y, et al. Mediation of dopamine D2 receptors activation in post-conditioning-attenuated cardiomyocyte apoptosis. Exp Cell Res. 2014;323:118–30.
10. Philipp S, Yang XM, Cui L, Davis AM, Downey JM, Cohen MV. Postconditioning protects rabbit hearts through a protein kinase C-adenosine A2b receptor cascade. Cardiovasc Res. 2006;70:308–14.
11. Zatta AJ, Kin H, Lee G, Wang N, Jiang R, Lust R, et al. Infarctsparing effect of myocardial postconditioning is dependent on protein kinase C signalling. Cardiovasc Res. 2006;70:315–24.
12. Hausenloy DJ, Tsang A, Yellon DM. The reperfusion injury salvage kinase pathway: a common target for both ischemic preconditioning and postconditioning. Trends Cardiovasc Med. 2005;15:69–75.
13. Boengler K, Schulz R, Heusch G. Loss of cardioprotection with ageing. Cardiovasc Res. 2009;83:247–61.
14. Jahangir A, Sagar S, Terzic A. Aging and cardioprotection. Appl Physiol. 2007;103:2120–8.
15. Chen Q, Ross T, Hu Y, Lesnefsky EJ. Blockade of electron transport at the onset of reperfusion decreases cardiac injury in aged hearts by protecting the inner mitochondrial membrane. J Aging Res. 2012;2012:753949.
16. Zhao K, Li H, Li S, Yang G. Regulation of cystathionine gamma-lyase/H2S system and its pathological implication. Front Biosci (Landmark Ed). 2014;19:1355–69.
17. Yang GD, Li HZ, Tang GH, Wu LY, Zhao KX, Cao QH, et al. Increased neointimal formation in cystathionine gamma-lyase deficient mice: role of hydrogen sulfide in α5β1-integrin and matrix metalloproteinase-2 expression in smooth muscle cells. J Mol Cell Cardiol. 2012;52:677–88.
18. Yang GD. Hydrogen sulfide in cell survival: a double-edged sword. Expert Rev Clin Pharmacol. 2011;4:33–47.
19. Meng QH, Yang G, Yang W, Jiang B, Wu L, Wang R. Protective effect of hydrogen sulfide on balloon injury-induced neointima hyperplasia in rat carotid arteries. Am J Pathol. 2007;170:1406–14.
20. Dayal S, Bottiglieri T, Arning E, Maeda N, Malinow MR, Sigmund CD, et al. Endothelial dysfunction and elevation of S-adenosylhomocysteine in cystathionine beta-synthase-deficient mice. Circ Res. 2001;88:1203–9.
21. Mani S, Li H, Untereiner A, Wu L, Yang G, Austin RC, et al. Decreased endogenous production of hydrogen sulfide accelerates atherosclerosis. Circulation. 2013;127:2523–34.
22. Wang R. Two's company, three's a crowd: can H_2S be the third endogenous gaseous transmitter? Faseb J. 2002;16:1792–8.
23. Wang R. The gasotransmitter role of hydrogen sulfide. Antioxid Redox Sig. 2003;5:493–501.
24. Yang G, Wu L, Jiang B, Yang W, Qi J, Cao K, et al. H_2S as a physiologic vasorelaxant: hypertension in mice with deletion of cystathionine gamma-lyase. Science. 2008;322:587–90.

25. Li HZ, Mani S, Cao W, Yang GD, Lai C, Wu LY, et al. Interaction of hydrogen sulfide and estrogen on the proliferation of vascular smooth muscle cells. PLoS One. 2012;7:e41614.
26. Zhao W, Zhang J, Lu Y, Wang R. The vasorelaxant effect of H_2S as a novel endogenous gaseous K_{ATP} channel opener. EMBO J. 2001;20:6008–16.
27. Li HZ, Wang YH, Wei C, Bai SZ, Zhao YJ, Li HX, et al. Mediation of exogenous hydrogen sulfide in recovery of ischemic post-conditioning-induced cardioprotection via down-regulating oxidative stress and up-regulating PI3K/Akt/GSK-3β pathway in isolated aging rat hearts. Cell Biosci. 2015;5:11.
28. Li HZ, Guo J, Gao J, Han LP, Jiang CM, Li HX, et al. Role of dopamine D2 receptors in ischemia/reperfusion induced apoptosis of cultured neonatal rat cardiomyocytes. J Biomed Sci. 2011;18:18.
29. Liu J, Wang J, Chen X, Guo C, Guo Y, Wang H. *Ginkgo biloba* extract EGB761 protects against aging-associated diastolic dysfunction in cardiomyocytes of D-galactose-induced aging rat. Oxid Med Cell Longev. 2012;2012:418748.
30. Chen B, Zhong Y, Peng W, Sun Y, Kong WJ. Agerelated changes in the central auditory system: comparison of D-galactose-induced aging rats and naturally aging rats. Brain Res. 2010;1344:43–53.
31. Li HZ, Han LP, Jiang CM, Li H, Zhao YJ, Gao J, et al. Effect of dopamine receptor 1 on apoptosis of cultured neonatal rat cardiomyocytes in simulated ischaemia/reperfusion. Basic Clin Pharmacol Toxicol. 2008;102:329–36.
32. Hausenloy D, Wynne A, Duchen M, Yellon D. Transient mitochondrial permeability transition pore opening mediates preconditioning-induced protection. Circulation. 2004;109:1714–7.
33. Dimri GP, Lee X, Basile G, Acosta M, Scott G, Roskelley C, et al. A biomarker that identifies senescent human cells in culture and in aging skin in vivo. Proc Natl Acad Sci USA. 1995;92:9363–7.
34. Li SY, Du M, Dolence EK, Fang CX, Mayer GE, Ceylan-Isik AF, et al. Aging induces cardiac diastolic dysfunction, oxidative stress, accumulation of advanced glycation endproducts and proteinmodification. Aging Cell. 2005;2:57–64.
35. Yang G, Wu L, Bryan S, Khaper N, Mani S, Wang R. Cystathionine gamma-lyase deficiency and overproliferation of smooth muscle cells. Cardiovasc Res. 2010;86:487–95.
36. Narula J, Pandey P, Arbustini E, Haider N, Narula N, Kolodgie FD. Apoptosis in heart failure: release of cytochrome c from mitochondria and activation of caspase-3 in human cardiomyopathy. Proc Natl Acad Sci. 1999;96:8144–9.
37. Zhong X, Wang L, Wang Y, Dong S, Leng X, Jia J, et al. Exogenous hydrogen sulfide attenuates diabetic myocardial injury through cardiac mitochondrial protection. Mol Cell Biochem. 2012;371:187–98.
38. Wang HC, Zhang HF, Guo WY, Su H, Zhang KR, Li QX, et al. Hypoxic post-conditioning enhances the survival and inhibits apoptosis of cardiomyocytes following reoxygenation: role of peroxynitrite formation. Apoptosis. 2006;11:1453–60.
39. Ji Y, Pang QF, Xu G, Wang L, Wang JK, Zeng YM. Exogenous hydrogen sulfide postconditioning protects isolated rat hearts against ischemia-reperfusion injury. Eur J Pharmacol. 2008;587:1–7.
40. Xia Z, Dickens M, Raingeaud J, Davis RJ, Greenberg ME. Opposing effects of ERK and JNK-p38 MAP kinases on apoptosis. Science. 1995;270:1326–31.
41. Hausenloy DJ, Yellon DM. Survival kinases in ischemic preconditioning and postconditioning. Cardiovasc Res. 2006;70:240–53.
42. Vinten-Johansen J. Postconditioning: a mechanical maneuver that triggers biological and molecular cardioprotective responses to reperfusion. Heart Fail Rev. 2007;12:235–44.
43. Gao X, Zhang H, Takahashi T, Hsieh J, Liao J, Steinberg GK, et al. The Akt signaling pathway contributes to postconditioning's protection against stroke; the protection is associated with the MAPK and PKC pathways. J Neurochem. 2008;105:943–55.
44. Pignataro G, Meller R, Inoue K, Ordonez AN, Ashley MD, Xiong Z, et al. In vivo and in vitro characterization of a novel neuroprotective strategy for stroke: ischemic postconditioning. J Cereb Blood Flow Metab. 2008;28:232–41.
45. Hausenloy DJ, Ong SB, Yellon DM. The mitochondrial permeability transition pore as a target for preconditioning and postconditioning. Basic Res Cardiol. 2009;104:189–202.

Complement C4 induces regulatory T cells differentiation through dendritic cell in systemic lupus erythematosus

Hong-Bin Cheng[1†], Rong-Yi Chen[2†], Jing-Ping Wu[1†], Li Chen[3], Yan-Hua Liang[4], Hai-Feng Pan[5], Zi-Feng Pan[2], Qing-Hua Zhang[2], Qing Li[6], Tian-Xi Du[3], Yong-Mei Lv[6*] and Jian-Qiang Shi[2*]

Abstract

Background: Systemic lupus erythematosus (SLE) is a prototypic systemic autoimmune disease. Complement component 4 (C4) has be proved to play a role in pathogenesis of SLE. In the present study, we investigated the effect of C4 on T cells differentiation.

Methods: Thirty SLE patients were included in this study. CD4+ T cells were isolated from healthy subjects, and dendritic cells (DCs) were isolated from healthy subjects or SLE patients. C4 was supplemented to co-incubate with T cells and DCs.

Results: Serum C4 concentration was positively correlated with regulatory T cell (Treg) percentage ($R^2 = 0.5907$, $p < 0.001$) and TGFβ concentration ($R^2 = 0.5641$, $p < 0.001$) in SLE patients. Different concentrations of C4 had no effect on T cells differentiation. Co-incubated T cells with DCs and C4 for 7 days, the Treg percentage and TGF-β concentration were significantly elevated. In addition, pre-treated DCs (from healthy subjects or SLE patients) with C4 and then co-incubated with T cells, the increases of Treg percentage and TGF-β concentration were also observed.

Conclusion: C4 takes part in T cells differentiation to Treg cells via DCs.

Keywords: Complement C4, Systemic lupus erythematosus, Treg cells, TGF-β

Background

Systemic lupus erythematosus (SLE), a severe multisystem autoimmune disease, is characterized by a loss of immune tolerance to self-antigens (Ags), which results in the persistent production of pathogenic autoantibodies, activation of lymphocyte and release of inflammatory mediators [1]. Many factors including genetic, environmental and hormonal contribute to initiate and drive SLE pathogenesis [2]. However, the exact pathogenic mechanisms remain to be elucidated.

Regulatory T cells (Tregs) are involved in inhibition process of CD4+ Th cells activation, cytotoxic CD8+ T cells differentiation and B cell activation [3–5]. The definitive role of Treg cells in SLE remains not fully clear. In SLE patients, the reduced number and function of CD4+CD25 Foxp3 Tregs have been observed [6]. The deficiencies of Tregs might contribute to the breakdown of self-tolerance and the development of the autoimmune response in SLE patients [7].

Complement component 4 (C4), a protein involved in complement system, takes part in multiple aspects of the immune system [8]. It has also be shown that complement system is implicated in pathogenesis of SLE and has important protective functions in SLE [9, 10]. SLE patients have decreased C4 copy number and serum C4 concentration [11], and low copy number of C4 is identified to be a risk factor for SLE susceptibility [12]. The mechanisms of the link between abnormal complement

*Correspondence: ymeilv@163.com; jianqshi@163.com
†Hong-Bin Cheng, Rong-Yi Chen and Jing-Ping Wu contributed equally to this work
[2] Department of Dermatology, Affiliated Hospital of Guangdong Medical College, No.57 Peoples Avenue South, Zhanjiang 524001, Guangdong, China
[6] Department of Dermatology, The Second Affiliated Hospital, Anhui Medical University Hefei, 678 Furong Road, Hefei 230601, Anhui, China
Full list of author information is available at the end of the article

system and SLE or SLE-like diseases have been partly proposed, including impaired clearance of immune complexes and apoptotic cells, abnormal development of B cell self-tolerance [8, 13]. In a recent study, it was shown that knockout C4 complement gene mice had a decreased frequency of Treg cells [14], which implies that C4 complement can promote differentiation of T lymphocyte to Tregs. C4-derived peptide has been demonstrated to inhibit Th1 cytokine production [15]. However, very few literatures have been emerging to elaborate the effects of C4 on Treg cells. Transforming growth factor-beta (TGF-β) is critical for the development and differentiation of Tregs, and it is an important indicator for reflecting the function and stabilization of Tregs [16]. In present study, we investigated whether C4 participated in T cells differentiation and the potential mechanism was also explored.

Methods

Subjects

Thirty SLE patients, with 10 female and 20 male, regularly followed up at the Second Affiliated Hospital of Anhui Medical University (from November 2012 to June 2014) were included in this study. The human study was approved by Ethics Committee of the Anhui Medical University and written informed consents were obtained from all patients. The clinical information including age, gender, duration of disease and concentrations of α-globulin, β-globulin, IgG, IgA and IgM were collected. The concentrations of α-globulin, β-globulin, IgG, IgA and IgM were detected.

Isolation and culture of T cells

The T cells were isolated from peripheral blood mononuclear cells (PBMCs) of healthy subjects. PBMCs were isolated by Ficoll density gradient centrifugation and collected to culture in RPMI1640 medium (Gibco, USA). Immuno-magnetic beads (Miltenyi Biotec, Germany) were used to isolate CD4+ T cells according to the manufacturer's instructions. The obtained T cells were cultured in RPIM1640 medium containing 10 % fetal bovine serum (Gibco, USA), penicillin–streptomycin (100 IU/ml and 100 μg/ml, Sigma, USA) and 2 mM L-glutamine (Sigma, USA). In addition, different concentrations (0, 250, 500 and 1000 μg/ml) of C4 were supplemented in medium to co-incubate with T cells for 7 days.

Isolation and culture of dendritic cells

The dendritic cells (DCs) were also isolated from peripheral blood of healthy subjects or SLE patients with C4 number <4 copies. Mononuclear cells were collected from the blood supernatant. RPMI1640 medium, containing 10 % autoserum (Gibco, USA) and 50 ng/ml rhIL-7 (R&D Systems, USA), was used to culture and induce differentiation of mononuclear cells for 24 h. In some experiments, 500 μg/ml complement C4 (Sigma-Aldrich, USA) was pre-treated with DCs for 48 h. Then C4 treated DCs were co-cultured with 2×10^4 freshly isolated CD4+ T cells in round-bottom 96-well culture plates for 7 days. In other experiments, DCs co-incubated with 2×10^4 freshly isolated CD4+ T cells in RPMI1640 medium containing 500 μg/ml complement C4 for 7 days.

Detection of serum complement C4 and TGFβ concentrations

The isolated serum from patients was stored at 80 °C. The serum C4 level was measured using a human ELISA kit (DRG-international, Germany). The TGF-β concentrations were also determined using commercial ELISA kit (R&D Systems, USA). All the experimental operations were performed according to the manufacturer's instructions.

Flow cytometry

T lymphocyte subsets were analyzed by flow cytometry (Beckman Coulter, USA). The cells were stained using PerCP-Cy5.5-labeled anti-human CD3 (eBioscience, USA) and fluorescein isothiocyanate (FITC)-labeled anti-human CD8 (eBioscience, USA). Treg cells were identified using FITC-labeled anti-human CD4 (eBioscience, USA). The various T lymphocyte subsets were calculated using the antibody signals of the specific proteins.

Real-time quantitative PCR

FlexiGene DNA Kit (Qiagen, Germany) was used to extract genomic DNA from human whole blood. TaqMan® Genotyping Master Mix (Applied Biosystems, USA) was used to quantify gene expression, with RNaseP (Applied Biosystems, USA) serving as reference genome. The C4 copy number was analyzed by CopyCaller™ Software.

The total mRNA of T cells was extracted with RNeasy kit (Invitrogen, USA). cDNA was synthesized using ImProm-II™ Reverse Transcription System (Promega, USA). The mRNA expression of FOXP3 was quantified by Applied Biosystems 7500 Real-Time PCR System (Applied Biosystems, USA) with Power SYBR® Green PCR Master Mix (Applied Biosystems, USA). The FOXP3 primers are as follows: forward 5′-AGGCTTCATCTG TGGCATCAT-3′; reverse 5′-CTTGCGGAACTCCAGC TCAT-3′. β-actin serves as the control gene to normalize the quantification of FOXP3. The primers of β-actin are as follows: forward 5′-CTCCATCCTGGCCTCGCTGT-3′; reverse 5′-GCTGTCACCTTCACCGTTCC-3′. $\Delta\Delta^{C_t}$ method was used to analyze the relative gene expression.

Statistical method

The results are given as mean ± standard error (SEM). Statistical significance among three experimental groups was assessed by ANOVO, and the difference between two experimental groups was assessed by independent-samples T test. Correlations between plasma complement C4 and Treg percentage/TGF-β were determined by Pearson correlation coefficient. All statistical analyses were performed using the SPSS 17.0. Significance was assumed at a p level of less than 5 %.

Results

Summary of study group characteristics and observed expressions

As shown in Table 1, the patients with C4 copy numbers <4 were matched with the patients with C4 copy numbers = 4 or C4 copy numbers >4 for sample number, and there were no significant differences in age, gender and duration of disease among three groups. The levels of α-globulin and γ-globulin in subjects with C4 copy numbers >4 were significantly decreased compared with subjects with C4 copy numbers <4. The concentrations of IgG, IgA and IgM were decreased with the increasing of C4 copy numbers. In addition, serum complement C4 concentrations were elevated with the increasing of C4 copy numbers.

Correlation of serum complement C4 concentration and Treg percentage

The serum Treg percentages of SLE patients were detected. As shown in Fig. 1a, the values of Treg percentage in patients with C4 < 4 copies, = 4 copies and >4 copies respectively were 0.62, 0.79 and 1.00. The Fig. 1b, c showed that peripheral serum C4 concentration was positively correlated with Treg percentage ($R^2 = 0.5907$, $p < 0.001$) and TGFβ concentration ($R^2 = 0.5641$, $p < 0.001$) respectively in SLE patients.

The effect of complement C4 on differentiation of T lymphocytes

Administrated T cells with complement C4 of different concentrations (DC:T = 1: 6) for 7 days, the CD4+CD25+FOXP3+Treg percentage was determined by Flow Cytometer. The results showed that there was no difference in CD4+CD25+FOXP3+Treg percentage between cells with or without complement C4 treatment (Fig. 2a, b). The differences of Foxp3 mRNA expression and TGFβ concentrations were not observed in cells treated with complement C4 of different dosages (Fig. 2c, d).

Complement C4 promotes T lymphocytes differentiation via DCs in healthy subjects

Isolated DCs from healthy subjects. Pre-incubated T lymphocytes with the DCs for 24 h, and then supplemented with 500 μg/ml complement C4 for 7 days. The results of Flow Cytometer showed that complement C4 significantly increased CD4+CD25+FOXP3+Treg percentage in cells pretreated with DCs. However, the effect was reversed by interference of CR1, a receptor of complement C4 (Fig. 3a, b). The concentration of TGFβ was also increased by complement C4 in T lymphocytes pre-incubated with DCs, and supplement of siRNA-CR1 decreased TGFβ concentration.

On the other hand, treated DCs (from healthy subjects) with 500 μg/ml complement C4 for 48 h, and then incubated with T lymphocytes for another 7 days. The data also shown that CD4+CD25+FOXP3+Treg cells

Table 1 Summary of study group characteristics and observed expressions

Variable	C4 copy numbers <4	C4 copy numbers = 4	C4 copy numbers >4
Number of samples (n)	10	10	10
Age (years)	52.4 ± 6.8	53.3 ± 4.9	51.8 ± 8.4
Gender, male/female (n)	7/3	6/4	7/3
Duration of disease (years)	3.5 ± 1.3	2.9 ± 0.9	2.7 ± 1.5
α-Globulin (g/cl)	0.72 ± 0.07	0.69 ± 0.05	0.59 ± 0.06*#
γ-Globulin (g/cl)	0.82 ± 0.11	0.71 ± 0.09*	0.70 ± 0.07*
IgG (mg/cl)	1459 ± 104	1302 ± 58*	1219 ± 49*#
IgA (mg/cl)	31.8 ± 4.9	26.5 ± 6.1*	20.6 ± 3.9*#
IgM (mg/cl)	32.5 ± 5.3	25.2 ± 4.18*	19.4 ± 2.0*#
Serum complement C4 (g/L)	49.3 ± 7.9	78.4 ± 12.3*	110.3 ± 15.2*#

Data are presented as the mean ± standard error of mean

Ig immunoglobulin

* $p < 0.05$, vs group (C4 copy numbers <4)

# $p < 0.05$, vs group (C4 copy numbers = 4)

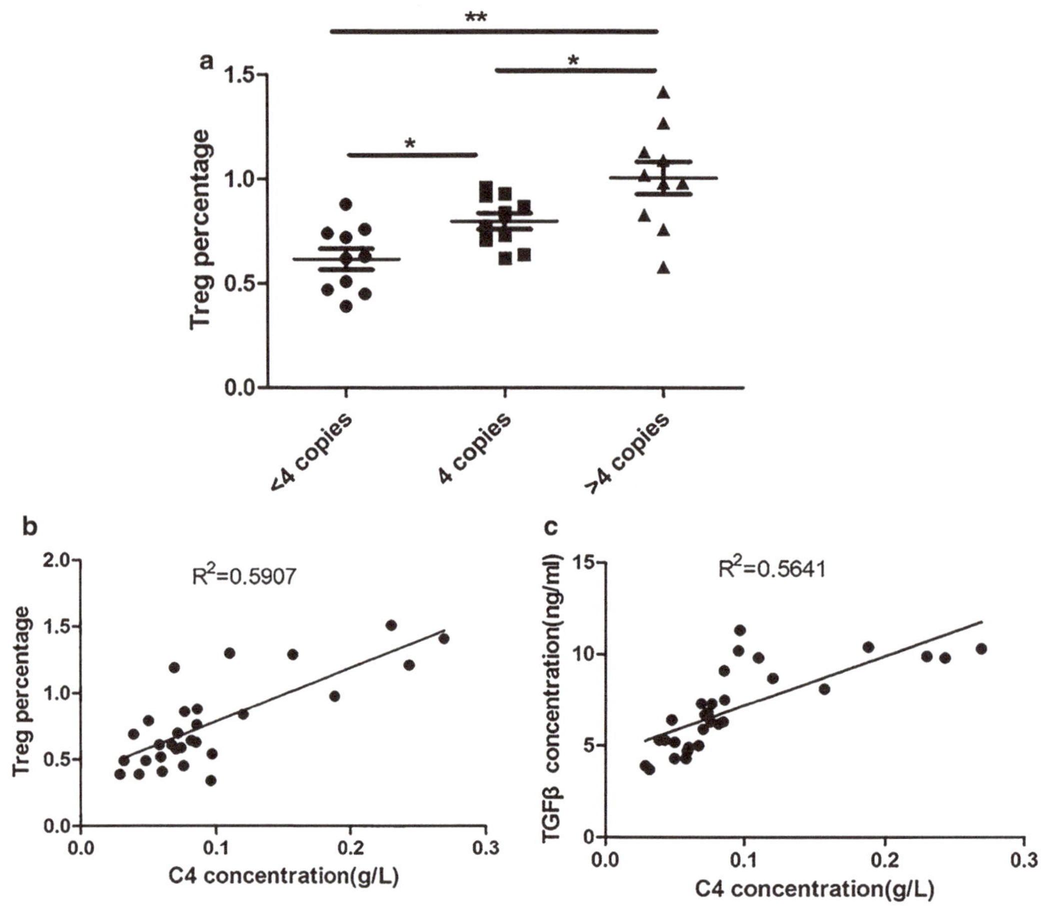

Fig. 1 The correlation between serum complement C4 concentration and Treg percentage. **a** The Treg percentage was detected by flow cytometry; n = 10; the data were expressed as mean ± standard error; *$p < 0.05$; **$p < 0.01$. **b** Spearman correlation was used to evaluate the relationship between Treg percentage and C4 concentration. **c** Spearman correlation was used to evaluate the relationship between Treg percentage and TGFβ concentration

percentage (Fig. 4a, b) and TGFβ concentration (Fig. 4c) were markedly elevated by DCs exposed to complement C4.

Complement C4 promotes T lymphocytes differentiation via DCs in SEL patients

Isolated DCs from SLE patients with C4 copy numbers <4. DCs were pre-treated with complement C4 before co-incubated with T lymphocytes. It was also observed that complement C4 significantly increased CD4+CD25+FOXP3+Treg cells percentage (Fig. 5a, b) and TGFβ concentration (Fig. 5c) via DCs.

Discussion

The complement system, exists in tissues and serum, is a part of immune system that helps or complements the ability of antibodies and phagocytic cells to clear pathogens from the organism [17]. C4 is one important component of complement system. The role of complement in SLE is complex. On one hand, complement is integral in the inflammatory reaction in SLE that results in tissue and organ damage. On another hand, the deficiency of complement is a strong risk factor to promote the development of SLE [8, 11, 13, 18]. However, it has been widely considered that complement system plays a protective role against the progression of SLE and other autoimmune disorders in normal subjects. In the present study, we found serum complement C4 concentrations were elevated with the increasing of C4 copy numbers. Waste disposal hypothesis, impaired immune complex processing and dysregulation of cytokines are proposed to explain the causal link between SLE and early classical pathway complement deficiencies [8, 19, 20]. While the exact mechanisms remain to be elucidated. We observed serum complement C4 in SLE patients was positively correlated with Treg percentage. The further studies confirmed that complement C4 modulated T cells differentiation by mediating DCs.

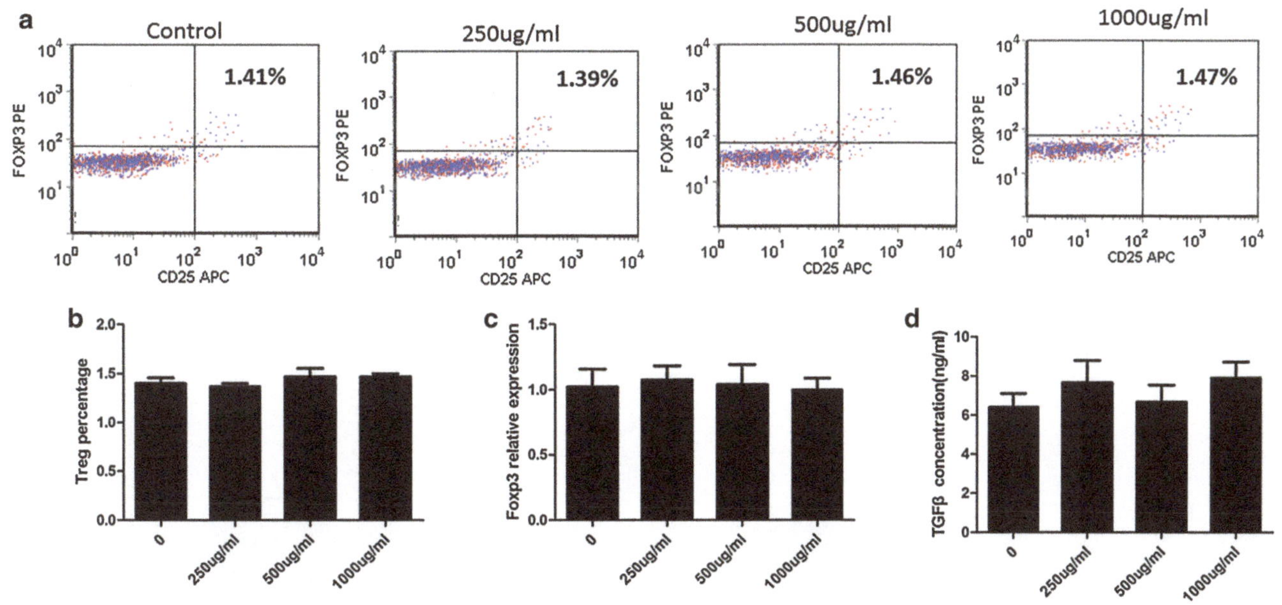

Fig. 2 The effect of complement C4 on differentiation of T lymphocytes. **a** Flow Cytometer was used to determine the CD4+CD25+FOXP3+Treg percentage. **b** The statistical result of Flow Cytometer was shown. **c** Real-time PCR was used to quantify Foxp3 relative mRNA expression. **d** TGFβ concentration of cells was determined by ELISA kit

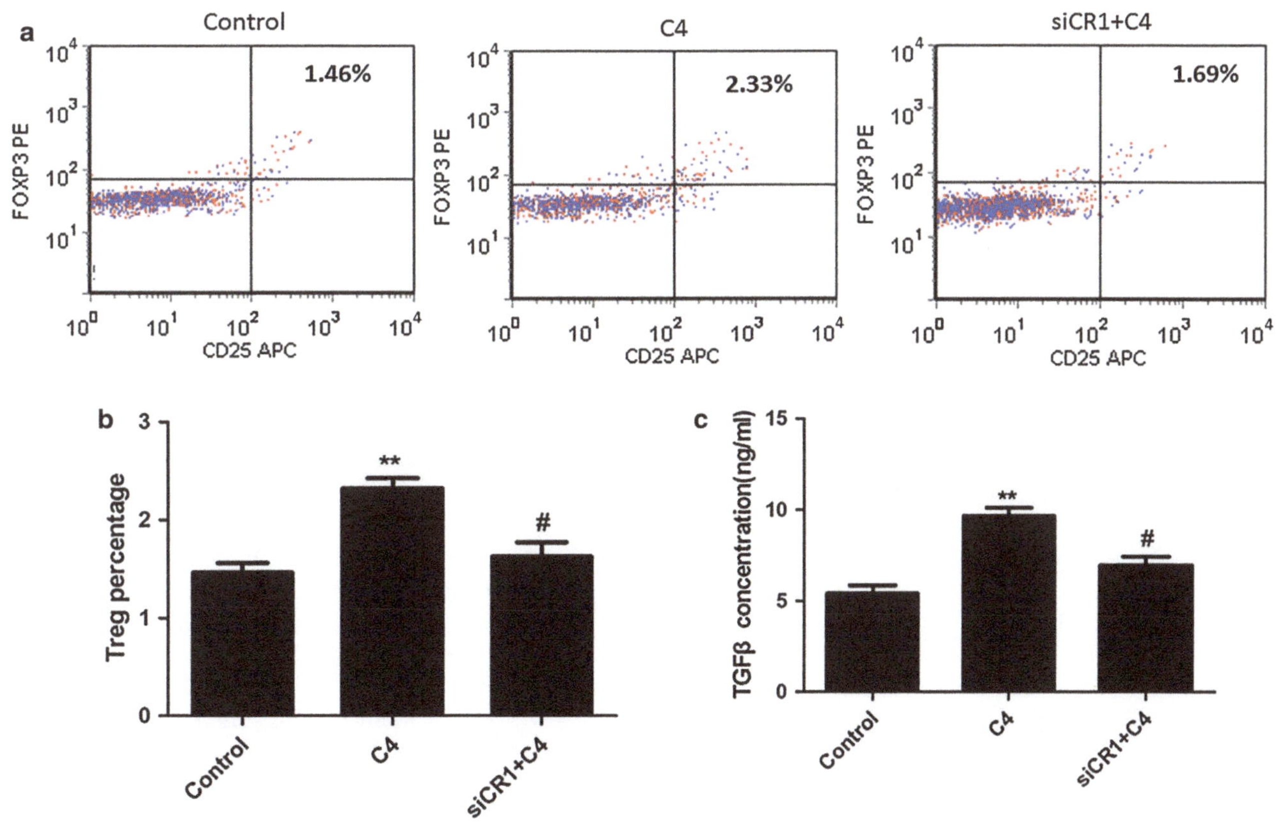

Fig. 3 Complement C4 promotes T lymphocytes differentiation via DCs. Pre-incubated T lymphocytes with DCs for 48 h, and then 500 µg/ml complement C4 was supplemented for 7 days. **a** Flow Cytometer was used to determine the CD4+CD25+FOXP3+Treg percentage. **b** The statistical result of Flow Cytometer was shown. **c** TGFβ concentration of cells was determined by ELISA kit. **$p < 0.01$ vs control; $^{\#}p < 0.05$ vs C4 group

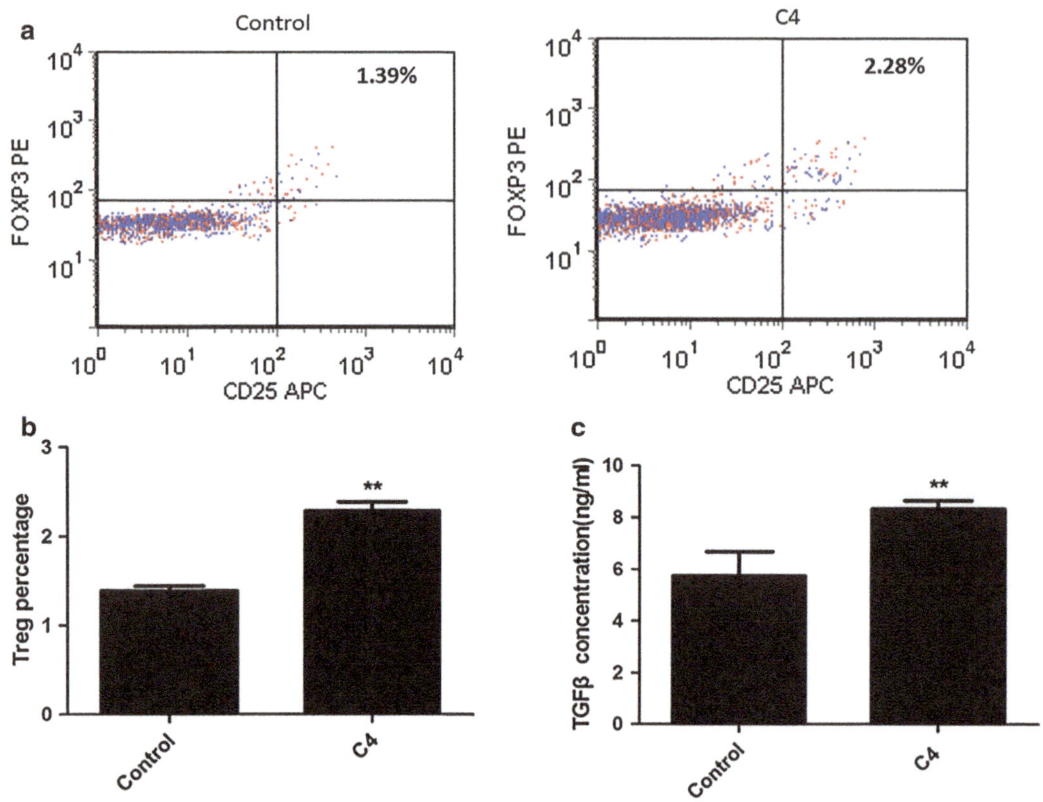

Fig. 4 Pretreating DCs from healthy subjects with complement C4 promotes T lymphocytes differentiation. Pre-incubated DCs (from healthy subjects) with 500 μg/ml complement C4 for 48 h, and then incubated with T lymphocytes for 7 days. **a** Flow Cytometer was used to determine the CD4+CD25+FOXP3+Treg percentage. **b** The statistical result of Flow Cytometer was shown. **c** TGFβ concentration of cells was determined by ELISA kit; $^{**}p < 0.01$ vs control

Tregs, commonly known as suppressor T cells, are a component of the immune system that suppress immune responses of other cells and prevent the onset of aberrant self-immune response [21, 22]. Recently, Tregs have been assessed in SEL patients [23–25]. The decreased Tregs number and impaired function are observed in SLE patients [26, 27]. However, it remains unknown whether Tregs are necessary for the pathophysiology of SLE, which is a very important topic for us and other investigators. In this study, the value of Treg percentage was elevated with the increase of serum C4 copy number in patients with SLE, which implied a close relationship between Treg cells and complement C4 level. However, administrated T cells with different concentrations of complement C4, no significant differences were observed in CD4+CD25+FOXP3+Treg population, FOXP3 mRNA and TGFβ concentrations compared with T cells without the treatment of complement C4. FOXP3 appears to function as a master regulator in the development and function of Treg cells [28]. TGFβ is known to be critical for the activation of Treg cells and the expression of FOXP3 [29], and it has been reported that low levels of TGFβ1 correlate with increased SLE disease activity [30]. The above results suggest that complement C4 is associated with Treg cells, but the role of complement C4 on Treg cells is not conducted directly.

There are two ways to have functions on Treg cells by complement, which including direct action and indirect action. William et al. demonstrated that targeting C3a/C3aR and C5a/C5aR interactions could facilitate iTreg-mediated tolerance to alloantigens in humans [31]. Our in vitro study demonstrated that it was not through direct action in C4 induced Treg cells differentiation. Sacks et al. found C5aR activates naïve CD4+ Th cells to undergo differentiation not only to IL-17 producing T helper (Th17) cells but also to Treg via a TGFβ dependent pathway [32]. Recent studies form human and animals provide the evidences for the role of IL-17 and Th17 cells in the pathogenesis of SLE [33, 34]. Therefore, we supposed C4 maybe have effect on promoting Treg cells differentiation via DCs. We found that T cells, co-incubated with DCs and then administrated with complement C4,

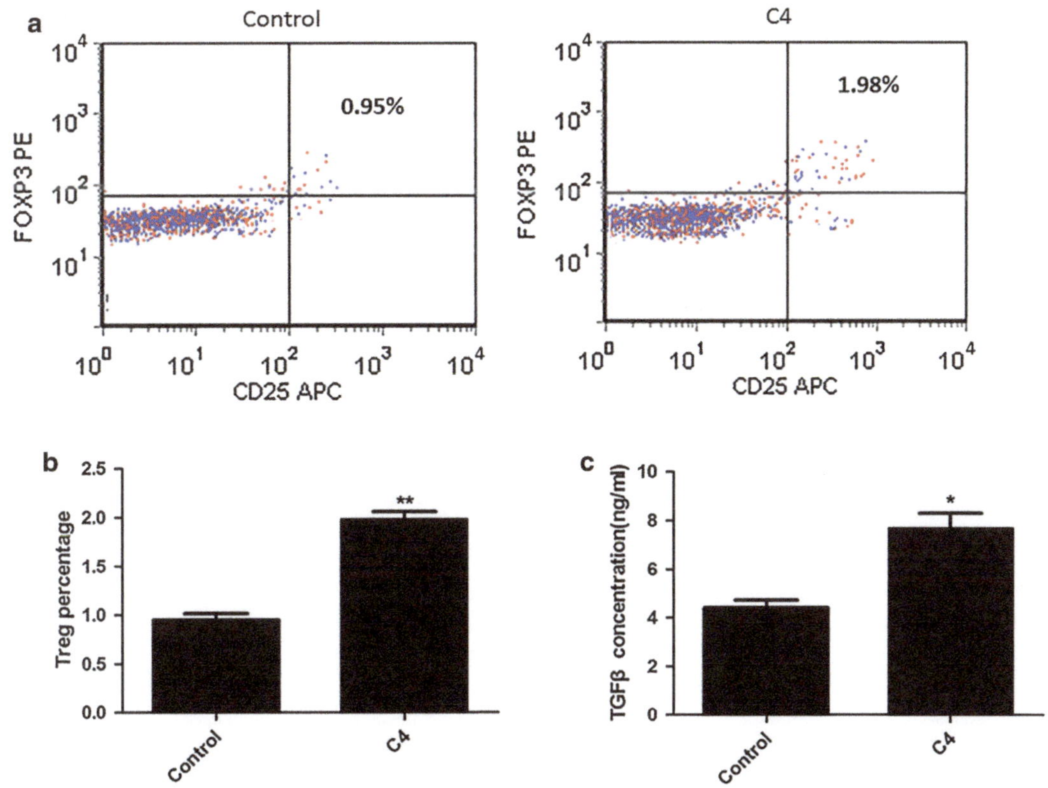

Fig. 5 Pretreating DCs from SLE patients with C4 copy numbers <4 with complement C4 promotes T lymphocytes differentiation. Pre-incubated DCs (from SLE patients with C4 copy numbers <4) with 500 μg/ml complement C4 for 48 h, and then incubated with T lymphocytes for 7 days. **a** Flow Cytometer was used to determine the CD4+CD25+FOXP3+Treg percentage; **b** the statistical result of Flow Cytometer was shown; **c** TGFβ concentration of cells was determined by ELISA kit; **p < 0.01 vs control

had a higher level of CD4+CD25+FOXP3+Treg percentage and TGFβ concentration. In addition, DCs pretreated with complement C4 before co-incubated with T cells, the similar results were observed. These data suggested that DCs took part in mediating T cells differentiation induced by complement C4. Complement receptor type 1 (CR1), the receptor of complement C4, serves as the main system for processing and clearance of complement opsonized immune complexes [35]. Inhibiting CR1 of T cells, which were co-incubated with DCs and then administrated with C4, showed the decreased levels of CD4+CD25+FOXP3+Treg percentage and TGFβ concentration. The data confirmed that C4 mediated the T cells differentiation.

In summary, we found C4 takes part in T cells differentiation to Treg cells via DCs, suggesting that Treg cells serve as the target therapy in preventing or controlling immune-mediated inflammatory disorders. Knowledge about Tregs and C4 and other regulatory cytokines provides new insights in the pathogenesis of SLE. The new lines of investigation for SLE treatment concerning Tregs and C4 will be opened in the near future.

Authors' contributions

HC and RC conceived and designed the experiments, carried out the molecular genetic studies. JW and LC carried out the immunoassays and participated in the sequence alignment. YL, HP and ZP participated in the design of the study and performed the statistical analysis. QZ, QL and TD conceived of the study, and contributed to reagents, and YL and JS drafted the manuscript. All authors read and approved the final manuscript.

Author details

[1] Teaching Hospital of Chengdu University of TCM, Chengdu 610072, Sichuan, China. [2] Department of Dermatology, Affiliated Hospital of Guangdong Medical College, No.57 Peoples Avenue South, Zhanjiang 524001, Guangdong, China. [3] Laboratory Animal Center, Anhui Medical University, Hefei 230032, Anhui, China. [4] Department of Dermatology, Nanfang Hospital, Southern Medical University, Guangzhou 510515, Guangdong, China. [5] Department of Epidemiology and Biostatistics, School of Public Health, Anhui Medical University, Hefei 230032, Anhui, China. [6] Department of Dermatology, The Second Affiliated Hospital, Anhui Medical University Hefei, 678 Furong Road, Hefei 230601, Anhui, China.

Acknowledgements

This work was supported by National Natural Science Foundation of China Grant 81201226 and 81472880.

Competing interests

The authors declare that they have no competing interests.

References

1. Poole BD, Niewold TB, Tsokos GC. Cytokines in systemic lupus erythematosus 2011. J Biomed Biotechnol. 2012;2012:427824.
2. Tsokos GC. Systemic lupus erythematosus. N Engl J Med. 2011;365:2110–21.
3. Thornton AM, Shevach EM. CD4+CD25+ immunoregulatory T cells suppress polyclonal T cell activation in vitro by inhibiting interleukin 2 production. J Exp Med. 1998;188:287–96.
4. McNally A, Hill GR, Sparwasser T, Thomas R, Steptoe RJ. CD4+CD25+ regulatory T cells control CD8+ T-cell effector differentiation by modulating IL-2 homeostasis. Proc Natl Acad Sci USA. 2011;108:7529–34.
5. Lim HW, Hillsamer P, Banham AH, Kim CH. Cutting edge: direct suppression of B cells by CD4+ CD25+ regulatory T cells. J Immunol. 2005;175:4180–3.
6. Lyssuk EY, Torgashina AV, Soloviev SK, Nassonov EL, Bykovskaia SN. Reduced number and function of CD4+CD25 high FoxP3+ regulatory T cells in patients with systemic lupus erythematosus. Adv Exp Med Biol. 2007;601:113–9.
7. Bonelli M, Savitskaya A, von Dalwigk K, Steiner CW, Aletaha D, Smolen JS, et al. Quantitative and qualitative deficiencies of regulatory T cells in patients with systemic lupus erythematosus (SLE). Int Immunol. 2008;20:861–8.
8. Bryan AR, Wu EY. Complement deficiencies in systemic lupus erythematosus. Curr Allergy Asthma Rep. 2014;14:448.
9. Sturfelt G. The complement system in systemic lupus erythematosus. Scand J Rheumatol. 2002;31:129–32.
10. Watanabe H, Sugimoto M, Asano T, Sato S, Suzuki E, Takahashi A, et al. Relationship of complement activation route with clinical manifestations in Japanese patients with systemic lupus erythematosus: a retrospective observational study. Mod Rheumatol Jpn Rheum Assoc 2015;25:205-9.
11. Hagen JP, Muller PC, Bredius RG, ten Cate R. Low complement levels in paediatric systemic lupus erythematosus and the risk of bacteraemia. BMJ Case Rep 2013;2013. doi:10.1136/bcr-2013-010378
12. Yang Y, Chung EK, Wu YL, Savelli SL, Nagaraja HN, Zhou B, et al. Gene copy-number variation and associated polymorphisms of complement component C4 in human systemic lupus erythematosus (SLE): low copy number is a risk factor for and high copy number is a protective factor against SLE susceptibility in European Americans. Am J Hum Genet. 2007;80:1037–54.
13. Sturfelt G, Truedsson L. Complement and its breakdown products in SLE. Rheumatology (Oxford, England). 2005;44:1227–32.
14. Leaungwutiwong P, Ittiprasert W, Saikhun K, Tong-Ngam P, Akapirat S, Chattanadee S, et al. Impairment of CD4+CD25+ regulatory T cells in C4-deficient mice. Asian Pacific J Allergy Immunol Launched Allergy Immunol Soc Thail. 2011;29:220–8.
15. Takeda Y, Kaneda K, Jimma F, Shiobara N, Saniabadi AR, Wakabayashi I. Suppression of Th1 cytokine production by a peptide derived from C4b. Inflamm Res. 2013;62:951–9.
16. Horwitz DA, Zheng SG, Wang J, Gray JD. Critical role of IL-2 and TGF-β in generation, function and stabilization of Foxp3+CD4+ Treg. Eur J Immunol. 2008;38:912–5.
17. Chen M, Daha MR, Kallenberg CG. The complement system in systemic autoimmune disease. J Autoimmun. 2010;34:J276–86.
18. Wu YL, Hauptmann G, Viguier M, Yu CY. Molecular basis of complete complement C4 deficiency in two North-African families with systemic lupus erythematosus. Genes Immun. 2009;10:433–45.
19. Gullstrand B, Mårtensson U, Sturfelt G, Bengtsson AA, Truedsson L. Complement classical pathway components are all important in clearance of apoptotic and secondary necrotic cells. Clin Exp Immunol. 2009;156:303–11.
20. Lood C, Gullstrand B, Truedsson L, Olin AI, Alm GV, Rönnblom L, Sturfelt G, et al. C1q inhibits immune complex-induced interferon-alpha production in plasmacytoid dendritic cells: a novel link between C1q deficiency and systemic lupus erythematosus pathogenesis. Arthritis Rheum. 2009;60(10):3081–90.
21. Sakaguchi S, Miyara M, Costantino CM, Hafler DA. FOXP3+ regulatory T cells in the human immune system. Nat Rev Immunol. 2010;10:490–500.
22. Shevach EM. Mechanisms of foxp3+ T regulatory cell-mediated suppression. Immunity. 2009;30:636–45.
23. Gerli R, Nocentini G, Alunno A, Bocci EB, Bianchini R, Bistoni O, et al. Identification of regulatory T cells in systemic lupus erythematosus. Autoimmun Rev. 2009;8:426–30.
24. Pan X, Yuan X, Zheng Y, Wang W, Shan J, Lin F, et al. Increased CD45RA+ FoxP3(low) regulatory T cells with impaired suppressive function in patients with systemic lupus erythematosus. PLoS One. 2012;7:e34662.
25. Tu H, Li Q, Xiang S, Jiang H, Mao Y, Shou Z, et al. Dual effects of statins therapy in systemic lupus erythematosus and SLE-related atherosclerosis: the potential role for regulatory T cells. Atherosclerosis. 2012;222:29–33.
26. Lyssuk EY, Torgashina AV, Soloviev SK, Nassonov EL, Bykovskaia SN. Reduced number and function of CD4+CD25highFoxP3+ regulatory T cells in patients with systemic lupus erythematosus. Adv Exp Med Biol. 2007;601:113–9.
27. Golding A, Hasni S, Illei G, Shevach EM. The percentage of FoxP3+Helios+ Treg cells correlates positively with disease activity in systemic lupus erythematosus. Arthritis Rheum. 2013;65:2898–906.
28. Zhang L, Zhao Y. The regulation of Foxp3 expression in regulatory CD4(+)CD25(+) T cells: multiple pathways on the road. J Cell Physiol. 2007;211:590–7.
29. Chen W, Jin W, Hardegen N, Lei K-J, Li L, Marinos N, et al. Conversion of peripheral CD4+CD25- naive T cells to CD4+CD25+ regulatory T cells by TGF-beta induction of transcription factor Foxp3. J Exp Med. 2003;198:1875–86.
30. Becker-Merok A, Eilertsen GO, Nossent JC. Levels of transforming growth factor-beta are low in systemic lupus erythematosus patients with active disease. J Rheumatol. 2010;37:2039–45.
31. van der Touw W, Cravedi P, Kwan W-h, Paz-Artal E, Merad M, Heeger PS. Cutting edge: Receptors for C3a and C5a modulate stability of alloantigen-reactive induced regulatory T cells. J Immunol (Baltimore, Md: 1950). 2013;190:5921–5.
32. Sacks SH. Complement fragments C3a and C5a: the salt and pepper of the immune response. Eur J Immunol. 2010;40:668–70.
33. Chen XQ, Yu YC, Deng HH, Sun JZ, Dai Z, Wu YW, et al. Plasma IL-17A is increased in new-onset SLE patients and associated with disease activity. J Clin Immunol. 2010;30:221–5.
34. Martin JC, Baeten DL, Josien R. Emerging role of IL-17 and Th17 cells in systemic lupus erythematosus. Clin Immunol (Orlando, Fla). 2014;154:1–12.
35. Singh V, Mahoney JA, Petri M. Erythrocyte C4d and complement receptor 1 in systemic lupus erythematosus. The Journal of rheumatology. 2008;35:1989–93.

21

Deoxyinosine repair in nuclear extracts of human cells

Chia-Chia Lee[1], Ya-Chien Yang[1,2], Steven D. Goodman[3], Shi Chen[1], Teng-Yung Huang[1], Wern-Cherng Cheng[2], Liang-In Lin[1,2] and Woei-horng Fang[1,2*]

Abstract

Background: Deamination of adenine can occur spontaneously under physiological conditions generating the highly mutagenic lesion, hypoxanthine. This process is enhanced by ROS from exposure of DNA to ionizing radiation, UV light, nitrous acid, or heat. Hypoxanthine in DNA can pair with cytosine which results in A:T to G:C transition mutations after DNA replication. In *Escherichia coli*, deoxyinosine (hypoxanthine deoxyribonucleotide, dI) is removed through an alternative excision repair pathway initiated by endonuclease V. However, the correction of dI in mammalian cells appears more complex and was not fully understood.

Results: All four possible dI-containing heteroduplex DNAs, including A-I, C-I, G-I, and T-I were introduced to repair reactions containing extracts from human cells. The repair reaction requires magnesium, dNTPs, and ATP as cofactors. We found G-I was the best substrate followed by T-I, A-I and C-I, respectively. Moreover, judging from the repair requirements and sensitivity to specific polymerase inhibitors, there were overlapping repair activities in processing of dI in DNA. Indeed, a hereditable non-polyposis colorectal cancer cell line (HCT116) demonstrated lower dI repair activity that was partially attributed to lack of mismatch repair.

Conclusions: A plasmid-based convenient and non-radioisotopic method was created to study dI repair in human cells. Mutagenic dI lesions processed in vitro can be scored by restriction enzyme cleavage to evaluate the repair. The repair assay described in this study provides a good platform for further investigation of human repair pathways involved in dI processing and their biological significance in mutation prevention.

Keywords: Deoxyinosine repair, Mismatch repair, Human cell extracts, In vitro assay, DNA repair deficiency

Background

Deoxyinosine (hypoxanthine deoxyribonucleotide, dI) in DNA can arise from spontaneous deamination of deoxyadenosine residue, and is also induced by ROS produced from normal aerobic respiration. In addition, exposure of DNA to ionizing radiation, UV light, nitrous acid, or heat can promote the formation of dI [1, 2]. Alternatively, dI can be introduced by misincorporation of dITP in the nucleotide pool during replication [3, 4]. Deoxyinosine derived from deamination of deoxyadenosine in DNA is potentially mutagenic since it prefers to pair with dCTP during replication, yielding A:T to G:C transition mutations at sites of adenine deamination [5].

In mammalian cells, base excision repair (BER) was thought to be the major pathway for dI repair. The excision of base damage is initiated by a specific DNA glycosylase: Hypoxanthine is bound and excised efficiently by human *N*-methylpurine-DNA glycosylase (MPG, also known as AAG, ANPG, APNG, or MDG) [6]. From radionucleotide incorporation fine mapping, the resulting apurinic/apyrimidinic (AP) sites are further processed by both the short patch pathway (1-nucleotide gap filling) with DNA polymerase (Pol) β and the long patch pathway (2-6 nucleotide resynthesis) with Pol δ and PCNA [7].

In *Escherichia coli*, early studies indicated that the DNA glycosylase encoded by *alkA* gene could recognize and release hypoxanthine residues from DNA [1]. However,

*Correspondence: whfang@ntu.edu.tw
[1] Department of Clinical Laboratory Sciences and Medical Biotechnology, College of Medicine, National Taiwan University, #7, Chung-Shan South Road, Taipei 10002, Taiwan, ROC
Full list of author information is available at the end of the article

subsequent in vivo and in vitro studies showed that DNA glycosylase initiated BER is not the major pathway to process dI in *E. coli* [8, 9]. The repair pathway initiated by endonuclease V (EndoV, encoded by *nfi* gene [10]) was shown to be the major pathway for dI processing both in vivo and in vitro [8, 9, 11]. A mutagenesis assay also showed that under HNO_2 treatment, which will promote hypoxanthine formation, that a *nfi* mutant demonstrated over a 200-fold increase in mutation frequency, while the *alkA* mutant did not significantly increase the mutation frequency under the same experimental conditions [12].

Endonuclease V (EndoV) in *E. coli* is active upon DNA exposed to UV light, OsO4, acids, or X-rays [10]. This enzyme was later characterized as 3′-deoxyinosine endonuclease that incises the DNA at the second phosphodiester bond 3′ to the dI lesion, leaving 3′-OH and 5′-P termini [13]. *Nfi* homologues from *Thermotoga maritima* possess 3′-exonuclease activity that might be used for removal of damaged bases [14], but similar exonuclease activities were not found in EndoV from *E. coli* and mammalian cells. Therefore, additional enzymes are required to excise the dI lesions in the EndoV-mediated repair process. In our previous study, we found DNA pol I played dual roles in both repair synthesis and using its 3′-5′ proofreading exonuclease to remove EndoV incised dI lesion [9, 11].

A mammalian homologue of *E. coli nfi* gene was identified and characterized [15]. The mouse EndoV seems to be active only on dI, while bacterial EndoV exhibits broad substrate spectrum. Furthermore, expression of mouse EndoV in an *alkA*, and *nfi* double mutant *E. coli* strain significantly suppresses the spontaneous mutagenesis frequency, which suggested that this eukaryotic EndoV initiates an alternative excision repair pathway for dI correction [15]. A biochemical analysis of purified human EndoV showed it favored dI-containing DNA but with only a minor preference on deoxyxanthosine-containing DNA [16]. Expression of hEndoV in *E. coli* cells deficient in *nfi, mug* and *ung* genes caused 3-fold reduction in mutation frequency [16]. However, recent reports demonstrated efficient cleavage of inosine-containing RNA by human EndoV [17] suggesting that hEndoV may involve in RNA editing [18]. Therefore, the full involvement of hEndoV in dI repair in human cells is still unknown.

The major function of mismatch repair (MMR) is its role in correction of nucleotide base misincorporation during replication [19–21], which requires that repair be directed to a newly synthesized DNA strand. A strand-specific nick or gap is sufficient to direct MMR in extracts of mammalian cell extracts, and an obvious possibility is that DNA termini that occur naturally at the replication fork serve as the strand signals that direct the reaction in the eukaryotic cell [19]. Several purified systems have been reconstituted using near homogeneous human proteins and support 3′- and/or 5′-directed mismatch-provoked excision or repair. According to the current model, the mismatch recognition activities MutS-α (MSH2·MSH6 heterodimer) or MutS-β (MSH2·MSH3 heterodimer), MutL-α (MLH1·PMS2 heterodimer), RPA (replication protein A), the 5′–3′ double-strand hydrolytic activity exonuclease 1 (Exo1) [19], the replication clamp proliferating cell nuclear antigen (PCNA) and the clamp loader replication factor C (RFC) yields a system that supports mismatch-provoked excision directed by a 3′ or 5′ strand break, and where hydrolysis is attenuated upon mismatch removal [19].

The roles and sequence events utilizing each of the aforementioned proteins have at least been partially elucidated. RPA plays a primary role in terminating excision by MutS-α-activated Exo1; additionally high mobility group protein B1 (HMGB1) was found to substitute for RPA [19]. MutL-α is a latent endonuclease that is activated in a manner that depends on a mismatch, MutS-α, RFC, PCNA, ATP and a strand break. While the function of RFC in MutL-α activation is apparently restricted to clamp loading, the PCNA loading orientation determines the strand direction of MutL-α incision, targeting endonuclease action to the heteroduplex strand that contains a preexisting break [22, 23]. Incision in this manner introduces additional breaks, providing a 5′ nick that serves as a loading site for MutS-α-activated Exo1, which removes the mismatch. Upon completion of the mismatch excision process [24], DNA pol δ synthesizes DNA in the place of the excised sequence and DNA ligase I then joining any nicks in the DNA sequence [21]. While this human mismatch repair pathway may recognize base analogs and damaged bases [25] our previous attempts to show in vitro processing of a dI containing heteroduplexes by bacterial MutHLS mismatch repair pathway was insignificant [9, 11]. However the possibility of overlapping repair activities for dI process in human mismatch repair was not tested.

In this study a convenient and non-radioisotopic method was used to study dI repair in mammalian cells. Specifically, we took advantage of a functional assay that uses DNA substrates containing a dI residing in the recognition site or cleavage site of restriction enzymes. Substrates processed by human cell-free extracts can be scored by restriction enzyme cleavage to evaluate the repair of dI. We found that all four dI lesions of A-I, C-I, G-I and T-I can be processed by human extracts with different efficiencies. We also performed a comparative examination of repair requirements of different dI containing substrates in vitro and the results indicated that there were overlapping activities of several repair pathways in processing of dI in DNA.

Results

Deoxyinosine-containing substrates are efficiently processed in Hela cell extracts

Previously, to evaluate EndoV repair system in *E. coli*, we constructed a set of dI-containing substrates A-I, G-I and T-I heteroduplexes [9, 11]. In these substrates, a dI resided in a disrupted restriction endonuclease recognition or cleavage site (Fig. 1). We employed a restriction endonuclease assay to score for the repair of dI. In the presence of dI lesion, heteroduplex DNA is refractory to restriction endonuclease cleavage. After in vitro repair the specific restriction endonuclease recognition sequence was restored and repair level can be scored by the extent of restriction digestion [9, 11]. In this study, we added newly constructed C-I substrate (Fig. 1) to this assay platform and extended our study to determine the dI repair efficiency in human nuclear extracts.

We first tested G-I repair in nuclear extracts from a HeLa cell line. In a preliminary trial, reaction conditions for both *E. coli* dI repair [9, 11] and human MMR [26] were tested. To our surprise, the G-I substrate was only marginally repaired by human nuclear extracts in reaction buffer for *E. coli* dI repair (Fig. 2a, 0 mM entry), but in human MMR reaction buffer, it was efficiently corrected (Fig. 2a, 1 mM entry). The major difference in these two reaction buffers was human MMR buffer contained 1 mM ATP while *E. coli* dI repair buffer contained no ATP. We therefore did an ATP titration experiment as shown in Fig. 2a. We found the presence of ATP could stimulate human dI repair. The highest level of correction occurred at a concentration of 2 mM ATP; higher ATP concentrations (>2 mM) caused extensive degradation of DNA and therefore inhibited the repair (Fig. 2a). We also performed a Mg^{2+} titration experiment as shown in Fig. 2b. The best repair level was at 2.5 mM, while higher Mg^{2+} concentrations were inhibitory.

A time course showing the amount of repaired products of a G-I heteroduplex when incubated with HeLa extracts is shown in Fig. 2c, d. Digestion of the unprocessed heteroduplex G-I with AlwNI and XhoI, whose recognition sequence for XhoI is blocked by the presence of dI lesion, will yield a 7.2-kb linear fragment only (Fig. 2c, 0 min). However, digestion of DNA with both enzymes in which the XhoI recognition sequence has been restored by repair will yield 4.1- and 3.1-kb fragments (Fig. 2c, 10–60 min). The repair efficiency can be determined by measurement of band intensity (Fig. 2d).

Although higher ATP concentrations (1.5–2 mM in Fig. 2a) and lower Mg^{2+} (2.5 mM in Fig. 1b) showed better dI repair activity, we decided using conventional human MMR reaction buffer containing 1 mM ATP and 5 mM Mg^{2+} for standard dI repair assay in order to compare dI correction versus human MMR activities described in the subsequent section. As shown in Table 1, in human MMR buffer, A-I, C-I, G-I and T-I can be repaired with different efficiencies. The G-I heteroduplex was most efficiently corrected, and followed by T-I, A-I, and C-I substrates. The levels of repair were about 25–60 % of our previous observed bacterial reactions [9, 11].

Reaction requirements of dI repair in human extracts

In human dI repair, we adopted reaction conditions of in vitro human mismatch repair for comparison. It is known that in vitro human mismatch repair requires the addition of $MgCl_2$, ATP and the four dNTPs [27]. In order to understand if all of these components are essential for dI repair, we systematically omitted the exogenous cofactors in separate reactions. As shown in Table 1, in the absence of Mg^{2+}, the repair efficiency of all four dI substrates were reduced below the level of detection in HeLa extracts, which is consistent with that Mg^{2+} being an essential cofactor for most DNA repair enzymes [7, 15, 27]. In the absence of exogenous dNTPs, the repair levels dropped to less than one-third of the standard reactions. The cell-free extracts prepared for this study may contain trace amount of dNTPs [26] and may contribute to these residual repair levels.

In the absence of exogenous ATP, the relative repair levels of each substrate showed variable degrees of decreasing activity when compared to standard ones (Table 1, HeLa entries). This is in contrast to our previous studies in *E. coli* where ATP was not required in bacterial dI repair [9, 11]. This effect might be caused by the fact that the human system employs multiple ATP-dependent repair proteins, for example, human uses ATP-dependent DNA ligase while *E. coli* uses NAD^+-dependent ligase, respectively. The low level repair in the absence of exogenous ATP might be due to trace amounts of ATP in the cell-free extracts we prepared. Thus the increase in repair by addition of exogenous ATP might be due to insufficient ATP levels for some of the repair proteins. To clarify the role of ATP in the reaction, ATPγS, an ATP analog that is resistant to hydrolysis, was included in the reactions. In the G-I repair reaction, omitting ATP and addition of ATPγS showed a similar limiting of repair (Table 1). However, the repair efficiency of T-I substrates with HeLa extracts showed an extensive reduction when exogenous ATP was replaced by ATPγS in the repair reactions, with the repair levels in ATPγS reactions being even lower than the reactions omitting ATP. Therefore, the presence of an ATP cofactor and its hydrolysis were likely both essential for human T-I lesion repair. To determine if the ATP dependence was nucleotide triphosphate specific, we also tested the effects of exogenous GTP addition from 0.5 to 2 mM to G-I repair reactions; no

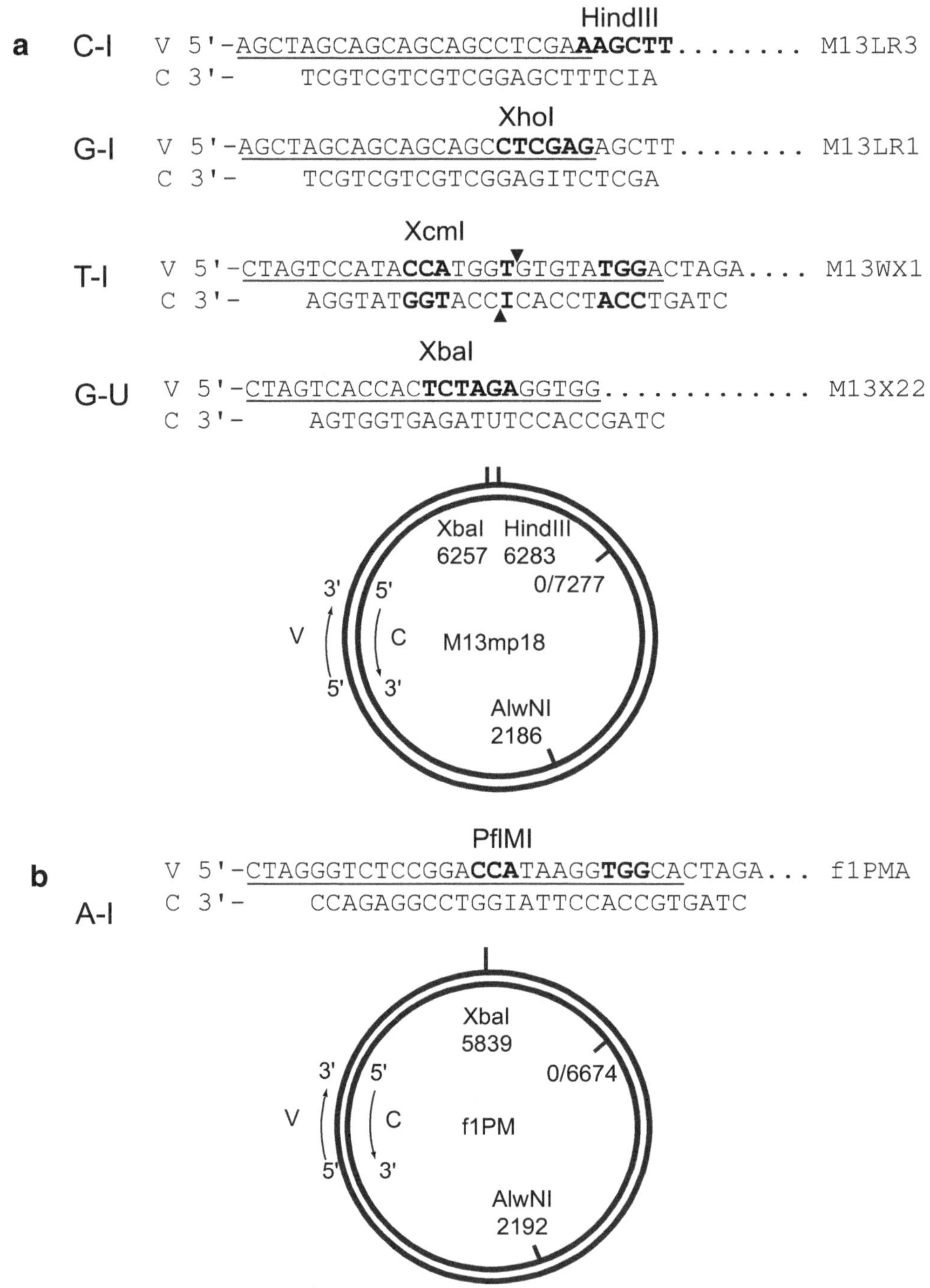

Fig. 1 Map of M13mp18 and f1PM based heteroduplex substrates. **a** The map of bacteriophage M13mp18 replicative form (RF) DNA shows restriction enzyme sites relevant to this study with derivatives M13LR1 and M13LR3 containing 22-bp insertions at the unique HindIII restriction site, and phage M13WX1 and M13X22 containing 26-bp and 22-bp insertions at *XbaI* site respectively. **b** The map of bacteriophage f1PM RF DNA with its derivative f1PMA with a 27-bp insertion at *XbaI*. 'V', phage viral strand. 'C', phage complementary strand. Underlines beneath each viral strand are the original insertion sequences. The C-strand from parental phage RF DNA was paired with viral strand of its insertion derivative to produce gapped duplex DNA, and the gap was sealed with dI or deoxyuridine containing synthetic oligodeoxyribonucleotide. A-I, C-I, G-I, T-I, and G-U are the resulting substrates and DNA sequence shown on each C-strand of the the synthetic linker used. In the presence of dI, the substrates were refractory to the restriction endonuclease scoring. After the repair, DNA products become sensitive to restriction endonuclease cleavage. The recognition sequence of corresponding restriction endonuclease markers for repair products are shown in bold on V-strands

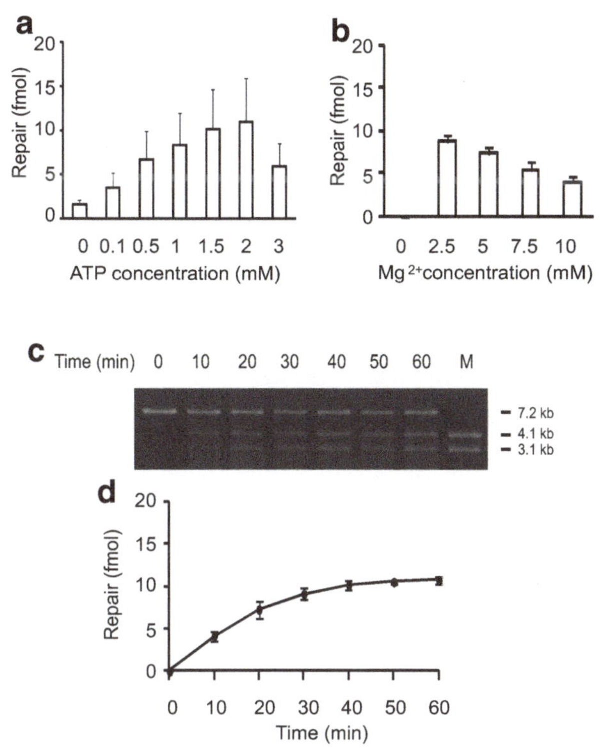

Fig. 2 ATP, Mg^{++} titrations and time course of G-I repair in human nuclear extracts. Each reaction contained 90 μg HeLa extracts and 21 fmol G-I substrate. **a** Repair reactions with HeLa extracts were determined as described in Methods except that where indicated ATP was added. **b** Repair reaction with HeLa extracts were performed as described in Methods except where indicated Mg^{2+} was added. **c** Reactions were performed under standard conditions and scaled; 10-μl samples were removed as indicated. DNA products were digested with AlwNI and XhoI and then subjected to agarose gel electrophoresis to score for the repair of dI lesion. The bar pointing to the 7.2-kb fragment represents unrepaired substrate linearized with AlwNI; size marker (M) of 4.1 and 3.1-kb fragments are indicative of repaired products that were generated by treatment of M13LR1 with AlwNI and XhoI. **d** Quantitative analysis of the time course reaction, the error bars represent S.D. from three determinations

obvious change of repair levels with GTP addition was observed compared to conditions without exogenous ATP (data not shown).

Both aphidicolin- and lithocholic acid-sensitive DNA polymerases were involved in correcting dI in mammalian cells

Several classes of DNA polymerases have been identified in different DNA repair pathways. For example, pol δ is involved in MMR [28, 29], nucleotide excision repair [30, 31] and long-patched BER [32] pathways. In classic mammalian short-patched BER pathway, pol β is responsible for the repair DNA synthesis [33, 34]. In order to evaluate the involvement of DNA polymerases in repairing dI, an inhibitor targeting pol α, δ and ε was added into the repair reactions. Aphidicolin has been found to block the repair DNA synthesis in MMR system [26, 27]. The repair of C-I was not sensitive to aphidicolin inhibition (Fig. 3a). The repair of G-I, T-I, and A-I were significantly reduced by addition of aphidicolin at the concentration of 30 μM in HeLa extract-containing repair reactions (Fig. 3a). However, as the concentration of aphidicolin increased to above 90 μM, at which pol δ dependent MMR should be abolished [26, 27], relatively high levels of residual dI repair remained. This observation suggested both aphidicolin-sensitive and aphidicolin-resistant DNA polymerases participating dI lesions repair, in addition to possible overlapping repair mechanisms for dI repair in human cells.

Deoxyinosine was thought to be repaired by base excision repair in mammalian cells [35, 36]. In classic mammalian short-patched BER pathway, pol β is responsible for the repair DNA synthesis. A bile acid derivative lithocholic acid (LCA) can bind to pol β and disrupts its AP lyase ability to block the DNA replication functions, with the *Ki* value of 10 μM [37]. We therefore introduced this DNA polymerase β inhibitor into dI repair reactions in human extracts. As shown in Fig. 3B, the repair levels

Table 1 Repair requirement of dI-containing heteroduplex in extracts from MMR-proficient and MMR-deficient mammalian cells

Reaction condition	Repair levels (fmol)							
	HeLaS3				HCT116			
	G-I	T-I	A-I	C-I	G-I	T-I	A-I	C-I
Standard	7.6 ± 1.3	3.8 ± 0.8	3.0 ± 0.6	2.4 ± 0.2	3.2 ± 0.5	2.3 ± 0.6	1.1 ± 0.3	0.9 ± 0.09
Mg^{2+} (-)	-***	-***	-***	-***	-***	-***	-***	-***
dNTP (-)	1.7 ± 0.1***	1.2 ± 0.2***	0.6 ± 0.1***	1.0 ± 0.1**	1.2 ± 0.4**	1.1 ± 0.8	-***	0.7 ± 0.09
ATP (-)	4.7 ± 0.2***	2.8 ± 1.0	2.0 ± 0.3**	1.1 ± 0.1**	2.2 ± 0.6	1.5 ± 0.2**	0.8 ± 0.02	0.7 ± 0.07*
ATPγS	4.3 ± 0.01***	1.0 ± 0.4***	0.7 ± 0.1***	1.1 ± 0.1**	2.9 ± 0.6*	0.3 ± 0.4***	1.0 ± 0.2	0.8 ± 0.02

Repair efficiency was determined as described in "Methods". Twenty-one fmol of dI-containing DNA was incubated with 90 μg of HeLaS3 or HCT116 cell-free extracts at 37 °C for 30 min. Repair level lower than 0.3 fmol was regarded as background (–). Each data corresponds to the average and standard deviation from at least three independent measurements. Statistical analysis: * $p < 0.05$, ** $p < 0.001$, *** $p < 0.001$ versus Standard reaction (Student's t-test)

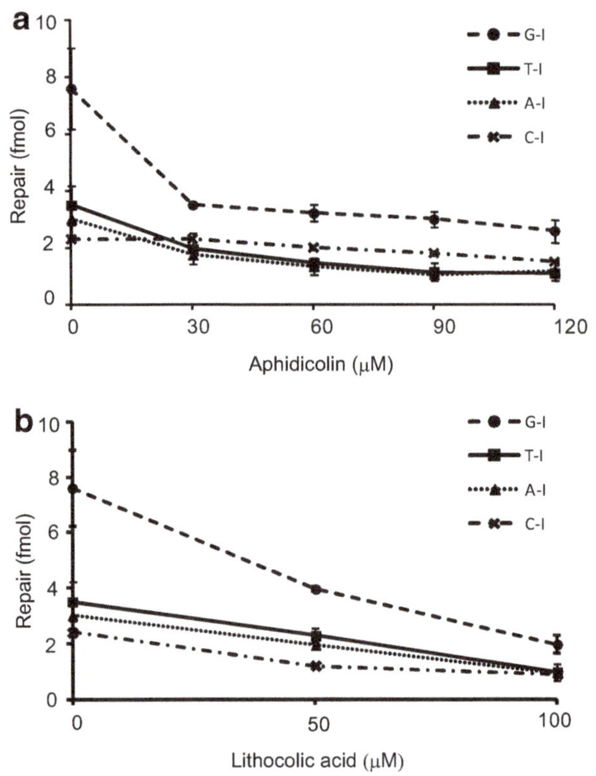

Fig. 3 Inhibitory effects of aphidicolin and lithocholic acid on dI correction in mammalian cell-free extracts. Heteroduplexes G-I, T-I, C-I and A-I (21 fmol) were incubated with 90 μg HeLa extracts containing indicated DNA polymerases inhibitors for 30 min at 37 °C. Reactions were analyzed by gel electrophoresis after restriction endonuclease digestion with AlwNI and the scoring enzymes. **a** Addition of aphidicolin. **b** Addition of Lithocolic acid. Each data corresponds to the average and standard deviation (*error bars*) from at least three independent reactions

of dI heteroduplex DNA were impaired with lithocholic acid treatments with a dose dependency. This observation suggested that pol β and possibly short-patched BER are involved in repairing dI lesions in mammalian cells. At the concentration of LCA at 50 μM, at which pol β activity should be near background level [37], relatively high levels of residual dI repair remained (more than 50 % of activity relative to standard reactions). Since pol δ and ε were not affected by 50 μM LCA [37], it's possible these LCA-resistant DNA polymerases participate in repair of dI lesions.

A hereditary non-polyposis colorectal cancer cell line showed lower repair activity toward certain dI lesions

It is known that mismatch repair activity not only can repair mismatches, but also may recognize base analogs as well. The A-I, C-I, G-I and T-I substrates we prepared share a great deal of similarity to mismatches. It is also known that ATP is required in the mismatch repair pathway and our exogenous ATP and ATPγS experimental data were strongly suggested possible involvement of mismatch repair in human dI lesion repair. In order to clarify this issue, we employed extracts from a mismatch repair deficient HCT116 cells in our dI repair assay.

To ensure the quality of both HeLa and HCT116 extracts were comparable, a G-U substrate (Fig. 1) was prepared to evaluate their BER activity. Using the repair assay conditions described above, both cell extracts could actively repair G-U substrate. In a reaction of 21 fmol G-U substrate, repair levels from HeLa was 17.9 ± 0.2 fmol and from HCT116 was 17.4 ± 0.3 respectively.

However, we found the repair levels of HCT116 decreased about 60 % in G-I, 35 % in T-I, 66 % in A-I, and 38 % in C-I substrates when compared to repair levels derived from HeLa cells (Table 1). We also determined the repair requirements for HCT116 extracts (Table 1). In the absence of exogenous dNTPs, the repair levels dropped to near background for A-I to less than half of the standard reactions for G-I and T-I (Table 1). In the absence of exogenous ATP, the repair levels of HCT116 for each substrate also showed variable degrees of decreasing repair when compared to standard ones (Table 1, HCT116 entries). It is very interesting to note that the repair efficiency of T-I showed an extensive reduction in both HeLa and HCT116 extracts when exogenous ATP was replaced by ATPγS in the repair reactions. This implies that the T-I specific repair mechanism exists in human cell relies on ATP hydrolysis.

Since HCT116 lacks functional MutL-α for mismatch repair, the observation described above prompted us to test the involvement of MutL-α in human dI repair. As shown in Fig. 4, supplemented purified human MutL-α to MMR proficient HeLa extracts showed no significant change in 5′G-T repair levels (Fig. 4, HeLa entries). However, supplementing of MutL-α to HCT116 extracts was able to restore its MMR activity for both 3′-G-T and 5′-G-T heteroduplexes. Addition of MutL-α to HCT116 extracts also increased the G-I repair level comparably to that of HeLa extract containing reactions (Fig. 4 and G-I entry in Table 1). However, the processing of A-I, C-I and T-I showed no significant change in the presence or absence of MutL-α (Fig. 4). This observation suggested human MMR enzymes can recognize and process G-I but not A-I, C-I and T-I lesions.

Discussion

Deamination of purine bases can occur spontaneously. The conversion rate of adenine to hypoxanthine in DNA under physiological condition is about 2 % of the rate of the conversion of cytosine to uracil [2], which in turn is about 2–5 times per human cell per day [38]. The resulting I-T mismatch in DNA is potentially mutagenic since

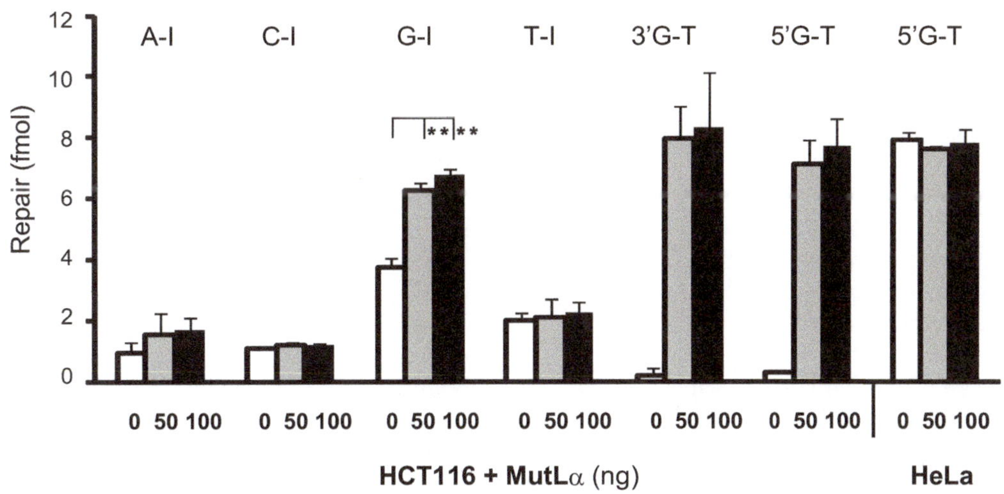

Fig. 4 MuL-α complementation assay for Hct116 extracts. Heteroduplex A-I, C-I, G-I, T-I, 3′G-T and 5′G-T (21 fmol) as indicated were incubated with 90 μg Hct116 extracts in the absence (*white bar*) or presence of 50 ng (*gray bar*) or 100 ng (*black bar*) of human MutL-α recombinant protein. Repair of 5′G-T with HeLa was included as a control. Each *data-bar* corresponds to the average and standard deviation (*error bars*) from at least three independent reactions. **p < 0.01 versus addition of exogenous MutL-α (Student's *t* test)

a dI in the DNA template prefers to pair with dCTP during replication, yielding A:T to G:C transition mutations at sites of adenine deamination [5]. Therefore dI in DNA should be removed by living organisms to maintain genome integrity.

Previously we developed an in vitro assay for bacterial repair and found that different dI-containing substrates were predominately repaired by the EndoV repair pathway [11]. In this study, we took advantage of our previously described bacterial dI in vitro repair assay to determine repair capabilities in human cell-free extracts for all four dI-containing A-I, C-I, G-I and T-I substrates. Similar to *E. coli*, we found that human cell extracts can also efficiently process dI lesions. However, some significant differences do exist between human and bacterial reactions. In the reactions withholding specific exogenous cofactors, we found that high concentrations of exogenous ATP was required for the human reaction (Table 1) but not in the bacterial reaction [11], This observation might be attributed to some of mammalian DNA processing proteins requirement for ATP for their enzymatic reactions. Mammalian DNA ligases, PCNA loader (RFC), MutS-α, MutL-α are among the likely ATP utilizing candidates involved in the reaction.

As to substrates specificity, under similar reaction conditions, we found G-I was the best substrate for human cell extracts followed by T-I, A-I and C-I. This hierarchy of repair specificity in human cells is different from what we previously reported in the bacterial system i.e. T-I is a better substrate than A-I and G-I [11]. In *E. coli*, both in vivo and in vitro studies suggested that EndoV pathway is the major system for processing dI lesions. All the mutagenic dI-containing DNA of A-I, G-I and T-I were repaired with similar biochemical process in vitro [11] and with the same genetic requirements for in vivo correction [8]. However, correction of dI in human extracts appears to be more complex. We suspect there are multiple overlapping dI repair activities judging from different repair responses for G-I, T-I, C-I and A-I with specific inhibitors.

It is not uncommon for repair proteins or pathways to demonstrate overlapping specificity toward the same DNA errors or lesions. For example, to deal with cytosine deamination, mammalian cells utilize four nuclear uracil DNA glycosylases (UDGs), namely, UNG2, SMUG1, TDG and MBD4 [39]. Likewise, BER was thought to be the major pathway for dI repair in mammalian cells. According to the model, hypoxanthine (Hx) would be bound and excised relatively efficiently by human *N*-methylpurine-DNA glycosylase (MPG, also known as AAG, ANPG, APNG, and MDG) [6]. The human MPG has a broad substrate specificity, excising a structurally diverse group of modified purines from DNA [40]. Single-turnover kinetics of excision of Hx paired with T showed that excision of Hx was very fast relative to any other damaged purines. However, the opposing pyrimidine base had a significant effect on the kinetics of excision and DNA binding affinity of Hx; replacing a T with a U opposite Hx dramatically reduced the excision rate [35]. In mammalian cells, pol β is responsible for the dominant 1-nucleotide replacement or so-called short-patch BER pathway. In long-patch BER pathway, DNA

Pol δ or ε, FEN1, PCNA and DNA ligase I are required for gap filling and deoxyribosephosphate removal.

An initial effort toward identifying the requirements in our human dI repair assay was to use DNA polymerase inhibitors. Using lithocholic acid or aphidicolin treatments, the repair of G-I, C-I, T-I, and A-I were partially inhibited in reactions containing HeLa extracts (Fig. 3). This observation implies the possible role for both a lithocholic acid sensitive polymerase (i.e. β) and aphidicolin sensitive polymerases (i.e. α, δ or ε) in dI repair. Different repair specificities toward A-I, C-I, G-I, and T-I substrates and involvement of both lithocholic acid sensitive and aphidicolin sensitive DNA polymerases are an indication of possible involvement of both short- and long- patch BER pathway. Our observation is consistent with a previous report that repair of a hypoxanthine residue initiated by the MPG utilizes both short- and long-patch repair synthesis [7].

The A-I, C-I, G-I and T-I mispairs share some similar features to base–base mismatches and cause protrusion of the DNA duplex [41]. However, in *E. coli*, both in vivo and in vitro studies showed the mismatch repair pathway plays little, if any role in processing dI lesions [8, 9, 11]. Using extracts from an MMR-deficient HNPCC cell line with a complementation assay demonstrated that G-I substrate could be partially processed by MMR pathway (Fig. 4). A notable finding from this study is that we found extracts of HCT116 showed lower dI processing capability compared to HeLa cell extracts. HCT116 is defective in mismatch repair due to a lack of human MutL-α activity indicating a possible role of the mismatch repair protein MutL-α in processing dI lesions. However, we found the deficiency was not completely due to mismatch repair since addition of recombinant MutL-α, which can restore HCT116's MMR activity, failed to significantly increase the repair levels of T-I, C-I and A-I substrates, while significantly improving G-I repair (more than 50 % increase as shown in Fig. 4). A single-strand break is required to initiate repair and to provide strand specificity for human MMR [26]. Structurally similar to mismatches, covalently-closed-circular G-I substrate may be detected by MutS-α which subsequently stimulates MutL-α nicking activity to initiate the repair [22, 23]. Alternatively, an incision created by an EndoV-like activity [42] might be sufficient to direct the repair. The interaction between EndoV and MMR enzymes for G-I processing remains to be determined.

EndoV from *E. coli* has been shown to have similar activity on oligodeoxynucleotides containing T-I, C-I, G-I or A-I pairs [13]. Recently, the human EndoV homologue was identified and characterized [16]. The mammalian EndoV showed lower endonucleolytic activity than *E. coli* homologues towards dI lesions [15, 16]. The activity of mammalian EndoV was most active on G-I followed by T-I>A-I>C-I [16]. In combination with the overlapping repair of G-I by MMR, this might explain our findings that G-I was most efficiently processed followed by T-I, A-I, and C-I (Table 1). Further study is required to clarify this issue.

Variations in DNA repair activities are connected to both individual and population disease susceptibilities [43, 44], Several DNA repair defects have been linked to cancers [43, 44]. Oxidatively damaged DNA and its repair are also positively correlated in colon carcinogenesis [45]. Increased risk of lung cancer is associated with a functionally impaired polymorphic variant of the human DNA glycosylase NEIL2 [46]. Thus, studying DNA repair activities in human cells is an important issue. A very interesting finding from this study is that we found that HNPCC cell line HCT116 showed lowered dI processing capability in part because of its MMR deficiency (for part of G-I repair) and possibly other mechanism(s) for T-I, C-I and A-I repair. Production of dI can be enhanced by exposure of DNA with nitrite ion. Nitrites are commonly used in the food production industry for curing meat. It's likely that the digestive tract e.g. the colon would be exposed and affected by nitrite when consuming preserved meat items. Patients of putative HNPCC families might be more susceptible to this mutagenic effect. The interrelationship of a MMR deficiency and other dI repair activities in HNPCC tumors needs to be determined. The dI repair assay described in this study provides a good platform for further investigation.

Conclusions

In this study a plasmid-based convenient and non-radioisotopic method was introduced to study dI repair in human cells. All four possible dI lesions of A-I, C-I, G-I and T-I processed by human cell-free extracts could be scored by restriction enzyme cleavage to evaluate the repair. In addition, repair derived from a MMR deficient cancer cell line was less efficient in dI repair that was partially attributed to lack of MutL-α. The repair assay described in this study provides a good platform for further investigation of human repair pathways involved in dI processing and their biological significance in mutation and cancer prevention.

Methods

Materials

Bacteriophage M13LR1 and M13LR3 were derivatives of M13mp18 with a 22-base pair (bp) insertion at HindIII site [47]. M13WX1 and M13X22 were derivatives of M13mp18 with 26 and 22-bp insertion at XbaI site, and phage f1PM-A was a derivative of f1PM with a 27-bp insertion at XbaI site [11] (Fig. 1). *E. coli* DNA ligase, T4 polynucleotide kinase, HindIII-HF^{TM} and other restriction endonucleases were obtained from New England Biolabs. RecBCD nuclease was purchased from EPICENTRE Biotechnologies. Aphidicolin and lithocolic acid were purchased from Sigma and dissolved in DMSO. Recombinant human MutL-α was kindly provided by Dr. Paul Modrich (Duke University).

Cell culture and preparation of human cell-free nuclear extracts

The human cell line HeLa S3 were grown in 10 % FBS supplemented DMEM/F12 medium (Sigma), and Hct116, a mismatch repair deficient colorectal carcinoma cell line were grown in 10 % FBS supplemented RPMI 1640 medium (Biological Industry) at 37 °C under a 5 % CO_2 atmosphere.

Human cell-free nuclear extracts was prepared as described [27]. In brief, human cell lines were cultured to a total cell number about 2×10^9 cells. Cells were washed twice with a buffer of 20 mM HEPES (pH7.5), 5 mM KCl, 0.2 M sucrose, 0.5 mM $MgCl_2$, 0.1 % PMSF, and 0.5 mM dithiothreitol, and then incubated in a hypotonic solution of 20 mM HEPES (pH7.5), 5 mM KCl, 0.5 mM $MgCl_2$, 0.1 % PMSF, and 0.5 mM dithiothreitol. Cells were lysed with a dounce homogenizer, nuclei were collected by centrifugation. Nuclear protein were extracted in 50 mM HEPES (pH7.5), 10 % sucrose, 0.1 % PMSF, 155 mM NaCl, and 0.5 mM dithiothreitol, and then concentrated by ammonium sulfate precipitation (0.42 g/ml). The pellet was dialyzed against 25 mM HEPES (pH7.5), 50 mM KCl, 0.2 % PMSF, and 1 mM dithiothreitol until the conductivity achieved a value equivalent to that of 0.1–0.2 M KCl. The soluble fraction was frozen in small aliquots in liquid nitrogen and stored at −80 °C.

Batch to batch variation of cell-free nuclear extracts for repair activity was quite high (up to 30 % differences for standard reaction). Higher S.D. in some data reflected using average of equal number measurements from different batch of extracts.

Deoxyinosine-containing heteroduplex DNA substrates

Preparation of heteroduplex DNA substrates was carried out by annealing a 5′-phosphorylated dI-containing oligonucleotides (Fig. 1) to a gap-duplex DNA and then sealed by T4 DNA ligase as described [11]. All the covalently-closed-circular dI containing substrates were purified by CsCl-Ethidium bromide density gradient centrifugation. The key feature of prepared A-I, C-I, G-I and T-I substrates were summarized in Fig. 1. All of the dI-containing substrates were confirmed to be refractory to respective diagnosis restriction endonuclease cleavage prior the repair reaction.

Repair assays using cell-free extracts

The deoxyinosine repair assay with human extracts was similar to a human mismatch repair assay as described [26]. Briefly, 21 fmol of DNA substrate was incubated with 90 to 105 μg of human nuclear extracts in a 20-μl reaction containing 20 mM Tris–HCl (pH 7.6), 50 μg/ml bovine serum albumin, 5 mM $MgCl_2$, 1 mM ATP, and 0.1 mM each of the four dNTPs. Reactions were incubated for 30 min at 37 °C and quenched by adding 40 μl of 40 mM EDTA (pH8.0). DNA was isolated by phenol extraction and ethanol precipitation, and was then digested with AlwNI and the indicated scoring restriction enzymes. The resulting products were separated by agarose gel electrophoresis, and detected by ethidium bromide staining. The gel-images were captured by a gel documentation CCD camera (UVP Ltd.) using Viewfinder 3.0, and band intensities were then measured by NIH Image J 1.45 s software.

A DNA mismatch repair assay using nicked 5′-GT and 3′-GT heteroduplex was as described [48]. In the MutL-α complementation assay, purified MuL-α protein was supplemented to the HCT116 nuclear extracts and the repair assay was as described above.

A G-U substrate (Fig. 1) was prepared to evaluate BER activity of Hela and Hct116 extracts. The G-U repair assay is similar to dI assay described above.

Abbreviations

dI: deoxyinosine; MMR: mismatch repair; RPA: replication protein A; Exo1: exonuclease 1; PCNA: proliferating cell nuclear antigen; RFC: replication factor C; BER: base excision repair; Pol: DNA polymerase; EndoV: endonuclease V; LCA: lithocholic acid.

Authors' contributions

CCL carried out the substrate preparation, in vitro assay and drafted the manuscript. SC and TYH carried out part of the assay. YCY, SDG, LIL and WCC participated the experiment design, data analysis and draft the manuscript. WHF conceived of the study, and participated in its design and coordination and helped to draft the manuscript. All authors read and approved the final manuscript.

Author details

[1] Department of Clinical Laboratory Sciences and Medical Biotechnology, College of Medicine, National Taiwan University, #7, Chung-Shan South Road, Taipei 10002, Taiwan, ROC. [2] Department of Laboratory Medicine, National Taiwan University Hospital, Taipei 10002, Taiwan, ROC. [3] Center for Microbial Pathogenesis, Nationwide Children's Hospital, Columbus, OH, USA.

Acknowledgements

We thank Dr. Paul Modrich and Dr. Jochen Genschel provided us MuL-α and critically reviewed this manuscript. This work was supported by grants MOST 103-2320-B-002-053 from Ministry of Science and Technology, Taiwan, ROC.

Compliance with ethical guidelines

Competing interests

The authors declare that they have no competing of interests.

References

1. Karran P, Lindahl T. Hypoxanthine in deoxyribonucleic acid: generation by heat-induced hydrolysis of adenine residues and release in free form by a deoxyribonucleic acid glycosylase from calf thymus. Biochemistry. 1980;19:6005–11.
2. Lindahl T. Instability and decay of the primary structure of DNA. Nature. 1993;362:709–15.
3. Myrnes B, Guddal PH, Krokan H. Metabolism of dITP in HeLa cell extracts, incorporation into DNA by isolated nuclei and release of hypoxanthine from DNA by a hypoxanthine-DNA glycosylase activity. Nucleic Acids Res. 1982;10:3693–701.
4. Pang B, McFaline JL, Burgis NE, Dong M, Taghizadeh K, Sullivan MR, Elmquist CE, Cunningham RP, Dedon PC. Defects in purine nucleotide metabolism lead to substantial incorporation of xanthine and hypoxanthine into DNA and RNA. Proc Natl Acad Sci USA. 2012;109:2319–24.
5. Hill-Perkins M, Jones MD, Karran P. Site-specific mutagenesis in vivo by single methylated or deaminated purine bases. Mutat Res. 1986;162:153–63.
6. O'Brien PJ, Ellenberger T. Dissecting the broad substrate specificity of human 3-methyladenine-DNA glycosylase. J Biol Chem. 2004;279:9750–7.
7. Fortini P, Parlanti E, Sidorkina OM, Laval J, Dogliotti E. The type of DNA glycosylase determines the base excision repair pathway in mammalian cells. J Biol Chem. 1999;274:15230–6.
8. Weiss B. Removal of deoxyinosine from the Escherichia coli chromosome as studied by oligonucleotide transformation. DNA Repair. 2008;7:205–12.
9. Lee CC, Yang YC, Goodman SD, Yu YH, Lin SB, Kao JT, Tsai K-S, Fang WH. Endonuclease V-mediated deoxyinosine excision repair in vitro. DNA Repair. 2010;9:1073–9.
10. Gates FT 3rd, Linn S. Endonuclease V of Escherichia coli. J Biol Chem. 1977;252:1647–53.
11. Lee C-C, Yang Y-C, Goodman SD, Lin C-J, Chen Y-A, Wang Y-T, Cheng W-C, Lin L-I, Fang W-H. The excision of 3′ penultimate errors by DNA polymerase I and its role in endonuclease V-mediated DNA repair. DNA Repair. 2013;12:899–911.
12. Schouten KA, Weiss B. Endonuclease V protects Escherichia coli against specific mutations caused by nitrous acid. Mutat Res. 1999;435:245–54.
13. Yao M, Hatahet Z, Melamede RJ, Kow YW. Purification and characterization of a novel deoxyinosine-specific enzyme, deoxyinosine 3′ endonuclease, from Escherichia coli. J Biol Chem. 1994;269:16260–8.
14. Feng H, Dong L, Klutz AM, Aghaebrahim N, Cao W. Defining amino acid residues involved in DNA-protein interactions and revelation of 3′-exonuclease activity in endonuclease V. Biochemistry. 2005;44:11486–95.
15. Moe A, Ringvoll J, Nordstrand LM, Eide L, Bjoras M, Seeberg E, Rognes T, Klungland A. Incision at hypoxanthine residues in DNA by a mammalian homologue of the Escherichia coli antimutator enzyme endonuclease V. Nucleic Acids Res. 2003;31:3893–900.
16. Mi R, Alford-Zappala M, Kow YW, Cunningham RP, Cao W. Human endonuclease V as a repair enzyme for DNA deamination. Mutat Res-Fund Mol M. 2012;735:12–8.
17. Morita Y, Shibutani T, Nakanishi N, Nishikura K, Iwai S, Kuraoka I: Human endonuclease v is a ribonuclease specific for inosine-containing RNA. *Nat Commun* 2013, 4.
18. Alseth I, Dalhus B, Bjørås M. Inosine in DNA and RNA. Curr Opin Genet Dev. 2014;26:116–23.
19. Modrich P. Mechanisms in eukaryotic mismatch repair. J Biol Chem. 2006;281:30305–9.
20. Li GM. Mechanisms and functions of DNA mismatch repair. Cell Res. 2008;18:85–98.
21. Jiricny J. Postreplicative mismatch repair. *CSH Perspect*. Biol. 2013;5:1–23.
22. Pena-Diaz J, Bregenhorn S, Ghodgaonkar M, Follonier C, Artola-Boran M, Castor D, Lopes M, Sartori AA, Jiricny J. Noncanonical Mismatch Repair as a Source of Genomic Instability in Human Cells. Mol Cell. 2012;47:669–80.
23. Pluciennik A, Burdett V, Baitinger C, Iyer RR, Shi K, Modrich P. Extrahelical (CAG)/(CTG) triplet repeat elements support proliferating cell nuclear antigen loading and MutL alpha endonuclease activation. Proc Natl Acad Sci U S A. 2013;110:12277–82.
24. Shao H, Baitinger C, Soderblom EJ, Burdett V, Modrich P. Hydrolytic function of Exo1 in mammalian mismatch repair. Nucleic Acids Res. 2014;42:7104–12.
25. Brierley DJ, Martin SA. Oxidative stress and the DNA mismatch repair pathway. Antioxid Redox Signal. 2013;18:2420–8.
26. Fang WH, Modrich P. Human strand-specific mismatch repair occurs by a bidirectional mechanism similar to that of the bacterial reaction. J Biol Chem. 1993;268:11838–44.
27. Holmes J Jr, Clark S, Modrich P. Strand-specific mismatch correction in nuclear extracts of human and Drosophila melanogaster cell lines. Proc Natl Acad Sci USA. 1990;87:5837–41.
28. Longley MJ, Pierce AJ, Modrich P. DNA polymerase delta is required for human mismatch repair in vitro. J Biol Chem. 1997;272:10917–21.
29. Dzantiev L, Constantin N, Genschel J, Iyer RR, Burgers PM, Modrich P. A defined human system that supports bidirectional mismatch-provoked excision. Mol Cell. 2004;15:31–41.
30. Nichols AF, Sancar A. Purification of PCNA as a nucleotide excision repair protein. Nucleic Acids Res. 1992;20:2441–6.
31. Shivji MKK, Kenny MK, Wood RD. Proliferating cell nuclear antigen is required for DNA excision repair. Cell. 1992;69:367–74.
32. Matsumoto Y, Kim K, Bogenhagen DF. Proliferating cell nuclear antigen-dependent abasic site repair in Xenopus laevis oocytes: an alternative pathway of base excision DNA repair. Mol Cell Biol. 1994;14:6187–97.
33. Dianov G, Price A, Lindahl T. Generation of single-nucleotide repair patches following excision of uracil residues from DNA. Mol Cell Biol. 1992;12:1605–12.
34. Matsumoto Y, Kim K. Excision of deoxyribose phosphate residues by DNA polymerase β during DNA repair. Science. 1995;269:699–702.
35. Abner CW, Lau AY, Ellenberger T, Bloom LB. Base excision and DNA binding activities of human alkyladenine DNA glycosylase are sensitive to the base paired with a lesion. J Biol Chem. 2001;276:13379–87.
36. Xia LQ, Zheng L, Lee HW, Bates SE, Federico L, Shen BH, O'Connor TR. Human 3-methyladenine-DNA glycosylase: effect of sequence context on excision, association with PCNA, and stimulation by AP endonuclease. J Biol Chem. 2005;346:1259–74.
37. Ogawa A, Murate T, Suzuki M, Nimura Y, Yoshida S. Lithocholic acid, a putative tumor promoter, inhibits mammalian DNA polymerase β. Jpn J Cancer Res. 1998;89:1154–9.
38. Friedberg EC, Walker GC, Siede W, Wood RD, Schultz RA, Ellenberger T. DNA repair and mutagenesis. 2nd ed. Washington, DC: ASM Press; 2006.
39. Visnes T, Doseth B, Pettersen HS, Hagen L, Sousa MML, Akbari M, Otterlei M, Kavli B, Slupphaug G, Krokan HE. Uracil in DNA and its processing by different DNA glycosylases. PHILOS T ROY SOC B. 2009;364:563–8.
40. O'Connor TR. Purification and characterization of human 3-methyladenine-DNA glycosylase. Nucleic Acids Res. 1993;21:5561–9.
41. Oda Y, Uesugi S, Ikehara M, Kawase Y, Ohtsuka E. NMR-studies for identification of DI-DG mismatch base-pairing structure in DNA. Nucleic Acids Res. 1991;19:5263–7.
42. Cao W. Endonuclease V: an unusual enzyme for repair of DNA deamination. Cell Mol Life Sci. 2013;70:3145–56.
43. Frosina G. The current evidence for defective repair of oxidatively damaged DNA in Cockayne syndrome. Free Radical Bio Med. 2007;43:165–77.
44. Frosina G. Tumor suppression by DNA base excision repair. Method Enzymol. 2007;7:727–43.
45. Tudek B, Speina E. Oxidatively damaged DNA and its repair in colon carcinogenesis. Mutat Res-Fund Mol M. 2012;736:82–92.
46. Dey S, Maiti AK, Hegde ML, Hegde PM, Boldogh I, Sarkar PS, Abdel-Rahman SZ, Sarker AH, Hang B, Xie J, et al. Increased risk of lung cancer associated with a functionally impaired polymorphic variant of the human DNA glycosylase NEIL2. DNA Repair. 2012;11:570–8.
47. Fang W, Wu JY, Su MJ. Methyl-directed repair of mismatched small heterologous sequences in cell extracts from Escherichia coli. J Biol Chem. 1997;272:22714–20.
48. Huang YM, Chen SU, Goodman SD, Wu SH, Kao JT, Lee CN, Cheng WC, Tsai KS, Fang WH. Interaction of nick-directed DNA mismatch repair and loop repair in human cells. J Biol Chem. 2004;279:30228–35.

Integrated transcriptional profiling and genomic analyses reveal *RPN2* and *HMGB1* as promising biomarkers in colorectal cancer

Jialing Zhang[1,2,3], Bin Yan[4], Stephan Stanislaw Späth[5], Hu Qun[6], Shaleeka Cornelius[3], Daogang Guan[7], Jiaofang Shao[8], Koichi Hagiwara[9], Carter Van Waes[3], Zhong Chen[3*], Xiulan Su[2*] and Yongyi Bi[1*]

Abstract

Colorectal cancer (CRC) is a heterogeneous disease that is associated with a gradual accumulation of genetic and epigenetic alterations. Among all CRC stages, stage II tumors are highly heterogeneous with a high relapse rate in about 20–25 % of stage II CRC patients following surgery. Thus, a comprehensive analysis of gene signatures to identify aggressive and metastatic phenotypes in stage II CRC is desired for a more accurate disease classification and outcome prediction. By utilizing a Cancer Array, containing 440 oncogenes and tumor suppressors to profile mRNA expression, we identified a larger number of differentially expressed genes in poorly differentiated stage II colorectal adenocarcinoma tissues, compared to their matched normal tissues. Ontology and Ingenuity Pathway Analysis (IPA) indicated that these genes are involved in functional mechanisms associated with several transcription factors. Genomic alterations of these genes were also investigated through The Cancer Genome Atlas (TCGA) database, utilizing 195 published CRC specimens. The percentage of genomic alterations in these genes was ranked based on their mRNA expression, copy number variations and mutations. This data was further combined with published microarray studies from a large set of CRC tumors classified based on prognostic features. This led to the identification of eight candidate genes including *RPN2*, *HMGB1*, *AARS*, *IGFBP3*, *STAT1*, *HYOU1*, *NQO1* and *PEA15* that were associated with the progressive phenotype. In particular, *RPN2* and *HMGB1* displayed a higher genomic alteration frequency in CRC, compared to eight other major solid cancers. Immunohistochemistry was performed on additional 78 stage I–IV CRC samples, where RPN2 protein immunostaining exhibited a significant association with stage III/IV tumors, distant metastasis, and poor differentiation, indicating that RPN2 expression is associated with poor prognosis. Further, our study revealed significant transcriptional regulatory mechanisms, networks and gene signatures, underlying CRC malignant progression and phenotype warranting future clinical investigations.

Keywords: Colorectal cancer, Gene signature, Genomic alterations, Transcription factor, Gene regulation

Background

Colorectal cancer (CRC) is the third most common cancer worldwide [1]. TNM staging is a standard pathology classification used for treatment strategy and outcome prediction, especially for most stage-I, -III, and -IV CRC patients. In the clinical setting, approximately 90 % of localized stage I CRC patients are cured by surgical removal of the tumor burden, so the prognosis and treatment plan for stage I CRC patients has been standardized [2, 3]. However, stage II CRC is highly heterogeneous, with 20–25 % of patients exhibiting recurrence or relapsed disease following surgery. The 5-year overall-survival of patients with stage II tumors ranges from 58 to 85 % [4–6]. Although a wide variety of potential clinical and pathological risk factors have been examined

*Correspondence: chenz@nidcd.nih.gov; xlsu@hotmail.com; yongyib@yahoo.com.cn
[1] School of Public Health, Wuhan University, Wuhan, China
[2] Clinical Medicine Research Center, The Affiliated Hospital, Inner Mongolia Medical University, Hohhot, China
[3] Tumor Biology Section, Head and Neck Surgery Branch, National Institute on Deafness and Other Communication Disorders, NIH, Bethesda, USA
Full list of author information is available at the end of the article

for improved outcome prediction, such as T4 lesions, poorly differentiated histology or intestinal obstruction [7], the molecular mechanisms underlining the heterogeneous characteristics of stage II CRC are still not well established. In fact, previous publications indicated that clinical outcome prediction and treatment of stage II CRC remains controversial, with a necessity for a better molecular classification utilizing gene signatures and biomarkers, in order to complement TNM staging [8–10].

Over the past few years, there has been a significant progress in identifying distinct molecular signatures to better define CRC subsets. The biological and clinical significance of overexpressed oncogenes (i.e. *EGFR* and *MYC*), and functional loss of tumor suppressor genes (i.e. *TP53* and *APC*) have been well characterized [11–15]. Better understanding of the oncogenes and related signaling pathways have led to successful CRC therapies, especially in targeting the *EGFR-RAS-MAPK* signaling pathway [16, 17]. Further discoveries on TP53 and APC have been utilized to predict poor CRC prognosis, with the presence of defective of APC expression or point mutations in *TP53* [18]. However, these gene signatures have not been successfully utilized as biomarkers to classify the heterogeneous stage II CRC for diagnosis and treatment. More comprehensive gene signatures and signaling transduction pathways related to stage II CRC are needed to understand the disease progression and for an improved prognosis, as well as treatment.

Recent development of high throughput technologies, such as gene expression profiling and genomic sequencing analysis, enabled us to identify comprehensive cancer gene signatures and related signaling pathways, based on the genetic and expression alterations in multiple cancers [19, 20]. Previously published gene signatures using gene profiling, RT-PCR, or sequencing technologies varied considerably in terms of their gene composition, with little gene overlap [21]. The lack of concordant gene signatures could be related to several issues, including differences: (1) in technological platforms, such as microarray, RT-PCR or sequencing technologies; (2) different sample types selected for analysis, and (3) the different analytical tools used to generate the gene signatures [22]. Hence, an integrative approach combining the information derived from different technological platforms, summarizing different categories of genetic and expression alterations from a large number of samples, may more accurately identify the associations of clinical phenotypes with genetic and expression alterations.

In the current study, we performed an integrated data analysis, combining gene expression profiles from our collected paired stage II CRC patient's samples, with genomic alteration data of 195 CRC samples, previously published by the Cancer Genome Atlas (TCGA) project, along with extracted results from more than 50 previously published microarray studies. This integrated approach has identified eight gene candidates, significantly associated with a progressive CRC phenotype. Among these genes, a significantly higher alteration profile for *Ribophorin II* (*RPN2*) and *High-mobility group protein B1* (*HMGB1*) was observed in CRC tumors, compared to other eight major human solid cancer types, currently available in the TCGA database. Immunohistochemistry was performed on 78 clinical stage I–IV CRC samples, where RPN2 exhibited a significant association with distant metastasis and poor differentiation. These gene signatures expand the current CRC biomarker pools for tumor progression and CRC outcome prediction. Further, these gene signatures warrant future validation as potential biomarkers in large clinical trials.

Results

Identification of gene expression signatures, related pathways and upstream regulators

To investigate important gene signatures in stage II CRC tissues with implications in aggressive malignant phenotypes, we utilized a cancer-specific array, containing known cancer related gene probes ($N = 440$) for mRNA expression profiling. A total of 92 genes, exhibiting at least 1.5-fold difference with $p < 0.05$ in mRNA level between tumor and normal samples were identified (Additional file 1: Table S1). Unsupervised hierarchical clustering algorithm was used to classify sub-populations based on the list of differentially expressed genes. As expected, tumor and normal samples were clearly separated into two subgroups (Fig. 1a). We further identified two characteristic clusters, including an over-expressed gene cluster A and an under-expressed gene cluster B in the tumor subgroup (Fig. 1b, c).

To investigate their functional relevance, we annotated differentially expressed genes in Fig. 1 according to Gene Ontology (GO) biological processes, by using the DAVID software. We observed significant enrichment in apoptosis, phosphorylation, cell proliferation, protein kinase cascade, colorectal cancer metastasis and intracellular signaling cascade in stage II CRC (Additional file 1: Table S2a). We further applied IPA (Ingenuity Pathway Analysis) to identify enriched pathways and unveil the functional relevance of our differentially expressed genes in stage II CRC. Using this approach, six enriched subnetworks were hence identified. They were associated with NFKB, AP1, STAT3, TP53, HSP90 and CTNNB1 signaling pathways (Additional file 2: Figure S1). Furthermore, utilizing the IPA tool, we also investigated upstream regulatory molecules that are responsible for identified pathways and altered gene expression in stage II CRC. As shown in Additional file 1: Table S2b, three

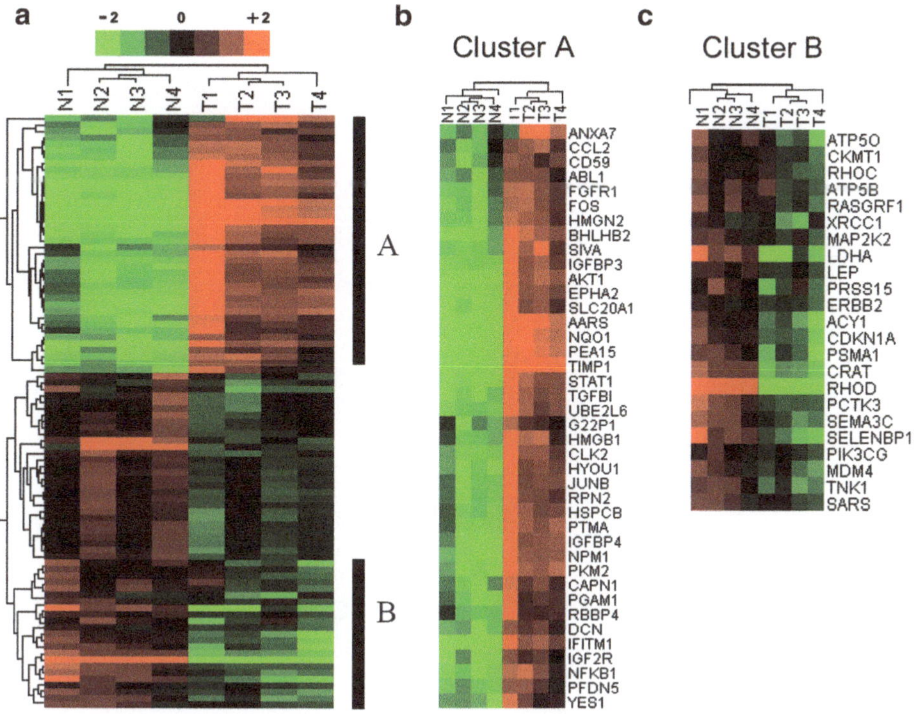

Fig. 1 Identification of CRC gene signatures using global expression profiles. Microarray analysis was performed using stage II CRC cancer specimens (T1-4), compared to matched mucosal tissue samples (N1-4). **a** Unsupervised hierarchical clustering of differentially expressed genes was used to identify differentially expressed genes (fold change 1.5, $p < 0.05$). Over-expressed and under-expressed genes are indicated by *red* and *green* colour. The expression level is proportional to colour brightness. *Black bars* on the *left* indicate gene *clusters A* and B, respectively. An expanded view of *cluster A* (over-expressed genes, **b**), or *cluster B* (under-expressed genes, **c**), with the indicated gene names is shown

top transcription regulators TP53, TP63 and TP73 were significantly enriched in stage II CRC. In addition, several transcription factors and oncogenes ranked top on the list, such as NFKB, AP1, STAT3 and MYC, as well as other regulators (i.e. E2F1, HIF1A and ANR). This data suggests that aberrant regulation of these TFs (NFKB, AP1, STAT3, TP53, TP63 and MYC) could potentially influence the stage II CRC progression.

Transcriptional regulatory gene network in CRC

To test the hypothesis on how upstream oncogenic and tumor suppressor TFs regulate gene expression in stage II CRC, we applied a previously developed bioinformatics model [24] able to predict these TFs regulation of their target genes. As shown in Additional file 1: Table S1, we generated a list of putative targets for the seven TFs, including NFKB1, RelA, TP53, TP63, STAT3, MYC and AP1. About 35–40 % of NFKB1 or TP53 targets were previously validated by experimental data (Additional file 1: Table S1). There were twenty-nine NFKB1 targeted genes, consisting of both predicted and validated gene candidates, as well as eight unique NFKB1 target genes, including RPN2 and HMGB1 (Additional file 1: Table S1). In addition, there were many genes under the regulation of multiple TFs (Additional file 1: Table S1). Subsequently, we constructed a transcriptional regulatory gene network, presented in Fig. 2. We predicated ten genes being co-targeted by all of the seven TFs, including under-expressed (*BAX*, *CDKN1A*, *CDKN2B*, *LDHA*, *MDM2*, *SLC16A1*, *WEE1*) and over-expressed (*HSP90AB*, *NQO*1 as well as *PTMA*) genes, respectively. These genes are known to be involved in biological processes, such as apoptosis, cell proliferation, and cell cycle. Our data suggests that the interaction of these seven TFs may participate alone or co-regulate the signaling pathways, associated with the progression of stage II CRC.

Genomic and expression alterations of identified CRC-related genes in the TCGA database

To identify the genomic alterations for the differentially expressed genes discovered in this project, we took the advantage of the TCGA database, containing recently published large mRNA expression and genomic alteration data, derived from 195 stage I–IV CRC patients [20]. We analyzed 92 differentially expressed genes identified in our study, using the TCGA database and determined that a total of 24 genes (22 over- and 2 under-expressed genes), exhibited consistent expression patterns with the TCGA

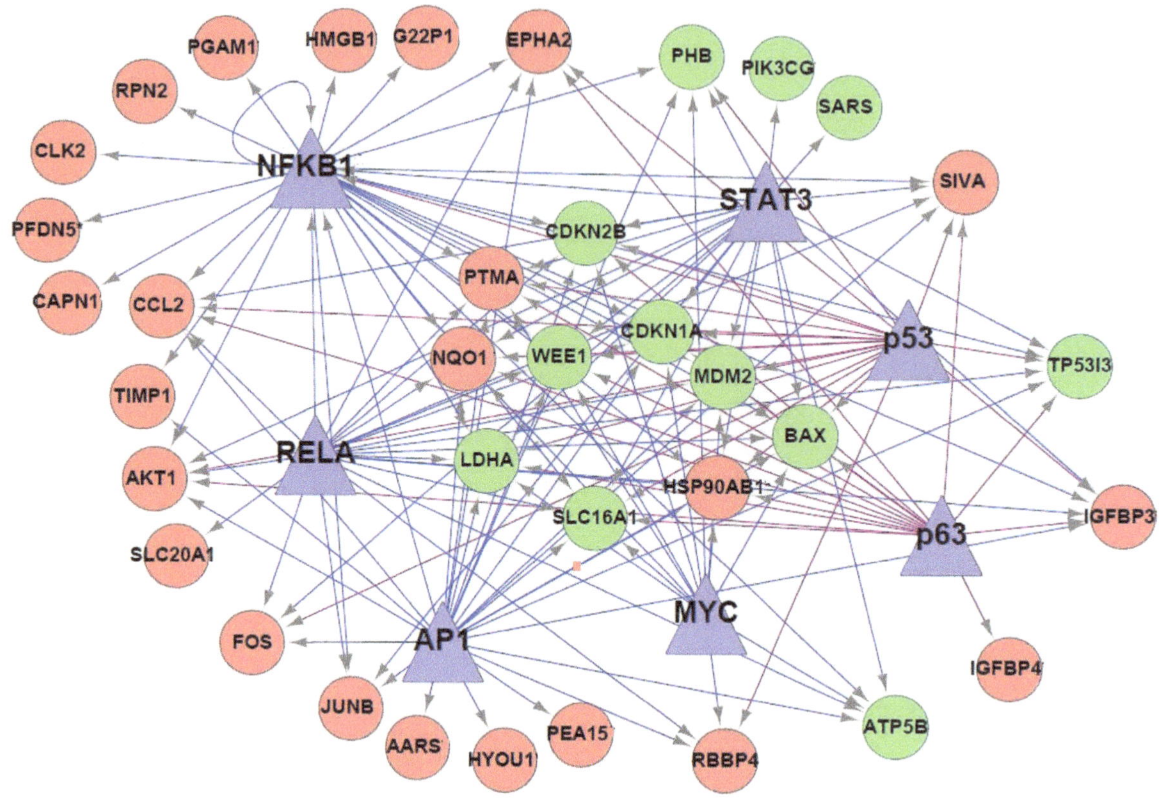

Fig. 2 Inferred transcriptional regulatory gene network in CRC. A newly developed computational model was utilized to identify target genes of seven cancer-related TFs and to construct gene regulatory networks. The *triangular nodes* represent corresponding TFs. *Circle nodes* refer to the target genes of TFs. *Arrow lines* show regulatory relationships from TFs to their target genes. *Purple* or *blue lines* stand for TFs that act as tumor suppressor or oncogene, respectively. *Red* and *green* nodes refer to over- and under-expressed genes, respectively

data (Additional file 2: Figure S2). Among the over-expressed genes, *RPN2* was altered most frequently in 87 out of 195 (37 %) CRC cases at stage II and III, including significant gene amplification and mRNA overexpression. The second most altered gene was *HMGB1* (13 %), which exhibited a significantly higher rate of mRNA up-regulation (Fig. 3a; Additional file 2: Figure S3). The remaining 19 over-expressed genes were altered similarly in 195 CRC cases (5–10 %) and across all stages (Fig. 3a; Additional file 2: Figure S3a). Alterations of *TNK1* included mRNA down-regulation or mutations in 22 out of 195 cases (13 %) across all tumor stages (Additional file 2: Figure S3). We further examined if copy number variations (CNVs) are associated with mRNA expression for the 24 genes, identified in the TCGA. The mRNA expression of 14 out of these 24 genes correlated significantly with CNVs (Fig. 3b). In addition, ≥25 % recurrent CNVs were observed as gains on chromosomes 20q, 13q, 6q, 16q, 10q, 11q, 12q, 14q, and 1q, as well as losses at 17p and 1p, respectively (Fig. 3b). Remarkably, *RPN2* and *HMGB1* had a higher percentage of CNV in these cases, including gains (*RPN2* and *HMGB1*) and amplifications (RPN2, Fig. 3b).

Identification of CRC-specific gene signatures across multiple data sets

Previous evaluation of 29 microarray studies, utilizing CRC tumor specimens, has identified 31 gene signatures with prognosis significance [31]. Out of these 31 genes, 28 were overlapping with our identified differentially expressed genes from our microarray data, of which 8 genes (*AARS, PEA15, NQO1, STAT1, IGFBP3, HYOU1, HMGB1* and *IGF2R*) were also matched genes, previously verified in the TCGA dataset (Table 1; Fig. 3; Additional file 2: Figure S3). Next, we manually searched for the presence of these 28 differentially expressed genes in 50 previously published microarray studies that were utilizing CRC tissues (Additional file 1: Table S3). The 50 published microarray studies were selected based on prognosis signature inclusion criteria. Sixteen out of these 28 genes were overlapping with the 50 published microarray experiments. Further investigation revealed

Table 1 Comparison of differentially expressed genes with published CRC microarray studies

Gene symbol	Fold change[a]	Tumors with prognosis gene signatures[b]	Tumors from other microarrays[c]
TIMP1	8.34	232	52
AARS[d]	4.48		30
PEA15[d]	4.23	215	22
CD59	1.61	232	
IFITM1	3.03		106
HMGB1[d]	2.07	215	496
RPN2[d]	1.91		15
IGF2R	1.75	215	107
IGFBP3[d]	2.29	232	706
NPM1	2.60	87	679
NQO1[d]	3.77	55	200
TGFB1	2.35		531
AKT1	3.33		43
HYOU1[d]	2.16		30
STAT1[d]	2.83	215	30

[a] The fold changes of differential gene expression between Stage II CRC tumor and normal tissues were extracted from the microarray data presented in Fig. 1

[b] Prognosis gene signatures were extracted from the publication of Sanz-Pamplona et al., which surveyed 29 microarray studies with patient's data of recurrence, metastasis and survival [25]

[c] Additional microarray data from 50 previous publications was extracted from CRC tumor and metastatic specimens (Additional file 1: Table S3). The indicated number stands for tumor specimens with increased gene expression

[d] Refers to genes that are involved in transcriptional regulation (Fig. 3; Additional file 1: Table S1) and an overlapping with TCGA data (Additional file 2: Figure S2)

that 10 out of these 16 genes (*RPN2, AARS, PEA15, NQO1, AKT1, STAT1, IGFBP3, HYOU1, HMGB1* and *IGF2R*) also matched with the identified genes in the TCGA database (Table 1).

Finally, we selected 8 out of the above 10 genes from above list (*RPN2, HMGB1, AARS, IGFBP3, STAT1, HYOU1, NQO1* and *PEA15*), based on the following criteria: (1) previously identified by CRC tumor microarray experiments; (2) previously published as a prognosis markers and (3) identified candidate within the transcriptional regulation network presented in Fig. 2. The genomic alterations of these selected genes appeared to be more evident in stage II, compared to stage I CRC tumors, as observed in the TCGA database (Fig. 4a). Furthermore, we analyzed these eight genes for alteration frequency in nine major solid cancer types, available in the TCGA database. A significantly higher alteration frequency for *RPN2* and *HMGB1* genes was observed in CRC tumors, when compared with other tumors (Fig. 4b).

Association of RPN2, HMGB1 and NFkB1 protein expression with CRC clinic-pathological features

Based on our observations, where a higher percentage of CRC cases exhibited an association between genetic alterations and expression profiles in *RPN2* and *HMGB1,* as well as *NFkB1,* a common transcriptional regulator of both genes, we performed immunohistochemistry to validate RPN2, HMGB1 and NFkB1 protein expression in a cohort of additional 78 CRC specimens (Fig. 5). A total of 29.5 % of stage I/II and 51.4 % of stage III/IV specimens were positive for cytoplasmic RPN2, with a significant association between tumor stages ($p = 0.047$). In addition, RPN2 staining was also strongly associated with distant metastasis ($p = 0.0007$) and histological differentiation ($p = 0.015$), but not with gender, age or tumor location (Fig. 5a, b). Characteristic cytoplasmic and nuclear staining was observed for NFkB1 in the majority of tumor specimens (stage I–IV). However, cases with positive staining were highest in stage III/IV tumors but barely reached statistical significance ($p = 0.055$, Fig. 5a, b). No significant association of NFkB1 protein expression was observed for distant metastasis or other clinic-pathological features (Fig. 5b). In addition, ~90 % of all examined CRC tumor samples exhibited HMGB1 immuno-reactivity, however no difference association with clinicopathological features was observed (Fig. 5b).

Discussion

In this study, we performed an integrated data analysis combining differentially expressed genes from microarray (Fig. 1), with published literature (Additional file 1: Table S3) and available genomic, as well as expression datasets from TCGA (Figs. 2, 4). The integrated analysis

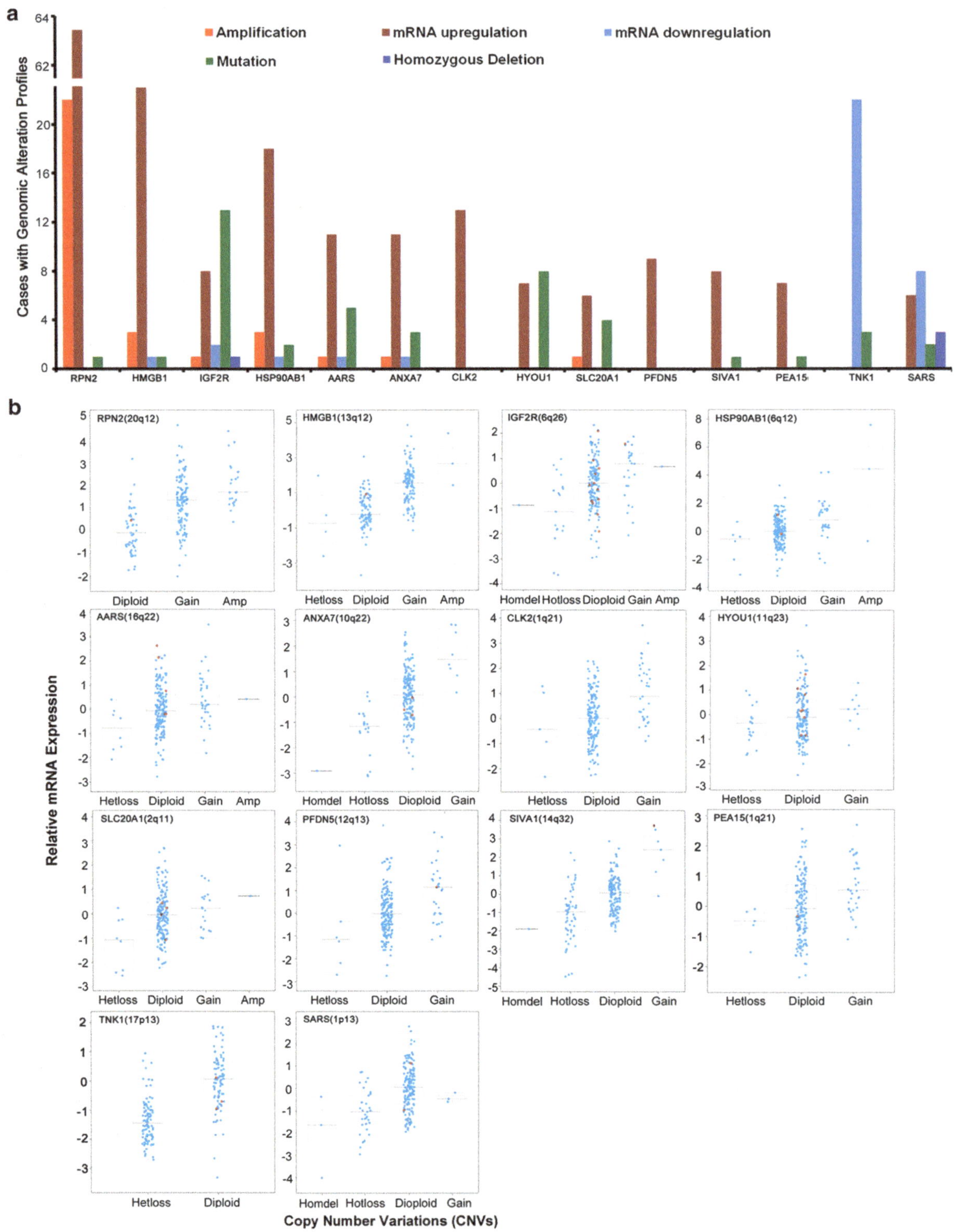

Fig. 3 Evaluation of genomic alterations in TCGA CRC dataset. **a** Genomic alterations, including copy number variations (CNVs), mutations and gene expression of each gene candidate were extracted from the TCGA colorectal cancer (CRC) database. The *X*- and *Y*-axis represent genomic alterations and case number, respectively. **b** Variations of mRNA expression versus CNVs and chromosomal locations for individual gene candidates are shown. CNV categories include homozygous deletions (Homodel), heterozygous deletions (Hetloss), diploid, gain and amplification (Amp). mRNA was expressed as 25th, 50th, and 75th percentile and *whiskers* represent minimal and maximal values, excluding the outliers. *Red circle* indicates missense mutations

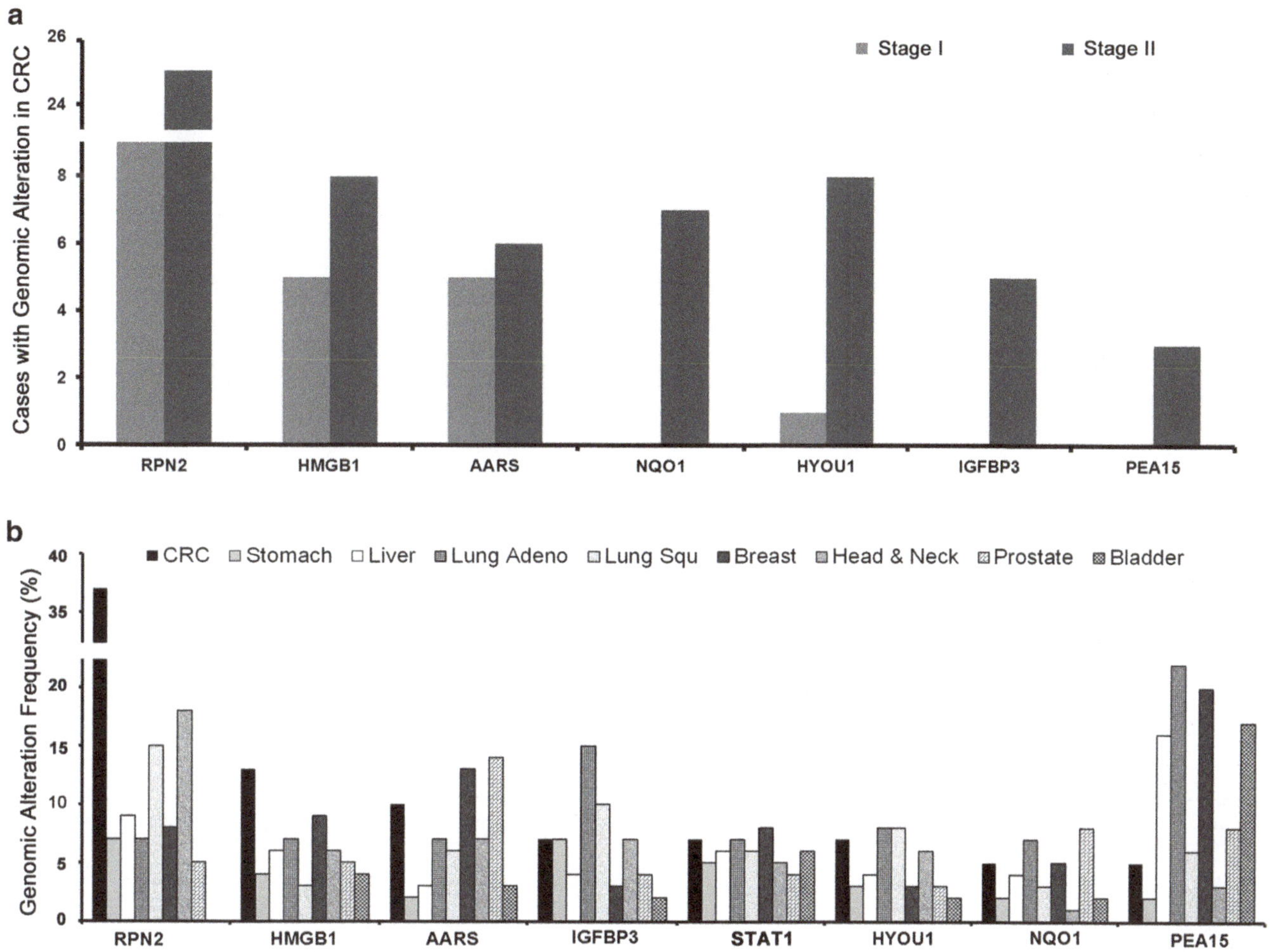

Fig. 4 Identification of CRC-specific gene signatures across most common solid tumors. **a** Case numbers with genomic alterations for each gene candidate, identified in stage I/II colorectal cancer from the TCGA dataset. **b** The frequency of genomic alterations for each gene candidates was analyzed across nine different solid cancer types (each with >150 tumor samples) from the TCGA database

identified novel gene signatures in stage II CRC tumors, with strong implications for late stage aggressive and metastatic phenotypes (Table 1; Fig. 5). Bioinformatics analysis indicated that these genes were regulated by seven TFs, including NFKB1, RelA, TP53, TP63, STAT3, MYC and AP1 (Fig. 3), and further enriched in NFKB, AP1, STAT3, TP53, HSP90 and CTNNB1 pathways, known to be important regulators for cell proliferation, cell cycle, apoptosis, and intracellular signaling (Additional file 1: Table S1; Additional file 2: Figure S1). Furthermore, integrated evaluation of large published CRC datasets from TCGA identified eight candidate genes that were associated with the progressive phenotype of CRC (Table 1; Fig. 4a). A significantly higher alteration frequency for *RPN2* and *HMGB1* was also observed in CRC tumors, compared to other eight common solid tumor types. Finally, immunohistochemistry of RPN2, HMGB1 and NFkB1, revealed a significant association of RPN2 with CRC stage, metastasis and differentiation, in a cohort of additional CRC samples (Fig. 5). Our data revealed an association of important gene signatures with aggressive stage II CRC and their underlining molecular regulatory mechanisms.

Among our differentially expressed gene list, we observed several overexpressed genes being tightly regulated by several critical TFs that control cell proliferation, survival and inflammation [32–34]. Using IPA analysis, to identify upstream regulators for the differentially expressed genes in stage II CRC samples used in this study, we observed a strong enrichment for tumor suppressor TP53 family members and oncogenic TFs (i.e.NFKB, AP1 and MYC) that either individually or combined regulate gene expression through shared or unique target genes (Fig. 2; Additional file 1: Table S1).

a

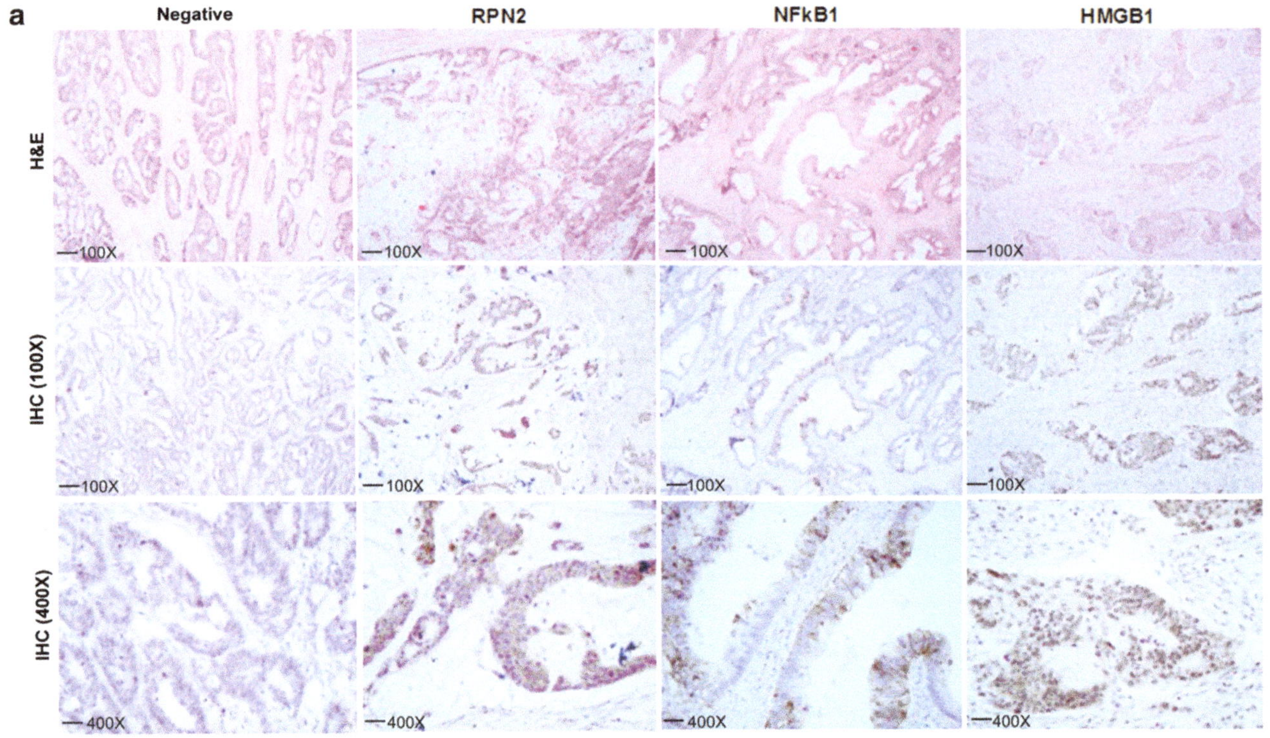

b

Features	Total (n)	RPN2 Positive (%)	RPN2 Negative (%)	RPN2 X^2	RPN2 p-value	NFkB1 Positive (%)	NFkB1 Negative (%)	NFkB1 X^2	NFkB1 p-value	HMGB1 Positive (%)	HMGB1 Negative (%)	HMGB1 X^2	HMGB1 p-value
Gender													
Male	46	18 (39.1)	28 (60.9)	0.018	0.894	10 (21.7)	36 (78.3)	0.103	0.748	41 (89.1)	5 (10.9)	0.689	0.406
Female	32	13 (40.6)	19 (59.4)			6 (18.8)	26 (81.2)			31 (96.9)	1 (3.1)		
Age (Years)													
≤55	38	16 (42.1)	22 (57.9)	0.173	0.687	9 (23.7)	29 (76.3)	0.156	0.692	34 (89.5)	4 (10.5)	0.241	0.624
≥55	40	15 (37.5)	25 (62.5)			7 (17.5)	33 (82.5)			38 (95.0)	2 (5.0)		
Stages													
I-II	41	12 (29.5)	29 (70.5)	3.96	0.047 *	5 (12.2)	36 (87.8)	3.667	0.055	39 (95.1)	2 (4.9)	0.309	0.578
III-IV	37	19 (51.4)	18 (48.6)			11 (29.7)	26 (70.3)			33 (89.2)	4 (10.8)		
Metastasis													
Lymph nodes	28	10 (35.7)	18 (64.28)	11.26	0.0007 *	7 (25.0)	21 (75)	0.477	0.489	24 (85.7)	4 (14.3)	0.34	0.559
Distant	9	9 (100)	0 (0)			4 (44.4)	5 (55.56)			9 (100)	0 (0)		
Location													
Colon	34	15 (44.1)	19 (55.9)	0.482	0.488	10 (29.4)	24 (70.6)	2.927	0.087	33 (97.1)	1 (2.9)	0.914	0.339
Rectal	44	16 (36.4)	28 (63.6)			6 (13.6)	38 (86.4)			39 (88.6)	5 (11.4)		
Histological Differentiation													
Well-moderate	57	18 (31.6)	39 (68.4)	5.893	0.015 *	9 (15.8)	48 (84.2)	2.897	0.089	53 (93.0)	4 (7.0)	0.012	0.912
Poorly	21	13 (61.9)	8 (38.1)			7 (33.3)	14 (66.7)			19 (90.5)	2 (9.5)		

*** Significant difference when p<0.05.**

Fig. 5 Association of RPN2, NFkB1 and HMGB1 protein expression with clinicopathological features in a cohort of CRC. **a** Immunohistochemical analysis of RPN2, HMGB1 and NFkB1 protein expression was performed in a cohort of additional 78 CRC specimens. H&E refers to Hematoxylin and Eosin staining. Microscope images were taken at either ×100 or ×400 magnifications. The *low-scale bar* represents 200 μm and *high-scale bar* corresponds to 50 μm. **b** Correlation analysis of RPN2, NFkB1 and HMGB1 expression by gender, age, stages, metastasis, tumor location, and histological differentiation in 78 CRC samples. The cases with metastasis were divided into lymph node only and distant metastasis. *Corresponds to a p value <0.05 (Fisher's exact test)

The tumor suppressor TP53 family members and oncogenic TFs (NFKB1, AP1 and MYC) are thought to play a crucial role in controlling CRC progression, consistent with the observed results in the published TCGA report [20]. Our data suggested an existing strong link between the regulatory programs of these TFs in CRC. In particular, this study unveiled several potentially unique target genes for each TF, such as *RPN2* and *HMGB1* being targeted by NFKB1. These findings are consistent with previous studies of these important TFs in carcinogenesis [35–37]. Our experimental data from microarray is supported by both computational analysis and literature searches, where differentially expressed gene signatures are shown to promote the malignant CRC process.

Additional support for our experimental data comes from the analysis of gene signature expression profiles across 195 CRC samples that are associated with different CRC stages from the TCGA database (Additional file 2: Figure S2). We found that about 55 % of identified over-expressed genes from our cancer array did overlap with published TCGA data. Interestingly, several genes exhibited recurrent CNVs (frequency > 25 %), which directly modulate their mRNA expression (Fig. 3b), hence providing a genetic mechanism for gene expression, showing consistency with previous reports [38, 39]. These findings highlight our observation that this subset of overexpressed genes may play a critical role in genomic instability, which is significantly associated with progressive CRC phenotypes. We further examined gene signatures with a prognostic CRC marker potential and by utilizing an integrated analysis approaches, we have identified eight gene candidates, including *RPN2, HMGB1, AARS, IGFBP3, STAT1, HYOU1, NQO1* and *PEA15*. Among this list, six out of eight genes have been previously implicated in deregulation of gene expression and associated with the prognosis of CRC and other cancer types [40–43]. Only *RPN2* and *AARS* were novel genes, with no previous publication describing their functional contribution to CRC. The genetic alteration and expression profiles for this eight candidate genes were compared across different cancer types. Only *RPN2*- and *HMGB1*-genes were found to be most altered in CRC (Fig. 4b), further supporting their biological significance in CRC pathogenesis. We used a cohort of 78 independent CRC specimens (stages I–IV) to validate RPN2, HMGB1 and NFkB1 protein expression and their association with several clinic-pathological features. We observed that only RPN2 expression was significantly associated with tumor stage, histological differentiation and distant metastasis (Fig. 5). HMGB1 was positively expressed in 90 % of cells in all tumor stages and across our selected CRC samples. HMGB1 has been previously implicated in CRC with controversial roles in cancer immunity and metastasis [44–48]. Although, it was not significantly associated with clinic-pathological features in our CRC samples (Fig. 5b), we still observed a consistent mRNA and protein over-expression of HMGB1 (Figs. 1, 5), as well as significant correlation between mRNA and CNV gains (Fig. 3b). Our data suggest that these gene markers can be identified in CRC samples, as early as stage II, but are not solely stage II specific. The consistent overexpression of these gene markers further supports their functional importance as oncogenes in tumor progression.

Our bioinformatics analysis suggests that *HMGB1* and *RPN2* are both targeted by an oncogenic TF, namely NFkB1 (Fig. 2). In fact, aberrant expression of NFkB1 expression was also observed in about 29.7 % of stage III/IV CRC cases (Fig. 5), which is consistent with previously published findings [43]. The *RPN2* gene, located on chromosome 20q13, encodes a proteasome scaffolding protein that inhibits *Bcl*-mediated apoptosis and stabilizes mutated *p53* protein expression through inactivation of *GSK3β* in breast cancer [49, 50]. Overexpression of *RPN2* in stage II CRC was also reported by another microarray that focused on CRC tumor metastasis (Table 1), supporting its implication beyond early staged tumors. In TCGA CRC dataset, *RPN2* up-regulation was observed in 65 out of 195 CRC cases (37 %) and was significantly associated with copy number gain (Fig. 3). This is consistent with previous findings, where >65 % of CRC cases have shown gains on chromosome and a strong association with liver metastasis and poor outcome [51–53]. In addition, we examined RPN2- and HMGB1 alteration profiles in 195 CRC staged patients, available in the TCGA database, by ranking them according to their alteration rates (Additional file 2: Figure S2). Further evaluation revealed a slightly longer survival of patients without RPN2 alteration, but that did not reach statistical significance ($p = 0.38$, data not shown). This survival data may be valid, because the marker was not originally identified as a predictor for CRC survival in all stage cancers. It will be interesting to complement the genetic alteration and differential expression profiles of these molecules as biomarkers in future clinical trials for stage II CRC patients.

Furthermore, the importance of *RPN2* in tumor prognosis and therapeutic implications has been documented in other solid cancers, including esophageal squamous cell carcinoma [54, 55], osteosarcoma [56, 57] and breast cancer [50]. We observed that *RPN2* is also highly altered in head and neck squamous cell carcinoma (HNSCC), as well as lung squamous cell carcinoma (Fig. 4b), consistent with previously published studies [55, 58]. In various human malignancies, silencing of *RPN2* was associated with increased apoptosis, reduced tumor growth and increased sensitivity of tumor cells to docetaxel response [49, 54]. The value of *RPN2*, both as a prognostic marker and as a therapeutic target is suggested for future validation. In this manuscript, we have shown that CRC cases with RPN2 staining were significantly higher in stage III/IV, in distant metastatic, and poorly differentiated tumors, indicating that its expression is associated with worse prognosis. In addition, NFkB1 protein expression was also associated with distant metastasis. Our data presents experimental evidence that RPN2 protein expression could serve as a potential biomarker to predict metastasis and worse prognosis. However, due to the lack of patient survival and outcome data in the current study, these molecules need to be further validated for their value as biomarkers in larger clinical trials.

Conclusions

In this manuscript, by utilizing mRNA profiling, we have identified a panel of differentially expressed gene signatures in stage II colorectal adenocarcinoma tissues. Through integrated analyses of the transcriptional regulation, The Cancer Genome Atlas database, and 50 published microarray studies of colorectal cancer specimens, we have identified eight candidate genes that are significantly associated with the aggressive phenotype, including *RPN2, HMGB1, AARS, IGFBP3, STAT1, HYOU1, NQO1* and *PEA15*. Among those genes, *RPN2* and *HMGB1* displayed higher frequencies of genomic alterations in colorectal cancer, compared to other solid tumors. Furthermore, RPN2 protein expression evaluated by immunohistochemistry in 78 independent (stage I–IV) colorectal cancer tissues, exhibited a significant association with stage III/IV tumors, distant metastasis, and poor differentiation. Our study identified important molecular signatures underlying malignant progression and phenotype of colorectal cancer, which warrants future clinical investigations.

Methods

Patients

This study was approved by the ethical committee at Inner Mongolia Medical University and a written informed patient consent was obtained. A total of 82 patients were diagnosed with pathological stages (Additional file 2: Figure S3) and underwent surgical resection for CRC at Inner Mongolia Medical University Hospital from 2002 to 2006 and were diagnosed with pathological stages. Patients with hereditary syndromes, e.g. familial adenomatous polyposis (FAP), Lynch syndrome or hereditary nonpolyposis colorectal cancer (HNPCC), or inflammatory syndromes were pre-screened and excluded from this study. The preoperational chemoradiotherapy or chemotherapy could significantly influence the expression of biomarkers. Hence none of the patients used in this study received treatment prior to surgery. Tumor staging was performed according to TNM classification criteria and guidelines of the International Union Against Cancer (UICC) guidelines [23]. Histological differentiation was evaluated, as poorly differentiated carcinomas are known to have a high-risk of recurrence or metastasis. Accordingly, we randomly selected 4 poorly differentiated adenocarcinoma (stage II) samples with matched adjacent normal mucosa tissues and performed microarray analysis. Histological evaluation confirmed the content of tumor- or normal colon epithelium cells to be more than 50 % (Additional file 2: Figure S1b).

RNA extraction and microarray profiling analysis

Total RNA was isolated from frozen tissue samples and extracted using the RNeasy Mini Kit (QIAGEN, Maryland, USA) according to manufacturer's instructions. Gene expression was analyzed using Oligo GEArray Human Cancer Microarray® (Cat# OHS-802SA, Biosciences, CA, USA), which contains a total of 480 probes for 440 genes, encoding for tumor suppressors, oncogenes, signal transduction molecules, growth factors and their corresponding receptors, as well as others associated with angiogenesis. Gene expression levels were normalized to the *beta-actin* housekeeping gene. The selection criterion of differentially expressed genes was based on at least 1.5-fold threshold between the CRC tumors and matched normal tissues.

Computational inference of transcription factor target genes

We have developed a mathematical model, capable to identify target genes of a particular transcription factor (TF) and thus to construct a gene network, regulated by that TF. By recursively applying this model to the identified network, multiple networks can be interconnected. Moreover, the model is able to infer how likely a gene is regulated by a particular TF, which has been successfully applied in other cancer datasets [24–28]. In this study, this model was applied to the above-obtained CRC differential gene expression data, in order to investigate target genes regulated by seven common cancer-related TFs, including NFKB1, RELA, AP1, TP53, TP63, STAT3 and MYC.

Genomic alterations from TCGA database

The cancer genome Atlas (TCGA) project has published the first "Marker" paper of colon cancer in 2012, which included genomic sequencing, epigenetic and mRNA expression profiling across 195 human colorectal cancer specimens [20]. The data is accessible through the cBio Cancer Genomics Portal (http://cbioportal.org) [29], a web resource designed for the visualization of oncogenomic datasets. Using the differentially expressed gene list in our current study, we extracted genomic alteration profiles from 195 CRC specimens, which have been published and deposited in the TCGA database. Since the first "Marker" paper of colon cancer was published [20], there is a constant submission of more colon cancer samples to the TCGA project, for continued generation of high throughput experimental data. However, not all of these data are complete or have gone through the confirmation and validation process, and thus are not included in this study.

Immunohistochemical analysis

Thin sections of 10 % formalin-fixed, paraffin-embedded tissue specimens were treated with goat anti-human RPN2 antibody (sc-12165, Santa Cruz), rabbit anti-human HMGB1 antibody (#6893S, Cell Signaling), or rabbit anti-human NFKB1 antibody (sc-1190, Santa Cruz), followed by a peroxidase-conjugated goat anti-rabbit (sc-2018, Santa Cruz) or rabbit anti-goat (sc-2023, Santa Cruz) secondary antibody. Color was developed using Avidin and Biotin-conjugated horseradish peroxidase (ABC reagents) and according to standard protocols. The percentage of positively stained cancer cells was determined under the microscope from more than four visual fields (at 400× magnification). Specimens were evaluated by two independent pathologists and classified into 2 groups: negative staining (no cells were intensely stained), and positive staining (at least 10 % cells were intensely stained) [30].

Statistical analysis

Correlation between gene expression and distinct clinicopathologic characteristic was analyzed by the Fisher's exact test. For all statistical analysis, a P value of <0.05 was considered significant.

Additional files

Additional file 1: Table S1. List of differentially expressed genes with transcriptional regulation. **Table S2**. Gene Ontology (GO) and Ingenuity Pathway Analysis (IPA) of differentially expressed genes based on biological processes, canonical pathways and upstream regulators. **a** GO biological processes enriched (P<0.01, FDR<5%). **b** Upstream regulator analysis using Ingenuity Pathway Analysis 2013 (P<0.00001) **Table S3**. Comparison of differentially expressed genes with published CRC microarray studies

Additional file 2: Figure S1. Ingenuity Pathway Analysis (IPA) identifies enriched top pathway networks in CRC.**Figure S2**. Oncoprint summary of genomic alterations in CRC from the TCGA database. **Figure S3**. Clinino-pathological characteristics of CRC samples

Abbreviations

CRC: colorectal cancer; GO: gene ontology; IPA: ingenuity pathway analysis; TCGA: The Cancer Genome Atlas; CNVs: copy number variations; TF: transcription factor; RPN2: ribophorin II; HMGB1: high-mobility group protein B1.

Authors' contributions

Conception and design: JLZ, ZC, XLS and YYB. Subject recruitment: JLZ, HQ, XLS, and YYB. Data acquisition: BY, DGG, JFS, HQ, XLS and YYB. Analysis and interpretation of data: JLZ, BY, SSS, HQ and ZC. Drafting of the manuscript: JLZ, BY, SSS, SC, YYB, XLS, CVW, QH and ZC. Study supervision: ZC, XLS and YYB. All authors read and approved the final manuscript.

Author details

[1] School of Public Health, Wuhan University, Wuhan, China. [2] Clinical Medicine Research Center, The Affiliated Hospital, Inner Mongolia Medical University, Hohhot, China. [3] Tumor Biology Section, Head and Neck Surgery Branch, National Institute on Deafness and Other Communication Disorders, NIH, Bethesda, USA. [4] Laboratory for Food Safety and Environmental Technology, Shenzhen Institutes of Advanced Technology, Chinese Academy of Sciences, Shenzhen, China. [5] Pediatric Endocrinology Unit, Department of Women's and Children's Health, Karolinska Institute and University Hospital, Stockholm, Sweden. [6] Department of Oncology, The Affiliated Hospital, Inner Mongolia Medical University, Hohhot, China. [7] Department of Biology, Hong Kong Baptist University, Hong Kong, China. [8] Department of Bioinformatics, School of Basic Medical Sciences, Nanjing Medical University, Nanjing, China. [9] Department of Respiratory Medicine, Saitama Medical Center, Jichi Medical University, Saitama, Japan.

Acknowledgements

This work was supported by the National Natural Science Foundation of China (Grant no. 81160253, China) and Natural Science Foundation of Inner Mongolia (Grant no. 2011MS1158, China). JLZ was supported by Natural Science Foundation of Inner Mongolia. ZC and CVW are supported by NIDCD intramural project ZIA-DC-00016. We thank Dr. Jiro Kato at NIH/NHLBI and Han Si at NIH/NEI for critical reading of the manuscript and for valuable discussions.

Compliance with ethical guidelines

Competing interests

The authors declare that they have no competing interests.

References

1. Kuipers EJ, Rosch T, Bretthauer M. Colorectal cancer screening–optimizing current strategies and new directions. Nature review. Clin Oncol. 2013;10(3):130–42.
2. Kuntz KM, Lansdorp-Vogelaar I, Rutter CM, Knudsen AB, van Ballegooijen M, Savarino JE, et al. A systematic comparison of microsimulation models of colorectal cancer: the role of assumptions about adenoma progression. Med Decis Mak Int J Soc Med Decis Mak. 2011;31(4):530–9.
3. Labianca R, Merelli B. Screening and diagnosis for colorectal cancer: present and future. Tumori. 2010;96(6):889–901.
4. Akiyoshi T, Kobunai T, Watanabe T. Recent approaches to identifying biomarkers for high-risk stage II colon cancer. Surg Today. 2012;42(11):1037–45.
5. Koelzer VH, Lugli A. The tumor border configuration of colorectal cancer as a histomorphological prognostic indicator. Front Oncol. 2014;18(4):29.
6. Lavery IC, De Campos-Lobato LF. How to evaluate risk and identify stage II patients requiring referral to a medical oncologist: a surgeon's perspective. Oncol N Y. 2010;24(1):14–6.
7. Fleming M, Ravula S, Tatishchev SF, Wang HL. Colorectal carcinoma: pathologic aspects. J Gastrointest Oncol. 2012;3(3):153–73.
8. Furlan D, Carnevali IW, Bernasconi B, Sahnane N, Milani K, Cerutti R, et al. Hierarchical clustering analysis of pathologic and molecular data identifies prognostically and biologically distinct groups of colorectal carcinomas. Mod Pathol. 2011;24(1):126–37.
9. Madhavan S, Gusev Y, Natarajan TG. Genome-wide multi-omics profiling of colorectal cancer identifies immune determinants strongly associated with relapse. Front Genet. 2013;20(4):236.
10. Sharif S, O'Connell MJ. Gene signatures in stage II colon cancer: a clinical review. Curr Colorectal Cancer Rep. 2012;8(3):225–31.
11. Chu D, Zhang Z, Li Y, Wu L, Zhang J, Wang W, Zhang J, et al. Prediction of colorectal cancer relapse and prognosis by tissue mRNA levels of NDRG2. Mol Cancer Ther Jan. 2011;10:47.
12. Vicuna B, Benson AB 3rd. Adjuvant therapy for stage II colon cancer: prognostic and predictive markers. J Nat Compr Cancer Net JNCCN. 2007;5(9):927–36.
13. Walther A, Johnstone E, Swanton C, Midgley R, Tomlinson I, Kerr D. Genetic prognostic and predictive markers in colorectal cancer. Nat Rev Cancer. 2009;9(7):489–99.

14. Roth AD, Tejpar S, Delorenzi M, Yan P, Fiocca R, Klingbiel D, et al. Prognostic role of KRAS and BRAF in stage II and III resected colon cancer: results of the translational study on the PETACC-3, EORTC 40993, SAKK 60-00 trial. J Clin Oncol Off J Am Soc Clin Oncol. 2010;28(3):466–74.
15. Ogino S, Nosho K, Irahara N, Shima K, Baba Y, Kirkner GJ, et al. CpG island methylator phenotype, microsatellite instability, BRAF mutation and clinical outcome in colon cancer. Gut. 2009;58(1):90–6.
16. Amado RG, Wolf M, Peeters M, Van Cutsem E, Siena S, Freeman DJ, et al. Wild-type KRAS is required for panitumumab efficacy in patients with metastatic colorectal cancer. J Clin Oncol. 2008;26(10):1626–34.
17. Razis E, Pentheroudakis G, Rigakos G, Bobos M, Kouvatseas G, Tzaida O, et al. EGFR gene gain and PTEN protein expression are favorable prognostic factors in patients with KRAS wild-type metastatic colorectal cancer treated with cetuximab. J Cancer Res Clin Oncol. 2014;140(5):737–48.
18. Smith FM, Stephens RB, Kennedy MJ, Reynolds JV. P53 abnormalities and outcomes in colorectal cancer: a systematic review. Br J Cancer. 2005;92(9):1813.
19. Ribic CM, Sargent DJ, Moore MJ, Thibodeau SN, French AJ, Goldberg RM, et al. Tumor microsatellite-instability status as a predictor of benefit from fluorouracil-based adjuvant chemotherapy for colon cancer. N Engl J Med. 2003;349(3):247–57.
20. Network Cancer Genome Atlas. Comprehensive molecular characterization of human colon and rectal cancer. Nature. 2012;487(7407):330–7.
21. Shibayama M, Maak M, Nitsche U, Gotoh K, Rosenberg R, Janssen KP. Prediction of metastasis and recurrence in colorectal cancer based on gene expression analysis: ready for the clinic? Cancers. 2011;3:2858–69.
22. Watanabe T. Biomarker for high-risk patients with stage II colon cancer. Lancet Oncol. 2013;14(13):1247–8.
23. Sobin LH, Fleming ID. TNM classification of malignant tumors, fifth edition (1997). Union Internationale Contre le Cancer and the American Joint Committee on Cancer. Cancer. 1997;80(9):1803–4.
24. Yan B, Li H, Yang X, Shao J, Jang M, Guan D, et al. Unraveling regulatory programs for NF-kappaB, p53 and microRNAs in head and neck squamous cell carcinoma. PLoS One. 2013;8(9):e73656.
25. Ethayathulla AS, Nguyen HT, Viadiu H. Crystal structures of the DNA-binding domain tetramer of the p53 tumor suppressor family member p73 bound to different full-site response elements. J Biol Chem. 2013;288(7):4744–54.
26. Martynova E, Pozzi S, Basile V, Dolfini D, Zambelli F, Imbriano C, et al. Gain-of-function p53 mutants have widespread genomic locations partially overlapping with p63. Oncotarget. 2012;3(2):132–43.
27. Kim J, Lee JH, Iyer VR. Global identification of Myc target genes reveals its direct role in mitochondrial biogenesis and its E-box usage in vivo. PLoS One. 2008;3(3):e1798.
28. Zeller KI, Jegga AG, Aronow BJ, O'Donnell KA, Dang CV. An integrated database of genes responsive to the Myc oncogenic transcription factor: identification of direct genomic targets. Genome Biol. 2003;4(10):R69.
29. Cerami E, Gao J, Dogrusoz U, Gross BE, Sumer SO, Aksoy BA, et al. The cBio cancer genomics portal: an open platform for exploring multidimensional cancer genomics data. Cancer Discov. 2012;2(5):401–4.
30. Huqun, Ishikawa R, Zhang J, Miyazawa H, Goto Y, Shimizu Y, et al. Enhancer of zeste homolog 2 is a novel prognostic biomarker in nonsmall cell lung cancer. Cancer. 2012;118(6):1599–606.
31. Sanz-Pamplona R, Berenguer A, Cordero D, Riccadonna S, Solé X, et al. Clinical value of prognosis gene expression signatures in colorectal cancer: a systematic review. PLoS One. 2012;7(11):e48877.
32. Oikawa T. ETS transcription factors: possible targets for cancer therapy. Cancer Sci. 2004;95(8):626–33.
33. Gronemeyer HJA. Gustafsson, and V. Laudet. Principles for modulation of the nuclear receptor superfamily. Nat Rev Drug Disc. 2004;3(11):950–64.
34. Sharma HW, Perez JR, Higgins-Sochaski K, Hsiao R, Narayanan R, et al. Transcription factor decoy approach to decipher the role of NF-kappa B in oncogenesis. Anticancer Res. 1996;16(1):61–9.
35. Hasselblatt P, Gresh L, Kudo H, Guinea-Viniegra J, Wagner EF. The role of the transcription factor AP-1 in colitis-associated and beta-catenin-dependent intestinal tumorigenesis in mice. Oncogene. 2008;27(47):6102–9.
36. Nakao K, Mehta KR, Fridlyand J, Moore DH, Jain AN, Lafuente A, et al. High-resolution analysis of DNA copy number alterations in colorectal cancer by array-based comparative genomic hybridization. Carcinogenesis. 2004;25(8):1345–57.
37. Gordziel C, Bratsch J, Moriggl R, Knösel T, Friedrich K. Both STAT1 and STAT3 are favourable prognostic determinants in colorectal carcinoma. Br J Cancer. 2013;109(1):138–46.
38. Camps J, Nguyen QT, Padilla-Nash HM, Knutsen T, McNeil NE, Wangsa D, et al. Integrative genomics reveals mechanisms of copy number alterations responsible for transcriptional deregulation in colorectal cancer. Genes Chromosom Cancer. 2009;48(11):1002–17.
39. Henrichsen CN, Chaignat E, Reymond A. Copy number variants, diseases and gene expression. Hum Mol Genet. 2009;18(R1):R1–8.
40. Yi JM, Dhir M, Van Neste L, Downing SR, Jeschke J, Glöckner SC, et al. Genomic and epigenomic integration identifies a prognostic signature in colon cancer. Clin Cancer Res Off J Am Assoc Cancer Res. 2011;17(6):1535–45.
41. Yao X, Zhao G, Yang H, Hong X, Bie L, Liu G. Overexpression of high-mobility group box 1 correlates with tumor progression and poor prognosis in human colorectal carcinoma. J Cancer Res Clin Oncol. 2010;136(5):677–84.
42. Slaby O, Sobkova K, Svoboda M, Garajova I, Fabian P, Hrstka R. Significant overexpression of Hsp110 gene during colorectal cancer progression. Oncol Rep. 2009;21(5):1235–41.
43. Southern SL, Collard TJ, Urban BC, Skeen VR, Smartt HJ, Hague A, et al. BAG-1 interacts with the p50-p50 homodimeric NF-kappaB complex: implications for colorectal carcinogenesis. Oncogene. 2012;31(22):2761–72.
44. Kang R, Zhang Q, Zeh HJ 3rd, Lotze MT, Tang D. HMGB1 in cancer: good, bad, or both? Clin Cancer Res Off J Am Assoc Cancer Res. 2013;19(15):4046–57.
45. Süren D, Yıldırım M, Demirpençe Ö, Kaya V, Alikanoğlu AS, Bülbüller N, et al. The role of high mobility group box 1 (HMGB1) in colorectal cancer. Med Sci Monit. 2014;31(20):530–7.
46. Ueda M, Takahashi Y, Shinden Y, Sakimura S, Hirata H, Uchi R, et al. Prognostic significance of high mobility group box 1 (HMGB1) expression in patients with colorectal cancer. Anticancer Res. 2014;34(10):5357–62.
47. Zhang CC, Gdynia G, Ehemann V, Roth W. The HMGB1 protein sensitizes colon carcinoma cells to cell death triggered by pro-apoptotic agents. nt. J Oncol. 2015;46(2):667–76.
48. Zhu L, Li X, Chen Y, Fang J, Ge Z. High-mobility group box 1: a novel inducer of the epithelial-mesenchymal transition in colorectal carcinoma. Cancer Lett. 2015;357(2):527–34.
49. Honma K, Iwao-Koizumi K, Takeshita F, Yamamoto Y, Yoshida T, Nishio K, et al. RPN2 gene confers docetaxel resistance in breast cancer. Nat Med. 2008;14(9):939–48.
50. Takahashi RU, Takeshita F, Honma K, Ono M, Kato K, Ochiya T. Ribophorin II regulates breast tumor initiation and metastasis through the functional suppression of GSK3 beta. Sci Rep. 2013;3:2474.
51. Vilar E, Gruber SB. Microsatellite instability in colorectal cancer-the stable evidence. Nature reviews. Clin Oncol. 2010;7(3):153–62.
52. Nanashima A, Yamaguchi H, Yasutake T, Sawai T, Kusano H, Tagawa Y, et al. Gain of chromosome 20 is a frequent aberration in liver metastasis of colorectal cancers. Dig Dis Sci. 1997;42:1388–93.
53. Loo LW, Tiirikainen M, Cheng I, Lum-Jones A, Seifried A, Church JM, et al. Integrated analysis of genome-wide copy number alterations and gene expression in microsatellite stable, CpG island methylator phenotype-negative colon cancer. Genes Chromosomes Cancer. 2013;52(5):450–66.
54. Kurashige J, Watanabe M, Iwatsuki M, Kinoshita K, Saito S, Nagai Y, et al. RPN2 expression predicts response to docetaxel in oesophageal squamous cell carcinoma. Br J Cancer. 2012;107(8):1233–8.
55. Lian M, Fang J, Han D, Ma H, Feng L, Wang R, et al. Microarray gene expression analysis of tumorigenesis and regional lymph node metastasis in laryngeal squamous cell carcinoma. PLoS One. 2013;8(12):e84854.
56. Fujiwara T, Takahashi RU, Kosaka N, Nezu Y, Kawai A, et al. RPN2 gene confers osteosarcoma cell malignant phenotypes and determines clinical prognosis. Molecular therapy. Nucleic Acids. 2014;3:e189.
57. Bielack SS, Kempf-Bielack B, Delling G, Exner GU, Flege S, Helmke K, et al. Prognostic factors in high-grade osteosarcoma of the extremities or trunk: an analysis of 1702 patients treated on neoadjuvant cooperative osteosarcoma study group protocols. J Clin Oncol. 2002;20(3):776–90.
58. Fujita Y, Takeshita F, Mizutani T, Ohgi T, Kuwano K, Ochiya T. A novel platform to enable inhaled naked RNAi medicine for lung cancer. Scientific Rep. 2013;3:3325.

Molecular characterization of HIV-1 genome in fission yeast *Schizosaccharomyces pombe*

Joseph Nkeze[1†], Lin Li[1,4†], Zsigmond Benko[1,5], Ge Li[1] and Richard Y Zhao[1,2,3*]

Abstract

Background: The human immunodeficiency virus type 1 (HIV-1) genome (~9 kb RNA) is flanked by two long terminal repeats (LTR) promoter regions with nine open reading frames, which encode Gag, Pol and Env polyproteins, four accessory proteins (Vpu, Vif, Vpr, Nef) and two regulatory proteins (Rev, Tat). In this study, we carried out a genome-wide and functional analysis of the HIV-1 genome in fission yeast (*Schizosaccharomyces pombe*).

Results: Each one of the HIV-1 genes was cloned and expressed individually in fission yeast. Subcellular localization of each viral protein was first examined. The effect of protein expression on cellular proliferation and colony formations, an indication of cytotoxicity, were observed. Overall, there is a general correlation of subcellular localization of each viral protein between fission yeast and mammalian cells. Three viral proteins, viral protein R (Vpr), protease (PR) and regulator of expression of viral protein (Rev), were found to inhibit cellular proliferation. Rev was chosen for further analysis in fission yeast and mammalian cells. Consistent with the observation in fission yeast, expression of HIV-1 *rev* gene also caused growth retardation in mammalian cells. However, the observed growth delay was neither due to the cytotoxic effect nor due to alterations in cell cycling. Mechanistic testing of the Rev effect suggests it triggers transient induction of cellular oxidative stress.

Conclusions: Some of the behavioral and functional similarities of Rev between fission yeast and mammalian cells suggest fission yeast might be a useful model system for further studies of molecular functions of Rev and other HIV-1 viral proteins.

Keywords: HIV-1, Viral genome, Gene expression, Functional analysis, Fission yeast, *Schizosaccharomyces pombe*, Subcellular localization, Cellular proliferation, Colony formation, Oxidative stress, Mammalian cell

Background

The human immunodeficiency virus type 1 (HIV-1), like other retroviruses, is made up of an RNA encoded genome of approximately 9.7 kilobases (kb). Both ends of the RNA genome are flanked by a long terminal repeat (LTR) promoter region (Fig. 1). Between the two LTR regions, there are three polyproteins (Gag, Pol, Env), four accessory proteins (Vpu, Vif, Vpr, Nef) and two regulatory proteins (Rev, Tat). HIV-1 RNA also contains regulatory regions which are important for transcription initiation and polyadenylation.

The polyprotein Gag is required for both virion assembly and maturation [1, 2]. The Gag protein is cleaved by viral protease into P17, P24, P7, and P6 proteins shortly after budding from the host cell [1]. P17 (MA) protein lies in the inner surface membrane of matured viral particles [3]. It is important for RNA targeting of the plasma membrane prior to viral assembly, incorporation of the Env glycoprotein into the viral particle [4, 5] and the particle release [6, 7]. P24 (Capsid domain, CA) protein forms a shell surrounding the viral RNA genome and core-associated proteins in mature virion. It plays various roles including incorporation of the Gag-Pol precursor into virions during viral assembly [8], recruitment of the

*Correspondence: rzhao@som.umaryland.edu
†Joseph Nkeze and Lin Li are co-first authors
[3] Institute of Human Virology, University of Maryland School of Medicine, Baltimore, MD 21201-1192, USA
Full list of author information is available at the end of the article

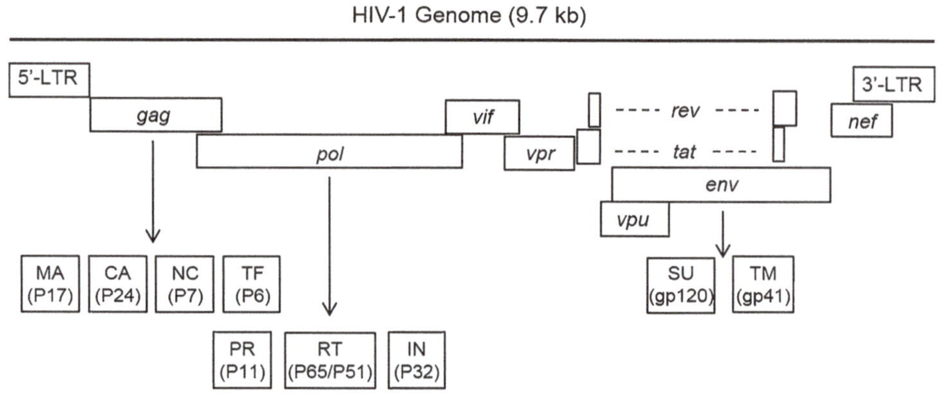

Fig. 1 Schematic diagram of HIV-1 genome. The total size of HIV-1 genome is approximately 9.7 kb. Each of the viral genes is drawing based on the relative orientation in the entire RNA genome. *Arrows* points to cleaved protein products. *Dashed lines* represent RNA splicing. The *number in parenthesis* is molecular weight of each protein. *LTR* long-term repeat, *Gag* group-specific antigen, *MA* matrix protein, *CA* capsid domain, *NC* nucleocapsid, *TF* trans-frame protein, *Pol* polymerases, *PR* protease, *RT* reverse transcriptase, *IN* integrase, *Env* envelope protein, *SU* surface membrane protein, *TM* trans-membrane protein, *Vif* viral infectivity factor, *Vpr* viral protein R, *Vpu* viral protein U, *Nef* negative regulatory factor, *Rev* regulator of expression of viral proteins, *Tat* trans-activator of transcription.

viral infectivity enhancing protein Cyclophilin A (CypA) [9–11], and early post entry [12]. P7 (Nucleocapsid, NC) plays important roles in the encapsulation and protection of viral RNA, promotion of viral assembly and in early post entry steps including reverse transcription [13]. P6 is important for Vpr packaging into the viral particle and virus budding from the cell membrane [14].

The Pol protein is expressed as a Gag–Pol fusion product since its gene lacks an initiation codon. It is subsequently cleaved by HIV-1 protease to produce MA, CA, NC, trans-frame protein (TF), viral enzymes protease (PR), reverse transcriptase (RT), and integrase (IN) [15]. PR cleaves the Gag and Pol precursors thus rendering the virion infectious [16]. RT is an asymmetric heterodimer with its main role to reverse transcribe viral RNA into pro-viral DNA prior to viral integration to host chromosomes [17]. Other functions of RT include RNA-directed DNA polymerase, DNA directed DNA polymerase and ribonuclease hybrid activities (RNase H) [18]. IN is active only as a tetramer and it is responsible for the integration of the linear double-stranded proviral DNA into the host cell chromosome [19].

The Env/gp160 protein is a precursor protein encoded by a spliced mRNA, which is subsequently cleaved by cellular proteases into the envelope gp120 surface membrane protein (SU) and gp41 trans-membrane protein (TM) [20]. The gp120 surface subunit harbors the N-terminal of the Gp160. It binds to cell receptors attaching virus to target cells and also regulates viral entry. Gp41 is the C-terminal 345-amino acid protein of gp160. It is also involved in the viral entry and mediation of fusion [21].

In addition to the retroviral Gag, Pol, and Env proteins, HIV-l produces four accessory proteins, i.e. Nef, Vif, Vpr and Vpu, and two regulatory protein, i.e. Tat, and Rev [22]. While Tat and Rev are required for viral replication, Nef, Vif, Vpr and Vpu are dispensable for viral proliferation in many of the in vitro systems [23, 24]. However, they are often necessary for viral replication and pathogenesis in vivo and for many of the essential viral functions during the viral life cycle.

The fission yeast *Schizosaccharomyces pombe* (*S. pombe*) is a unicellular eukaryote of the Division Ascomycota. It is cylindrical and rounded at both ends. It reproduces meiotically by ascospores and proliferates asexually by cell division (fission). Its length and diameter are about 7–12 μm and 3–4 μm, respectively [25, 26]. It has a relative small genomic size of about 1.5×1 0^7 bp in the haploid state [27]. *S. pombe* has many of the same fundamental cellular features as larger multicellular organisms which makes it very useful in many of the molecular-biological studies [25–28]. It contains gene slicing mechanism that is able to remove introns from genes of higher eukaryote and mammals [25, 27, 29]. Its signal-transduction system is able to transmit signals from the mating factor receptor through a G-protein-coupled system to the effectors [25]. The cell cycle is also similar to that in higher eukaryotes [27, 31]. For more than three decades, fission yeast has been used in many studies to investigate the structures, functions and expression of eukaryotic genes, especially from mammalian origins [25, 27, 29, 31]. It should also be mentioned that our laboratory has been using fission yeast as a model system to study the effect of HIV-1 Vpr on basic cellular functions in the past 20 years, which includes cell cycle G2/M regulation, nuclear transport and induction of cell death and apoptosis [31–36]. Results of those earlier studies have demonstrated the effects of Vpr are resembled, most of the time, to those of found in mammalian cells. Furthermore, this simple model system allowed us to discover new Vpr-specific activities that are otherwise difficult to uncover solely based on mammalian studies [37–41]. Our intention in this study was therefore to expand and to test whether we could also use fission yeast as a host system to study other HIV-1 proteins.

It should be mentioned that both fission yeast and budding yeast (*Saccharomyces cerevisiae*) have long been used to study various HIV-1 proteins. Some specific examples include HIV-1 Gag [31], Tat [32], Rev [33], Vpr [34], Vpx [35], Vpu [36], Integrase [42] and Protease [43], respectively. A number of reviews have also described the use of yeast as a model system for HIV-1 studies [44–47]. However, none of those early yeast studies has studied the whole HIV-1 genome all at once. Therefore our goal here was to carry out a genome-wide and functional analysis by cloning and expressing every viral gene encoded by the HIV genome in fission yeast. Subcellular localizations and effects of these viral proteins on fission yeast cell proliferation and colony formation, an indication of cytotoxicity, were observed and analyzed.

Results

Subcellular localizations of HIV-1 proteins in fission yeast

In order to determine the subcellular localization of HIV-1 proteins in fission yeast, SP223 cells were transformed with a fission yeast expression pYZ3N plasmid producing each of the HIV-1 viral protein sequences in fusion with an N-terminal GFP [48]. The fission yeast strains containing different viral proteins expressing plasmids were inoculated into liquid selective medium and the protein expression was induced following the removal of thiamine from the growth medium as described previously [34, 49]. After cultured for 24–30 h (depending on the intensity of green fluorescence), the GFP-viral fusion protein products were observed under a fluorescence microscope. As shown in Fig. 2a, GFP alone disperses throughout the cells indicating no preference of subcellular location. In contrast, the Gag protein aggregated in the cytoplasm of unknown sites. P17 protein was excluded from the nucleus and localized exclusively in the cytoplasm. P24 protein was localized both in the nucleus and cell membrane, while the P7 protein was predominantly localized in the nucleus. P6 was found distributed throughout the cell. The localizations of Pol proteins (P66, P51, IN, PR) and Env proteins (including Gp120 and Gp41) were monitored and shown in Fig. 2b. P66 was found more in the nucleus than in the cytoplasm; whereas P51 proteins were found exclusively in the cytoplasm. Consistent with the role of HIV-1 integrase, IN was indeed found more in the nucleus than in the cytoplasm. PR was distributed evenly throughout the cell, while Gp120 and Gp41 were localized more in the nucleus than in the cytoplasm. The subcellular distribution of HIV-1 accessory proteins (Vpr, Vpu, Vif, Nef, Rev, and Tat) was shown in Fig. 2c. Consistent with previous findings with Vpr [48], it localizes predominantly in the nucleus. Similarly, Vif, Rev, and Tat all accumulated in the nucleus of yeast cells. Nuclear localization of Tat has also been reported in budding yeast previously [50]. Vpu in cytoplasm but Nef was distributed throughout the cell. Finally, the subcellular location patterns observed in fission yeast were compared with that reported from mammalian cell studies. As summarized in Table 1, overall, there is a general correlation of the subcellular localization of each viral protein between fission yeast and that of previously reported in mammalian cells.

Effects of HIV-1 gene expression on yeast colony formation

To determine potential cytotoxic effect of HIV-1 viral protein expression on fission yeast, yeast colony formation, an indication of cellular growth and potential cytotoxicity, was measured. Fission yeast cells that were transformed with each one of the viral proteins via the inducible pYZ1N plasmids [48] were plated on selected agar plates under the gene-repressing (gene-Off) or gene-inducing (gene-On) conditions (Fig. 3). Correct nucleotide sequence of each viral gene carried on the pYZ1N plasmid was confirmed by Sanger sequencing. *S. pombe* cells transformed with pYZ1N-Vpr or an empty pYZ1N plasmid were used as positive and negative controls, respectively. We have reported previously that Vpr prevents colony formation whereas pYZ1N plasmid has no cytotoxic effect on cells [34, 64]. As shown in Fig. 3, all HIV-1 viral gene-repressing (gene-Off) cells formed colonies as anticipated. On the gene-inducing (gene-On) plates, as expected, cells containing the empty pYZ1N plasmid formed colonies but HIV-1 Vpr prevented colony formation. Most of the HIV-1 viral gene expressions in fission yeast did not show any cytotoxic effects as they formed the same sizes of colony as the pYZ1N control. In contrast, however, the fission yeast strains expressing *rev* and *PR* showed much reduced or no colony formation indicating inhibition of cell growth or possible cytotoxic effects following expression of the respective genes.

Effects of HIV-1 *rev* gene expression on yeast cell growth

To further differentiate the inhibitory effect of HIV-1 Rev protein on the cellular growth or toxicity of yeast cells, we measured the growth kinetics of *S. pombe* cells

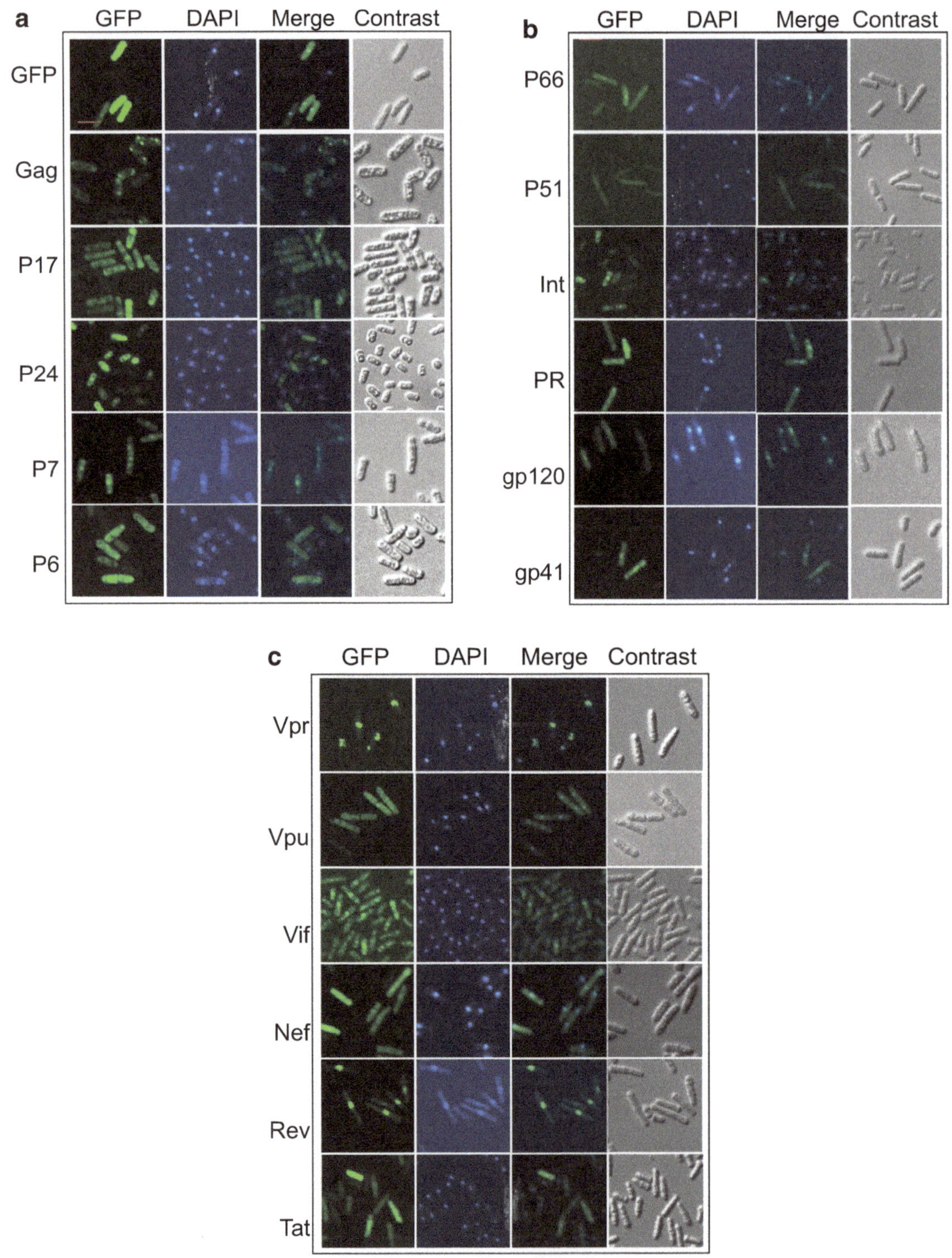

Fig. 2 Subcellular localization of HIV-1 proteins in fission yeast. Fission yeast strains expressing normal GFP or N-terminally GFP-tagged HIV-1 proteins were grown to a log phase in EMM selective media. The cells were re-inoculated into fresh media without thiamine (to induce gene expression) and grown for 24–30 h. The nuclei were stained with DAPI. The cells were examined using fluorescence microscopy for subcellular localizations of the GFP-tagged proteins with stained cellular nuclei. *Each column* represents different microscopic views: GFP, for protein subcellular location; DAPI, for localization of the nucleus; Merge, merging images of GFP and DAPI; and the "Contrast" is for the overall view of the cell. The Gag gene products are shown in **a**, the Pol and Env gene products in **b**, and the auxiliary and regulatory proteins in **c**. The *scale bar* represents 10 μm.

Table 1 Subcellular localization of HIV-1 proteins in mammalian and fission yeast cells

HIV-1 protein	Subcellular localization	
	Mammalian (references)	Fission yeast (this study)
Gag	Cytoplasmic membrane [51]	Cytoplasm
P17	Cytoplasm, membrane [52]	Cytoplasm
P24	Cytoplasmic membrane [53]	Nucleus and cell membrane
P7	Nucleus [54]	Nucleus
P6	Cytoplasmic membrane [55]	Throughout cell[a]
P66	Cytoplasm [56]	Nuclear > cytoplasm
P51	Cytoplasm [56]	Cytoplasm
Integrase	Nucleus [57]	Nuclear > cytoplasm
Protease	No report found	Throughout cell
Gp120	No report found	Nuclear > cytoplasm
Gp41	No report found	Nuclear > cytoplasm
Vpr	Nucleic membrane [48]	Nucleus [58]
Vpu	Cytoplasm [59]	Cytoplasm
Vif	Nucleus [60]	Nucleus
Nef	Cytoplasm [61]	Throughout cell[a]
Rev	Nucleus [62]	Nucleus
Tat	Nucleus [63]	Nucleus

[a] Different subcellular localization pattern was observed.

with and without *rev* gene expression. *S. pombe* cells containing pYZ1N-*rev* and pYZ1N control vectors were grown under gene-repressing (+T) and gene-inducing (−T) conditions in liquid minimal and selective EMM medium. Cellular growth was measured by the optical density (OD) over time from 0 to 122 h (5 days). At the first 24 h, both cells grown at the same pace with a doubling time of approx. 24 h. After 24 h of gene induction when the *rev* gene expression was fully expressed [34, 65], the growth velocity of Rev-producing cells became slower than those without *rev* gene expression that was grown actively in a logarithmic fashion (Fig. 4a). By 48 h, i.e., 2 days after *rev* gene induction, the difference in growth between *rev*-expressing and *rev*-repressing cells reached to the maximum level. As control, the pYZ1N transformed yeast cells showed no difference in growth of neither gene-repressing nor gene-inducing condition.

Rev causes growth delay but not cell death

Retarded cell growth could be an indication of cell death due to cytotoxicity. So we checked whether the growth delay caused by Rev was due to cell death. A semi-quantitative colony dot dilution assay was used, which quantified the ability of individual cells to form colonies on agar plate. All of the cells expressing *rev* formed colonies with expected numbers on each agar plate although the colony sizes were much smaller (Fig. 4b). This observation suggested that Rev causes growth delay but not cell death. Therefore, Rev causes growth delay but not cell death.

Rev does not affect cell cycling of fission yeast

Because Rev affects cellular growth of fission yeast cells, we were interested in testing whether it affects the distribution of cell cycles. The cell cycle profile of *S. pombe* cells containing *rev*-expressing plasmid was monitored by flow cytometry. In standard EMM medium, *S. pombe* cells normally reside predominantly in the G2 phase of the cell cycle [66]. If Rev induces G1 delay, we should expect a shift of the predominantly G2 cell population to G1 after the production of Rev protein. Similarly, Rev-induced G2 delay should be represented by no shift of G2 cell population to G1 in the EMM medium. In this experiment, production of HIV-1 Rev protein did not change the cell cycle profile (Fig. 4c). Consistently, the pYZ1N vector was used as a control and showed no cell cycle difference between gene-repressing (+T) and gene-inducing (−T) conditions.

Rev stimulates the production of reactive oxygen species (ROS)

To further explore the possible molecular mechanism underlying Rev-induced growth delay, possible intracellular stress induced by Rev was measured by probable production of ROS. A ROS-specific dye, DHE that produces red fluorescence in the presence of ROS, was used to measure possible cellular oxidative stress in *rev*-expressing cells. A ROS scavenger TMPO that can specifically remove free radicals by forming stable complexes [67], was also used as a control to verify the specific production of ROS. Expression of HIV-1 *rev* was induced in a fission yeast strain carrying the pYZ1N-*rev* plasmid, and the level of ROS was subsequently detected in cells at 21, 24, and 30 h after *rev* gene induction (Fig. 5). At 21 h, strong red fluorescence was detected in the *rev*-expressing cells; whereas little or no red fluorescence was observed in the *rev*-repressing cells (Fig. 5a). Consistently, treatment of the same *rev*-expressing cells with the ROS scavenger TMPO significantly reduced intensity of the red fluorescence suggesting the observed ROS production is Rev specific. Interestingly, Rev-induced ROS production faded away very quickly (Fig. 5b). About half of the *rev*-expressing cells produced the ROS signals 21 h after *rev* gene induction. Less than 30% of the cells showed ROS production 3 h later and a little more than 10% of those cells were DHE-positive by 30 h after gene induction. Together these data suggest expression of HIV-1 *rev* gene in fission yeast triggers intracellular oxidative stress. However, such a cellular stress response

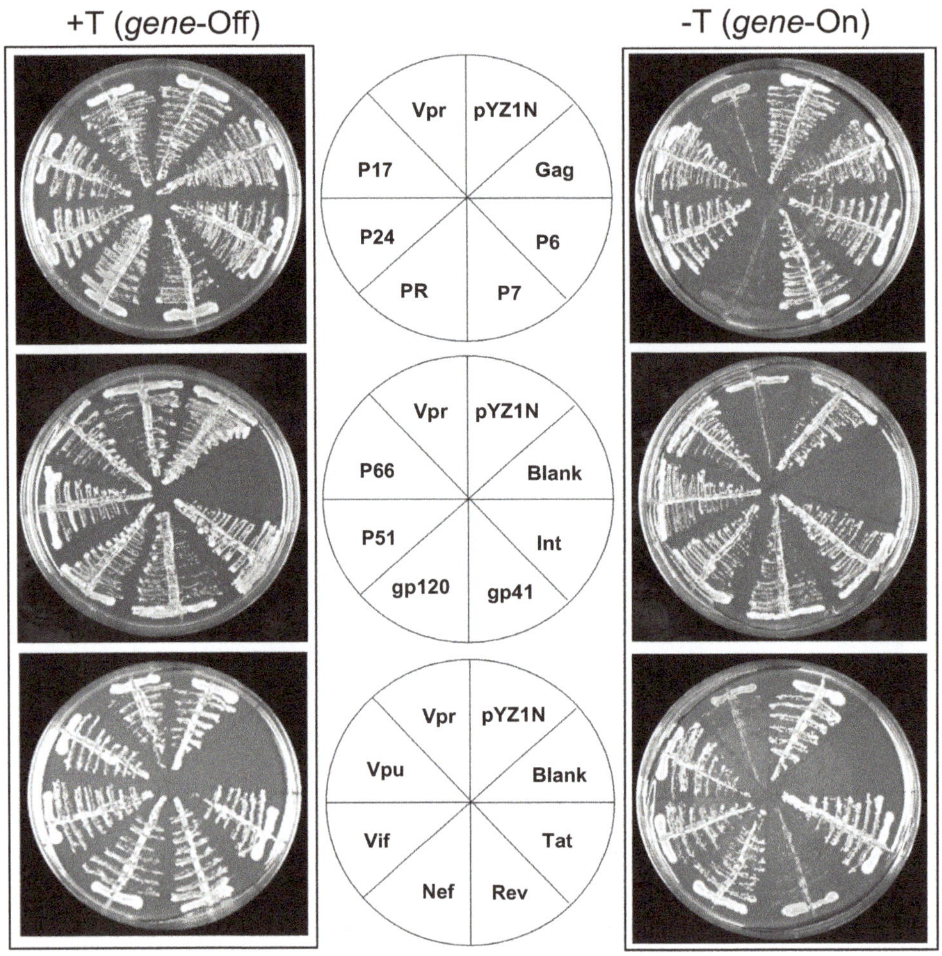

Fig. 3 Effects of HIV-1 viral proteins on colony formation. Wild type *S. pombe* cells containing HIV-1 viral gene-expressing plasmids were grown overnight in EMM liquid medium supplemented with thiamine to mid-log phase. The following day, cells were recovered, re-suspended in fresh media and streaked onto the minimal selection EMM agar plates with thiamine (*left* +T plates; no gene expression) or without thiamine (*right* −T plates; with gene expression). The plates were incubated at 30°C for 6 days before observation. The pYZ1N-*vpr* and pYZ1N plasmids were used as positive and negative controls, respectively [34].

might be transient, which could potentially explain at least in part why those *rev*-expressing cells slowed cell growth but did not die.

Effect of Rev protein on mammalian cell growth

Since HIV-1 Rev caused growth delay in *S. pombe*, we were interested in whether the same effect could also be observed in mammalian cells. In order to observe the effect of Rev protein on mammalian cellular growth, we created a mammalian gene inducible system to produce Rev. The HIV-1 *rev* gene was cloned into the mammalian cell expressing vector pZH-1 and transfected into 293VE632 cells [68]. The transfected cells were selected with hygromycin. After exerting drug selection for 2 weeks, Rev protein production was tested by inducing its expression with muristerone A. The cell lysate were collected and monoclonal anti-Rev antibody was used to confirm the expression of Rev protein (Fig. 6a). It was anticipated that if Rev affects mammalian cell growth, there should be a difference of cell numbers between *rev*-expressing and *rev*-repressing cells. The cell numbers of *rev*-containing 293VE632 cells were counted with Trypan blue staining under *rev*-repressing and *rev*-inducing conditions, and growth curves were generated. Indeed, there was a diverging growth differences between *rev*-expressing and *rev*-repressing cells after 5 days of culture (Fig. 6b). Finally, we tested whether the Rev-induced growth delay was due to, or at least partially due to alteration in cell cycling. To test this, 293VE632 cells containing pZH-1 and pZH-*rev* were

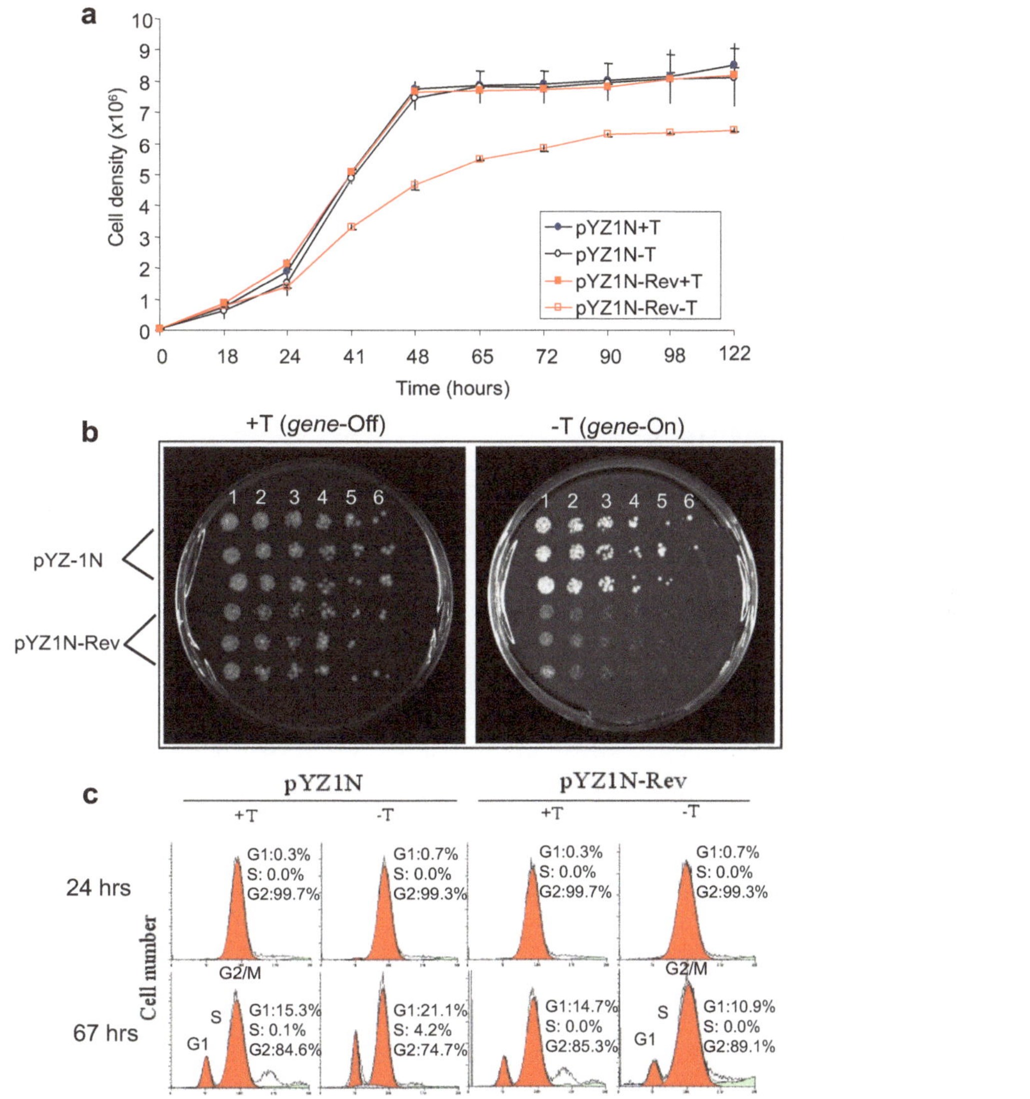

Fig. 4 Effect of HIV-1 Rev protein production on fission yeast. **a** Expression of HIV-1 *rev* delays cellular growth of *S. pombe*. *S. pombe* cells containing pYZ1N-*rev* was grown under gene-repressing (+T) and gene-inducing (−T) conditions in liquid minimal selection EMM at 30°C. The cell density was measured over time and growth curves were plotted. *S. pombe* cell containing pYZ1N was used as a control. The experiment was repeated three times and the standard errors of each time point were calculated. **b** Rev delays colony formation in fission yeast cells. A semi-quantitative colony dot dilution assay was use to evaluate the ability of individual *rev*-expressing *S. pombe* cells to form colonies on agar plates. The pYZ1N-*rev* transformed *S. pombe* cells were grown in liquid EMM medium to log phase with thiamine. Thiamine was then removed from cells by washing and equal number of cells transferred to EMM supplemented plates with (gene-off, *left plate*) and without (gene-on, *right plate*) thiamine. The plates were incubated at 30°C for 5 days. Each colony on a plate from *left* to *right* (1–6) represents cells plated from approximately 1,000 to 3 cells following threefold dilutions. The pYZ1N plasmid was used as a control. **c** Rev does not affect cell cycle of fission yeast. Cell cycle profiles were measured in the pYZ1N-*rev* and pYZ1N control *S. pombe* cells by flow cytometric analysis. The data show analyses after 24 and 67 h of cell culture in EMM selective media with (gene-off) and without (gene-on) thiamine. The cell cycle stages were monitored after staining with propidium iodide. The *up-right numbers* are the percentage of cells in G1, S and G2 phases of the cell cycle.

cultured under the *rev*-repressing and *rev*-inducing conditions. Following gene induction for 5 days, the cells were harvested and the DNA contents were measured by flow cytometry as described in the materials and methods. No significant differences in cell cycle distributions were seen between *rev*-expressing and other control 293VE632 cells (Fig. 6c). Therefore, consistent with our observations in fission yeast, Rev also reduces mammalian cellular growth but does not affect its cell cycle distribution.

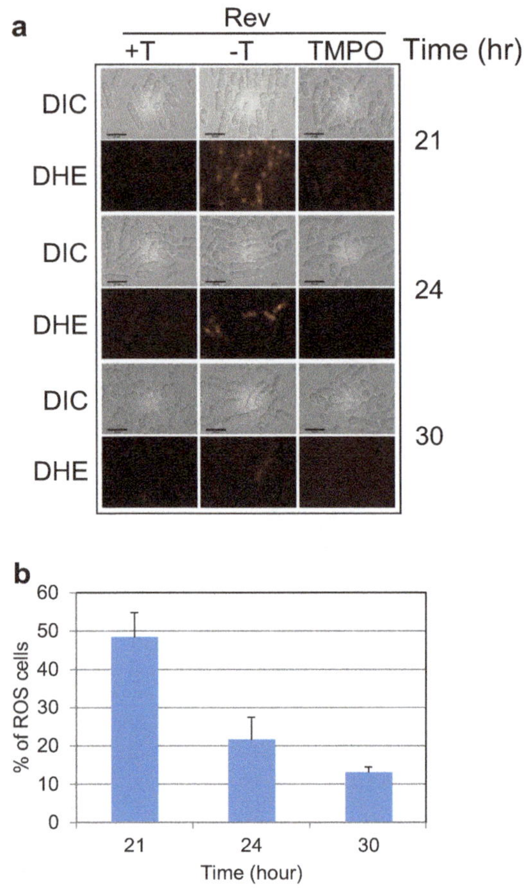

Fig. 5 Expression of *rev* stimulates production of reactive oxygen species (ROS) in *S. pombe* cells. Fission yeast strain carrying pYZ1N-*rev* was grown in selective EMM either in the presence (+T) or absence (−T) of thiamine to suppressor or induce *rev* gene induction, respectively. **a** ROS production was detected by addition of a ROS indicator dye (DHE) to the culture medium right before microscopic observation overtime at different times as indicated. An oxygen radical scavenger (TMPO) was also added in separate test tubes but concurrently to test the specific production of ROS. TMPO was added twice during the course of the *rev* expression. TMPO was first added to the culture at the time of cell inoculation when *rev* gene expression was induced, and cells were treated again with TMPO when DHE was added to the culture to detect ROS production. *DHE* DHE-positive cells, *DIC* cells shown by differential interference contrast. *Scale bar* 10 μm. **b** Percentage of ROS-producing cells induced by HIV-1 Rev decreases over time. The % of ROS-producing cells induced by HIV-1 Rev was quantified by counting the numbers of DHE-positive cells over the entire cell population of three independent experiments.

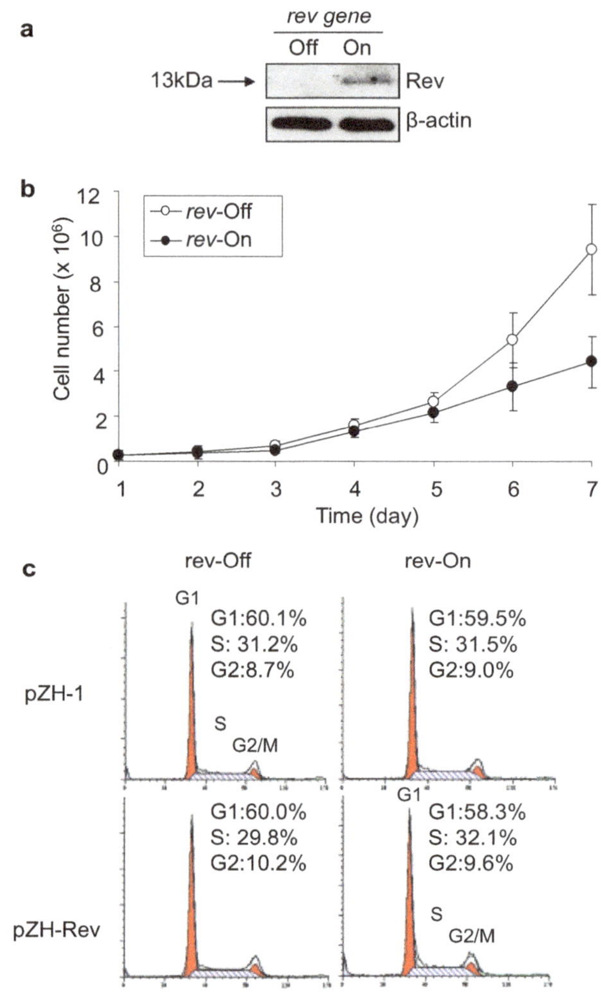

Fig. 6 Effect of HIV-1 Rev in mammalian cells. **a** Stable expression of HIV-1 *rev* gene in 293VE632 cells. The inducible pZH-1-*rev* plasmid was transfected into 293VE632 cells. The *rev* gene was expressed following addition of muristerone A and confirmed by Western blot analysis using a HIV-1 Rev monoclonal antibody. Lane "Off", *rev*-repressing 293VE632 cells; lane "On", *rev*-expressing 293VE632 cells. Western blot shows a 13 kDa protein band that was reacted to the anti-Rev antibody. β-actin was used as a loading control. **b** The 293VE632 cells containing the pZH-1-*rev* plasmid were grown under gene-repressing (*rev*-Off) and gene-inducing (*rev*-On) conditions for up to 7 days. The cells were collected every 24 h, and the cell numbers were counted with Tryptan blue staining (Sigma-Aldrich) [69]. The growth curves were generated with an average of three different experiments. **c** Rev does not affect mammalian cell cycle. The 293VE632 cells transfected with pZH-1 and pZH-1-*rev* plasmids were cultured without muristerone A (*rev*-Off) or with muristerone A (*rev*-On). DNA contents of the cells were determined by flow cytometric analyses after 5 days of culture. The *upright numbers* are the percentage of cells in the G1, S and G2 phases of the cell cycle. The 293VE632 cells containing pZH-1 plasmid was used as a control (*upper row*).

Discussion

Maintaining faithful viral production during HIV-1 infection requires highly coordinated production of each individual viral protein and orchestration of the entire protein complexes. Each viral protein has to interact with host cellular proteins at defined subcellular sites to ensure successful completion each step of the viral life cycle. Identification of subcellular localization of all viral proteins encoded by HIV-1 is therefore a key step towards a comprehensive understanding of viral production and their potential effects on basic cellular functions. Here, we demonstrated the subcellular localizations of all HIV-1 viral proteins in fission yeast cells. This might be the first effort to illustrate the subcellular localizations of the entire HIV-1 genome all at once in a single cellular system. The use of GFP tagging allows the selective and specific detection of HIV-1 proteins at very low concentrations with good signal-to-background ratio. Combined information on HIV-1 viral protein subcellular localization with genome-wide protein–protein interaction data will be instrumental in establishing the interrelationships between the viral and host cellular proteins that determine virologic functions of the virus [70].

In fission yeast, we observed that HIV-1 P24, P7, P66, P51, IN, Gp120, Gp41, Vpr, Vif, Rev and Tat are all predominantly localized in the nuclei (Fig. 2). Please note that nuclear localization of Vpr has long been established in our laboratory [48]. It was used as a positive control here to confirm appropriate experimental conditions. The P17 and Vpu are primarily localized in the cytoplasm, which is consistent with previous findings in mammalian cells [59]. Also, the Gag precursor protein was seen to aggregate in the cytoplasm of unknown sites that resembles mammalian report [51]. The PR and Nef did not seem have any preference but distributed throughout the cell. Based on the previous reports on subcellular localizations of HIV-1 viral proteins in mammalian cells, there is a general correlation between fission yeast and mammalian cells (Table 1).

We further examined the potential growth or cytotoxic effects of the viral gene expressions on fission yeast cells. While most of the HIV-1 viral protein productions have no inhibitory effects on colony formation in fission yeast, Vpr, PR and Rev showed significant inhibitory effects (Fig. 3). The effect of Vpr has been studied extensively before [34, 37–40, 48]. Rev was chosen here for further analysis (Note: we have carried out subsequent and extensive studies on PR that will be described elsewhere).

HIV-1 Rev is an 18 kD phosphoprotein with 116 amino acids that contains a nuclear localization signal (NLS) and nuclear export signal (NES) [71, 72]. Thus it is capable of shutting between the cytoplasm and nucleus where it also specifically bind to the Rev responsive element (RRE) for nuclear transport of HIV-1 RNAs. In HIV-infected cells, HIV-1 Rev protein is located predominantly in the nucleus/nucleolus [73–75]. In addition, Rev is also a shutting protein between the nucleus and cytoplasm [75]. Thus it was not surprising that Rev was found to localize predominantly in the nucleus but also in the cytoplasm of the fission yeast cells (Fig. 2c, 5th row). Rev is a "nuclear regulatory protein" [76]. Mechanistically, Rev was found in the nucleus of mammalian and budding yeast cells where they both interact with a small nucleoporin-like protein hRIP/RAB1 and yRip1p, respectively [62, 77]. Thus it would be interesting in the future to test whether Rev also interact with a similar nucleoporin-like protein in fission yeast. In addition, we found that the production of HIV-1 Rev protein appeared to slow down cellular growth in both fission yeast and mammalian cells. However, Rev does not appear to induce cell death in proliferating cells but reduced the size of yeast colony formation (Fig. 4b) and the number of mammalian cells (Fig. 6b) presumably due to growth retardation. Consistently, there has been no report of Rev causing death in actively dividing mammalian cells. Interestingly, however, overproduction of Rev has been reported to cause death of non-dividing human cells [78]. In an attempt to resolve this potential discrepancy, we have explored possible molecular mechanism underlying Rev-induced growth delay revealed that expression of HIV-1 *rev* gene in fission yeast triggers transient production of ROS indicating fission yeast cells were experiencing intracellular oxidative stress upon Rev production (Fig. 5). Typically, upon induction of cellular oxidative stress, large amounts of ROS are released from mitochondria within the cell that often cause cell death [79, 80]. Paradoxically, no cell death was observed in the *rev*-producing cells. One possible explanation could be due to the rapid dissipation of the cellular stress response in continue dividing cells. Conceivably, possible accumulation of ROS production in non-dividing cells could potentially contribute to the cell death caused by Rev [78]. Test of this possibility will be our future goal of the study.

Even though Rev causes significant growth delay in fission yeast (Fig. 4a) and mammalian cells (Fig. 6b), it does not affect distributions of neither cell cycles (Figs. 3c, 6c). Altogether, our data suggested that Rev is a nuclear protein that reduces cellular proliferation in both fission yeast and mammalian cells. However, it does not affect cell cycling with minimal or no cytotoxic effect at least in proliferating cells. Future studies on molecular actions of HIV-1 Rev are important because expression of HIV-1 Rev protein is essential for completion of the viral life cycle [78, 81]. In particular, by localizing in the nucleus, Rev mediates nuclear export of partially spliced and unspliced viral transcripts and its nuclear export signal allows nucleocytoplasmic shuttling [78, 81]. Therefore, Rev plays a pivotal role in viral replication. Conceivably, inhibition of its activities should block HIV-1 viral replication thus infection.

In summary, we successfully cloned and expressed all of the HIV-1 viral genes in *S. pombe.* By using a fission yeast inducible *nmt1* promoter, we were able to demonstrate the specific effects of viral proteins on fission yeast. In particular, we observed that, most of the viral proteins localized at the same or similar subcellular sites to human cells, suggesting fission yeast could be used as a simple and suitable model for future analysis of some of the HIV-1 proteins. Interestingly, besides HIV-1 Vpr, we found that HIV-1 PR and Rev also inhibit colony formation of fission yeast. Additional analysis of Rev suggested that there are a number of functional resemblances of the Rev effect between fission yeast and mammalian cells. These physical and similar effects on cellular functions suggest similar molecular mechanism of actions for HIV-1 Rev in yeast and mammalian cells, despite their evolutionary distance. Therefore, fission yeast might be suited as a model system for further investigation of this viral protein.

Methods

Cell and growth media

SP223, a wild-type *S. pombe* strain (*h-*, *ade6-216*, *leu1-32*, *ura4-294*), was used in this study [27, 34]. Standard YES complete and EMM minimal media supplemented with adenine, uracil, leucine or thiamine (20 μM) when necessary, were used for yeast cell culture and growth. Solid Luria–Bertani (LB) medium supplemented with Ampicillin (100 μg/ml) was used for competent *E. coli* Top 10 cell transformation. Mammalian 293VE632 cell was used to create a *rev*-inducible gene expression system. This is a stable zeocin-resistant mammalian cell line [68] expressing a heterodimer of the modified ecdysone receptor (VgEcR) and the retinoid X receptor. The heterodimer binds to a hybrid ecdysone response element (ECRE) only in the presence of the synthetic analogue of ecdysone, muristerone A, thus leading to induction of HIV-1 *rev* gene expression [82, 83]. The mammalian cell lines were maintained in Dulbecco's modified Eagle (DMEM) medium containing 10% FBS, 100 μg/ml Zeocin (Invitrogen).

Plasmids

pYZ1N and pYZ3N were used as previously described [48] for inducible viral gene expressions in fission yeast cells. These plasmids carry a *no message in thiamine* (*nmtl*) promoter. Under this inducible gene expression system, viral gene expression can be repressed or induced in the presence or absence of thiamine, respectively [65, 84]. These plasmids carry the *leu2* gene as a selection marker. In pYZ3N, GFP is fused to the viral gene at its 5′ end that was used to visualize intracellular location of each viral protein. For mammalian studies, a muristerone A-inducible gene expression pZH-1 plasmid was used as described previously [68].

Molecular cloning of HIV-1 genes in fission yeast and mammalian cells

The plasmid pNL4-3, which carries an entire HIV-1 genome, was used as a template for viral gene cloning with the exception of *rev* and *tat* genes. The PSV-Rev plasmid, which carries a *rev* cDNA and originated from a HIV-1 cDNA clone pCV1, was used and obtained from the NIH AIDS Reagent Program [85]. The ptatC6H plasmid carrying the *tat* cDNA was used, which was a gift from Dr. David Pauza and originated from [86]. For mammalian studies, the *rev* gene was cloned in pZH-1 and gene expression was induced in 293VE632 cells by adding 1 μM muristerone A to the growth medium [68].

Recombinant DNA transformation and gene expression

Each of the viral genes was PCR amplified, cloned and confirmed by Sanger DNA sequencing. The confirmed recombinant DNA was transformed into SP223 cells by electroporation using the BTX ECM600 protocol 0226 [87]. The transformants were selected on a minimal selective medium. For viral gene expression, a single yeast colony, which carries viral gene-containing plasmids, was grown to log phase on specific EMM liquid medium supplemented with 20 μM thiamine. The cells were then harvested and washed to remove the thiamine. Finally, 2×10^5 cells/ml were grown and tested in fresh specific EMM liquid medium with thiamine (gene-Off) and without thiamine (gene-On). The cell suspensions were incubated at 30°C with constant shaking before observations.

Subcellular localization of HIV-1 viral proteins in fission yeast

The HIV-1 viral proteins fused to GFP at their 5′ ends in pYZ3N were expressed and their subcellular localizations were visualized by fluorescent microscopy. Prior to visualization, the nucleus of the cells were stained with a nuclear dye 4′,6′ diamino-2-phenylindole (DAPI). Briefly, thiamine was washed out of a log phase culture with distilled water. The cells were inoculated in a thiamine free minimal media and incubated for at least 14 h for gene expression. The cells were then collected by spinning at 3,000 rpm for 5 min and re-suspended in suitable EMM medium. For DAPI staining, 5 μl of the cell suspension was pipetted onto a glass slide. The cells were heat fixed for 1 min at 70°C on a hot plate. The slide was then cooled down for a few seconds before counterstained with 1 μg/ml final concentration of DAPI. A coverslip was applied and the cells visualized under a fluorescence microscopy. A Leica DMR fluorescence microscope equipped with a high performance charge-coupled device camera (Hamamatsu) and Open-Lab software (Improvision, Inc., Lexington, MA, USA) was used for all imaging analysis. For DAPI, the cells were observed with a Leica A8 filter with an excitation of 360 nm (ranged from 340 to 380 nm) and emission of 470 nm (range, 450 to 490 nm). For the observation of GFP, a Leica L5 filter, which has an excitation of 480 nm (ranged from 460 to 500 nm) and emission of 527 nm (ranged from 512 to 542 nm), was used.

Effect of HIV-1 viral proteins on yeast colony formation

A single yeast colony, which carries viral gene-containing plasmids, was picked from a selective minimal plate and inoculated overnight in specific EMM liquid medium supplemented with thiamine. The following day, 1 ml of a mid-log phase culture was spin down, washed three times with distilled water and the cells re-suspended in appropriate volume of water. About 1–5 µl were streaked onto selective EMM plates with and without thiamine. The plates were incubated at 30°C for 6 days to observe for colony formation and numbers of cells within each colony (at low dilutions) as a semi-quantitative indicator of the viral effect on cellular growth or cytotoxicity.

Characterization of HIV-1 Rev protein activities in fission yeast

Apart from the colony formation assay on agar plates, the effect of Rev on yeast cell proliferation was also determined by growth kinetics analyses as previously described [34]. Cell cycle profile of *r*ev-expressing cells was measured by flow cytometry using a previously described method [31, 49]. A semi-quantitative growth and colony dot test was also used to quantify the effect of Rev on yeast cellular growth and colony formation. Briefly, the cells were grown to a log phase in liquid EMM as previously described and washed to remove thiamine. Cell suspension of 5×10^5 cells/ml was made on a 96 well plate and five consecutive threefold dilutions were made. Using a multiple pipette, 2 µL spots were generated on EMM supplemented media with (gene-off) and without (gene-on) thiamine. The plates were incubated at 30°C for 5 days to observe for colony formation. Fission yeast cells that were transformed with an empty pYZ1N vector were used as control. Potential effect of Rev on cellular oxidative stress was measured by production of reactive oxygen species (ROS), which can be detected by a ROS-specific dye, dihydroethidium (DHE) that produces red fluorescence in the presence of ROS as described previously [39]. A ROS scavenger, 3,3,5,5-tetramethylpyrroline N-oxyde (TMPO) was used as a control to specifically remove ROS [71].

Characterization of Rev-specific activities in mammalian cells

A Rev protein-inducible mammalian system was created and used for growth kinetics measurement as well as for analysis of cell cycle profile. For growth kinetics measurement, the Rev protein was expressed in transfected 293VE632 cells following the addition of muristerone A. Protein expression was confirmed by Western Blot analysis using a monoclonal anti-Rev antibody as previously described [40]. Viable cells were grown in equal numbers in both *rev*-inducing and *rev*-repressing conditions for 7 days. The number of viable cells were counted by observation of differential stainings of the Trypan Blue (Sigma-Aldrich) [69]. Finally, for cell cycle profile measurement, 293VE632 cells containing pZH-1 (control cells) and pZH-1-*rev* were cultured under *rev*-repressing and *rev*-inducing conditions as mentioned before. Following gene induction of 5 days, the cells were harvested and prepared for flow cytometry as described [40, 41]. The DNA contents of the cells were analyzed on a FACScan flow cytometry device (Becton–Dickinson) using the Cell Quest software.

Authors' contributions

JN participated in data analyses and writing the manuscript. LL carried out most of the initial experiments. ZB carried out some of the fission yeast experiments. GL conducted the ROS tests. RYZ designed the experiments and participated in writing of the manuscript. All authors read and approved the final manuscript.

Author details

[1] Division of Molecular Pathology, Department of Pathology, University of Maryland School of Medicine, Baltimore, MD 21201-1192, USA. [2] Department of Microbiology and Immunology, University of Maryland School of Medicine, Baltimore, MD 21201-1192, USA. [3] Institute of Human Virology, University of Maryland School of Medicine, Baltimore, MD 21201-1192, USA. [4] AIDS Research Department, Beijing Institute of Microbiology and Epidemiology, Beijing 100071, China. [5] Department of Chromosome Biology, Max F. Perutz Laboratories, University of Vienna, Vienna, Austria.

Acknowledgements

The authors would like to thank Dong Liang for critical reading and comments on this manuscript, Jianneng Dai for assistance in figure preparation. The mammalian expression vectors pZH-1 was a gift from Lee Ratner at the Department of Medicine and Molecular Microbiology, Washington University School of Medicine, St. Louis, Missouri. The plasmids PSV-Rev and PtatC6H were gifts from the NIH AIDS Reagent Program and Dr. David Pauza (UMB), respectively. This work was also submitted in partial fulfillment of Lin Li's Doctoral Dissertation.

Compliance with ethical guidelines

Competing interests

The authors declare that they have no competing interests.

References

1. Freed EO. HIV-1 gag proteins: diverse functions in the virus life cycle. Virology. 1998;251(1):1–15.
2. Gottlinger HG. The HIV-1 assembly machine. Aids. 2001;15(Suppl 5):S13–20.
3. Wilk T, Geiselhart V, Frech M, Fuller SD, Flugel RM, Lochelt M. Specific interaction of a novel foamy virus Env leader protein with the N-terminal Gag domain. J Virol. 2001;75(17):7995–8007
4. Freed EO, Martin MA. The role of human immunodeficiency virus type 1 envelope glycoproteins in virus infection. J Biol Chem. 1995;270(41):23883–6.

5. Mammano F, Kondo E, Sodroski J, Bukovsky A, Gottlinger HG. Rescue of human immunodeficiency virus type 1 matrix protein mutants by envelope glycoproteins with short cytoplasmic domains. J Virol. 1995;69(6):3824–30
6. Deora A, Spearman P, Ratner L. The N-terminal matrix domain of HIV-1 Gag is sufficient but not necessary for viral protein U-mediated enhancement of particle release through a membrane-targeting mechanism. Virology. 2000;269(2):305–12.
7. Gallay P, Swingler S, Song J, Bushman F, Trono D. HIV nuclear import is governed by the phosphotyrosine-mediated binding of matrix to the core domain of integrase. Cell. 1995;83(4):569–76
8. Accola MA, Strack B, Gottlinger HG. Efficient particle production by minimal Gag constructs which retain the carboxy-terminal domain of human immunodeficiency virus type 1 capsid-p2 and a late assembly domain. J Virol. 2000;74(12):5395–402.
9. Braaten D, Ansari H, Luban J. The hydrophobic pocket of cyclophilin is the binding site for the human immunodeficiency virus type 1 Gag polyprotein. J Virol. 1997;71(3):2107–13.
10. Kootstra NA, Munk C, Tonnu N, Landau NR, Verma IM. Abrogation of postentry restriction of HIV-1-based lentiviral vector transduction in simian cells. Proc Natl Acad Sci USA. 2003;100(3):1298–303
11. Thali M, Bukovsky A, Kondo E, Rosenwirth B, Walsh CT, Sodroski J, et al. Functional association of cyclophilin A with HIV-1 virions. Nature. 1994;372(6504):363–5
12. von Schwedler UK, Stemmler TL, Klishko VY, Li S, Albertine KH, Davis DR, et al. Proteolytic refolding of the HIV-1 capsid protein amino-terminus facilitates viral core assembly. EMBO J. 1998;17(6):1555–68
13. Carroll SS, Olsen DB, Bennett CD, Gotlib L, Graham DJ, Condra JH, et al. Inhibition of HIV-1 reverse transcriptase by pyridinone derivatives. Potency, binding characteristics, and effect of template sequence. J Biol Chem. 1993;268(1):276–81
14. Lu M, Blacklow SC, Kim PS. A trimeric structural domain of the HIV-1 transmembrane glycoprotein. Nat Struct Biol. 1995;2(12):1075–82.
15. Hill M, Tachedjian G, Mak J. The packaging and maturation of the HIV-1 Pol proteins. Curr HIV Res. 2005;3(1):73–85.
16. Pearl LH, Taylor WR. A structural model for the retroviral proteases. Nature. 1987;329(6137):351–4.
17. Hoffman AD, Banapour B, Levy JA. Characterization of the AIDS-associated retrovirus reverse transcriptase and optimal conditions for its detection in virions. Virology. 1985;147(2):326–35.
18. Oude Essink BB, Das AT, Berkhout B. HIV-1 reverse transcriptase discriminates against non-self tRNA primers. J Mol Biol. 1996;264(2):243–54.
19. Chiu TK, Davies DR. Structure and function of HIV-1 integrase. Curr Top Med Chem. 2004;4(9):965–77.
20. McCune JM, Rabin LB, Feinberg MB, Lieberman M, Kosek JC, Reyes GR, et al. Endoproteolytic cleavage of gp160 is required for the activation of human immunodeficiency virus. Cell. 1988;53(1):55–67
21. Weiss CD. HIV-1 gp41: mediator of fusion and target for inhibition. AIDS Rev. 2003;5(4):214–21.
22. Li L, Li HS, Pauza CD, Bukrinsky M, Zhao RY. Roles of HIV-1 auxiliary proteins in viral pathogenesis and host–pathogen interactions. Cell Res. 2005;15(11–12):923–34
23. Fan L, Peden K. Cell-free transmission of Vif mutants of HIV-1. Virology. 1992;190(1):19–29.
24. Strebel K, Klimkait T, Martin MA. A novel gene of HIV-1, vpu, and its 16-kilodalton product. Science. 1988;241(4870):1221–3.
25. Giga-Hama Y, Kumagai H. Expression system for foreign genes using the fission yeast *Schizosaccharomyces pombe*. Biotechnol Appl Biochem. 1999;30(Pt 3):235–44.
26. Piel M, Tran PT. Cell shape and cell division in fission yeast. Curr Biol. 2009;19(17):R823–7.
27. Zhao Y, Lieberman HB. *Schizosaccharomyces pombe*: a model for molecular studies of eukaryotic genes. DNA Cell Biol. 1995;14(5):359–71.
28. Chino A, Watanabe K, Moriya H. Plasmid construction using recombination activity in the fission yeast *Schizosaccharomyces pombe*. PLoS One. 2010;5(3):e9652.
29. Lu Q, Bauer JC, Greener A. Using *Schizosaccharomyces pombe* as a host for expression and purification of eukaryotic proteins. Gene. 1997;200(1–2):135–44.
30. Takegawa K, Tohda H, Sasaki M, Idiris A, Ohashi T, Mukaiyama H, et al. Production of heterologous proteins using the fission-yeast (*Schizosaccharomyces pombe*) expression system. Biotechnol Appl Biochem. 2009;53(Pt 4):227–35
31. Jacobs E, Gheysen D, Thines D, Francotte M, de Wilde M. The HIV-1 Gag precursor Pr55gag synthesized in yeast is myristoylated and targeted to the plasma membrane. Gene. 1989;79(1):71–81
32. Toyama R, Bende SM, Dhar R. Transcriptional activity of the human immunodeficiency virus-1 LTR promoter in fission yeast *Schizosaccharomyces pombe*. Nucleic Acids Res. 1992;20(10):2591–6.
33. Stutz F, Rosbash M. A functional interaction between Rev and yeast pre-mRNA is related to splicing complex formation. EMBO J. 1994;13(17):4096–104.
34. Zhao Y, Cao J, O'Gorman MR, Yu M, Yogev R. Effect of human immunodeficiency virus type 1 protein R (vpr) gene expression on basic cellular function of fission yeast *Schizosaccharomyces pombe*. J Virol. 1996;70(9):5821–6
35. Zhang C, Rasmussen C, Chang LJ. Cell cycle inhibitory effects of HIV and SIV Vpr and Vpx in the yeast *Schizosaccharomyces pombe*. Virology. 1997;230(1):103–12.
36. Herrero L, Monroy N, Gonzalez ME. HIV-1 Vpu protein mediates the transport of potassium in *Saccharomyces cerevisiae*. Biochemistry. 2013;52(1):171–7.
37. Benko Z, Liang D, Agbottah E, Hou J, Chiu K, Yu M, et al. Anti-Vpr activity of a yeast chaperone protein. J Virol. 2004;78(20):11016–29
38. Elder RT, Yu M, Chen M, Edelson S, Zhao Y. Cell cycle G2 arrest induced by HIV-1 Vpr in fission yeast (*Schizosaccharomyces pombe*) is independent of cell death and early genes in the DNA damage checkpoint. Virus Res. 2000;68(2):161–73
39. Huard S, Chen M, Burdette KE, Fenyvuesvolgyi C, Yu M, Elder RT, et al. HIV-1 Vpr-induced cell death in *Schizosaccharomyces pombe* is reminiscent of apoptosis. Cell Res. 2008;18(9):961–73
40. Li G, Park HU, Liang D, Zhao RY. Cell cycle G2/M arrest through an S phase-dependent mechanism by HIV-1 viral protein R. Retrovirology. 2010;7:59
41. Iordanskiy S, Zhao Y, Dubrovsky L, Iordanskaya T, Chen M, Liang D, et al. Heat shock protein 70 protects cells from cell cycle arrest and apoptosis induced by human immunodeficiency virus type 1 viral protein R. J Virol. 2004;78(18):9697–704
42. Caumont AB, Jamieson GA, Pichuantes S, Nguyen AT, Litvak S, Dupont C. Expression of functional HIV-1 integrase in the yeast *Saccharomyces cerevisiae* leads to the emergence of a lethal phenotype: potential use for inhibitor screening. Curr Genet. 1996;29(6):503–10
43. Blanco R, Carrasco L, Ventoso I. Cell killing by HIV-1 protease. J Biol Chem. 2003;278(2):1086–93.
44. Zhao Y, Elder RT. Yeast perspectives on HIV-1 Vpr. Front Biosci. 2000;5:905–16.
45. Zhao RY, Bukrinsky M, Elder RT. HIV-1 viral protein R (Vpr) and host cellular responses. Indian J Med Res. 2005;121(4):270–86.
46. Li G, Bukrinsky M, Zhao RY. HIV-1 viral protein R (Vpr) and its interactions with host cell. Curr HIV Res. 2009;7(2):178–83.
47. Andreola ML, Litvak S. Yeast and the AIDS virus: the odd couple. J Biomed Biotechnol. 2012;2012:549020.
48. Zhao Y, Elder RT, Chen M, Cao J. Fission yeast expression vectors adapted for positive identification of gene insertion and green fluorescent protein fusion. Biotechniques. 1998;25(3):438–40, 42, 44
49. Maundrell K. Thiamine-repressible expression vectors pREP and pRIP for fission yeast. Gene. 1993;123(1):127–30.
50. Braddock M, Chambers A, Wilson W, Esnouf MP, Adams SE, Kingsman AJ, et al. HIV-1 TAT "activates" presynthesized RNA in the nucleus. Cell. 1989;58(2):269–79
51. Ono A. HIV-1 assembly at the plasma membrane: gag trafficking and localization. Future Virol. 2009;4(3):241–57.
52. Zhou W, Resh MD. Differential membrane binding of the human immunodeficiency virus type 1 matrix protein. J Virol. 1996;70(12):8540–8.
53. Dennin RH, Beyer A. Application of scanning electron microscopy (SEM) and microbead techniques to study the localization of p24 and p18 antigens of HIV-1 on the surface of HIV-1-infected H9-lymphocytes. J Microsc. 1991;164(Pt 1):53–60.
54. Haffar OK, Popov S, Dubrovsky L, Agostini I, Tang H, Pushkarsky T, et al. Two nuclear localization signals in the HIV-1 matrix protein regulate nuclear import of the HIV-1 pre-integration complex. J Mol Biol. 2000;299(2):359–68

55. Salgado GF, Vogel A, Marquant R, Feller SE, Bouaziz S, Alves ID. The role of membranes in the organization of HIV-1 Gag p6 and Vpr: p6 shows high affinity for membrane bilayers which substantially increases the interaction between p6 and Vpr. J Med Chem. 2009;52(22):7157–62
56. Ansari-Lari MA, Gibbs RA. Analysis of HIV type 1 reverse transcriptase expression in a human cell line. AIDS Res Hum Retroviruses. 1994;10(9):1117–24.
57. Levin A, Armon-Omer A, Rosenbluh J, Melamed-Book N, Graessmann A, Waigmann E, et al. Inhibition of HIV-1 integrase nuclear import and replication by a peptide bearing integrase putative nuclear localization signal. Retrovirology. 2009;6:112
58. Chen M, Elder RT, Yu M, O'Gorman MG, Selig L, Benarous R, et al. Mutational analysis of Vpr-induced G2 arrest, nuclear localization, and cell death in fission yeast. J Virol. 1999;73(4):3236–45
59. Schubert U, Bour S, Ferrer-Montiel AV, Montal M, Maldarell F, Strebel K. The two biological activities of human immunodeficiency virus type 1 Vpu protein involve two separable structural domains. J Virol. 1996;70(2):809–19
60. Wichroski MJ, Ichiyama K, Rana TM. Analysis of HIV-1 viral infectivity factor-mediated proteasome-dependent depletion of APOBEC3G: correlating function and subcellular localization. J Biol Chem. 2005;280(9):8387–96.
61. Fackler OT, Kienzle N, Kremmer E, Boese A, Schramm B, Klimkait T, et al. Association of human immunodeficiency virus Nef protein with actin is myristoylation dependent and influences its subcellular localization. Eur J Biochem. 1997;247(3):843–51
62. Boe SO, Bjorndal B, Rosok B, Szilvay AM, Kalland KH. Subcellular localization of human immunodeficiency virus type 1 RNAs, Rev, and the splicing factor SC-35. Virology. 1998;244(2):473–82
63. Yang Y, Ma J, Song Z, Wu M. HIV-1 TAT-mediated protein transduction and subcellular localization using novel expression vectors. FEBS Lett. 2002;532(1–2):36–44
64. Zhao Y, Yu M, Chen M, Elder RT, Yamamoto A, Cao J. Pleiotropic effects of HIV-1 protein R (Vpr) on morphogenesis and cell survival in fission yeast and antagonism by pentoxifylline. Virology. 1998;246(2):266–76
65. Maundrell K. nmt1 of fission yeast. A highly transcribed gene completely repressed by thiamine. J Biol Chem. 1990;265(19):10857–64.
66. Mitchison DO. Physiological and cytological methods for *Schizosaccharomyces pombe*. Methods Cell Physiol. 1970;4:131–65.
67. Hardy M, Rockenbauer A, Vasquez-Vivar J, Felix C, Lopez M, Srinivasan S, et al. Detection, characterization, and decay kinetics of ROS and thiyl adducts of mito-DEPMPO spin trap. Chem Res Toxicol. 2007;20(7):1053–60
68. Zhou Y, Ratner L. A novel inducible expression system to study trans-dominant mutants of HIV-1 Vpr. Virology. 2001;287(1):133–42.
69. Frei M. Cell viability and proliferation-trpan blue, in centrifugation. St. Louis: Sigma-Aldrich; 2001.
70. Zhao, RY. Interactions of Vpr with host cellular proteins. Reactome. 2006;19. http://dx.doi.org/10.3180/REACT_6288.4.
71. Sodroski J, Goh WC, Rosen C, Dayton A, Terwilliger E, Haseltine W. A second post-transcriptional trans-activator gene required for HTLV-III replication. Nature. 1986;321(6068):412–7
72. Pollard VW, Malim MH. The HIV-1 Rev protein. Annu Rev Microbiol. 1998;52:491–532.
73. Malim MH, Bohnlein S, Hauber J, Cullen BR. Functional dissection of the HIV-1 Rev trans-activator—derivation of a trans-dominant repressor of Rev function. Cell. 1989;58(1):205–14
74. Cochrane AW, Perkins A, Rosen CA. Identification of sequences important in the nucleolar localization of human immunodeficiency virus Rev: relevance of nucleolar localization to function. J Virol. 1990;64(2):881–5.
75. Suhasini M, Reddy TR. Cellular proteins and HIV-1 Rev function. Curr HIV Res. 2009;7(1):91–100.
76. Malim MH, Hauber J, Le SY, Maizel JV, Cullen BR. The HIV-1 rev trans-activator acts through a structured target sequence to activate nuclear export of unspliced viral mRNA. Nature. 1989;338(6212):254–7
77. Stutz F, Neville M, Rosbash M. Identification of a novel nuclear pore-associated protein as a functional target of the HIV-1 Rev protein in yeast. Cell. 1995;82(3):495–506.
78. Levin A, Hayouka Z, Friedler A, Loyter A. Over-expression of the HIV-1 Rev promotes death of nondividing eukaryotic cells. Virus Genes. 2010;40(3):341–6.
79. Hockenbery DM, Oltvai ZN, Yin XM, Milliman CL, Korsmeyer SJ. Bcl-2 functions in an antioxidant pathway to prevent apoptosis. Cell. 1993;75(2):241–51
80. Kane DJ, Sarafian TA, Anton R, Hahn H, Gralla EB, Valentine JS, et al. Bcl-2 inhibition of neural death: decreased generation of reactive oxygen species. Science. 1993;262(5137):1274–7
81. Fineberg K, Fineberg T, Graessmann A, Luedtke NW, Tor Y, Lixin R, et al. Inhibition of nuclear import mediated by the Rev-arginine rich motif by RNA molecules. Biochemistry. 2003;42(9):2625–33
82. No D, Yao TP, Evans RM. Ecdysone-inducible gene expression in mammalian cells and transgenic mice. Proc Natl Acad Sci USA. 1996;93(8):3346–51.
83. Thomas HE, Stunnenberg HG, Stewart AF. Heterodimerization of the Drosophila ecdysone receptor with retinoid X receptor and ultraspiracle. Nature. 1993;362(6419):471–5.
84. Basi G, Schmid E, Maundrell K. TATA box mutations in the *Schizosaccharomyces pombe* nmt1 promoter affect transcription efficiency but not the transcription start point or thiamine repressibility. Gene. 1993;123(1):131–6.
85. Lewis N, Williams J, Rekosh D, Hammarskjold ML. Identification of a *cis*-acting element in human immunodeficiency virus type 2 (HIV-2) that is responsive to the HIV-1 rev and human T-cell leukemia virus types I and II rex proteins. J Virol. 1990;64(4):1690–7
86. Patki AH, Lederman MM. HIV-1 Tat protein and its inhibitor Ro 24-7429 inhibit lymphocyte proliferation and induce apoptosis in peripheral blood mononuclear cells from healthy donors. Cell Immunol. 1996;169(1):40–6.
87. BXT, Electro Cell Manipulator: ECM 600 protocol 0226. 2001.

The role of alpha-actinin-4 in human kidney disease

Di Feng[1], Clark DuMontier[2] and Martin R Pollak[1*]

Abstract

Mutations in the Alpha-actinin-4 gene (ACTN4) cause a rare form of familial focal segmental glomerulosclerosis in humans. Individuals with kidney disease-associated ACTN4 mutations tend to have mild to moderate proteinuria, with many developing decreased kidney function progressing to end stage kidney disease. All of the disease-causing ACTN4 mutations identified to date are located within the actin-binding domain of the encoded protein, increasing its binding affinity to F-actin and leading to abnormal actin rich cellular aggregates. The identification of ACTN4 mutations as a cause of human kidney disease demonstrates a key cellular pathway by which alterations in cytoskeletal behavior can mediate kidney disease. Here we review the studies relevant to ACTN4 and its role in mediating kidney disease.

Keywords: Focal segmental glomerulosclerosis, Alpha-actinin-4, Kidney, Podocytes, Cytoskeleton protein

Background

Focal segmental glomerulosclerosis (FSGS) is a common histologic pattern of kidney injury, often associated with progressive chronic kidney disease and overt kidney failure. FSGS is defined histologically by sclerosis occurring in a portion of the glomerulus and affecting a subset of glomeruli. While these biopsy features define a pattern of injury, they do not define the underlying etiology [1]. Electron microscopy typically shows fusion of epithelial cell foot processes, or so-called foot process effacement. Common features of FSGS patients include proteinuria, edema, hypertension and hypercholesterolemia.

FSGS is found in about 20–25% of all renal biopsies [2, 3]. However, the incidence and prevalence of FSGS in children may be underestimated [4]. This is because many children with nephrotic syndrome (NS), defined as heavy proteinuria, hypoalbuminemia, and peripheral edema, are generally assumed to have minimal change syndrome and not subjected to renal biopsy. Even when a biopsy is performed, the characteristic lesion necessary for diagnosis might not be captured in the sample. It is estimated that the incidence of NS in children is between 2 and 4 new cases per 100,000 children per year, with biopsy-confirmed FSGS comprising 15–20% [4, 5]. The prevalence of FSGS continues to increase for unknown reasons [2, 5, 6]. FSGS is seen in approximately 2–5% of cases of end stage renal disease (ESRD) in adults and about 10% in children [7].

A number of etiologies have been associated with FSGS and are often used as the basis for further classification. Broadly, FSGS is divided into primary (idiopathic) and secondary forms. Secondary FSGS is thought to result from a wide range of systemic conditions, including reflex nephropathy, heroin use, decreased renal mass, hypertension, diabetes, obesity, and HIV infection [8, 9]. In comparison with secondary FSGS, primary FSGS is more likely to present with nephrotic-range proteinuria and have a poorer prognosis, with 50% progressing to ESRD over 3–8 years ([9, 10]. For FSGS patients with nephrotic-range proteinuria, the use of corticosteroids is associated with an increased likelihood of a remission [9, 11]. However, steroid resistance can be present in up to 50% of patients, and a prolonged steroid treatment is associated with significant side effects [9]. Therefore, there is great interest in understanding the molecular mechanisms underlying different forms of FSGS and kidney injury. Mutations in several genes are associated with

*Correspondence: mpollak@bidmc.harvard.edu
[1] Division of Nephrology, Department of Medicine, Beth Israel Deaconess Medical Center, Boston, MA 02215, USA
Full list of author information is available at the end of the article

familial forms of FSGS or nephrotic syndrome, including α-actinin-4 (here we use ACTN4 to designate the human gene or protein and Actn4 to designate the mouse gene or protein) [12], inverted formin 2 (INF2) [13], canonical transient receptor potential 6 (TRPC6) [14, 15], nephrin (NPHS1) [16], and podocin (NPHS2) [17]. This review will focus on ACTN4 and its role in mediating human FSGS.

The α-actinins are 100 kD rod shaped proteins that form head-to-tail homodimers [18]. α-Actinin monomers contain three distinct domains: an N-terminal actin binding domain (ABD), four spectrin-like repeats (SRs), and a C-terminal EF hands (calmodulin like domain). There are four human α-actinin (ACTN1-4) family members, encoding closely related actin crosslinking proteins. ACTN2 and ACTN3 (calcium insensitive) show sarcomere-limited expression [19]. The non-muscle cytoskeletal ACTN1 (highly calcium sensitive) and ACTN4 (moderately calcium sensitive), appear to be widely expressed [20, 21]. However, for unclear reasons, the human phenotype associated with ACTN4 mutations is apparent only in the kidney [12]. Additionally, ACTN1 mutations were identified as a cause of congenital macrothrombocytopenia, an inherited disorder showing low platelet counts [22]. ACTN2 mutations have been found in rare families with hypertrophic cardiomyopathy [23]. The ACTN3 R577X variant, leading to absence of ACTN3 protein due to an early stop-codon, is absent in 18% of healthy white individuals [24]. There is no apparent disease phenotype as a result of this variant. However, the homozygous genotype appears with very low frequency in elite sprint athlete [25]. The loss of ACTN3 is associated with reduced skeleton high velocity contraction. Altogether, these studies revealed unique roles of different α-actinin isoforms different tissues.

In addition to bundling F-actin, ACTN4 interacts with various other proteins, consistent with multiple roles in cell function. Some of these studies were conducted either using crude extraction of α-actinin or anti-α-actinin antibodies that are not specific for ACTN4. For example:

1. *Cell adhesion* α-actinins interact directly with β1-integrin [26, 27], vinculin [28, 29], zyxin [30], kindlin-1 [31] to modulate focal adhesion, and to link the cytoskeleton to the extracellular matrix.
2. *Cell junction* The glomerular slit diaphragm between podocyte foot processes shares many morphologic features with the adherens junction seen in epithelial cells. The glomerular slit diaphragm composes of P-cadherin, α-catenin, β-catenin, γ-catenin, and ZO-1 [32]. α-actinins have been shown to interact directly with α-catenin [33]. Moreover, the slit-diaphragm protein nephrin appears to form a major structural component of the slit diaphragm between adjacent podocytes. ACTN4, together with five other cell junction proteins, including the membrane-associated guanylate kinase inverted 2_synaptic scaffolding molecule (MAGI-2/S-SCAM), IQ motif-containing GTPase activating protein1 (IQGAP1), αII spectrin, and βII spectrin was detected as part of the neprhin multiprotein complex [34]. Therefore, ACTN4 could serve as a linker between F-actin and other adherens junction proteins.
3. *Cell signaling* One of the key signaling molecules phosphatidylinositol 4,5-bisphosphate (PIP2) was shown to bind α-actinin at the plasma membrane. Upon PI3 Kinase (PI3K) activation, PIP2 is converted to phosphatidylinositol 3,4,5-trisphosphate (PIP3), which decreases the association of α-actinin to actin filament within stress fibers, as well as the association rate to integrin within focal adhesions [35, 36]. Moreover, ACTN4 can interact PI3K downstream kinase Akt to mediate cell proliferation [37]. Finally, PIP3 binding ACTNs also increases their susceptibility to calpain-1 and -2-mediated proteolysis [38].
4. *Nuclear transcription activator* ACTN4 was reported to be present in cell nuclei in 1998 [39]. Notably, PI3K inhibition and actin depolymerization both promote nuclear accumulation of ACTN4. Since then, ACTN4 has been reported to be a transcription activator of the estrogen receptor (ERα) [40, 41], the retinoic acid receptor (RAR) [42], the myocyte enhancer factor (MEF) [43, 44], the vitamin D receptor [41], the androgen receptor [45], NF-ḳB transcription factors [46], thus potentially regulating transcription activity of multiple genes.

ACTN4 mutations in humans with FSGS

Positional cloning approaches identified three different point mutations in ACTN4 as the cause of FSGS in three unrelated families [12]. These families show autosomal dominant inheritance of disease, with high but incomplete penetrance and variable expressivity. Most of the affected individuals initially presented with low-grade proteinuria mainly in early adulthood with declining kidney function that slowly progressed to ESRD. The K255E, T259I, and S262P mutations identified in these families are all located within the evolutionarily conserved ABD of ACTN4. As assessed by actin filament co-sedimentation assays, all mutations are associated with increased ACTN4 binding affinity to F-actin. ACTN4, but not ACTN1, is expressed at high levels (as detected by western blot) in human kidney. By immunofluorescence staining, it was found that ACTN4 is most prominently distributed in podocytes, with some distribution in other vasculature in the renal cortex. These findings are consistent with previous reports, suggesting that ACTN4 is highly expressed in podocytes, and with less expression elsewhere within the kidney [47, 48].

Two additional missense mutations in the ABD, W59R and I149del, were subsequently defined as disease-causing based on the following criteria: (1) mutants formed abnormal cellular aggregates with F-actin within the cell; (2) these mutations increased binding affinity of ACTN4 to F-actin, (3) ACTN4 with these mutations co-segregated with affected individuals within families; (4) the mutations occur in evolutionarily-conserved ABD domain [49]. ACTN4 mutations (five total disease-causing mutations including the three previously discovered) accounted for approximately 3.5% of 141 familial FSGS cases screened in this study. The W59R substitution identified in this study was of particular interest as it was a de novo mutation not present in the proband's parent. This individual exhibited proteinuria at age 5 and progressed to ESRD within 3 years, much earlier than other families with ACTN4 mutations. In addition, this individual developed recurrent proteinuria and FSGS after transplantation, the only such case reported to date.

Another clinical report documented a germline mosaicism ACTN4 mutation at S262F in the father of two affected siblings [50]. This mutation occurs at the same location as the previously reported heterozygous mutation S262P. Both patients developed FSGS in early childhood (3–4 years old) and rapidly progressed to ESRD. Renal biopsy showed a collapsing variant of FSGS in one affected sibling, a histological subtype of FSGS associated with a poorer prognosis. All of the disease causing ACTN4 mutations and their location in ABD has been summarized in Fig. 1 [51, 52].

Actn4 mouse models

Kos et al. generated Actn4 knockout (Actn4 KO) mice [53]. A significant percentage of homozygous Actn4 KO mice suffer perinatal death. The remaining survivors go on to develop albuminuria and FSGS at about 10 weeks of age. Transmission electron microscopy of these Actn4 KO mice shows podocyte foot-process effacement. There is no clear alteration in podocin, nephrin, or type IV collagen expression in homozygous Actn4 KO mice by immunofluorescence staining. Even though strong expression of both Actn1 and Actn4 are detected in wild type (WT) mouse podocytes, the loss of Actn4 alone leads to a significant renal phenotype, suggesting that Actn4 plays a nonreduntant role in the mouse kidney. Additionally, homozygous Actn4 KO mice also show a decrease in the number of podocytes in the glomeruli, and a significant increased number of podocytes shedding in the urine as indicated by the presence of podocyte marker WT-1 protein [54]. Podocytes isolated from homozygous Actn4 KO mice showed decreased phosphorylation of β1-integrin and weaker integrin-cytoskeleton linkages. Consequently, They also showed decreased attachment in response to shear stress in culture. Altogether, homozygous Actn4 KO mice demonstrated the importance of the expression level of Actn4 in kidney disease. Indeed, Liu et al. reported that decreased expression of ACTN4 could occur in humans with primary glomerulopathies including sporadic FSGS, minimal change disease, and IgA nephropathy [55].

Yao et al. generated Actn4 K256E (a mutation analogous to the FSGS-causing K255E mutation in humans) knock-in (Actn4 KI) mice in an effort to mimic the human phenotype [56]. Homozygous Actn4 KI mice also showed perinatal lethality, albuminuria, and podocyte

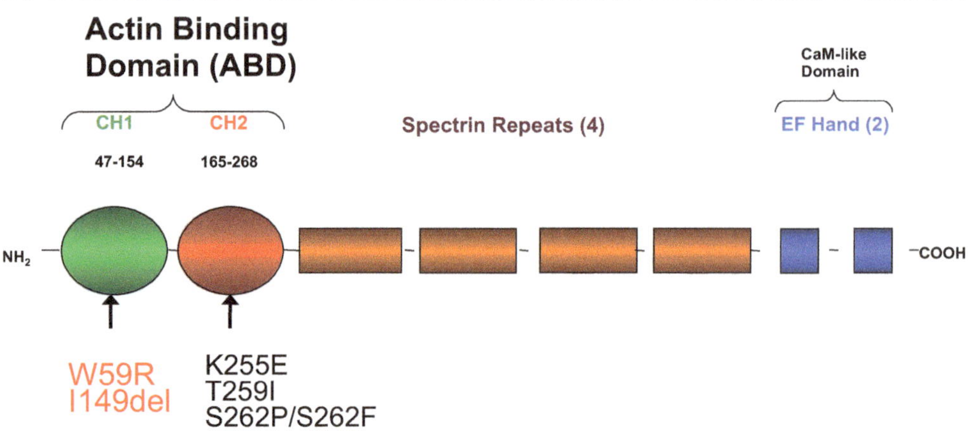

Fig. 1 Functional domains of the human ACTN4 protein. The actin-binding domain (ABD) consists of CH1 (amino acid 47–154) and CH2 domain (amino acid 165–268). Mutations within ACTN4 including W59R and I149del in the CH1 domain and K255E, T259I, S262P and S262F in the CH2 domain have been associated with human FSGS.

foot enfacement as seen in the Actn4 KO mice. Henderson et al. further examined the pathological characterization of both K256E and KO mice [57]. Both homozygous KI and KO mice exhibit the phenotype of collapsing glomerulopathy. Actn4 KI and KO mice did not survive past 21 and 15 weeks respectively. Homozygous KI mice and all KO mice show decreased expression of podocyte differentiation markers, including WT-1 and synaptopodin, and increased proliferation markers, including cyclin D1 and KI-67. Heterozygous Actn4 KI mice represent a more genetically faithful model for the autosomal-dominant ACTN4-mediated FSGS in humans. These mice did not develop glomerulosclerosis during the 70-week study period. However, they did exhibit focal glomerular hypertrophy and mild glomerular ultrastructural abnormalities, including mild podocyte cell body abnormalities, glomerular basement membrane (GBM) thickening and redundancy, and diffuse electron-dense aggregate accumulation. These abnormalities in heterozygous Actn4 KI mice may increase susceptibility to injury caused by other genetic or environmental stressors.

Michaud et al. generated podocyte-specific (driven by murine nephrin promoter) transgenic mice that overexpressed the K256E mutation (homologus to the human K255E mutation) [58]. Podocyte specific K256E mutant (K256E-Actn4^{pod}) mice show heterogeneity, potentially due to variation in the expression of the transgene. The transgenic mice that had higher expression of mutant Actn4 exhibited significant albuminuria, glomerulosclerosis, and foot process enfacement at 10 weeks of age. These proteinuric transgenic mice also showed reduced expression of nephrin. Both proteinuric and non-proteinuric Actn4 transgenic mice exhibited increased average systolic BP measured by tail-cuff plethysmography. Michaud et al. also generated podocyte-specific transgenic mice overexpressing the wild-type Actn4 (WT-Actn4^{pod}) as a control line of mice. They showed that WT-Actn4^{pod} mice are indistinguishable from their non-transgenic littermates [59]. These mice do not develop albuminuria, glomerulosclerosis, foot process enfacement, or elevated systemic blood pressure. The authors concluded that it is the K256E Actn4 mutation, not the overexpression of Actn4, underlies the FSGS phenotype in K256E-Actn4^{pod}.

Mechanisms by which ACTN4 mutations lead FSGS

Several studies have examined the effect of ACTN4 mutations on protein function in vitro. Weins et al. found that K255E mutant ACTN4 (full length or ABD) shows greater binding affinity to F-actin compared to WT ACTN4 based on co-sedimentation studies [60]. The addition of Ca^{2+} decreased the binding affinity of WT ACTN4 to F-actin, but not K255E ACTN4. These results suggest that K255E mutant ACTN4 binding to F-actin is not subject to Ca^{2+} regulation in vitro. One hypothesis proposed in this study is that a conformational change occurs when mutant K255E binds to F-actin, resulting in greater binding affinity. Interestingly, the crystal structure of the ABD of mutant K255E ACTN4 in absence of actin shows the same conformation as the WT protein [52]. Perhaps, the F-actin bound form of ACTN4 adopts a different structural conformation than ACTN4 alone. Galkin et al. used cryo-electron microscopy reconstruction (relative low resolution) of F-actin cross-linked by ABD of ACTN4 to build a model. They predicted that the bound form of ACTN4 would adopt a different conformation than the unbound ACTN4 crystal structure to enable binding to F-actin [61]. Therefore, the high-resolution cryo-electron microscopy structure of F-actin cross-linked by mutant ACTN4 is needed to better explain how mutations lead to binding affinity changes of ACTN4 to F-actin, and to visualize the exact conformational changes.

Weins et al. used electron microscopy to examine the appearance of actin filaments cross-linked either by WT or K255E mutant ACTN4 in vitro [60]. They showed that WT ACTN4 crosslinks actin filaments into thick parallel bundles with defined spacing. On the other hand, mutant ACTN4 induces the formation of a disordered and entangled network of thin filament bundles. Similarly, under fluorescent microscopy, actin filaments (fluorescently labeled) cross-linked by WT ACTN4 form an evenly spaced and finely reticulated actin network. In comparison, actin filaments cross-linked by K255E mutant ACTN4 form a more coarsely reticulated network with a smaller mesh size [62]. Based on bulk rheology experiments, Ward et al. suggested that the dissociation of mutant K255E ACTN4 from actin is much slower than the WT ACTN4. Additionally, Yao et al. observed that the actin network cross-linked by K255E mutant ACTN4 is more brittle, with a lower breaking stress in comparison to networks cross-linked with WT [63]. Together, these in vitro studies reflect how mutations within ACTN4 change the intrinsic biochemical and biophysical properties of the protein.

The effects of K255E mutant ACTN4 on cellular functions have also been examined. Using immortalized lung fibroblasts and podocytes isolated from homozygous Actn4 KI mice, Weins et al. observed that mutant Actn4 aggregates with F-actin [60]. Biopsies from patients with ACTN4 mutations also show segmental weak linear, irregular granular, and punctuate appearance of ACTN4 staining surrounding the glomerular capillary wall [64]. These abnormalities could potentially be direct results of increased binding affinity to F-actin of mutant actn4, resulting in disruption of actin reorganization or assembly. Additionally, Weins et al. also reported that two other known interacting proteins cortactin and synaptopodin were also present in the mutant Actn4/F-actin aggregates [60]. The sequestration of these binding partners, which play important roles in podocyte function, could alter the response of podocytes to environmental stressors. Michaud et al. used conditionally immortalized mouse podocytes infected with adenoviral constructs containing WT or K256E murine Actn4 to assess the functional consequence of mutations on subcellular localization, adhesion, spreading, migration, and formation of foot process-like peripheral projections [65]. They found that mutant K256E Actn4 was detected predominantly in the Triton-insoluble fraction of cellular extraction, and localizes almost exclusively along actin stress fibers. On the other hand, WT Actn4 was detected primarily in the Triton-soluble fraction of cellular extraction, localized to membrane-associated cortical actin and focal adhesions, with some expression along stress fibers. Podocytes overexpressing WT or mutant K256E Actn4 show similar adhesion to the extracellular matrix (collagen-I). However, podocytes overexpressing mutant K256E Actn4 exhibit significantly reduced ability to spread and migrate on collagen-I, and have a reduced mean number of actin-rich peripheral projections (reminiscent of podocyte foot processes in cell culture) compared to WT, perhaps all due to mutant Actn4/F-actin aggregates formation.

The sequestration of mutant ACTN4 together with F-actin in cellular aggregates can prevent ACTN4 to serve as transcriptional co-regulator. ACTN4 harbors a functional nuclear receptor interaction motif LXX LL (where L is leucine, X can be any amino acids) [41]. Khurana el al reported that a portion of WT ACTN4 can move to the podocyte nucleus and stimulate nuclear RARα [42] and NF-ķB [46] mediated transcription. When the LXXLL motif is mutated to LXXAA, WT ACTN4 (LXX AA) exhibits significant loss of the ability to potentiate RARα mediated transcription. On the other hand, disease-causing mutant ACTN4, predominantly cytoplasmic, failed to translocate to the nucleus and show an inability to stimulate RARα-mediated transcription.

Mutations within ABD of ACTN4 could lead to greater degradation of the protein in the cell [56]. Yao et al. reported that homozygous Actn4 KI mice showed markedly decreased expression of Actn4 protein in homozygous KI mice, and moderately decreased expression in heterozygous KI mice. Conditionally immortalized fibroblasts isolated from WT and homozygous K256E mice were used to compare actn4 protein synthesis and degradation rates in the cell. They found that the protein degradation rate of mutant Actn4 is much faster that WT Actn4. There is no difference in protein synthesis rates. The greater Actn4 degradation rate could potentially explain the lower level of Actn4 protein in homozygous KI mice compared to WT mice in kidney, lung, liver and brain. Rapid degradation of Actn4 in mutant fibroblasts can be reversed by the treating of a selective proteasome inhibitor lactacystin. This result suggests that mutant Actn4 may be degraded through the ubiquitin–proteasome pathway. Interestingly, it was reported that ubiquitin C-terminal hydrolase L1 (UCHL1) is up regulated in a subset of human glomerulopathies, including primary FSGS [66]. Reed et al. intercrossed K256E-Actn4^{pod} with heterozygous UCHI1 KO mice [67]. They found that mice that are heterozygous for an Actn4 transgene but homozygous for UCHL1 KO (K256E-Actn4^{pod+}/UCHL1$^{-/-}$) exhibited significantly ameliorated albuminuria, glomerulosclerosis, and foot process enfacement at 10 weeks of age. This result suggested that preserving K255E/WT Actn4 heterodimers from proteolysis might help to maintain podocyte function.

Recently, Grgic et al. used translating ribosome affinity purification (TRAP) to isolate and compare podocyte-specific mRNA expression between heterozygous Actn4 KI mice and WT [68]. They found that among other up-regulated genes in heterozygous Actn4 KI mice, myotonic dystrophy protein kinase (Dmpk), a Rho-associated serine-threonine protein kinase, is also upregulated at the protein level in human FSGS kidney biopsies. The role of DMPK in the development of FSGS in humans has yet to be elucidated.

Conclusions

Mutations in the ACTN4 gene cause a highly penetrant, autosomal dominant form of familial FSGS in humans. Studies in Actn4 KO, Actn4 KI, and transgenic Actn4 mouse models confirm the importance of this gene in kidney function. Even though several studies have shown that ACTN4 mutations lead to biochemical, biophysical, and cellular functional changes, more research is needed to elucidate the exact pathways by which these mutations lead to podocyte injury, which may provide insights into therapeutic development. Since highly penetrant Mendelian forms of kidney disease caused by mutations in ACTN4 and other genes are rare examples where we can unequivocally identify the cause, the development of the specific therapies treating these diseases will be a proof of concept to advance individualized treatment in nephrology.

Abbreviations

ACTN4: alpha-actinin-4 gene; FSGS: familial focal segmental glomerulosclerosis; ABD: actin-binding domain; NS: nephrotic syndrome; ESRD: end stage renal disease; INF2: inverted formin 2; TRPC6: canonical transient receptor potential 6; NPHS1: nephrin; NPHS2: podocin; SRs: spectrin-like repeats; MAGI-2/S-SCAM: membrane-associated guanylate kinase inverted 2_synaptic scaffolding molecule; IQGAP1: IQ motif-containing GTPase activatingprotein1; PIP2: phosphatidylinositol 4,5-bisphosphate; PI3K: PI3 kinase; PIP3: phosphatidylinositol 3,4,5-trisphosphate; Actn4 KO: actn4 knockout; WT: wild type; Actn4 KI: actn4 K256E knock-in; GBM: glomerular basement membrane; K256E-Actn4^{pod}: podocyte specific K256E mutant; UCHL1: ubiquitin C-terminal hydrolase L1; TRAP: translating ribosome affinity purification; Dmpk: myotonic dystrophy protein kinase.

Authors' contributions

All authors participated in the writing of the review. All authors read and approved the final manuscript.

Author details

[1] Division of Nephrology, Department of Medicine, Beth Israel Deaconess Medical Center, Boston, MA 02215, USA. [2] Department of Medicine, Boston University School of Medicine, Boston, MA 02118, USA.

Acknowledgement

Work in our laboratory on the topic of this review is supported by NIH grant DK59588.

Compliance with ethical guidelines

Competing interests

The authors declare that they have no competing interests.

References

1. Jefferson JA, Shankland SJ. The pathogenesis of focal segmental glomerulosclerosis. Adv Chron Kidney Dis. 2014;21(5):408–16. doi:10.1053/j.ackd.2014.05.009.
2. Swaminathan S, Leung N, Lager DJ, Melton LJ 3rd, Bergstralh EJ, Rohlinger A, et al. Changing incidence of glomerular disease in Olmsted County, Minnesota: a 30-year renal biopsy study. Clin J Am Soc Nephrol CJASN. 2006;1(3):483–7. doi:10.2215/CJN.00710805.
3. Braden GL, Mulhern JG, O'Shea MH, Nash SV, Ucci AA Jr, Germain MJ. Changing incidence of glomerular diseases in adults. Am J Kidney Dis Off J Natl Kidney Found. 2000;35(5):878–83.
4. Hogg R, Middleton J, Vehaskari VM. Focal segmental glomerulosclerosis–epidemiology aspects in children and adults. Pediatr Nephrol. 2007;22(2):183–6. doi:10.1007/s00467-006-0370-5.
5. Eddy AA, Symons JM. Nephrotic syndrome in childhood. Lancet. 2003;362(9384):629–39. doi:10.1016/S0140-6736(03)14184-0.
6. Haas M, Spargo BH, Coventry S. Increasing incidence of focal-segmental glomerulosclerosis among adult nephropathies: a 20-year renal biopsy study. Am J Kidney Dis Off J Natl Kidney Found. 1995;26(5):740–50.
7. Kitiyakara C, Eggers P, Kopp JB. Twenty-one-year trend in ESRD due to focal segmental glomerulosclerosis in the United States. Am J Kidney Dis Off J Natl Kidney Found. 2004;44(5):815–25.
8. Ichikawa I, Fogo A. Focal segmental glomerulosclerosis. Pediatr Nephrol. 1996;10(3):374–91.
9. Bose B, Cattran D. Toronto Glomerulonephritis R. Glomerular diseases: FSGS. Clin J Am Soc Nephrol CJASN. 2014;9(3):626–32. doi:10.2215/CJN.05810513.
10. Korbet SM. Clinical picture and outcome of primary focal segmental glomerulosclerosis. Nephrol Dial Transplant Off Publ Eur Dial Transplant Assoc Eur Ren Assoc. 1999;14(Suppl 3):68–73.
11. Korbet SM. Treatment of primary FSGS in adults. J Am Soc Nephrol JASN. 2012;23(11):1769–76. doi:10.1681/ASN.2012040389.
12. Kaplan JM, Kim SH, North KN, Rennke H, Correia LA, Tong HQ, et al. Mutations in ACTN4, encoding alpha-actinin-4, cause familial focal segmental glomerulosclerosis. Nat Genet. 2000;24(3):251–6. doi:10.1038/73456.
13. Brown EJ, Schlondorff JS, Becker DJ, Tsukaguchi H, Tonna SJ, Uscinski AL, et al. Mutations in the formin gene INF2 cause focal segmental glomerulosclerosis. Nat Genet. 2010;42(1):72–6. doi:10.1038/ng.505.
14. Reiser J, Polu KR, Moller CC, Kenlan P, Altintas MM, Wei C, et al. TRPC6 is a glomerular slit diaphragm-associated channel required for normal renal function. Nat Genet. 2005;37(7):739–44. doi:10.1038/ng1592.
15. Winn MP, Conlon PJ, Lynn KL, Farrington MK, Creazzo T, Hawkins AF, et al. A mutation in the TRPC6 cation channel causes familial focal segmental glomerulosclerosis. Science. 2005;308(5729):1801–4. doi:10.1126/science.1106215.
16. Kestila M, Lenkkeri U, Mannikko M, Lamerdin J, McCready P, Putaala H, et al. Positionally cloned gene for a novel glomerular protein—nephrin—is mutated in congenital nephrotic syndrome. Mol Cell. 1998;1(4):575–82.
17. Boute N, Gribouval O, Roselli S, Benessy F, Lee H, Fuchshuber A, et al. NPHS2, encoding the glomerular protein podocin, is mutated in autosomal recessive steroid-resistant nephrotic syndrome. Nat Genet. 2000;24(4):349–54. doi:10.1038/74166.
18. Otey CA, Carpen O. Alpha-actinin revisited: a fresh look at an old player. Cell Motil Cytoskelet. 2004;58(2):104–11. doi:10.1002/cm.20007.
19. Beggs AH, Byers TJ, Knoll JH, Boyce FM, Bruns GA, Kunkel LM. Cloning and characterization of two human skeletal muscle alpha-actinin genes located on chromosomes 1 and 11. J Biol Chem. 1992;267(13):9281–8.
20. Burridge K, Feramisco JR. Non-muscle alpha actinins are calcium-sensitive actin-binding proteins. Nature. 1981;294(5841):565–7.
21. Nikolopoulos SN, Spengler BA, Kisselbach K, Evans AE, Biedler JL, Ross RA. The human non-muscle alpha-actinin protein encoded by the ACTN4 gene suppresses tumorigenicity of human neuroblastoma cells. Oncogene. 2000;19(3):380–6. doi:10.1038/sj.onc.1203310.
22. Kunishima S, Okuno Y, Yoshida K, Shiraishi Y, Sanada M, Muramatsu H, et al. ACTN1 mutations cause congenital macrothrombocytopenia. Am J Hum Genet. 2013;92(3):431–8. doi:10.1016/j.ajhg.2013.01.015.
23. Chiu C, Bagnall RD, Ingles J, Yeates L, Kennerson M, Donald JA, et al. Mutations in alpha-actinin-2 cause hypertrophic cardiomyopathy: a genome-wide analysis. J Am Coll Cardiol. 2010;55(11):1127–35. doi:10.1016/j.jacc.2009.11.016.
24. North KN, Yang N, Wattanasirichaigoon D, Mills M, Easteal S, Beggs AH. A common nonsense mutation results in alpha-actinin-3 deficiency in the general population. Nat Genet. 1999;21(4):353–4. doi:10.1038/7675.
25. Yang N, MacArthur DG, Gulbin JP, Hahn AG, Beggs AH, Easteal S, et al. ACTN3 genotype is associated with human elite athletic performance. Am J Hum Genet. 2003;73(3):627–31. doi:10.1086/377590.
26. Pavalko FM, Otey CA, Simon KO, Burridge K. Alpha-actinin: a direct link between actin and integrins. Biochem Soc Trans. 1991;19(4):1065–9.
27. Otey CA, Vasquez GB, Burridge K, Erickson BW. Mapping of the alpha-actinin binding site within the beta 1 integrin cytoplasmic domain. J Biol Chem. 1993;268(28):21193–7.
28. Bois PR, Borgon RA, Vonrhein C, Izard T. Structural dynamics of alpha-actinin-vinculin interactions. Mol Cell Biol. 2005;25(14):6112–22. doi:10.1128/MCB.25.14.6112-6122.2005.
29. Kroemker M, Rudiger AH, Jockusch BM, Rudiger M. Intramolecular interactions in vinculin control alpha-actinin binding to the vinculin head. FEBS Lett. 1994;355(3):259–62.
30. Li B, Trueb B. Analysis of the alpha-actinin/zyxin interaction. J Biol Chem. 2001;276(36):33328–35. doi:10.1074/jbc.M100789200.
31. Has C, Herz C, Zimina E, Qu HY, He Y, Zhang ZG, et al. Kindlin-1 Is required for RhoGTPase-mediated lamellipodia formation in keratinocytes. Am J Pathol. 2009;175(4):1442–52. doi:10.2353/ajpath.2009.090203.
32. Reiser J, Kriz W, Kretzler M, Mundel P. The glomerular slit diaphragm is a modified adherens junction. J Am Soc Nephrol JASN. 2000;11(1):1–8.
33. Nieset JE, Redfield AR, Jin F, Knudsen KA, Johnson KR, Wheelock MJ. Characterization of the interactions of alpha-catenin with alpha-actinin and beta-catenin/plakoglobin. J Cell Sci. 1997;110(Pt 8):1013–22.
34. Lehtonen S, Ryan JJ, Kudlicka K, Iino N, Zhou H, Farquhar MG. Cell junction-associated proteins IQGAP1, MAGI-2, CASK, spectrins, and alpha-actinin are components of the nephrin multiprotein complex. Proc Natl Acad Sci USA. 2005;102(28):9814–9. doi:10.1073/pnas.0504166102.
35. Fraley TS, Tran TC, Corgan AM, Nash CA, Hao J, Critchley DR, et al. Phosphoinositide binding inhibits alpha-actinin bundling activity. J Biol Chem. 2003;278(26):24039–45. doi:10.1074/jbc.M213288200.
36. Fraley TS, Pereira CB, Tran TC, Singleton C, Greenwood JA. Phosphoinositide binding regulates alpha-actinin dynamics: mechanism for modulating cytoskeletal remodeling. J Biol Chem. 2005;280(15):15479–82. doi:10.1074/jbc.M500631200.
37. Ding Z, Liang J, Lu Y, Yu Q, Songyang Z, Lin SY, et al. A retrovirus-based protein complementation assay screen reveals functional AKT1-binding partners. Proc Natl Acad Sci USA. 2006;103(41):15014–9. doi:10.1073/pnas.0606917103.

38. Sprague CR, Fraley TS, Jang HS, Lal S, Greenwood JA. Phosphoinositide binding to the substrate regulates susceptibility to proteolysis by calpain. J Biol Chem. 2008;283(14):9217–23. doi:10.1074/jbc.M707436200.
39. Honda K, Yamada T, Endo R, Ino Y, Gotoh M, Tsuda H, et al. Actinin-4, a novel actin-bundling protein associated with cell motility and cancer invasion. J Cell Biol. 1998;140(6):1383–93.
40. Khurana S, Chakraborty S, Zhao X, Liu Y, Guan D, Lam M, et al. Identification of a novel LXXLL motif in alpha-actinin 4-spliced isoform that is critical for its interaction with estrogen receptor alpha and co-activators. J Biol Chem. 2012;287(42):35418–29. doi:10.1074/jbc.M112.401364.
41. Khurana S, Chakraborty S, Cheng X, Su YT, Kao HY. The actin-binding protein, actinin alpha 4 (ACTN4), is a nuclear receptor coactivator that promotes proliferation of MCF-7 breast cancer cells. J Biol Chem. 2011;286(3):1850–9. doi:10.1074/jbc.M110.162107.
42. Khurana S, Chakraborty S, Lam M, Liu Y, Su YT, Zhao X, et al. Familial focal segmental glomerulosclerosis (FSGS)-linked alpha-actinin 4 (ACTN4) protein mutants lose ability to activate transcription by nuclear hormone receptors. J Biol Chem. 2012;287(15):12027–35. doi:10.1074/jbc.M112.345421.
43. Chakraborty S, Reineke EL, Lam M, Li X, Liu Y, Gao C, et al. Alpha-actinin 4 potentiates myocyte enhancer factor-2 transcription activity by antagonizing histone deacetylase 7. J Biol Chem. 2006;281(46):35070–80. doi:10.1074/jbc.M602474200.
44. An HT, Kim J, Yoo S, Ko J. Small leucine zipper protein (sLZIP) negatively regulates skeletal muscle differentiation via interaction with alpha-actinin-4. J Biol Chem. 2014;289(8):4969–79. doi:10.1074/jbc.M113.515395.
45. Jasavala R, Martinez H, Thumar J, Andaya A, Gingras AC, Eng JK, et al. Identification of putative androgen receptor interaction protein modules: cytoskeleton and endosomes modulate androgen receptor signaling in prostate cancer cells. Mol Cell Proteom MCP. 2007;6(2):252–71. doi:10.1074/mcp.M600169-MCP200.
46. Zhao X, Hsu KS, Lim JH, Bruggeman LA, Kao HY. alpha-Actinin 4 potentiates nuclear factor kappa-light-chain-enhancer of activated B-cell (NF-kappaB) activity in podocytes independent of its cytoplasmic actin binding function. J Biol Chem. 2015;290(1):338–49. doi:10.1074/jbc.M114.597260.
47. Smoyer WE, Mundel P, Gupta A, Welsh MJ. Podocyte alpha-actinin induction precedes foot process effacement in experimental nephrotic syndrome. Am J Physiol. 1997;273(1 Pt 2):F150–7.
48. Kurihara H, Anderson JM, Farquhar MG. Increased Tyr phosphorylation of ZO-1 during modification of tight junctions between glomerular foot processes. Am J Physiol. 1995;268(3 Pt 2):F514–24.
49. Weins A, Kenlan P, Herbert S, Le TC, Villegas I, Kaplan BS, et al. Mutational and biological analysis of alpha-actinin-4 in focal segmental glomerulosclerosis. J Am Soc Nephrol JASN. 2005;16(12):3694–701. doi:10.1681/ASN.2005070706.
50. Choi HJ, Lee BH, Cho HY, Moon KC, Ha IS, Nagata M, et al. Familial focal segmental glomerulosclerosis associated with an ACTN4 mutation and paternal germline mosaicism. Am J Kidney Dis Off J Natl Kidney Found. 2008;51(5):834–8. doi:10.1053/j.ajkd.2008.01.018.
51. Franzot G, Sjoblom B, Gautel M, Djinovic Carugo K. The crystal structure of the actin binding domain from alpha-actinin in its closed conformation: structural insight into phospholipid regulation of alpha-actinin. J Mol Biol. 2005;348(1):151–65. doi:10.1016/j.jmb.2005.01.002.
52. Lee SH, Weins A, Hayes DB, Pollak MR, Dominguez R. Crystal structure of the actin-binding domain of alpha-actinin-4 Lys255Glu mutant implicated in focal segmental glomerulosclerosis. J Mol Biol. 2008;376(2):317–24. doi:10.1016/j.jmb.2007.11.084.
53. Kos CH, Le TC, Sinha S, Henderson JM, Kim SH, Sugimoto H, et al. Mice deficient in alpha-actinin-4 have severe glomerular disease. J Clin Investig. 2003;111(11):1683–90. doi:10.1172/JCI17988.
54. Dandapani SV, Sugimoto H, Matthews BD, Kolb RJ, Sinha S, Gerszten RE, et al. Alpha-actinin-4 is required for normal podocyte adhesion. J Biol Chem. 2007;282(1):467–77. doi:10.1074/jbc.M605024200.
55. Liu Z, Blattner SM, Tu Y, Tisherman R, Wang JH, Rastaldi MP, et al. Alpha-actinin-4 and CLP36 protein deficiencies contribute to podocyte defects in multiple human glomerulopathies. J Biol Chem. 2011;286(35):30795–805. doi:10.1074/jbc.M111.255984.
56. Yao J, Le TC, Kos CH, Henderson JM, Allen PG, Denker BM, et al. Alpha-actinin-4-mediated FSGS: an inherited kidney disease caused by an aggregated and rapidly degraded cytoskeletal protein. PLoS Biol. 2004;2(6):e167. doi:10.1371/journal.pbio.0020167.
57. Henderson JM, Al-Waheeb S, Weins A, Dandapani SV, Pollak MR. Mice with altered alpha-actinin-4 expression have distinct morphologic patterns of glomerular disease. Kidney Int. 2008;73(6):741–50. doi:10.1038/sj.ki.5002751.
58. Michaud JL, Lemieux LI, Dube M, Vanderhyden BC, Robertson SJ, Kennedy CR. Focal and segmental glomerulosclerosis in mice with podocyte-specific expression of mutant alpha-actinin-4. J Am Soc Nephrol JASN. 2003;14(5):1200–11.
59. Michaud JL, Stitt-Cavanaugh E, Endlich N, Endlich K, De Repentigny Y, Kothary R, et al. Mice with podocyte-specific overexpression of wild type alpha-actinin-4 are healthy controls for K256E-alpha-actinin-4 mutant transgenic mice. Transgenic Res. 2010;19(2):285–9. doi:10.1007/s11248-009-9305-9.
60. Weins A, Schlondorff JS, Nakamura F, Denker BM, Hartwig JH, Stossel TP, et al. Disease-associated mutant alpha-actinin-4 reveals a mechanism for regulating its F-actin-binding affinity. Proc Natl Acad Sci USA. 2007;104(41):16080–5. doi:10.1073/pnas.0702451104.
61. Galkin VE, Orlova A, Salmazo A, Djinovic-Carugo K, Egelman EH. Opening of tandem calponin homology domains regulates their affinity for F-actin. Nat Struct Mol Biol. 2010;17(5):614–6. doi:10.1038/nsmb.1789.
62. Ward SM, Weins A, Pollak MR, Weitz DA. Dynamic viscoelasticity of actin cross-linked with wild-type and disease-causing mutant alpha-actinin-4. Biophys J. 2008;95(10):4915–23. doi:10.1529/biophysj.108.131722.
63. Yao NY, Becker DJ, Broedersz CP, Depken M, Mackintosh FC, Pollak MR, et al. Nonlinear viscoelasticity of actin transiently cross-linked with mutant alpha-actinin-4. J Mol Biol. 2011;411(5):1062–71. doi:10.1016/j.jmb.2011.06.049.
64. Henderson JM, Alexander MP, Pollak MR. Patients with ACTN4 mutations demonstrate distinctive features of glomerular injury. J Am Soc Nephrol JASN. 2009;20(5):961–8. doi:10.1681/ASN.2008060613.
65. Michaud JL, Chaisson KM, Parks RJ, Kennedy CR. FSGS-associated alpha-actinin-4 (K256E) impairs cytoskeletal dynamics in podocytes. Kidney Int. 2006;70(6):1054–61. doi:10.1038/sj.ki.5001665.
66. Meyer-Schwesinger C, Meyer TN, Munster S, Klug P, Saleem M, Helmchen U, et al. A new role for the neuronal ubiquitin C-terminal hydrolase-L1 (UCH-L1) in podocyte process formation and podocyte injury in human glomerulopathies. J Pathol. 2009;217(3):452–64. doi:10.1002/path.2446.
67. Read NC, Gutsol A, Holterman CE, Carter A, Coulombe J, Gray DA, et al. Ubiquitin C-terminal hydrolase L1 deletion ameliorates glomerular injury in mice with ACTN4-associated focal segmental glomerulosclerosis. Biochim Biophys Acta. 2014;1842(7):1028–40. doi:10.1016/j.bbadis.2014.03.009.
68. Grgic I, Hofmeister AF, Genovese G, Bernhardy AJ, Sun H, Maarouf OH, et al. Discovery of new glomerular disease-relevant genes by translational profiling of podocytes in vivo. Kidney Int. 2014;86(6):1116–29. doi:10.1038/ki.2014.204.

Permissions

All chapters in this book were first published in Cell & Bioscience, by BioMed Central; hereby published with permission under the Creative Commons Attribution License or equivalent. Every chapter published in this book has been scrutinized by our experts. Their significance has been extensively debated. The topics covered herein carry significant findings which will fuel the growth of the discipline. They may even be implemented as practical applications or may be referred to as a beginning point for another development.

The contributors of this book come from diverse backgrounds, making this book a truly international effort. This book will bring forth new frontiers with its revolutionizing research information and detailed analysis of the nascent developments around the world.

We would like to thank all the contributing authors for lending their expertise to make the book truly unique. They have played a crucial role in the development of this book. Without their invaluable contributions this book wouldn't have been possible. They have made vital efforts to compile up to date information on the varied aspects of this subject to make this book a valuable addition to the collection of many professionals and students.

This book was conceptualized with the vision of imparting up-to-date information and advanced data in this field. To ensure the same, a matchless editorial board was set up. Every individual on the board went through rigorous rounds of assessment to prove their worth. After which they invested a large part of their time researching and compiling the most relevant data for our readers.

The editorial board has been involved in producing this book since its inception. They have spent rigorous hours researching and exploring the diverse topics which have resulted in the successful publishing of this book. They have passed on their knowledge of decades through this book. To expedite this challenging task, the publisher supported the team at every step. A small team of assistant editors was also appointed to further simplify the editing procedure and attain best results for the readers.

Apart from the editorial board, the designing team has also invested a significant amount of their time in understanding the subject and creating the most relevant covers. They scrutinized every image to scout for the most suitable representation of the subject and create an appropriate cover for the book.

The publishing team has been an ardent support to the editorial, designing and production team. Their endless efforts to recruit the best for this project, has resulted in the accomplishment of this book. They are a veteran in the field of academics and their pool of knowledge is as vast as their experience in printing. Their expertise and guidance has proved useful at every step. Their uncompromising quality standards have made this book an exceptional effort. Their encouragement from time to time has been an inspiration for everyone.

The publisher and the editorial board hope that this book will prove to be a valuable piece of knowledge for researchers, students, practitioners and scholars across the globe.

List of Contributors

Fatih Kocabas
Department of Internal Medicine, Division of Cardiology, UT Southwestern Medical Center at Dallas, Dallas, TX 75390, USA
Department of Genetics and Bioengineering, Faculty of Engineering, Yeditepe University, Istanbul 34755, Turkey

Li Xie, Zhuo Yu and Junke Zheng
Hongqiao International Institute of Medicine, Shanghai Tongren Hospital / Faculty of Basic Medicine, Shanghai Jiao Tong University School of Medicine, Shanghai 200025, China
Key Laboratory of Cell Differentiation and Apoptosis of Chinese Ministry of Education, Shanghai Jiao Tong University School of Medicine, Chongqing South Road 280, Shanghai 200025, China

Jingjing Xie
Bingzhou Medical University, Taishan Scholar Program, Yantai 264003, China

Ralph J. DeBerardinis
Departments of Pediatrics and Genetics, UT Southwestern Medical Center at Dallas, Dallas, TX 75390, USA

Wataru Kimura, SuWannee Thet, Hesham A. Sadek and Shalini Muralidhar
Department of Internal Medicine, Division of Cardiology, UT Southwestern Medical Center at Dallas, Dallas, TX 75390, USA

Ahmed F. Elshamy
Department of Clinical Pathology, El Galaa Hospital, Cairo, Egypt

Hesham Abouellail
Faculty of Medicine Ain Shams University, El Abbaseya, Cairo, Egypt

Xiaoye Liu
Key Laboratory of Cell Differentiation and Apoptosis of Chinese Ministry of Education, Shanghai Jiao Tong University School of Medicine, Chongqing South Road 280, Shanghai 200025, China

Chiqi Chen
Hongqiao International Institute of Medicine, Shanghai Tongren Hospital / Faculty of Basic Medicine, Shanghai Jiao Tong University School of Medicine, Shanghai 200025, China

Cheng Cheng Zhang
Departments of Physiology and Developmental Biology, UT Southwestern Medical Center at Dallas, 5323 Harry Hines Blvd, Dallas, TX 75390, USA

Anita C.H. Murphy and Paul W. Young
School of Biochemistry and Cell Biology, University College Cork, Cork, Ireland

Ying Liu and Johnny J He
Department of Cell Biology and Immunology, Graduate School of Biomedical Sciences, University of North Texas Health Science Center, 3500 Camp Bowie Blvd., Fort Worth, TX 76107, USA
Department of Infectious Diseases, The First Affiliated Hospital of Medical College, Xi'an Jiaotong University, Xi'an 710061, Shaanxi, China.
Department of Forensic Science, College of Medicine, Xi'an Jiaotong University, Xi'an 710061, Shaanxi, China

Jinfeng Liu
Department of Cell Biology and Immunology, Graduate School of Biomedical Sciences, University of North Texas Health Science Center, 3500 Camp Bowie Blvd., Fort Worth, TX 76107, USA
Department of Infectious Diseases, The First Affiliated Hospital of Medical College, Xi'an Jiaotong University, Xi'an 710061, Shaanxi, China.

Zenyuan Wang
Department of Cell Biology and Immunology, Graduate School of Biomedical Sciences, University of North Texas Health Science Center, 3500 Camp Bowie Blvd., Fort Worth, TX 76107, USA
Department of Forensic Science, College of Medicine, Xi'an Jiaotong University, Xi'an 710061, Shaanxi, China

Wei Cui
College of Life Sciences, Beijing Normal University, 100875 Beijing, China
Institute of Biochemistry I, Faculty of Medicine, Goethe-University Frankfurt, 60590 Frankfurt, Germany

Jie Zhou
College of Life Sciences, Beijing Normal University, 100875 Beijing, China

Nathalie Dehne and Bernhard Brüne
Institute of Biochemistry I, Faculty of Medicine, Goethe-University Frankfurt, 60590 Frankfurt, Germany

Arvind Thakkar, Sushma Chenreddy, Jeffrey Wang and Sunil Prabhu
Department of Pharmaceutical Sciences, College of Pharmacy, Western University of Health Sciences, 309 E Second Street, Pomona, CA 91766, USA

Dietmar Zechner, Florian Bürtin, Jonas Amme, Tobias Radecke and Brigitte Vollmar
Institute for Experimental Surgery, Rostock University Medical Center, University of Rostock, Schillingallee 69a, 18057 Rostock, Germany

Tobias Lindner
Core Facility Small Animal Imaging, Rostock University Medical Center, Schillingallee 69a, 18057, Rostock, Germany

Stefan Hadlich and Jens-Peter Kühn
Department of Diagnostic Radiology and Neuroradiology, University Medicine Greifswald, Sauerbruchstr. 1, 17489 Greifswald, Germany

Wei Zhou
Hongqiao International Institute of Medicine, Shanghai Tongren Hospital / Faculty of Basic Medicine, Shanghai Jiao Tong University School of Medicine, Shanghai 200025, China
Key Laboratory of Cell Differentiation and Apoptosis of Chinese Ministry of Education, Shanghai Jiao Tong University School of Medicine, Shanghai 200025, China

Hongfang Shao and Yincheng Teng
Centre for Reproductive Medicine, Shanghai Jiao Tong University Affiliated Sixth People Hospital, Shanghai 200233, China

Di Zhang
Key Laboratory of Cell Differentiation and Apoptosis of Chinese Ministry of Education, Shanghai Jiao Tong University School of Medicine, Shanghai 200025, China
Institute of Genetics and Developmental Biology, Chinese Academy of Sciences, Beijing 100101, China

Jian Dong, Lu Wang and Zhuo Yu
Key Laboratory of Cell Differentiation and Apoptosis of Chinese Ministry of Education, Shanghai Jiao Tong University School of Medicine, Shanghai 200025, China

Wei Cheng
College of Public Health, Shanghai Jiao Tong University School of Medicine, Shanghai 200025, China

Yu-Wei Chou
Tissue Bank and BioBank, Kaohsiung Chang Gung Memorial Hospital, No. 123, Da-Pi Road, Niao-Song District, Kaohsiung 833, Taiwan, ROC
Department of Biochemistry and Molecular Biology, College of Medicine, 985870 Nebraska Medical Center, University of Nebraska Medical Center, Omaha, NE 68198-5870, USA

Fen-Fen Lin
Department of Biochemistry and Molecular Biology, College of Medicine, 985870 Nebraska Medical Center, University of Nebraska Medical Center, Omaha, NE 68198-5870, USA

Sakthivel Muniyan
Department of Biochemistry and Molecular Biology, College of Medicine, 985870 Nebraska Medical Center, University of Nebraska Medical Center, Omaha, NE 68198-5870, USA

Frank C Lin
Department of Biochemistry and Molecular Biology, College of Medicine, 985870 Nebraska Medical Center, University of Nebraska Medical Center, Omaha, NE 68198-5870, USA
Division of Urology, Department of Surgery, University of Arizona Medical Center, Tucson, AZ, USA

Ching-Shih Chen
Division of Medicinal Chemistry and Pharmacology, College of Pharmacy, The Ohio State University, Columbus, OH, USA

Jue Wang
Division of Oncology/Hematology, Department of Internal Medicine, University of Nebraska Medical Center, Omaha, NE, USA
University of Arizona Cancer Center, St. Joseph's Hospital and Medical Center, Phoenix, AZ, USA

Chao-Cheng Huang
Tissue Bank and BioBank, Kaohsiung Chang Gung Memorial Hospital, No. 123, Da-Pi Road, Niao-Song District, Kaohsiung 833, Taiwan, ROC
Department of Pathology, Kaohsiung Chang Gung Memorial Hospital, and Chang Gung University College of Medicine, Kaohsiung, Taiwan, ROC

Ming-Fong Lin
Department of Biochemistry and Molecular Biology, College of Medicine, 985870 Nebraska
Eppley Institute for Research in Cancer and Allied Diseases, University of Nebraska Medical Center, Omaha, NE, USA
Department of Surgery/ Urology, University of Nebraska Medical Center, Omaha, NE, USA School of Pharmacy, Kaohsiung Medical University, Kaohsiung, Taiwan, ROC

Se Hee Han, Soo-Hyun Hahm and An Hue Vy Tran
Department of Advanced Technology Fusion, Konkuk University, 120 Neungdong-ro, Gwangjin-gu, Seoul 143-701, Republic of Korea

Ji Hyung Chung
Department of Applied Bioscience, College of Life Science, CHA University, 120 Haeryong-ro, Pocheon, Gyeonggi-do 463-836, Republic of Korea

Myoung-Ki Hong
Department of Biological Sciences, Konkuk University, 120 Neungdong-ro, Gwangjin-gu, Seoul 143-701, Republic of Korea

Hyun-Dong Paik
Department of Food Science and Biotechnology of Animal Resources, Konkuk University, 120 Neungdong-ro, Gwangjin-gu, Seoul 143-701, Republic of Korea

Key-Sun Kim
Center for Neuroscience, Korea Institute of Science and Technology, 5 Hwarang-ro 14-gil, Seongbuk-gu, Seoul, Republic of Korea

Ye Sun Han
Department of Advanced Technology Fusion, Konkuk University, 120 Neungdong-ro, Gwangjin-gu, Seoul 143-701, Republic of Korea
College of Global Integrated Studies, Division of Interdisciplinary Studies, Konkuk University, 120 Neungdong-ro, Gwangjin-gu, Seoul 143-701, Republic of Korea

Qing Li, Bin Hu, Shang-chun Guo, Yang Wang and Xin Niu
Institute of Microsurgery on Extremities, Shanghai Jiao Tong University Affiliated Sixth People's Hospital, Shanghai 200233, China

Shou-fu Tian
Department Nephrology and Rheumatology, Shanghai Jiao Tong University Affiliated Sixth People's Hospital, Shanghai 200233, China
Department of Integration of Traditional Chinese and Western Medicine, The First Affiliated Hospital of Soochow University, Suzhou 215006, China

Ye Guo
Department of Neurosurgery, Shandong Jining No. 1 People's Hospital, Jining 272011, China

Nian-song Wang
Department Nephrology and Rheumatology, Shanghai Jiao Tong University Affiliated Sixth People's Hospital, Shanghai 200233, China

Kazufumi Honda
Department of Chemotherapy and Clinical Research, National Cancer Center
Research Institute, 5-1-1 Tsukiji Chuoku, Tokyo 104-0045, Japan
AMED-CREST AMED, Japan Agency for Medical Research and Development, 1-7-1 Otemachi, Chiyoda, Tokyo 100-0004, Japan

Dan-Dan Yu, Shi-Wei Guo, Ying-Ying Jing, Yu-Long Dong and Li-Xin Wei
Tumor Immunology and Gene Therapy Center, Eastern Hepatobiliary Surgery Hospital, The Second Military Medical University, 225 Changhai Road, 200438 Shanghai, China

Hisham A. Alhadlaq
Department of Physics and Astronomy, College of Science, King Saud University, Riyadh 11451, Saudi Arabia

Mohd Javed Akhtar and Maqusood Ahamed
King Abdullah Institute for Nanotechnology, King Saud University, Riyadh 11451, Saudi Arabia

Xiao Xu, Liang Li, Cheng Wang, Yang Liu, Chong Chen, Junling Yan, Hong Ding and Su-yang Tang
Skin and Reconstructive Medicine Department, The General Hospital of Chinese People's Armed Police Forces, Beijing, People's Republic of China

Yunlan Tang, Yi Lin, Chuang Li, Xunwu Hu, Yi Liu, Mingyang He, Wenxin Li and Mingxiong Guo
College of Life Sciences and State Key Laboratory of Virology, Wuhan University, 430072 Wuhan, People's Republic of China

Jun Luo
Department of Pathology, Zhongnan Hospital, Wuhan University, 430071 Wuhan, People's Republic of China

Guihong Sun
School of Basic Medical Sciences, Wuhan University, 430071 Wuhan, People's Republic of China

Tao Wang
Department of Respiratory and Critical Care Medicine, Tongji Hospital, Tongji Medical College, Huazhong University of Science and Technology, 430030 Wuhan, China

Benjamin Yang, Andrew Yang and Shiwen Peng
Departments of Pathology, School of Medicine, Johns Hopkins University, CRBII Room 307, 1550 Orleans Street, Baltimore, MD 21231, USA

Xiaowu Pang
Department of Oral Pathology, College of Dentistry, Howard University, Washington, DC, USA

Richard B.S. Roden
Departments of Pathology, School of Medicine, Johns Hopkins University, CRBII Room 307, 1550 Orleans Street, Baltimore, MD 21231, USA
Obstetrics and Gynecology, Johns Hopkins Medical Institutions, Baltimore, MD, USA
Oncology, Johns Hopkins Medical Institutions, Baltimore, MD, USA

T.-C. Wu
Departments of Pathology, School of Medicine, Johns Hopkins University, CRBII Room 307, 1550 Orleans Street, Baltimore, MD 21231, USA
Obstetrics and Gynecology, Johns Hopkins Medical Institutions, Baltimore, MD, USA
Molecular Microbiology and Immunology, Johns Hopkins Medical Institutions, Baltimore, MD, USA
Oncology, Johns Hopkins Medical Institutions, Baltimore, MD, USA

Chien-Fu Hung
Departments of Pathology, School of Medicine, Johns Hopkins University, CRBII Room 307, 1550 Orleans Street, Baltimore, MD 21231, USA
Oncology, Johns Hopkins Medical Institutions, Baltimore, MD, USA

Michelle Helen Visagie, Thandi Vuyelwa Mqoco and Anna Margaretha Joubert
Department of Physiology, University of Pretoria, Private Bag X323, Arcadia 0007, South Africa

Leon Liebenberg, Edward Henry Mathews and George Edward Mathews
Centre for Research and Continued Engineering Development, North-West University, Lynnwood Ridge, South Africa

Yongfang Yang, Liwei Wen and Hongliang Zhu
Department of Food Biotechnology, College of Food Science and Nutritional Engineering, China Agricultural University, 100083 Beijing, China

Hongzhu Li, Changqing Xu and Xin Zhong
Department of Pathophysiology, Harbin Medical University, Baojian Road, Harbin 150081, China
The Key Laboratory of Cardiovascular Medicine Research (Harbin Medical University), Ministry of Education, Harbin 150086, China

Chao Zhang
Department of Emergency, Heilongjiang Provincia Hospital, Harbin 150036, China

Weiming Sun, Lina Li, Bo Wu, Shuzhi Bai and Hongxia Li
Department of Pathophysiology, Harbin Medical University, Baojian Road, Harbin 150081, China

Rui Wang
Department of Biology, Lakehead University, Thunder Bay, ON P7B 5E1, Canada

Lingyun Wu
Department of Health Science, Lakehead University, Thunder Bay, ON P7B 5E1, Canada

Hong-Bin Cheng and Jing-Ping Wu
Teaching Hospital of Chengdu University of TCM, Chengdu 610072, Sichuan, China

Rong-Yi Chen, Zi-Feng Pan, Qing-Hua Zhang and Jian-Qiang Shi
Department of Dermatology, Affiliated Hospital of Guangdong Medical College, No.57 Peoples Avenue South, Zhanjiang 524001, Guangdong, China

Li Chen and Tian-Xi Du
Laboratory Animal Center, Anhui Medical University, Hefei 230032, Anhui, China

Yan-Hua Liang
Department of Dermatology, Nanfang Hospital, Southern Medical University, Guangzhou 510515, Guangdong, China

Hai-Feng Pan
Department of Epidemiology and Biostatistics, School of Public Health, Anhui Medical University, Hefei 230032, Anhui, China

Qing Li and Yong-Mei Lv
Department of Dermatology, The Second Affiliated Hospital, Anhui Medical University Hefei, 678 Furong Road, Hefei 230601, Anhui, China

Chia-Chia Lee, Shi Chen and Teng-Yung Huang
Department of Clinical Laboratory Sciences and Medical Biotechnology, College of Medicine, National Taiwan University, #7, Chung-Shan South Road, Taipei 10002, Taiwan, ROC

Ya-Chien Yang, Liang-In Lin and Woei-horng Fang
Department of Clinical Laboratory Sciences and Medical Biotechnology, College of Medicine, National Taiwan University, #7, Chung-Shan South Road, Taipei 10002, Taiwan, ROC
Department of Laboratory Medicine, National Taiwan University Hospital, Taipei 10002, Taiwan, ROC

Steven D. Goodman
Center for Microbial Pathogenesis, Nationwide Children's Hospital, Columbus, OH, USA

Wern-Cherng Cheng
Department of Laboratory Medicine, National Taiwan University Hospital, Taipei 10002, Taiwan, ROC

Jialing Zhang
School of Public Health, Wuhan University, Wuhan, China
Clinical Medicine Research Center, The Affiliated Hospital, Inner Mongolia Medical University, Hohhot, China
Tumor Biology Section, Head and Neck Surgery Branch, National Institute on Deafness and Other Communication Disorders, NIH, Bethesda, USA

Bin Yan
Laboratory for Food Safety and Environmental Technology, Shenzhen Institutes of Advanced Technology, Chinese Academy of Sciences, Shenzhen, China

Stephan Stanislaw Späth
Pediatric Endocrinology Unit, Department of Women's and Children's Health, Karolinska Institute and University Hospital, Stockholm, Sweden

Hu Qu
Department of Oncology, The Affiliated Hospital, Inner Mongolia Medical University, Hohhot, China

Daogang Guan
Department of Biology, Hong Kong Baptist University, Hong Kong, China

Jiaofang Shao
Department of Bioinformatics, School of Basic Medical Sciences, Nanjing Medical University, Nanjing, China

Koichi Hagiwara
Department of Respiratory Medicine, Saitama Medical Center, Jichi Medical University, Saitama, Japan

Carter Van Waes, Zhong Chen and Shaleeka Cornelius
Tumor Biology Section, Head and Neck Surgery Branch, National Institute on Deafness and Other Communication Disorders, NIH, Bethesda, USA

Xiulan Su
Clinical Medicine Research Center, The Affiliated Hospital, Inner Mongolia Medical University, Hohhot, China

Yongyi Bi
School of Public Health, Wuhan University, Wuhan, China

Joseph Nkeze
Division of Molecular Pathology, Department of Pathology, University of Maryland School of Medicine, Baltimore, MD 21201-1192, USA

Lin Li
Division of Molecular Pathology, Department of Pathology, University of Maryland School of Medicine, Baltimore, MD 21201-1192, USA AIDS Research Department, Beijing Institute of Microbiology and Epidemiology, Beijing 100071, China

Zsigmond Benko
Division of Molecular Pathology, Department of Pathology, University of Maryland School of Medicine, Baltimore, MD 21201-1192, USA
Department of Chromosome Biology, Max F. Perutz Laboratories, University of Vienna, Vienna, Austria

Ge Li
Division of Molecular Pathology, Department of Pathology, University of Maryland School of Medicine, Baltimore, MD 21201-1192, USA

Richard Y Zhao
Division of Molecular Pathology, Department of Pathology, University of Maryland School of Medicine, Baltimore, MD 21201-1192, USA
Department of Microbiology and Immunology, University of Maryland School of Medicine, Baltimore, MD 21201-1192, USA
Institute of Human Virology, University of Maryland School of Medicine, Baltimore, MD 21201-1192, USA

Di Feng, and Martin R Pollak
Division of Nephrology, Department of Medicine, Beth Israel Deaconess Medical Center, Boston, MA 02215, USA

Clark DuMontier
Department of Medicine, Boston University School of Medicine, Boston, MA 02118, USA